PEDIATRIC FOOT & ANKLE SURGERY

PEDIATRIC FOOT & ANKLE SURGERY

RICHARD M. JAY, D.P.M., F.A.C.F.A.S.

Professor and Director of Pediatric Orthopedics
Temple University School of Podiatric Medicine
Director of Foot and Ankle Surgical Residency Program
The Graduate Hospital
Philadelphia, Pennsylvania

W.B. SAUNDERS COMPANY
A Division of Harcourt Brace & Company
Philadelphia London Toronto Montreal Sydney Tokyo

W.B. SAUNDERS COMPANY
A Division of Harcourt Brace & Company

The Curtis Center
Independence Square West
Philadelphia, Pennsylvania 19106

Library of Congress Cataloging-in-Publication Data

Jay, Richard M.
Pediatric foot and ankle surgery / Richard M. Jay.—1st ed.

p.   cm.

ISBN 0–7216–7445–3

1. Pediatric orthopedics. 2. Orthopedic surgery. 3. Foot—Surgery.
    4. Ankle—Surgery. 5. Children—Surgery.   I. Title.

[DNLM: 1. Orthopedic Procedures—in infancy & childhood. 2. Foot—surgery.
    3. Ankle—surgery. WS 270 J42p 1999]

RD732.3.C48J39 1999   618.92′0975059—dc21

DNLM/DLC   98–31651

PEDIATRIC FOOT AND ANKLE SURGERY   ISBN 0–7216–7445–3

Printed in the United States of America

Last digit is the print number: 9   8   7   6   5   4   3   2   1

Contributors

Scott A. Alter, D.P.M.

Barry University School of Graduate Medical Sciences, Miami Shores; Attending, South Shores Hospital, Miami Beach, Florida

Brodie's Abscess

Michael A. Bailey, R.P.H., D.P.M.

University Hospital, Augusta, Georgia

Subcapital Talar Osteotomy for Transverse Plane Structural Deformities

John Beaupied, D.P.M.

Staff, Holy Cross Hospital and Mercy Hospital and Medical Center, Chicago; Little Company of Mary Hospital, Evergreen Park, Illinois

Brachymetatarsia

Troy J. Boffeli, D.P.M.

Director of Podiatric Residency Training, Regions Hospital, St. Paul; Lecturer, Department of Surgery, University of Minnesota Medical School, Minneapolis, Minnesota; Adjunct Clinical Associate Professor, Podiatric Medicine, University of Osteopathic Medical and Health Services, Des Moines, Iowa

Triplane Correction of the Flexible Flatfoot

Lloyd E. Brotman, Ph.D.

Private practice; Principal, Periscope; Clinical Director, North, Clawson, Bolt, Ltd., Philadelphia, Pennsylvania

The Human Factor: Treatment of Children

Alan R. Catanzariti, D.P.M.

Director, Foot and Ankle Surgical Residency Training Program, The Western Pennsylvania Hospital, Pittsburgh, Pennsylvania

Medial Displacement Osteotomy of the Posterior Calcaneus for Flatfoot Deformity

Michael Chung, D.P.M.

Surgical Staff, The Graduate Hospital, Philadelphia, Pennsylvania

Nail Procedures; Kohler's Disease

Diane Collier, D.P.M.

Private Practice, Alabama South Family Podiatry, Dothan, Alabama

Soft Tissue Calcaneonavicular Coalition

Robert Cornfield, D.P.M.

Staff Physician, Straith Hospital, Southfield; Kern Hospital, Warren; St. John Oakland Hospital, Madison Heights, Michigan

Brachymetatarsia

Gary L. Dockery, D.P.M.

Director and Chairman, Northwest Podiatric Foundation for Education and Research, Seattle, Washington

Symptomatic Juvenile Flatfoot Condition

Gary Feldman, D.P.M.

Private Practice, Rockville, Maryland

Brachymetatarsia; Soft Tissue Calcaneonavicular Coalition

Renato J. Giorgini, D.P.M.

Professor of Podiatric Surgery, Division of Surgical Sciences, New York College of Podiatric Medicine; Director, Foot and Ankle Surgery, North General Hospital and Good Samaritan Hospital, New York; Brunswick Hospital, Amityville, New York

Correction of Spastic Equinus

Steven Glickman, D.P.M.

Chief of Podiatric Surgery, Straith Hospital, Southfield; William Beaumont Hospital, Troy, Michigan

Brachymetatarsia

John G. Goode, M.D., D.A.B.P.M.

Anesthesiologist, The Graduate Hospital, Philadelphia, Pennsylvania

Pediatric Anesthesia

Donald R. Green, D.P.M.

Clinical Professor, Temple University School of Podiatric Medicine, Philadelphia, Pennsylvania; Assistant Clinical Professor, Department of Orthopedics, University of California, San Diego, School of Medicine; Podiatric

Residency Director, Mercy Hospital and Hospital of the Scripps Clinic, San Diego, California
Epiphysiodesis for Juvenile Hallux Abducto Valgus

Richard M. Green, D.P.M.

Clinical Faculty, Department of Orthopedics, University of California, San Diego, School of Medicine; Orthopedic Supervisory Committee, Mercy Hospital and Hospital of the Scripps Clinic, San Diego, California
Epiphysiodesis for Juvenile Hallux Abducto Valgus

Jason Hanft, D.P.M.

Residency Director, South Miami Hospital, Baptist Hospital, Doctors Hospital, Miami, Florida
Brachymetatarsia

Bruce D. Harley, D.P.M., D.A.B.P.S.

Cincinnati, Ohio
Medial Column Soft Tissue Release for Metatarsus Adductus Correction in Infants; Abductory Midfoot Osteotomy for Metatarsus Adductus; Cole Midfoot Osteotomy

Edwin J. Harris, D.P.M.

Associate Clinical Professor, Department of Orthopaedics and Rehabilitation, Loyola University of Chicago Stritch School of Medicine, Maywood, Illinois
Pediatric Digital Deformities; An Approach to Toe-Walking: Appropriate Decision Making

Richard M. Jay, D.P.M., F.A.C.F.A.S.

Professor and Director of Pediatric Orthopedics, Temple University School of Podiatric Medicine; Director of Foot and Ankle Surgical Residency Program, The Graduate Hospital, Philadelphia, Pennsylvania
Metatarsus Adductus; Neuromuscular Disorders and Reflexes in the Child; Surgery for Metatarsus Adductus; Juvenile Hallux Abducto Valgus; Polydactyly; Brachymetatarsia; Macrodactyly; Nail Procedures; Introduction to the Flatfoot; Calcaneovalgus; Subtalar Extra-articular Arthrodesis; Arthroereisis-Subtalar; Evans Procedure; Cavus Deformity; Soft Tissue Calcaneonavicular Coalition; Equinus—Anterior Advancement of the Tendo Achillis; Osteoid Osteoma; Iselins Apophysitis; Freiberg's Infraction; Calcaneal Apophysitis; Internal Tibial Torsion; Equinus; Kohler's Disease; Orthotic Control of the Pediatric Patient; Pediatric Corrective Casting

J. Barry Johnson, D.P.M.

Adjunct Clinical Faculty, Barry University School of Podiatric Medicine, Miami Shores, Florida; Chairman, The Foot Surgery Center of North Carolina, LLC,

Greensboro, North Carolina; Vice President, Podiatry Insurance Company of America, Brentwood, Tennessee
Cotton Osteotomy

Elisa M. Kavanagh, D.P.M.

Temple University School of Podiatric Medicine; The Graduate Hospital, Philadelphia, Pennsylvania
Juvenile Hallux Abducto Valgus

Charles G. Kissel, D.P.M.

Chief, Section of Podiatric Surgery, Director, Podiatric Residency Training, Detroit Medical Center, Detroit, Michigan; Clinical Assistant Professor, Podiatric Medicine, University of Osteopathic Medicine and Health Services, Des Moines, Iowa
Tibialis Anterior Transfer "Into Talus" for Control of Severe Pes Planus; Triplane Correction of the Flexible Flatfoot

Stephen D. Lasday, D.P.M.

Private Practice, West Coast Podiatry Center, Sarasota and Bradenton, Florida
Tarsal Coalition

Leon Lenchik, M.D.

Assistant Professor, Department of Radiology, Bowman Gray School of Medicine of Wake Forest University, Winston-Salem, North Carolina
Imaging

William H. Mason, D.P.M.

Chief, Podiatric Medicine and Surgery, Sonoma Developmental Center, Eldridge, California
Congenital Cleft Foot Deformity (Split Foot or Lobster-Claw)

Nicholas Pachuda, D.P.M.

Private Practice, Bradenton, Florida
Tarsal Coalition

Mitchell Pokrassa, D.P.M.

Co-Director, Baja Project for Crippled Children; Associate Clinical Professor, California College of Podiatric Medicine, San Francisco; Attending Staff, Los Angeles County/University of Southern California Hospital, Los Angeles, California
Clubfoot

David C. Puleo, D.P.M.

Core Faculty, The Western Pennsylvania Hospital, Division of Podiatric Medical/Surgical Services; Pittsburgh, Pennsylvania
Syndactyly and Desyndactylization

Katherine M. Richman, M.D.

Body Imaging Fellow, Department of Radiology, University of California, San Diego, Medical Center, San Diego, California

Imaging

Kevin D. Roberts, D.P.M., R.Ph.

Research Director, The Graduate Hospital, Philadelphia, Pennsylvania

Management of the Pediatric Patient

Greg Rock, D.P.M.

St. Clair's Hospital, Cabrini Medical Center, Medical Arts Center Hospital, Fifth Avenue Surgery Center, New York, New York

Brachymetatarsia

David J. Sartoris, M.D.

Professor of Radiology, Musculoskeletal Imaging Section; Chief, Quantitative Bone Densitometry, University of California, San Diego, Medical Center, San Diego, California

Imaging

Michael Seiberg, D.P.M.

Desert Orthopedic Center, Rancho Mirage, California

Juvenile Fracture of Tillaux: A Distal Tibial; Epiphysiodesis for Juvenile Hallux Abducto Valgus

William H. Simon, D.P.M.

Clinical Instructor, Department of Internal Medicine, Eastern Virginia Medical School of the Medical College

of Hampton Roads, Norfolk; Department of Surgery, Virginia Beach General Hospital, Virginia Beach, Virginia

Epiphyseal Fracture

Ellen Sobel, D.P.M., Ph.D.

Associate Professor of Orthopedics, New York College of Podiatric Medicine, New York, New York

Correction of Spastic Equinus

Raymond K. Tsukuda, D.P.M.

Podiatric Surgical Resident, Encino-Tarzana Regional Medical Center, Encino, California

Clubfoot

Russell G. Volpe, D.P.M.

Professor and Chairman, Department of Pediatrics, New York College of Podiatric Medicine, New York; East Coast Medical Director, The Langer Biomechanics Group, Deer Park, New York

Ankle-Foot Orthoses Following Surgery

John H. Walter, Jr., D.P.M.

Professor and Chairman, Department of Podiatric Orthopedics, Temple University School of Podiatric Medicine, Philadelphia, Pennsylvania

Subcapital Talar Osteotomy for Transverse Plane Structural Deformities; Aneurysmal Bone Cyst

Jeanean Willis, D.P.M.

Assistant Clinical Professor, Temple University School of Podiatric Medicine, Philadelphia, Pennsylvania

Neuromuscular Disorders and Reflexes in the Child

Preface

The students who graduate from our institutions today are better educated and have a greater wealth of knowledge than ever before. They are the new leaders of our profession, but with this greater knowledge comes greater responsibility.

The adage first do no harm is paramount when treating children. Only when physicians have exhausted all conservative methods can they apply these surgical options. This practice ensures our profession's continued growth in the right direction.

Pediatric foot and ankle surgery has developed into a distinct specialty within the practice of podiatric and orthopedic surgery. This text is dedicated to the latest pediatric foot and ankle surgical techniques. The surgical procedures for treating adults do not necessarily apply for treating children. In this text, I have included new surgical techniques along with modifications of old ones. An attempt is made to provide an orderly approach to the structural and functional management of the pediatric patient.

The writing of a text on pediatric foot and ankle surgery is a monumental task, and I have no doubt omitted some topics and procedures. I have included surgical options and opinions that have proved successful in my treatment of children over the past 20 years. I have also provided the insights of my colleagues to present a well-rounded pediatric surgical text.

I would like to thank the contributors for their patience and admirable additions to this text. The graphic artists, Duke Yoo, D.P.M., and Melanie Newman, D.D.S., and the computer artist, Brian Rell, D.P.M., adeptly converted the printed word to a visual configuration. David Secord, D.P.M., and Jodai Serami, D.P.M., were an integral part of the process during early editorial work. Karen Gooden aided in the development of the photographic material.

I especially wish to thank Stephanie Donley and her staff at W.B. Saunders Company for their ability to sift through endless reams of paper and make them into an orderly manuscript.

Most importantly, I would like to thank my wife Roz and my daughter Kate for permitting me the time to write and edit this text.

RICHARD M. JAY, D.P.M., F.A.C.F.A.S.

NOTICE

Podiatric Medicine is an ever-changing field. Standard safety precautions must be followed, but as new research and clinical experience broaden our knowledge, changes in treatment and drug therapy become necessary or appropriate. Readers are advised to check the product information currently provided by the manufacturer of each drug to be administered to verify the recommended dose, the method and duration of administration, and the contraindications. It is the responsibility of the treating physician, relying on experience and knowledge of the patient, to determine the dosages and the best treatment for the patient. Neither the publisher nor the editor assumes any responsibility for any injury and/or damage to persons or property.

THE PUBLISHER

Contents

One

Medical Aspects

1

The Human Factor: Treatment of Children

Lloyd E. Brotman, Ph.D.

How and why do patients choose their treating physicians? Some go through a careful process of selection, while others call their managed care company for a referral to a physician who practices nearby. For some, clinical expertise is paramount; these patients focus on training and experience. Other patients are less concerned. They believe that if the doctor is licensed and in practice, he must be acceptable. The shared expectation held by both of these groups is that the doctor chosen will possess the necessary technical knowledge to diagnose and treat the presented problem effectively. In simple terms, the doctor will know what is wrong and will fix it!

How and why do patients decide to change or reject a treating physician? This is an easier question to answer. Patients often leave physicians because they do not like how they are treated. The term treated in this case does not refer to the technical but rather to the social aspects of the treatment process.

George Engel, an internist, suggested that the biomedical model used to approach the treatment of disease was too narrow and did not recognize the important systemic relationship that existed between biologic and psychosocial processes.[6] Engel's biopsychosocial model suggested that clinicians should recognize that treatment affects the whole person in a social context, not just the organ system under study.

Although the biopsychosocial model is acknowledged as relevant in the training of physicians, little serious structured attention is paid to it on an ongoing basis. The concept that doctors need to attend more to the whole person is generally accepted at face value, but few training programs approach it aggressively. This article attempts to sensitize treating podiatrists to a few aspects of the child patient's phenomenology.

Doctors tend to forget that patients are usually unfamiliar with all that doctors encounter each day. The sights, sounds, smells, and jargon that clinicians take for granted are new and unusual to most patients. Doctors are clear about the role they play, but patients are unclear about their own role. Patients may develop anticipatory anxiety from the time they discover that a problem exists, and that anxiety can build while they wait for an appointment date. Patients wonder about the diagnosis, the treatment intervention, the cost, and whether the doctors will treat them well. When the patients meet their doctors in consultation, they may often be surprised that they act like real persons, genuinely expressing concern. They feel they have been given something extra! Patients speak in amazement when they say, "My doctor called me," or "He said I should have called him sooner about my problem."

I recently saw a prominent orthopedic surgeon about a shoulder problem. I was less than pleased with my treatment, not because of the examination or the diagnosis, but because of the human contact that took place. Simple courtesy would have made all the difference in the world. No one who entered the examining room bothered to introduce himself or differentiate his role. I read the embroidery on the lab coat to distinguish the treating physician from the resident. Important people forget that not everyone can identify them on sight. A simple introduction means a great deal.

The abuse of patient time is a common complaint. I wondered whether my time was so much less important than the doctor's time when, after waiting for more than an hour, neither information nor apology was offered. "I'm sorry I'm running late" is a simple statement that shows social grace and respect. Then there is the experience of being examined in a teaching hospital where the treating physician often pays more attention to the students in the room than to the patient. I would have appreciated having the treating physician occasionally look my way or address me directly.

I suggest that you think of a new situation in which your power and control are taken away. How do you feel? Many doctors forget or, even worse, have never known how to empathize. They are unaware or don't care about such things or are so desensitized to the process that they forget the basics of human contact and respect. Physicians need to pay attention to how patients feel in various situations.

Clinicians are often overwhelmed by the medical issues they face in dealing with patients' problems. Some of them believe that these human issues are not important as long as the patient is treated with the appropriate medical procedure. Podiatrists need to be reminded that a head and a body are attached to the foot being treated. Treating the whole person does not slow down or complicate the day. In fact, by learning to manage people rather than control them, one's efficiency increases.

DEVELOPMENT

Children are often treated like smaller, younger adults. This type of treatment assumes that children's thinking is somewhere on the same continuum as adult thinking but that maturation has not yet taken place. It assumes that the difference is quantitative. The difference between adult and child thinking, however, is not quantitative but qualitative. Depending on the stage of development, children think in a qualitatively different manner than adults.

The work of Piaget (1952) suggests how this qualitative shift in cognitive development takes place.[25] Despite the fact that others have challenged, amplified, or elaborated on this theoretical position, this theory can still be used to illustrate important aspects of the developmental process. Piaget identified four main periods of development within which lie a number of substages. The sensorimotor period extends from birth to the twenty-first month. During this period, the child starts to recognize his interaction with the environment and begins to think and experiment with his impact on his world. During the preoperational thought period beginning at age 2 to 4 years, the addition of language changes the thought process because language provides representational thought. This period of development continues until the age of 7 or 8. The thought process in this period becomes more adaptable and logical, but these apparent flashes of clear thinking are riddled with distortion and inconsistency, and the child is highly egocentric. The concrete operational thought period beginning around age 8 brings more reasoning ability with abstract understanding that did not exist previously. Between the ages of 11 and 14, the formal operational thought period occurs. The child develops the capacity to think in more abstract terms about second-order relationships.

A look at the understanding that children have about death[30] reveals the shift that takes place as the cognitive process develops. Prior to age 2, despite the common display of separation anxiety when they are away from their primary caretakers, children do not understand the concept of death. Between the ages of 3 and 5, children gradually see that death occurs in their environment as they see pets, plants in the garden, and even people around them die. It is unclear to them, however, that unlike sleep, death is final. Children in this group do not connect with death as it pertains to themselves. Around the age of 6 to 7, the permanency of death is more clearly understood, and the child recognizes that he and those close to him will die sometime. This is believed to be something that will happen but will occur far in the future. Not until the preadolescent period does the concept of death become clearly understood as a result of life experiences and the more logical thought processes that accompany this period.

It is important to understand the child's concept of health-related matters and to recognize that the misconceptions children often have about these matters are a function of the cognitive process, not simply the amount of information available. With an understanding of and sensitivity to the level of a child's cognitive development, a sophisticated clinician can avoid describing anesthesia induction as being "put to sleep" because a young child may have heard this description used when a pet was put down. Young children have an extremely concrete understanding of language that can often lead to miscommunication.[34] The word *dye*, mentioned in a passing reference to a diagnostic test, could be understood as *die* by a listening child. Similarly, a child may believe he could die of betes if he overhears a discussion regarding the possibility that he has diabetes. Sheridan[29] points out that at some stages of cognitive development a child may be afraid of bleeding to death as a result of a blood test puncture. The podiatrist must think about the child's perspective and frame of reference. What might a child imagine about foot surgery? Could a toe be removed? Will a nail grow back? The real problem lies in the fact that children do not always display their confusion and give the doctor a chance to clarify. The sensitive, enlightened clinician recognizes that it is part of his job to understand the process of cognitive development and to anticipate these reactions. This requires a proactive, not a reactive, approach.

In addition to having some understanding of cognitive development or how a child thinks and perceives, it is helpful to have a grasp of the basics of psychosocial development or the development of a sense of self. Familiarity with the model of development expressed by Erik Erikson may be helpful.[35] Briefly, Erikson believed that children develop strengths and skills in stages. In the first stage, identified as basic trust, the highly dependent newborn evolves into the 18-month-old toddler, who shows early signs of independence. Early separation anxiety is reduced as the child becomes more tolerant of separation later in this stage. From 18 months to 3 years, during the autonomy stage, the child progresses in his capacity to manipulate the world. Language develops, affording the use of the word *NO*, and the child takes greater control of his eating habits, as well as bowel and bladder functions. Erikson labels the stage from 3 to 6 years old as that of initiative, during which the child's social skills develop. Identification with the body occurs, and physical appearance and bodily functions are highlighted. Next, during the industry stage, from age 6 until the preteen years, the influence of forces outside the home, such as peers and teachers, becomes significant. Self-concept is shaped by the ability to succeed in school and in the social context. During the fifth stage, adolescence, the child truly separates from the parents as he attempts to resolve conflicts about how his own value system fits or clashes with parents, peers, and cultures. Issues of independence are most significant.

The skilled clinician is mindful of the patient's developmental stage in attempting to communicate effectively. The clinician assesses whether the child is struggling with issues of trust or expressions of autonomy or is highly focused on his or her body and appearance. This understanding and anticipation will facilitate the doctor–patient relationship. Furthermore, the clinician's skillful handling of a child, based on his or her recognition of the level of cognitive and psychosocial development, may help the parents understand their child's behavior and increase their cooperation and compliance. A simple explanation that a toddler who is restricted from normal movement due to an injury or treatment intervention may display increased oppositional behavior may help the parents reduce their overprotectiveness, which only serves to worsen such problems.[17]

ESTABLISHING RAPPORT

When my daughter was 9 years old, she complained of a mysterious foot and ankle pain. She usually called attention to this pain at bedtime. It was hard to know whether this was a bedtime delaying tactic or truly an issue of concern. She identified and described the pain well at home and asked if we would call our friend, a podiatric surgeon, to discuss the problem. The next day we planned to spend time with this friend's family and to make time to look at my daughter's foot. I felt the same way I feel when I take the car to the mechanic and it fails to make the noise for him that it makes for me! I noticed that even though we were in the kitchen, a place with which we are all familiar, we all assumed different roles. Our friend became the Doctor, and although he had a wonderful relationship with my daughter, he had to establish rapport as a professional. My daughter became the patient. The symptoms became harder to describe than at home. Her anxiety interfered with her capacity to help in the diagnostic process. Perhaps she began to imagine a catastrophe as she did the night before when she asked, "What if I have to use crutches?" I noticed that I assumed the role of the concerned parent. I wanted to help my daughter and the doctor communicate more effectively, but I didn't want to get in the way. We all assumed the roles that doctors, patients, and parents assume every day in consultation.

Establishing rapport is a skill and an art. Relating to a child requires the clinician to focus on the child and pay attention to what makes him or her unique. Establishing rapport does not mean becoming best friends with the child. In fact, some children may be uncomfortable with behavior that is invasive and overly friendly. Establishing rapport requires the use of various tactics; the same ice breaker cannot be used with every child. As in social conversation, it is important to be aware of the cues, both verbal and nonverbal, coming from the patient and parent.

No matter what level of skill the doctor displays in dealing with children and establishing rapport, parents can facilitate or undermine the examination and treatment process. In one study, children and parents were studied while waiting for treatment at an outpatient clinic.[3] A correlation was noted between crying and other expressions of fear by children and visible agitation combined with anxious attempts to reassure the children by the parents. In addition, parents who reported having the most fear and anxiety themselves had the most fearful and tearful children. Children of parents who used distraction tactics displayed less crying and fewer expressions of fear. This study suggests that poorly prepared parents not only can make the treatment process more difficult for their children but also can make the examination process more difficult for the doctors by raising the level of patient anxiety. More aware parents, in contrast, can exert a positive impact on the treatment process because of the parental style they display prior to the examination. It may be useful to aid poorly prepared parents by making toys and books available for the children. In addition, a handout offering tips to parents could be made available to help them prepare the child for the examination.

Parents differ in their beliefs about appropriate child behavior and preparation. Mothers and children were interviewed prior to a clinic visit.[11] Mothers were labeled suppressive if they believed that it was unacceptable for children to cry or nonsuppressive if they thought that crying was acceptable when the child was hurt or upset. Suppressive mothers were more likely to have a highly anxious child and less likely to be aware that the child was anxious compared to nonsuppressive mothers. The same study went on to discuss the interaction between the level of preparation, anxiety, and curiosity about the medical procedure. Children who asked for preparatory information were less anxious if the mother offered detailed information about the procedure. However, if the mother initiated the discussion rather than the child, children displayed lower levels of anxiety if less detailed information was offered. In another study, however, children who were given more information prior to medical procedures displayed lower levels of behavioral upset.[22] The important difference here seemed to have more to do with the parents than the child. Some parents play out their own anxiety as they give information, while other parents teach their children how to cope more effectively by using available information. The coping capacity of the parents may be one of the most important variables affecting children in treatment. Doctors must recognize that each child may have a different need for information and that each family may use a different coping style; they should respond to the individual need rather than using the same strategy for all patients.

Parental presence is an issue that elicits various opinions. For hospitalized children, the conventional wisdom is that visits by family members and parental rooming-in aid the child in terms of emotional adjustment. Separation anxiety is minimized, and the child retains a sense of control, which is important for stability.[21] Furthermore, visible parents maintain their child's level of trust.[18] Despite studies reporting that 1 year after surgery, parents stated that the most stressful part of hospitalization for the child was remaining alone in the hospital and that remaining alone was rated as more stressful than vomiting blood or receiving injections, not all parents choose to stay with their children.[24]

In outpatient situations, the parental presence is not always viewed as positively as it is with hospitalized patients. Dentists, as a group, prefer that parents wait out of sight while children are being treated.[9] Dentists report that parents frequently express their own fears during the child's treatment, covering their eyes and showing fearful expressions, thus increasing the child's fears.[32]

Children's reactions were studied while they received injections.[28] Children were more likely to express distress when their parents were present. This may simply mean, however, that children are more comfortable in expressing themselves in the presence of parents rather than that parents are the source of distress. In fact, although the absence of expressions of distress may appear to be more positive to the treating clinician, not expressing distress might have a more negative impact in the long term. Each child's reaction to a procedure may be affected by factors such as age, preparation for the procedure, type of procedure, or familiarity with the procedure or other medical procedures.[20] Because no consensus about parental presence exists, it is important to have no set rule governing all situations. Each clinician should be aware of and honest about his own comfort level while working in the presence of parents. Attention should be given to the nature of the particular parent–child relationship and to each parent's capacity to support and calm the child. Parents may respond well to suggestions about the role they may play during the procedure. Making parents aware of the importance of their own actions can be an important intervention. Both parents and children can benefit from training in coping skills to be used before and after surgery.[24]

INTERVENTIONS

Some medical procedures cause sensations perceived as painful by the patient. As medical interventions become more sophisticated, the equipment utilized often triggers feelings of anxiety in patients. Thus, patients must at times cope with pain, anxiety, or both.[19] Some procedures may be threatening but not painful, like magnetic resonance imaging (MRI) or removal of a cast, and require the patient to cope with anxiety. Other procedures are both threatening and painful and require the child to cope with acute physical distress while remaining cooperative, managing emotional distress. Surgery causes no pain during the procedure, but pain may be experienced during recovery. In addition, presurgical anticipatory anxiety must be addressed. Settings such as the emergency room or intensive care may stimulate anxiety and require special intervention.

Peterson and Harbeck (1988) discuss cast removal as a painless but potentially anxiety-producing procedure.[19] Use of a saw on a previously injured part of the body may be very frightening. The child is unfamiliar with the noise and vibration caused by the saw. Regardless of the amount of reassurance, children may fear being cut by the tool. As cast removal proceeds, the smell of the burning cast is unfamiliar. Finally, the wrinkled, gray appearance of the skin may produce anxiety. Appropriate preparation can make this experience easier for children. The sequence of events should be described, emphasizing the importance of remaining still and reassuring the child that the saw will not touch the skin and that the foot or leg will appear a bit different from the healthy foot and leg. The anxious child can be helped by being given distracting thoughts to repeat to himself. For example, the child can be told to say to himself, "All I have to do is sit still. This will be over soon." For highly anxious, more frightened children, relaxation exercises may be

helpful. Procedures with unusual but nonpainful sensations, such as cast removal, are suitable for the use of sensory information techniques. These techniques address sensory issues like the sound of the saw, the smell of the cast, and the look of the skin. In a study involving 6- to 11-year-old children, sensory information reduced distress more effectively than general information about the procedure.[13]

Anesthesia induction is a process that most children find threatening. The idea of being "put to sleep" is very frightening to an unprepared child. There are reports of crying, screaming children being restrained and feeling suffocated, resulting in long-term complications such as stuttering or nightmares.[14, 15] A few simple strategies have been suggested that may be effective. By wearing a Mickey Mouse doll on the stethoscope or around his neck during the presurgical meeting and then again in the operating room (OR), the doctor may help the child recognize him as a friend, and the child is then more likely to cooperate.[36] Carrying a small child into the OR and actually performing the induction while the child remains in an adult's arms has been shown to increase cooperation and reduce anxiety.[8] Children who have been given an opportunity to view a film of a smooth, successful anesthesia induction have reportedly been less anxious and more cooperative.[33] With adequate preparation, children are not only less distressed but also assist in the procedure.

Highest on the list of fear-provoking treatments for children are probably the most frequently used interventions, injections and venipunctures.[26] No consensus exists on the best approach to use with children in performing these treatments. At one extreme is the report that during mass immunizations, children who received direct, no-nonsense instructions to "stand on their feet and not be silly" were less likely to vomit or faint than children who were given no instructions. Most clinicians, however, utilize a more sensitive approach. Again, preparation that identifies the sensory experience in an empathetic manner seems most effective.[7] In one report, the technician said to the child, "I'll bet the alcohol feels cold. In a moment, I'm going to stick you. You're probably feeling scared." This approach elicited less crying, wincing, and noncompliance than a cold direct approach like, "Act big and brave. Remain very still." Techniques using mental imagery,[2] sensory relabeling,[5] and coping techniques of relaxation exercises and distracting imagery[23] are all useful in helping children deal with both injections and chronic pain control.

Parents often ask, "What should I tell my child about coming to the hospital for surgery?" Presurgical interventions have progressed from the time when children were taken on what they believed was to be a fun outing only to end up being admitted at the hospital.[4] Some professionals, however, still believe that children should simply be brought in for treatment unprepared. They believe that any discussion will simply serve to increase anxiety.[19] More pediatric specialists, however, now believe that children should receive honest matter-of-fact information about any procedure they will face.[27]

Pretreatment interventions that have been shown to be highly effective for both inpatient and outpatient procedures can be quite simple or more involved. Simple instructions in deep breathing techniques, muscle relaxation, and coping with feelings, which take only a few minutes, can give a child the sense of control he needs.[37] More formal programs involving behavioral rehearsal and instructional videotapes are also useful.[23] Hypnosis appears to be useful for highly anxious patients. Contrary to popular misconceptions, use of hypnosis does not have to be time-consuming and formal. Hypnotic techniques can be woven into the standard approach used with every patient, and often the techniques of suggestion can be a natural part of the ongoing doctor–patient interaction.[1] A training course given by the American Society of Clinical Hypnosis can prepare physicians from all specialties in methods of incorporating hypnosis into daily practice. Doctors usually opt to use pharmacologic methods such as Valium rather than psychological coping interventions to deal with pain and anxiety. Evidence is mounting, however, that behavioral interventions outperform mild sedatives in reducing distress,[12] and that a combination of medication and behavioral strategies might be most effective.[19]

RECOMMENDATIONS

The information offered in this chapter may have generated more questions than answers for the treating doctor about appropriate techniques to be used with children. This was actually the intention of this article. Physicians need to be armed with a variety of techniques when dealing with the psychological needs of patients and must tailor the approach to each patient. Time should be spent in evaluating the child's level of cognitive and psychosocial development as an attempt is made to communicate with the child. Approaches in building rapport must become a natural part of the clinical strategy. Doctors should consider the possibility of using the energy of parents by letting them help with the treatment process. Parents need the doctor's help with this role. The skilled clinician can enlist parents as helpers and can train them to make the examination and intervention easier. Prepared children will feel more motivated to work with rather than against their doctor. The greater sense of control they feel makes them more likely to comply with the treatment. Thus, a positive outcome is more likely. Paying attention to the human factor results in a pay-off for both the patient and the doctor. The child and parents perceive the doctor as more caring, concerned, and in tune with their needs. They see the clinician as more in control because he helps them feel more in control. Thus, their level of trust in the physician and his or her judgment increases. There is great value in becoming as adept with compassion and empathy as with technology and jargon.

It may be helpful to offer coaching to parents in the form of an office handout. Often parents are happy to play a positive role but are not clear about what form this role should take. By offering this advice, the doctor allows the parents to feel more control over part of the treatment process. The following tip sheet may be used for this purpose.

Tips to Parents

Help your doctor and your child by keeping in mind that your role in the examination and treatment process is very important. Below are a few helpful tips.

Be careful not to "telegraph" your own anxiety to your child. Try to be upbeat, positive, and supportive. Parents who display the most fear and anxiety by words or actions often have the most fearful children.

While waiting, help distract your child by reading to him or encouraging him to play quietly with a toy. Help your child refocus anxiety by coming to the office prepared with a favorite book or toy from home.

Don't try to stop your child from crying if he or she is hurt or upset. This is a natural release. Just support your child by touch and quiet reassurance.

If your child asks for information in preparation for the examination or treatment, offer detailed information that is available to you. If, however, you initiate the discussion, offer minimal information. Don't give too much "reassuring" information to children who do not ask for it!

Do not misinform your child about the appointment to see the doctor. Don't tell the child you will be doing a few errands and then end up at the doctor's office. Children should receive accurate, honest, matter-of-fact information.

Teach your child how to cope by telling him or her your own experience in getting through a difficult, stressful medical procedure.

If your child needs to be hospitalized, consider rooming in if the hospital will allow you to do so and if this is possible. Staying in the hospital alone may be the most stressful part of the hospital experience for the child.

Your doctor is concerned with providing the proper care for your child not only technically but also psychologically. If you are aware of any special needs that your child may have, please inform your doctor or the office assistant.

References

1. American Society of Clinical Hypnosis: A Syllabus on Hypnosis and a Handbook of Therapeutic Suggestions. Des Plaines, IL, ASCH Education and Research Foundation, 1973.
2. Ayer WA: Use of visual imagery in needle phobic children. J Dent Child 1973; 28:41–43.
3. Bush JP, Melamid BG, Sheras PL: Mother-child patterns of coping with anticipatory medical stress. Health Psychol 1986; 5:137–157.
4. Chapman AH, Loeb DG, Gibbons MJP: Psychiatric aspects of hospitalizing children. Arch Pediatr 1956; 73:77–88.
5. Eland JM: Minimizing pain associated with prekindergarten intramuscular injections. Issues Comprehensive Pediatr Nurs 1981; 5:361–372.
6. Engel GL: The need for a new medical model: A challenge for biomedicine. Science 1977; 196:129–136.
7. Fernald CD, Corry JJ: Empathetic versus directive preparation of children for needles. J Assoc Care Child Health 1981; 10:44–47.
8. Gatch G: Caring for children needing anesthesia. AORN J 1982; 35:218–226.
9. Gershen JA: Maternal influence on the behavior patterns of children in the dental situation. J Dent Child 1976; 4:28–32.
10. Ginsburg H, Opper S: Piaget's Theory of Intellectual Development: An Introduction. Englewood Cliffs, NJ, Prentice-Hall, 1969.
11. Heffernan M, Azarnoff P: Factors in reducing children's anxiety about clinic visits. Health Services Ment Health Admin Health Rep 1971; 8:1131–1135.
12. Jay SM, Elliott CH, Katz E, et al: Cognitive behavioral and pharmacologic interventions for children's distress during painful medical

procedures: A treatment outcome study. J Consult Clin Psychol 1987; 5:860–865.

13. Johnson JE, Kirchoff KT, Endress MD: Altering children's distress behavior during orthopedic cast removal. Nurs Res 1975; 2:404–410.

14. Jones ST: Reducing children's psychological stress in the operating suite. Ophthal Plast Reconstr Surg 1985; 1:199–203.

15. Jones ST: Unnecessary psychological complications in children after surgery. J Pediatr Ophthalmol Strabismus 1985; 22:218–220.

16. Lovell K, Elkind D: An Introduction to Human Development. Glenview, IL, Scott, Foresman 1971.

17. Magrab PR, Calcagno PL: Psychological impact of chronic pediatric conditions. In Magreb PR (ed): Psychological Management of Pediatric Problems. Baltimore, University Park Press, 1978, vol 1, pp. 3–14.

18. Mason EA: Hospital and family cooperating to reduce psychological trauma. Community Ment Health J 1978; 14:153–159.

19. Peterson L, Harbeck C: The Pediatric Psychologist: Issues in Professional Development and Practice. Champaign, IL, Research Press, 1988.

20. Peterson L, Mori L: Preparation for hospitalization. In Routh DK (ed): Handbook of Pediatric Psychology. New York, Guilford, 1988, pp. 460–491.

21. Peterson L, Mori L, Carter P: The role of the family in children's responses to stressful medical procedures. J Clin Child Psychol 1985; 14:98–104.

22. Peterson L, Ridley-Johnson R, Tracy K, Mullins LL: Developing cost-effective presurgical preparation: A comparative analysis. J Pediatr Psychol 1984; 9:274–296.

23. Peterson L, Shigetomi C: The use of coping techniques to minimize anxiety in hospitalized children. Behav Ther 1981; 12:1–14.

24. Peterson L, Shigetomi C: One-year follow-up of elective surgery child patients receiving preoperative preparation. J Pediatr Psychol 1982; 7:43–48.

25. Piaget J: The Origins of Intelligence in Children. London, Routledge and Kegan Paul, 1952.

26. Poster EC: Stress immunization: Techniques to help children cope with hospitalization. Matern Child Nurs J 1983; 12:119–134.

27. Prugh DG, Jordan K: Physical illness or injury: The hospital as a source of emotional disturbances in child and family. In Berlin IN (ed): Advocacy for Child Mental Health. New York, Brunner/Mazel, 1975, pp. 208–249.

28. Shaw EG, Routh DK: Effect of mother presence on children's reaction to adverse procedures. J Pediatr Psychol 1982; 7:33–42.

29. Sheridan MS: Talk time for hospitalized children. Social Work 1975; 20:40–44.

30. Spinetta JJ: The dying child's awareness of death: A review. Psychol Bull 1974; 81:256–260.

31. Taylor SE, Aspinwall LG: Psychosocial aspects of chronic illness. In Costa PT Jr, VandenBos GR (eds): Psychological Aspects of Serious Illness: Chronic Conditions, Fatal Diseases, and Clinical Care. Washington, DC, American Psychological Association, 1990, pp. 3–60.

32. Venham LL: The effect of the mother's presence on the child's response to a stressful situation. Unpublished manuscript, University of Connecticut, Storrs, CT. In Peterson L, Harbeck C: The Pediatric Psychologist: Issues in Professional Development and Practice. Champaign, IL, Research Press, 1988.

33. Vernon DTA, Bailey WC: The use of motion pictures in the psychological preparation of children for the induction of anesthesia. Anesthesiology 1974; 40:68–74.

34. Whitt JK, Dykstra W, Taylor CA: Children's conceptions of illness and cognitive development: Implications for pediatric practitioners. Clin Pediatr 1979; 18:327–339.

35. Willis DJ, Elliott CH, Jay SM: Psychological effects of physical illness and its concomitants. In Tuma J (ed): Handbook for the Practice of Pediatric Psychology. New York, Wiley, 1982, pp. 28–66.

36. Wilson AM: A familiar face. Anaesthesia 1982; 37:1225.

37. Zastowny TR, Kirschenbaum DS, Meng AL: Coping skills training for children: Effects on distress before, during, and after hospitalization for surgery. Health Psychol 1986; 5:231–247.

2

Imaging

Katherine M. Richman, M.D., Leon Lenchik, M.D.,
and David J. Sartoris, M.D.

IMAGING TECHNIQUES

Conventional Radiography

Examination of the pediatric foot should include weight-bearing anteroposterior (AP) and lateral radiographs (Fig. 2–1). Infants may require an external support device to simulate weight-bearing positions. Oblique views assist in the evaluation of fractures, foreign bodies, and tarsal coalition.

Examination of the pediatric ankle should include AP and lateral radiographs as well as oblique views obtained for specific indications (Fig. 2–2). For evaluation of congenital deformities in infants, the tibias must be parallel to the sagittal plane. Lateral views must have the ankle rather than the foot in the true lateral position to avoid oblique views of the talus. Radiographs of the ankle in a stressed dorsiflexion position can reveal articular abnormalities.

Tomography of the foot and ankle, although rarely indicated, may provide useful information in patients with complex ankle fractures.

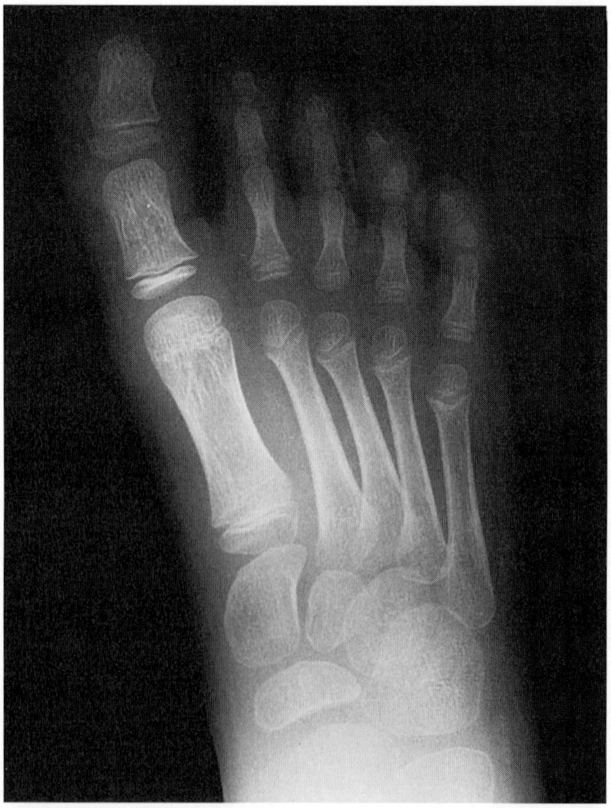

Computed Tomography

Computed tomography (CT) is an excellent modality that allows additional evaluation of the foot and ankle. It provides visualization of the soft tissues as well as excellent detail of the osseous anatomy. Images obtained in the coronal and axial planes allow accurate diagnosis, and, if necessary, surgical planning. CT surpasses magnetic resonance imaging (MRI) for evaluating the bony cortex and is often necessary in the assessment of fractures, tumors, and subtalar tarsal coalitions (Fig. 2–3).

Magnetic Resonance Imaging

MRI involves the magnetic alignment and excitement of hydrogen protons in tissue. Protons in various structures gain and lose signal at different time intervals; thus, different sequences allow differentiation of tissues and

Figure 2–1. Routine anteroposterior (AP) radiograph of the foot.

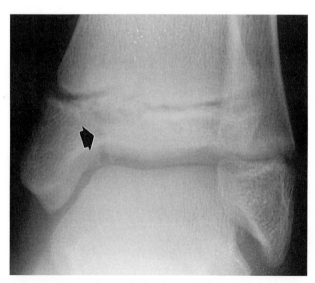

Figure 2–2. Anteroposterior (AP) radiograph of the ankle in a 13-year-old male. Note the Salter-Harris III fracture of the distal tibia (*arrow*) extending from the tibial epiphysis to the physis.

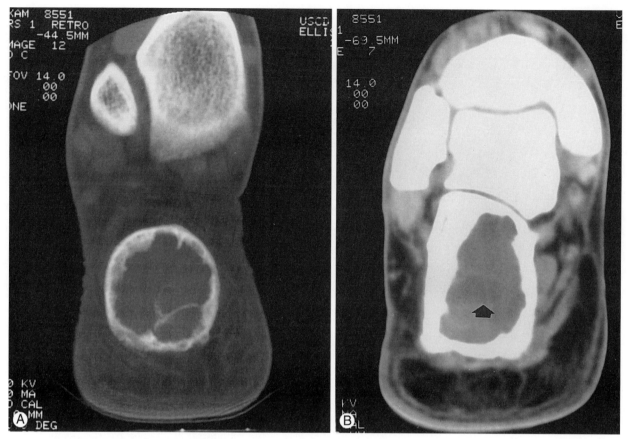

Figure 2–3. Computed tomography (CT) scan of an aneurysmal bone cyst. *A,* Coronal CT scan filmed with bone window setting shows an expansile, trabeculated, lytic lesion in the calcaneus. *B,* Coronal CT scan obtained with patient supine and filmed with soft tissue window setting shows multiple fluid levels *(arrow)* within the lesion.

can narrow the diagnostic possibilities in abnormal areas. The benefits of MRI include the availability of multiplanar imaging, excellent assessment of bone marrow for determination of the extent of a tumor or infection, lack of radiation, and evaluation of soft tissue abnormalities (Fig. 2–4). For example, MRI is ideal for evaluating ischemic necrosis of the talus and osteochondritis dissecans of the talus. The limitations of MRI include the need to refrain from all movement by the patient (which often requires sedation or general anesthesia in young children), high cost, and poor visualization of calcifications and cortical bone.

On T1-weighted images, the bone marrow is bright because of fat. The cortex forms a signal void around the bone marrow in all sequences. Articular cartilage has a low to intermediate signal, whereas tendons uniformly produce a dark signal.

Gadolinium-DTPA, the MR contrast agent, is an inert metal chelate. It is used only with T1-weighted fat-saturated sequences. As with the intravenous contrast agents used in CT, it delineates the vascular structures and highlights areas of inflammation, infection, and neoplasm. Unlike iodinated CT intravenous contrast agents, however, it rarely causes allergic reactions. Very few people (except patients with severe chronic obstructive pulmonary disease [COPD]) have had adverse responses to gadolinium.

Nuclear Scintigraphy

Several different nuclear scintigraphic examinations are useful for evaluating the pediatric foot and ankle. The three-phase bone scan with ^{99m}Tc-MDP assesses blood flow, initial radiopharmaceutical uptake, and delayed radiopharmaceutical uptake in bone. This scan is commonly used in the diagnosis of osteomyelitis. Indium-111 and gallium-67 citrate scintigraphy, used in combination with three- or four-phase bone scans, can help differentiate infections from other abnormalities.

Ultrasound

Ultrasound can help evaluate soft tissue masses, differentiating cystic from solid components. In neonates, ultrasound may show nonossified epiphyses. When septic arthritis is suspected, ultrasound demonstrates the presence of joint effusions and provides guidance for joint aspiration.

Arthrography

Although it is rarely used in children, arthrography may show unossified epiphyses and can thus delineate the extent of fractures.

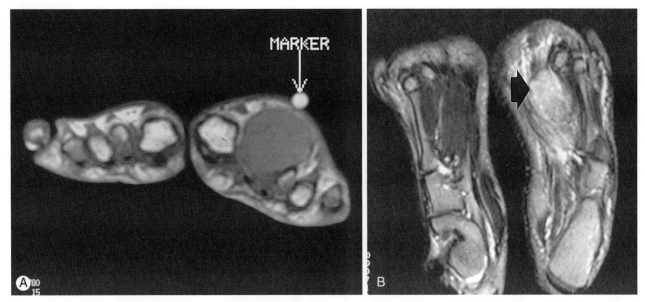

Figure 2–4. MR image of Ewing's sarcoma in an 11-year-old female. A, Axial T1-weighted MR image of both feet with a marker over a palpable mass shows a large low signal intensity lesion centered in the second metatarsal. B, Coronal T2-weighted MR image of both feet shows high signal intensity (arrow) in the lesion.

NORMAL VARIANTS

Ossification Patterns

At birth, three ossification centers are present in the foot: the talus, the calcaneus, and the cuboid. By the end of the first year, the distal tibia and the lateral cuneiform ossification centers become visible. Metatarsal, proximal phalangeal, and middle phalangeal ossification centers appear by the end of the second year; the distal phalanges, the navicular, and the medial and intermediate cuneiform centers ossify by the end of the third year. In general, male development in certain ossification centers lags behind female development by about a year (Table 2–1).

Accessory ossification centers are frequently seen on foot and ankle images (Fig. 2–5). Occasionally they may

be confused with fractures. In particular, the ossification center at the base of the fifth metatarsal should not be mistaken for a fracture. In general, avulsion fractures of the fifth metatarsal are oriented perpendicular to the long axis of the metatarsal bone, whereas the ossification center physis runs parallel to it (see Fig. 2–43).

Sesamoid bones lie within tendons and are always present along the first ray, occur commonly along the fifth ray, and nearly never arise along the second to fourth rays. The sesamoids may be bifid and are occasionally mistaken for fractures.

Common Anatomic Variants

Epiphyses

Epiphyses, especially epiphyses of the phalanges, can vary in shape from one individual to another. Some chil-

Table 2–1. **Timetable of Ossification**

Centers Present	Females	Fusion (yr)	Males	Fusion (yr)
At Birth	Calcaneus		Calcaneus	
	Talus		Talus	
	Cuboid		Cuboid	
End of 1 yr	Distal tibia (1–7 mo)	16 to 17	Distal tibia (1–7 mo)	17 to 19
	Distal fibula (1–7 mo)	15 to 17	Distal fibula (1–7 mo)	17 to 19
	Cuneiform III (3 mo)		Cuneiform III (6 mo)	
End of 2 yr	Metatarsals	17 to 20	Prox. phalanges (1–2.5 yr)	17 to 18
	Prox. phalanges (1–2.5 yr)	18		
	Mid. phalanges (.5–2.5 yr)	18		
End of 3 yr	Cuneiform I and II (0.5–2.5 yr)		Metatarsals	18 to 20
	Tarsal navicular (1–3 yr)		Mid. phalanges (1–4 yr)	18
	Dist. phalanges (1.5–4 yr)	18	Cuneiform I and II (1–3.5 yr)	
End of 4 yr			Tarsal navicular (1.5–5.5 yr)	
End of 6 yr			Dist phalanges (3.5–6.5 yr)	18
End of 8 yr	Calcaneal apophysis (5–12 yr)	12 to 22		
End of 10 yr			Calcaneal apophysis (5–12 yr)	12 to 22

Modified from Juhl JH, Crummy AB (eds): Paul and Juhl's Essentials of Radiologic Imaging, 6th ed. Philadelphia, J.B. Lippincott, 1993.

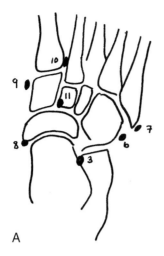
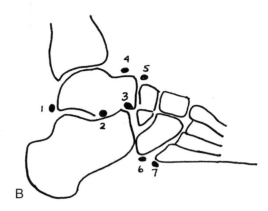

Figure 2–5. Accessory ossification centers of the foot and ankle. *A*, Diagram of the foot in the AP projection showing the various accessory ossification centers. *B*, Diagram of the ankle in lateral projection. (1, os trigonum; 2, os sustentaculi; 3, os calcaneus secondarius; 4, secondary astragalus; 5, supranavicular; 6, os peroneum; 7, os vesalianum; 8, os tibiale externum; 9, sesamoid tibiale anterius; 10, os intermetatarsum; 11, os intercuneiforme.)

A

B

dren have cone-shaped epiphyses, which are a variant of normal and do not portend a histologic or metabolic abnormality (Fig. 2–6).

Os Trigonum

The os trigonum occurs in 10% of the population, serves as the site of talofibular ligament attachment, and may show complete or incomplete separation from the talus. It should not be confused with a talar fracture.

Apophysis of the Os Calcis

The apophysis of the calcaneus develops along the posterior margin. In many skeletally immature individu-

als, the apophysis of the calcaneus often appears denser than the remainder of the calcaneus ("ivory epiphysis"), and it may be fragmented (Fig. 2–7). It should not be confused with a calcaneal fracture. Previously, some authors thought that a form of calcaneal apophyseal osteochondrosis, Sever's disease, could occur if apophyseal density or fragmentation and pain were present. The term is no longer valid; the variable appearance of the apophysis merely reflects the wide spectrum of normal variation. If the child has calcaneal pain, disease entities such as Achilles tendinitis should be considered.

Bipartite Navicular

The navicular may be bipartitite and may cause pain in the adolescent. Bone scintigraphy occasionally may help in differentiating a fractured navicular from a bipartite one because both can have similar radiographic appearances.

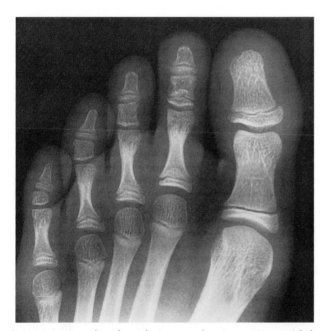

Figure 2–6. Cone-shaped epiphysis: normal variant. AP view of the forefoot shows multiple cone-shaped epiphyses, which are most apparent in the proximal phalanges of the third and fourth toes. The findings were bilateral.

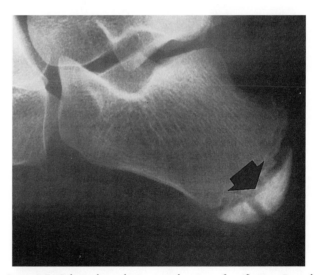

Figure 2–7. Calcaneal apophysis: normal variant of ossification. Lateral view of the ankle shows dense sclerosis and fragmentation *(arrow)* of the calcaneal secondary ossification center. The findings in this asymptomatic child were bilateral.

Accessory Navicular Bone

Children with an accessory navicular may have pain over the medial midfoot in their teens. The posterior tibialis tendon passes across and often inserts a portion of its fibers into the accessory bone. Conventional radiographs can detect its presence.[29] MRI, if needed, can determine the position and insertion of the posterior tibialis tendon.[2]

Osteochondroses

For the podiatrist, two osteochondroses are noteworthy: tarsal navicular (Koehler's disease) and metatarsal head (Freiberg's infraction). For each of these entities, conventional radiographs reveal increased density initially, and then fragmentation followed by gradual reossification.[29]

Tarsal Navicular Osteochondrosis (Koehler's Disease)

An uncommon, often asymptomatic disease, osteochondrosis of the tarsal navicular causes radiographic findings including subchondral sclerosis, fragmentation, and flattening of the navicular (Fig. 2–8). The physician should be aware that irregular ossification of the navicular can be a normal variant.[29]

Freiberg's Infraction

Freiberg's infraction can involve any of the metatarsal heads but most commonly affects the second, followed

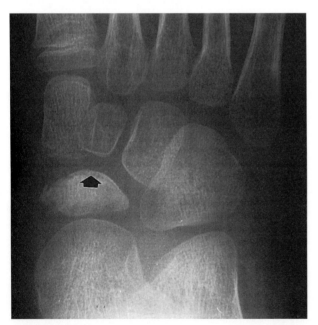

Figure 2–8. Koehler's disease in a 6-year-old girl. AP view of the foot shows sclerosis and fragmentation of the tarsal navicular bone. Subchondral lucency (*arrow*) represents an associated subchondral fracture.

by the third and first metatarsals. Girls are affected more often than boys, usually in their teens and twenties, and often give a history of new or increased use of high-heeled shoes. Radiographs show flattening or irregularity of the metatarsal head, followed by sclerosis and thickening of the metatarsal cortical shaft. Some authors consider Freiberg's infraction a type of stress fracture.

CONGENITAL ANOMALIES

1. Talipes equinovarus (clubfoot)
2. Talipes calcaneovalgus
3. Congenital vertical talus
4. Metatarsus adductus
5. Tarsal coalition
6. Toe deformities
7. Fibrodysplasia ossificans progressiva
8. Malformation syndromes
9. Amniotic band syndrome

General Comments

Evaluation of congenital anomalies on foot radiographs requires examination of the axis of the calcaneus, the relationship of the talar and calcaneal axes, and the metatarsal to talar axes. On lateral radiographs, the long axis of the calcaneus bisects the bone into superior and inferior segments. Plantar angulation of the distal portion of the calcaneal axis suggests that the calcaneus is in an equinus position. Dorsal angulation of the distal calcaneal axis indicates a calcaneus position. The AP radiograph shows the talocalcaneal relationship best. Lines that parallel the long axis of the calcaneus and the talus bisect the talus and calcaneus into medial and lateral segments. The normal heel has 5 to 10 degrees of calcaneal valgus. In calcaneal varus the calcaneal axis runs more parallel to the talar axis. In calcaneal valgus more than 10 degrees of hindfoot valgus is present.

Talipes Equinovarus (Clubfoot)

Clubfoot affects males more than females, may be unilateral or bilateral, and may arise from idiopathic or neurologic causes. This condition involves the hindfoot, forefoot, and midfoot. An equinovarus talocalcaneal relationship coexists with metatarsus adductus and medial rotation. AP foot radiographs show the long axis of the second metatarsal bone medial to the long axis of the talus (Figs. 2–9 and 2–10).

Talipes Calcaneovalgus

The most common neonatal deformity, talipes calcaneovalgus results from uterine confinement and frequently resolves without treatment. In one study, none of the children with calcaneovalgus required treatment.[33] On physical examination, the foot dorsiflexes easily, folds against the anterolateral surface of the tibia, and exhibits

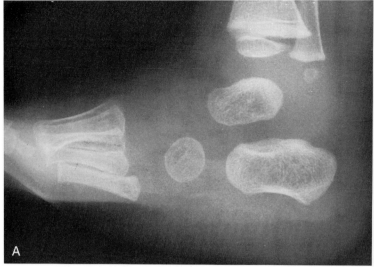

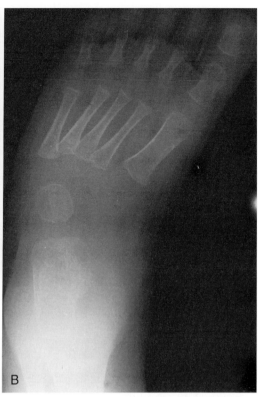

Figure 2–9. Congenital equinovarus (clubfoot) in an 18-month-old girl. *A*, Lateral view shows a more parallel configuration of the talar and calcaneal axes than normal. *B*, AP view shows marked hindfoot varus with superimposition of the talus and the calcaneus.

a long and stretched (but not tight) heel cord. The sole has a "banana" shape.

Severe cases of this condition may mimic vertical talus. As the name of the condition implies, AP radiographs of a child with calcaneovalgus demonstrate calcaneus position of the calcaneus and valgus angulation of the calcaneal axis. In contrast, in vertical talus the hindfoot is in equinus. Also, in vertical talus the heel cord is tight.[32]

Vertical Talus (Congenital Pes Valgus)

Congenital vertical talus is associated with neurologic disorders such as spina bifida, myelomeningocele, and arthrogryposis multiplex congenita. In this condition the peroneus longus and posterior tibial tendons act as dorsiflexors rather than plantar flexors. Since these tendons are more anterior than usual, they pull the talus into a vertical position. The condition is bilateral in 50% of cases.

Radiographs show vertical alignment of the talus with its long axis paralleling that of the tibia. The calcaneus is in equinus and valgus position with a widely divergent talocalcaneal angle. The child has a convex arch and dorsiflexed toes. Once ossified, the navicular is dislocated anterior to the talar neck. MRI can help in evaluating the talar axis and the position of the nonossified navicular.

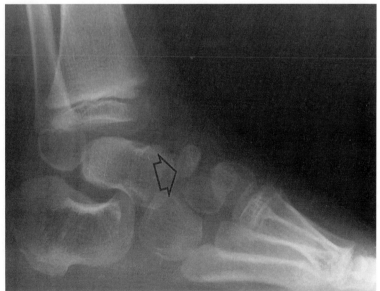

Figure 2–10. Congenital equinovarus. Postoperative appearance in a 4-year-old girl. Lateral weight-bearing radiograph shows talar deformity and a dislocated navicular *(arrow)*.

Sagittal images can show both the vertical orientation of the talus parallel to the axis of the tibia and the abnormal anterior position of the navicular.[2]

Metatarsus Adductus

Ten times more common than congenital clubfoot, unilateral or bilateral in distribution, metatarsus adductus often results from intrauterine confinement and is a self-limited condition in 85% of cases. Radiographs show a normal configuration of the hindfoot and midfoot with adduction of the forefoot.

Tarsal Coalition

Most fusions are congenital. Fusions can also arise after infection, surgery, or arthritis.[25] They can be fibrous, cartilaginous, osseous, or mixed. Fusion occurs in 1% to 3% of children and is bilateral in 60% of cases.[29] Calcaneonavicular fusion is the most common entity (53%), followed closely by talocalcaneal fusion (37%). Calcaneocuboid and talonavicular fusions are much less common.[25, 27]

The calcaneonavicular coalition typically ossifies between 8 and 12 years of age; the talocalcaneal coalition ossifies between 12 and 16 years. The less mobile ossified coalition often changes an asymptomatic fusion to one that causes pain.[31] In children with peroneal spasm or pes planus a coalition is frequently the cause of pain. Nonetheless, the clinical examination and radiographic studies must rule out infection, trauma, and juvenile chronic arthritis, all of which can induce similar symptoms.[19]

The initial radiographic procedure should include standing AP, lateral, and oblique conventional radiographs of the foot.[29] Primary radiographic findings demonstrate the actual coalition, whereas secondary radiographic findings suggest its presence because of the typical adaptive changes that occur (Table 2–2).

Calcaneonavicular Coalition

Calcaneonavicular coalition is the most common type of tarsal fusion. Most coalitions are visible on a 45-degree medial-oblique view, which demonstrates widening of the

Table 2–2. **Secondary Signs of Tarsal Coalition**

Calcaneonavicular Coalition
Hypoplasia of the talar head
Talocalcaneal Coalition
Narrowing of the posterior talocalcaneal joint space
Broadening or rounding of the lateral talar process
Ball-in-socket tibiotalar articulation
Osseous excrescence at dorsal aspect of talus
Concave undersurface of talar neck
Failure to visualize middle facet of anterior subtalar joint
Dorsal subluxation of navicular
Periosteal elevation at talonavicular ligament attachment site
Calcaneal valgus

anterior calcaneus and narrowing or obliteration of the fat plane between the calcaneus and the navicular[25] (Fig. 2–11). The lateral film demonstrates beaking of the calcaneus ("anteater" appearance) extending toward the navicular. Secondary radiographic findings include hypoplasia of the talar head and sclerosis at the talonavicular joint.[25] Under normal circumstances, no articulation exists between the calcaneus and the navicular. CT scanning is rarely indicated and can miss the plane of fusion, leading to a false-negative result. If CT is needed (perhaps to screen for other abnormalities), the foot should be in the oblique position to increase the chances of imaging along the plane of coalition.[19] CT or MRI scanning can help identify fibrous fusions.[27]

Talocalcaneal Coalition

Talocalcaneal coalition occurs in men more often than women and is bilateral in up to 25% of cases.[25] This type of coalition usually occurs between the middle talar facet and the sustentaculum tali of the calcaneus. Primary radiographic signs include absence of the middle subtalar joint and subchondral sclerosis and narrowing of the posterior subtalar joint.[10] These signs are absent in as many as 50% of patients.[10] In addition, the coalition produces other subtle findings on plain films, including anterior beaking of the talus, pes planus, and a ball-in-socket appearance of the tibiotalar joint. The lateral view is particularly helpful. Lateur and colleagues described a C sign that was visible on the lateral view in patients with subtalar fusion. The C-shaped line consists of the medial outline of the talar dome and the inferior outline of the sustentaculum tali when coalition is present. They found a rate of 90% sensitivity and specificity for diagnosis using

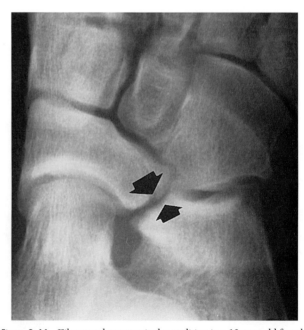

Figure 2–11. Fibrous calcaneonavicular coalition in a 12-year-old female. Oblique view of the foot shows subchondral sclerosis and irregularity of both the calcaneus and the navicular in the region of the coalition (*arrows*). The findings were bilateral.

this sign.[10] Comparison with the contralateral foot may help in identifying secondary signs of coalition.[10, 25] In some cases, the axial or Harris-Beath view can reveal the bony coalition.[19]

Scintigraphy with ^{99m}Tc-MDP leads to increased tracer uptake along the sustentaculum tali. This nonspecific finding can help in localizing the abnormality.[5] In children, however, normal epiphyseal uptake may render interpretation difficult.[31] Talonavicular arthrography using contrast agent and Xylocaine can indicate a coalition when the injected contrast agent does not flow between the sustentaculum tali of the calcaneus and the middle talar facet and the patient experiences pain relief.[19] CT scanning through the subtalar joint can both document the coalition and assist in surgical planning[29] (Fig. 2–12). In addition, it images the other foot at the same time; thus, bilateral coalitions can be discovered without extra time or cost.[19] At this time, CT is the most definitive imaging procedure[19] with scans taken in the angled coronal and sagittal projections.[30] CT shows osseous bridging in bony coalitions (synostosis) and joint space narrowing and hypertrophied reactive cortical bone in fibrous or cartilaginous coalitions (syndesmosis and synchondrosis, respectively).[30]

Nonetheless, in a few cases, conventional radiographs and CT scans fail to reveal the coalition. MRI can uncover bridging of the talus and calcaneus and absence of the joint space between the sustentaculum tali and the talus.[2] Rarely, proliferative synovitis can cause a false-positive result on MRI.[31] In children, MRI can display the coalition prior to ossification, thus allowing early treatment.[31]

Other Coalitions

Talonavicular and calcaneocuboid fusions occur rarely, can cause peroneal spasm, and may be associated with

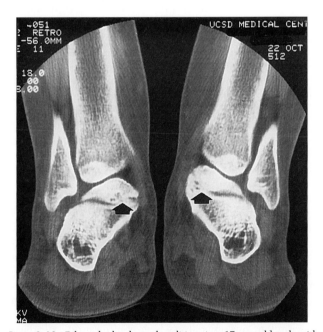

Figure 2–12. Bilateral talocalcaneal coalitions in a 17-year-old male with foot pain. Coronal CT scan of both ankles shows the osseous coalitions (arrows). The case is unusual in that the coalitions are posterior to the sustentaculum tali.

other congenital anomalies. Both are readily diagnosed on conventional radiographs.[25]

Amniotic Band Syndrome

This devastating anomaly occurs when a focal portion of the amnion separates from the chorion and adheres to the fetus. Amputations of fingers, toes, or entire extremities are common. Some authors consider amniotic bands part of a complex known as ADAM: amniotic deformity, adhesion, and mutilation. Radiography is rarely needed for diagnosis but can aid in surgical planning.

Fibrodysplasia Ossificans Progressiva

This rare hereditary mesodermal disorder causes progressive ossification of muscles, tendons, ligaments, and, occasionally, skin. The cause is unknown, but the disease affects men and women equally. Seventy-five to ninety percent of affected children have short first toes bilaterally, short thumbs, and valgus deformity. Often the phalanges are fused. Symptoms arise during the first decade and progress caudally from the neck down to the lower extremities. Complications include inability to ambulate (hip joint ankylosis), hearing loss (conductive), and respiratory failure (limited chest wall expansion).

On conventional radiographs, nearly 90% of affected persons have short first toes bilaterally with broad, square, often fused phalanges. They develop hallux valgus and thickening of the medial tibial cortices. Soft tissue masses arise and ossify over time. The differential diagnosis includes dermatomyositis (which causes calcification but not ossification) and dystrophic myositis from paraplegia or burns. The digital abnormalities distinguish fibrodysplasia ossificans progressiva from other entities.[21]

INFECTION

Osteomyelitis

Infection reaches the bones and joints through three routes: direct inoculation (foreign body puncture), hematogenous spread, and direct extension from a contiguous process (secondary osteomyelitis). Hematogenous spread accounts for nearly all cases of osteomyelitis in children. The blood supply to the epiphyses differs among infants, children, and adults. Whereas the nutrient artery extends from the diaphysis to the epiphysis in infants less than 18 months of age and in adults, the artery ends at the physis in children. Thus, in infants and adults, hematogenous osteomyelitis may begin in the epiphysis and extend into the joint or into the metaphysis. In children, hematogenous infection originates in the metaphysis and rarely extends into the epiphysis or the joint.

Hematogenous infection begins within the medullary space. The pus and subsequent edema destroy the trabeculae and cause vascular stasis, leading to bone infarction and necrosis. The infection breaks through the cortex and extends between the periosteum and the bone shaft, causing periosteal elevation.

Osteomyelitis has three stages: acute, subacute, and chronic, with different radiographic findings in each. It commonly affects more than one bone. Although the femur and humerus are the two most commonly affected bones, the tibia and calcaneus also are frequent sites of infection.[20]

Acute Osteomyelitis

During the first week of osteomyelitis, plain radiographs are often negative. Soft tissue swelling and loss of normal intermuscular fat planes account for the initial plain film findings. If allowed to progress, osteomyelitis can cause lytic bone lesions (Fig. 2–13). Periosteal elevation is consistent with but not specific for osteomyelitis (Fig. 2–14). Differential diagnosis includes metastatic neuroblastoma, Ewing's sarcoma, leukemia, and eosino-

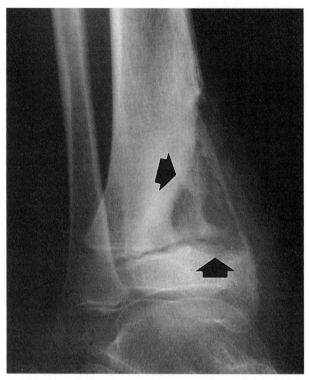

Figure 2–14. Osteomyelitis from coccidioidomycosis in a 12-year-old boy. AP view of the ankle shows a large lytic lesion *(arrows)* associated with periosteal reaction involving the medial metaphysis of the distal tibia.

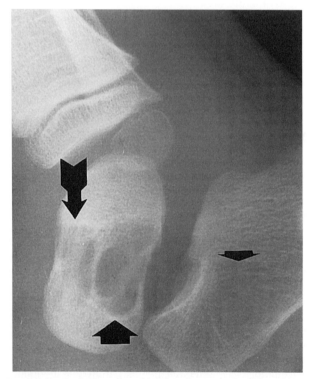

Figure 2–13. Disseminated osteomyelitis from coccidioidomycosis in a 3-year-old boy. Lateral view of the ankle shows a well-demarcated multilocular, lytic lesion *(arrows)* in the talus and a subtle lytic lesion *(arrow)* in the calcaneus.

philic granuloma. Osteomyelitis is more common in long bones than in flat bones, vertebral bodies, or small bones. Periosteal elevation occurs in long bone osteomyelitis, but in the short bones and vertebral bodies, one sees lysis of bone without periosteal elevation.

Bone scans and MRI provide definitive information during the first few days of osteomyelitis. On multiphase bone scans, areas of infection show increased blood flow and increased uptake. Areas of cellulitis may show initial radiopharmaceutical uptake and increased blood flow but no residual uptake. Osteomyelitis, on the other hand, demonstrates increased uptake on delayed images. Areas of bone that have infarcted will show decreased uptake. If multiphase bone scanning is insufficient, scintigraphy using indium-111 oxine-labeled white blood cells can help identify foci of infection. Also, gallium-67 citrate scintigraphy will show increased uptake in areas of infection.

MRI can reveal areas of cellulitis in the soft tissues through inhomogeneous signal and enhancement. If the child has not had surgery or trauma, MRI can accurately assess the bone marrow for osteomyelitis. Low signal intensity on T1-weighted images and high signal intensity on T2-weighted images indicate osteomyelitis. Some authors have reported greater sensitivity using fat-suppressed, contrast-enhanced T1-weighted images.[15] In children with cellulitis, foreign bodies in soft tissues, or abscesses, MRI can help decide whether the child has concomitant osteomyelitis, which is often a difficult diagnostic dilemma. Of note, previous surgery, neuropathy, or prior trauma can cause findings similar to osteomyelitis, rendering differentiation difficult.

Subacute and Chronic Osteomyelitis

Depending on the virulence of the organism and the timing of antibiotic treatment, conventional radiographs may show a Brodie's abscess. This lesion is characterized by dense sclerotic margins with an inhomogeneous center extending down to the growth plate along the long axis of the bone. It occurs most commonly in the tibia and femur. Chronic osteomyelitis may progress to form a sequestrum (a fragment of necrotic bone that appears very dense with a surrounding lucency known as a cloaca) and an involucrum (dense new bone and periosteum that occurs around the sequestum and cloaca).

On MRI, abscesses have low signal intensity on T1-weighted images and high signal intensity on T2-weighted images, as well as rim enhancement with gadolinium.

Specific Forms of Osteomyelitis

Tuberculosis. Skeletal tuberculosis (TB) affects adults more often than children. Nonetheless, tuberculous infection of the hands and feet is more common in children than adults. Less than 50% of those with skeletal tuberculosis have concomitant pulmonary TB.

Radiographs usually reveal findings similar to pyogenic osteomyelitis: soft tissue swelling, periostitis, and more gradual bone destruction.[34] TB involves the metaphyses and can spread across the physis, whereas pyogenic infections generally respect the physis. Spina ventosa refers to the specific cyst-like expansion of the affected metatarsals, metacarpals, and phalanges. Sinus tracts, sequestration, and diffuse trabecular involvement may all develop as part of tuberculous dactylitis.

The differential diagnosis includes other infections (pyogenic, fungal, and syphilitic dactylitis), metabolic abnormalities (hyperparathyroidism), and systemic diseases (anemias, sarcoid). Biopsy or aspiration is often required for specific diagnosis.

Meningococcemia. Disseminated meningococcemia in children causes severe mortality and morbidity. Radiographic findings during the acute stage of disease include extensive epiphyseal destruction. Meningococcemia can result in disseminated intravascular coagulopathy, which in turn causes necrosis of skin and other tissues. Digital sloughing may occur. In the chronic phase, premature central growth plate closure leads to ball-in-socket joint deformities. Premature fusion of epiphyses occurs in a bilateral and symmetrical distribution.

Syphilis. Caused by *Treponema pallidum*, syphilis can affect infants owing to transplacental spread. Six to eight weeks of infection are necessary before radiographic abnormalities become visible. The child may have a rash, anemia, and hepatosplenomegaly in addition to marked periostitis. In the first 3 months of life, the child may refuse to move because of bone pain resulting from osteochondritis (chondroepiphysitis). Radiographs reveal the periosteal reaction as well as areas of lytic destruction and sclerosis in the the metaphysis (Fig. 2–15). The tibial

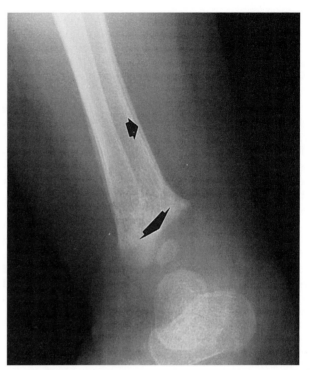

Figure 2–15. Osteomyelitis from congenital syphilis in a 6-month-old boy. Note the periosteal reaction along the diaphysis (*arrow*) and irregularity of the metaphysis (*arrow*) of the distal tibia.

metaphyses often exhibit characteristic periosteal thickening known as "saber shins."

Septic Arthritis

Septic arthritis affects children more often than adults; children less than 3 years of age account for 50% of cases. Septic arthritis in neonates differs somewhat from that in older children. Before 18 months of age, the vasculature crosses the physis, permitting metaphyseal infections to enter the epiphysis and the joint. In older children, however, the vasculature does not cross the physeal plate. *Haemophilus influenzae* causes most septic arthritis cases in toddlers (*Escherichia coli* is the most common cause in neonates). After 2 years of age, *Staphylococcus aureus* becomes the most likely organism.

Conventional radiographs may reveal joint effusions, bone destruction, osteopenia, and joint space narrowing if the infection is allowed to progress. Since infection causes hyperemia, septic arthritis can cause premature bone maturation and early closure of the physis.

Scintigraphy has limited usefulness in assessing septic arthritis without osteomyelitis. At times, arthrography is needed to assess the amount of epiphyseal bone and cartilage destruction. Ultrasound can locate the joint effusion and help guide joint aspiration for culture. MRI can detect the presence of effusion and can help in evaluating the epiphysis for erosion and the bone marrow for osteomyelitis complicating septic arthritis.

Differential diagnosis includes other infections (tuberculous arthritis), inflammatory arthritis (juvenile rheumatoid arthritis), articular abnormalities (pigmented villonodular synovitis, synovial osteochondromatosis), and systemic diseases (hemophilia).

Soft Tissue Infections

Soft tissue infections commonly result from trauma with direct inoculation. Puncture wounds most commonly result from stepping on a nail. Cellulitis and osteomyelitis develop in approximately 10% and 1% of punctures, respectively. The puncture typically occurs at the metatarsal-phalangeal junction. *Pseudomonas,* which frequently inhabits the soles of shoes, is the most common offending organism.

Puncture wounds and foreign bodies can incite abscess formation. Plain films show edema and loss of normal fat planes. CT and MRI both provide a better demonstration of the location and characteristics of the abscess. Wood particles have a density equal to air and can be difficult to assess using CT. At times, ultrasound allows detection of foreign bodies within the foot.

Chronic Recurrent Multifocal Osteomyelitis

Chronic recurrent multifocal osteomyelitis (CRMO) affects children aged 7 to 14 who present with palmar and plantar rash and pain. Radiographs show multiple areas of osteolysis intermingled with, and usually dominated by, areas of intense sclerosis.[20] In addition, exuberant periostitis is often present. Despite an appearance similar to osteomyelitis, bone biopsies in patients with this condition are usually negative.[17] The lesions show a predilection for symmetrical lower extremity metaphyseal involvement and typically occur in the tibia and femur, as well as in many other sites. Periosteal reaction may be present. The differential diagnosis includes osteomyelitis, chronic granulomatous disease, and vitamin D-resistant rickets. Antibotics have no effect; the condition often is self-limited.

METABOLIC DISORDERS

1. Rickets
2. Hyperparathyroidism
3. Hypothyroidism
4. Renal osteodystrophy
5. Pseudohypoparathyroidism and pseudopseudohypoparathyroidism
6. Lesch-Nyhan syndrome

Rickets

Rickets results from a deficiency or unresponsiveness to vitamin D. A variety of disorders—nutritional deficiencies or intestinal, hepatic, or renal abnormalities—can lead to rickets. A few cases result from familial vitamin D resistance or hypophosphatemia.

The classic radiographic findings include metaphyaseal widening and irregularity (particularly at the zone of provisional calcification) and osteopenia (Fig. 2–16). The findings are most prominent at areas of maximal bone growth: the wrists and knees. The radiographs show metaphyseal cupping, demineralization of the bones, and indistinct epiphyseal margins.[9] Incomplete ossification of the physis causes a false appearance of metaphyseal widening.[9]

Hyperparathyroidism

Hyperparathyroidism (HPT) has primary, secondary, and tertiary forms. Primary HPT usually results from a parathyroid adenoma releasing abnormally high hormone levels. Secondary HPT results from renal failure causing chronic hypocalcemia. Tertiary HPT arises from unresponsiveness of the parathyroid glands to serum calcium levels. The three forms have radiographic changes that overlap.

All forms of hyperparathyroidism cause bone resorption, of which there are six types: subperiosteal, intracortical, endosteal, intramedullary, subchondral, and subligamentous.[21] Table 2–3 lists those forms that commonly affect the foot. Subperiosteal resorption is the most helpful abnormality in diagnosing HPT. It creates erosions along the margins of joints similar in appearance to those of rheumatoid arthritis. In addition, subperiosteal resorption can cause band-like acro-osteolysis of the phalangeal tufts. Subchondral absorption causes weakening and collapse of the subchondral bone and depression of the articular cartilage. Thus, subperiosteal and subchondral resorption are the two most common articular changes noted with HPT. Irregularity along the physis due to

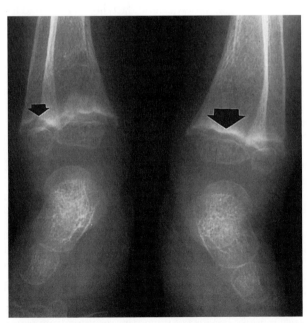

Figure 2–16. Treated rickets in a 2-year-old girl. AP view of both ankles shows generalized osteopenia as well as bilateral and symmetrical widening, cupping, and irregularity involving the metaphyses of the distal tibiae and fibulae *(arrows).*

Table 2–3. **Sites of Hyperparathyroid Bone Resorption in the Foot**

Subperiosteal bone resorption:	Acro-osteolysis; irregular cortex along phalanges, along the margin of joints, creating erosions (most useful sign)
Subchondral resorption:	Along the metatarsals, creating weakening and collapse
Subligamentous resorption:	Along the calcaneus just inferior to the Achilles tendon; along the inferior calcaneus at the planar fascial insertion
Subphyseal resorption:	Creates an irregular metaphysis, tubular bones of the foot, especially in children with primary or secondary HPT

subphyseal resorption, usually along the tubular bones of the foot, occurs especially in children with secondary or primary HPT. The three forms of HPT cause osteopenia, with ligamentous laxity and/or rupture (especially of the infrapatellar tendon).[21]

Primary hyperparathyroidism can also cause calcium pyrophosphate deposition and brown tumors. Brown tumors appear as cystic bone lesions resulting from intraosseous localized fibrous tissue accumulation. In infants, primary hyperparathyroidism can lead to such severe bone resorption and erosions of tubular bones that the child develops pathologic fractures. Severe cases of infantile HPT have been mistaken for congenital syphilis. In older children, the findings include genu valgum, osteopenia, bone resorption, and cystic bone lesions.[21] These children may also suffer from fractures and phalangeal clubbing.[21]

Secondary hyperparathyroidism may cause osteosclerosis (usually in the spine, producing a diffuse or "rugger jersey" spinal appearance). Periosteal new bone formation (periosteal neostosis) occurs in the pelvis, femur, and metatarsals.

Renal Osteodystrophy

Chronic renal insufficiency or renal failure in a child often creates skeletal changes typical of both rickets and hyperparathyroidism. Conventional radiographs may show bowing of the long bones, osteopenia, metaphyseal irregularity, and various types of bone resorption. In addition, ischemic necrosis may develop, usually in the femoral heads, but it can occur in the talar dome as well. Other complications include a slipped or separated epiphysis (of the long bones or, rarely, the hands and feet), amorphous soft tissue calcifications, and vascular calcifications (prominent in the hands and feet).

Hypothyroidism

Thyroid hormone plays a critical role in bone growth and maturation. Congenital deficiency of thyroid hormone (cretinism) affects girls more than boys (3:1), arises spo-

radically or from autosomal recessive transmission (uncommon), and frequently affects children with trisomy 21.

Radiographic findings include severe bone age delay along with epiphyseal fragmentation and irregularity. Epiphyseal irregularity results from disordered endochondral bone formation.[9] The differential diagnosis includes chondrodysplasia punctata, congenital warfarin exposure, and multiple epiphyseal dysplasia. Newborns may lack a cuboid ossification center; toddlers develop marked metaphyseal and, later, epiphyseal irregularities. Bone maturation should resume within 2 months of beginning thyroid hormone replacement.[9]

Pseudohypoparathroidism and Pseudopseudohypoparathyroidism

Most authors consider pseudopseudohypoparathyroidism (PPH) to be incomplete expression of pseudohypoparathyroidism (PH). Those with complete expression of the disease, or PH, have hypocalcemia and hyperphosphatemia resulting from insensitivity to parathyroid hormone. Those with PPH have normal serum calcium levels. The children usually are short, obese, and mentally retarded.[21]

Children with either entity have the same radiographic findings: short tubular bones of the hands and feet with particular shortening of the fourth metatarsal bone (Fig. 2–17). Less frequent radiographic findings include bowing of the long bones and exostoses.

Lesch-Nyhan Syndrome

This syndrome results from abnormalities in amino acid metabolism. Affected children have hyperuricosuria,

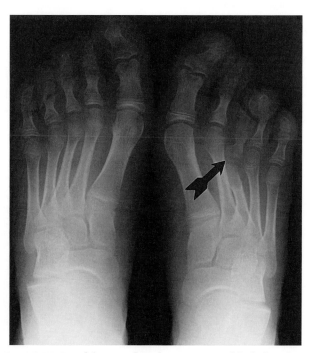

Figure 2–17. Pseudohypoparathyroidism. AP view of both feet shows shortening of the right third metatarsal (*arrow*).

uric acid stones, arthritis, evidence of juvenile gout, and self-mutilation. Decreased sensitivity to pain is present, which induces severe mutilating deformities of the hands and feet. Radiographic findings are similar to those resulting from other causes of pain insensitivity (see later Trauma section).

NEOPLASMS

1. Benign
2. Malignant
3. Dysplasia epiphysealis hemimelica

Plain films serve as a valuable screening tool for bone tumors. Scintigraphy, CT, and MRI can all contribute critical diagnostic information. As each lesion is discussed, the relative value of each imaging modality will be addressed. In general, scintigraphy allows detection of distant metastasis, and CT provides excellent evaluation of the cortical bone. MRI should never supplant conventional radiographs as the initial imaging modality for a bone lesion. Nonetheless, MRI far surpasses other modalities in determining soft tissue involvement and the extent of marrow involvement. MRI is invaluable in staging tumors and planning surgical intervention.[16]

Tumors can destroy bone (lytic lesions), produce bone (sclerotic or blastic lesions), or induce a mixed pattern. The borders of a lesion may be distinct (geographic or well-marginated lesion) or indistinct (moth-eaten, poorly marginated, or permeative lesion). Tumors can expand bone, creating a bubbly appearance. Many tumors produce a matrix with either calcification (chondroid tumors) or ossification (osteogenic tumors).

The location of the tumor (metaphyseal, diaphyseal, epiphyseal) is critical in narrowing the differential diagnosis. Tumors can extend from one area to another but usually have similar sites of origin from one patient to the next.[16]

Benign Tumors

Solitary or Unicameral Bone Cyst

The most common benign bone tumor, solitary bone cysts arise in children and adolescents and have a 2:1

Pearls

1. Always assess each possible tumor by location, number of lesions, soft tissue invasion, and growth characteristics.
2. Always begin with conventional radiographs.
3. Check both what the lesion does to the bone and how the bone responds.[16]
4. Typical locations

Epiphysis	Metaphysis	Diaphysis
Chondroblastoma	Fibrous cortical defect	Osteoblastoma
Giant cell tumor	Osteosarcoma	Osteoid osteoma
	Chondromyxoid fibroma	Aneurysmal cyst

Adapted from Mott MP, Gebhardt MC: Pediatric bone tumors. Comprehensive Ther 1993; 19(2):73–81.

---

male predominance. In the foot, most occur in the anterior calcaneus and often are asymptomatic. Radiographs reveal a well-demarcated, eccentric, metaphyseal, lucent lesion that does not disrupt the cortex. The "fallen fragment sign" occurs after a pathologic fracture, in which a fracture fragment falls to the base of the lesion. This sign is pathognomonic for a unicameral bone cyst.[16]

The differential diagnosis includes pseudotumor and intraosseous lipoma. CT or MRI provides definitive diagnosis if needed. Further work-up for lesions not located in the calcaneus should include bone scintigraphy and possibly a bone biopsy to rule out malignancy.[35]

Aneurysmal Bone Cyst

Unlike solitary bone cysts, aneurysmal bone cysts (ABC) frequently cause pain. They develop in young adults aged 20 to 30, most commonly in the tarsals and metatarsals. Plain radiographs demonstrate diaphyseal, eccentric, expansile, lytic lesions that may thin or erode the overlying cortex. These benign lesions may have a surprisingly aggressive appearance.[35] Thus, these lesions should undergo biopsy to rule out the presence of fibrosarcoma or osteosarcoma.[35] CT and MRI can demonstrate fluid-fluid levels; fluid-fluid levels commonly occur in aneurysmal bone cysts but are not specific because they can also occur in osteosarcoma (see Fig. 2–3).[16]

Enchondroma

This benign tumor has a matrix of cartilage that may or may not calcify. Enchondromas are the most common lytic lesions in the phalanges of the hands and feet. They rarely cause symptoms unless they are associated with pathologic fractures. On conventional radiographs, an enchondroma appears as a slow-growing lucency that respects the overlying cortex but causes a periosteal reaction (Fig. 2–18).[35]

Enchondromas are usually solitary but may be multiple. Multiple enchondromas are associated with Ollier's disease (familial enchondromatosis) or Maffucci's syndrome (multiple enchondromas and hemangiomas). Since each enchondroma has approximately a 1% risk of becoming malignant (chondrosarcoma), children and adults with familial syndromes have an increased risk of malignant transformation.

Osteochondroma

The most common primary bone neoplasm in children, osteochondromas typically occur at the knee or scapula. Children with multiple osteochondromas may have osteochondromas of the tibia. Osteochondromas have a cartilaginous cap and a cortex that is contiguous with that of the adjacent bone. Rarely, these lesions can become malignant, changing into a chondrosarcoma. Conventional radiographs are usually sufficient for diagnosis[16] (Fig. 2–19). MRI can help in those few cases in which malignancy is suspected.

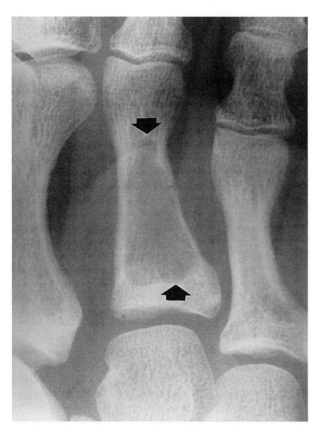

Figure 2–18. Enchondroma in a 17-year-old female. AP view of the foot shows a well-defined osteolytic lesion with a lobulated contour and endosteal erosions *(arrows)* involving the proximal phalanx of the second toe.

Osteoid Osteoma and Osteoblastoma

These lesions have the same histologic appearance and thus are grouped together. The size of the lesion determines the diagnosis: lesions less than 2 cm in diameter are osteoid osteomas; lesions greater than 2 cm in diameter are osteoblastomas. Men are affected more frequently than women, usually in their twenties, and often present complaining of nocturnal pain that is relieved by aspirin. In the foot, osteoid osteoma is much more common; osteoblastoma prefers the spine and long bones.

Osteoid osteomas are frequently tarsal and expansile, with sharp zones of transition and no cortical erosion. The sine qua non is the central radiolucent nidus surrounded by a region of sclerotic new bone (Figs. 2–20 to 2–22).

Scintigraphy shows focal increased tracer uptake in a "double intensity" fashion at the site of the lesion, which distinguishes osteoma from chronic osteomyelitis.[16] Some surgeons use scintigraphy for preoperative or intraoperative localization.[17] Rarely, conventional radiographs and scintigraphy fail to reveal the presence of the lesion. In such cases, CT with thin slices through the lesion can localize the nidus.[16] MRI shows calcified portions of the nidus and surrounding sclerosis as areas of low signal intensity on all pulse sequences.[8] In some cases, the treating physician may use percutaneous CT-guided heat

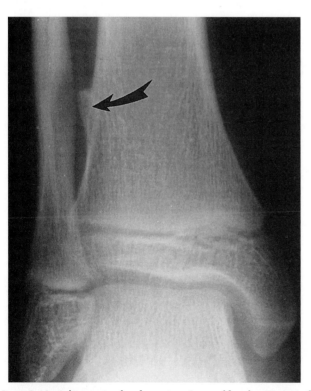

Figure 2–19. Solitary osteochondroma in a 9-year-old male. AP view of the ankle shows a sessile osteochondroma *(arrow)* arising from the medial metaphysis of the distal tibia.

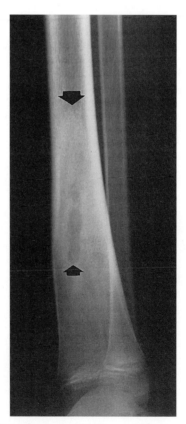

Figure 2–20. Osteoid osteoma. This 11-year-old boy presented with the classic history of pain that was worse at night and was relieved by aspirin. Lateral view of the distal tibia shows an elongated lytic lesion representing the nidus *(arrow)*, which is surrounded by an extensive reactive sclerosis *(arrow)*.

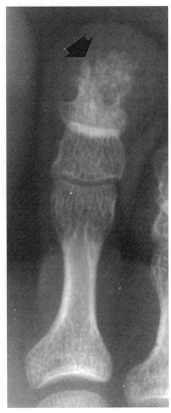

Figure 2–21. Osteoid osteoma. AP view of the second toe shows soft tissue swelling, erosions, and sclerosis of the distal phalanx *(arrow)*.

ablation or removal of the nidus rather than surgical resection.[16]

Differential diagnosis includes chronic osteomyelitis, reactive stress lesion, and juvenile rheumatoid arthritis (if the osteoid osteoma causes a reactive synovitis).[17]

Nonossifying Fibroma

This benign lesion commonly occurs around the knee and often arises from points of ligamentous or tendinous

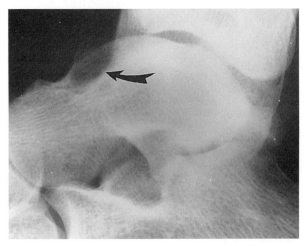

Figure 2–22. Osteoid osteoma. Lateral view of the ankle shows a well-defined lytic lesion, representing the nidus *(arrow)*, in the dome of the talus.

insertion. On conventional radiographs, the lesion is round or oval and lytic and often has sclerotic margins (Fig. 2–23). Usually there is no periosteal reaction. Small, nonossifying fibromas are called benign cortical defects; the term nonossifying fibromas refers to lesions that expand to greater than 2 cm and grow into the medullary canal. The abnormality is uncommon before 18 months and peaks at 5 years of age. As the child grows, the defect may enlarge and expand the cortical margin. As the child matures, sclerotic bone fills and eventually replaces the abnormality so that the lesion disappears.[17]

Chondromyxoid Fibroma

This uncommon fibrous lesion arises in the proximal tibia, distal femur, and the tarsal bones and phalanges of the foot. Patients, males more than females, usually present as young adults (Figs. 2–24 and 2–25). Conventional radiographs demonstrate a diaphyseal, geographic, eccentric, lucent lesion causing cortical expansion and significant endosteal sclerosis. The endosteal sclerosis helps to differentiate chondromyxoid fibroma from enchondroma. Calcification and periosteal reaction are both rare. Differential diagnosis includes aneurysmal bone cyst, giant cell tumor, nonossifying fibroma, and enchondroma.

Fibrous Dysplasia

This benign hamartomatous condition occurs at any age but typically affects adolescents and young adults. The abnormality may be monostotic or polyostotic. Polyostotic fibrous dysplasia affects males and females equally. None-

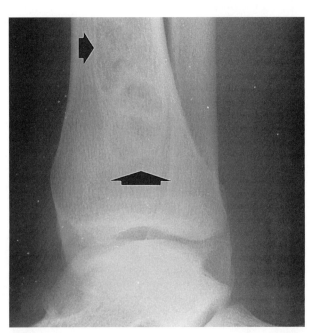

Figure 2–23. Nonossifying fibroma in an asymptomatic 16-year-old male. Lateral view of the ankle shows a well-demarcated radiolucent lesion with a sclerotic margin *(arrows)* located in the metaphysis of the distal tibia.

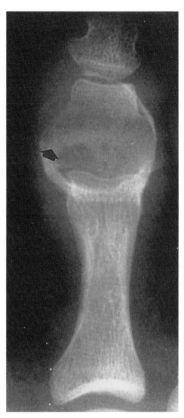

Figure 2–24. Chondromyxoid fibroma in a child with foot pain. AP view of the second toe shows an expansile lesion involving most of the middle phalanx and associated with a pathologic fracture *(arrow)*.

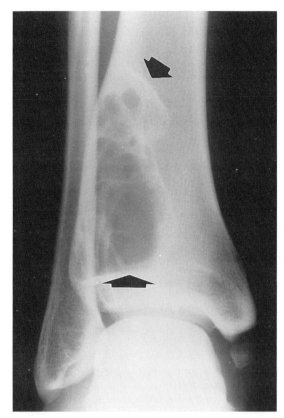

Figure 2–25. Chondromyxoid fibroma in a 20-year-old male with foot pain. AP view of the ankle shows an eccentric, slightly expansile, trabeculated, lytic lesion *(arrows)* involving the metaphysis of the distal tibia.

theless, the polyostotic form is associated with a syndrome in which children have café-au-lait spots on the skin and precocious puberty. This triad constitutes the McCune-Albright syndrome, which affects girls much more often than boys. Polyostotic fibrous dysplasia often comes to clinical attention before the child is 10 years of age.

Monostotic fibrous dysplasia arises in metadiaphyseal regions. It is common in the tibia. Polyostotic fibrous dyplasia, on the other hand, can occur in the epiphysis, diaphysis, or metaphysis. Radiographs demonstrate a ground-glass, sclerotic, or lytic appearance (Fig. 2–26). Typically, the lesions are expansile, well-defined, and without periosteal reaction. Polyostotic fibrous dysplasia may be a bilateral process but frequently prefers one side of the body (in 90% of cases), creating an asymmetrical distribution. T2-weighted MRI images show high signal intensity marrow in fibrous dysplasia lesions. Complications include pathologic fractures (in 40% of cases).

Malignant Lesions

Osteosarcoma

Osteosarcoma occurs in children 10 to 25 years of age, causes pain and swelling, and usually occurs in the metaphyseal region. It is the most common primary bone malignancy but rarely occurs in the foot. It metastasizes to lung; 10% to 20% of patients have metastases at the

time of diagnosis. Overall survival is 70% in those without metastases. Approximately 10% of patients have local recurrences.[16]

The lesion has an aggressive appearance on plain films

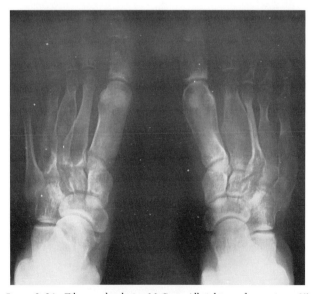

Figure 2–26. Fibrous dysplasia. McCune-Albright syndrome in a 15-year-old female with precocious puberty and café-au-lait spots. AP view of both feet shows bilateral expansile lytic lesions with ground-glass matrix involving predominantly the metatarsals. These findings are consistent with the diagnosis of polyostotic fibrous dysplasia.

with a wide zone of transition, cortical erosion, frequent invasion of adjacent soft tissues, and rapid growth. The periosteal response may occur in a sunburst pattern or Codman's triangle. Ten percent of children have multicentric or synchronous lesions. Bone scanning, though useful, may miss skip metastases. MRI provides much better evaluation of soft tissue and bone marrow extent as well as neurovascular involvement; the involved marrow is dark on T1-weighted images and bright on T2-weighted images.

Differential diagnosis includes stress fracture, chronic osteomyelitis, and, rarely, osteoid osteoma.[9]

Ewing's Sarcoma

An uncommon tumor in general, Ewing's sarcoma nonetheless remains the most common primary bone malignancy in the foot. It affects children aged 5 to 15 years old and causes pain and swelling. As with osteosarcoma, Ewing's sarcoma sends hematogenous metastases to the lungs. The overall survival rate at 5 years has been reported to be 60% to 70%.[16]

Ewing's sarcoma creates a permeative pattern of bone destruction with a wide zone of transition, frequent invasion into the soft tissues, and lysis of the cortex (Fig. 2–27). It arises in the metaphysis or diaphysis (rarely the epiphysis) and commonly affects the tarsal bones. An

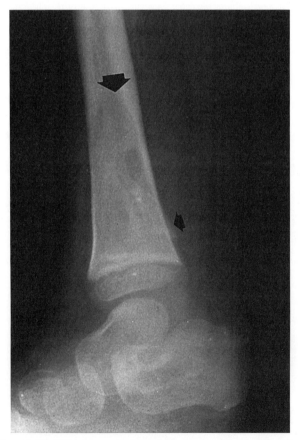

Figure 2–27. Ewing's sarcoma. Lateral view of the ankle shows an elongated lytic lesion *(arrow)* with periosteal reaction *(arrow)* involving the metadiaphysis of the distal tibia.

onion-skin type of periosteal reaction may occur, a sensitive but not specific finding. The differential diagnosis includes infection, and, rarely, osteosarcoma.[16]

MRI delineates the marrow and soft tissue extent of the tumor. The larger the lesion, the worse the prognosis. Some authors have reported using dynamic gadolinium-enhanced MRI to assess the patient's response to chemotherapy.[7]

Chondroblastoma

This tumor affects males twice as often as females. It typically occurs in young adults but may accompany an aneurysmal bone cyst in younger patients (Fig. 2–28). Radiographs demonstrate an epiphyseal, expansile, lytic lesion with sclerotic borders. In the foot and ankle, it can appear in the tibia or tarsal bones. Fifty percent of the lesions cross the physis; just as many have a calcified matrix. Treatable with curettage, chondroblastoma is more likely to recur if the child has a coexisting aneurysmal bone cyst.

Metastatic Tumors

Tumors rarely metastasize to the foot. Leukemia, lymphoma, neuroblastoma, Wilms' tumor, retinoblastoma, medulloblastoma, Ewing's sarcoma, and rhabdomyosarcoma all metastasize to bone. Most metastatic bone lesions are lytic in nature and have no clear zone of transition; pathologic fractures are frequent. Initial evaluation with plain films should be followed by a general skeletal scintigraphic survey. Some metastatic tumors are seen better on plain film skeletal surveys as opposed to scintigraphy.[28] Tumors with potentially poor visibility on scintigraphy include eosinophilic granuloma and lymphoma. Chemotherapy and severe illness can cause sporadic bone growth that is reflected in growth recovery lines within the bone (Fig. 2–29).

Dysplasia Epiphysealis Hemimelica

This benign tumor, also known as Trevor's disease, arises from cartilage. An osteochondromatous lesion, it grows out from an epiphysis or epiphyseal equivalent. Affecting boys more often than girls, usually between ages 2 and 8 years, the epiphyseal dysplasia occurs primarily in the talus.[17] The lesion behaves similarly to a metaphyseal exostosis, causing mechanical interference and pain. The child presents with a hard mass in the knee or ankle. Hemimelica refers to the propensity for second or multiple lesions to occur in the same extremity, often along the same side (medial or lateral) of that extremity.

Plain films show a focal epiphyseal projection with irregular calcifications; the lesion can cause pressure erosion on neighboring bones (Fig. 2–30). MRI and arthrography both reveal enlarged epiphyses.

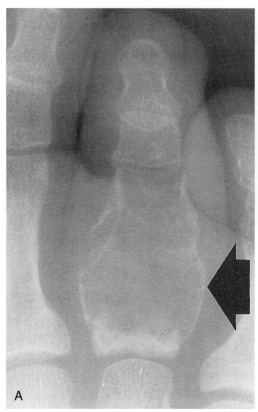

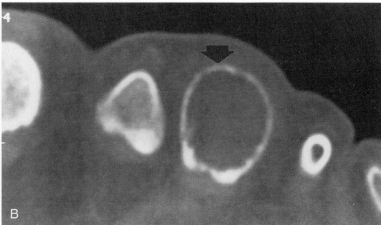

Figure 2–28. Chondroblastoma with associated aneurysmal bone cyst in a 15-year-old male. *A*, AP view of the third toe shows a lobulated, expansile, osteolytic lesion *(arrow)* involving the proximal phalanx. *B*, Axial CT scan shows the expansile lesion *(arrow)*.

VASCULAR

1. Avascular necrosis
2. Infarcts
3. Sickle cell disease
4. Collagen vascular diseases

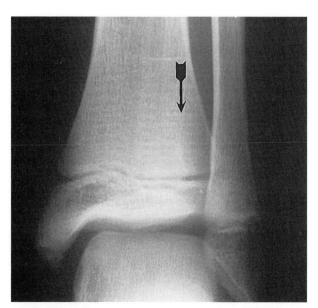

Figure 2–29. Growth recovery lines in an 11-year-old female with leukemia. AP view of the left ankle shows multiple transverse radiodense lines *(arrow)* in the metadiaphyses of the distal tibia and fibula.

Avascular Necrosis

A variety of insults can lead to avascular necrosis (AVN), also known as ischemic necrosis of bone. In children, AVN may be idiopathic or may result from a variety of causes, including trauma, renal failure, steroid use, sickle cell anemia, collagen vascular diseases, Gaucher's disease, and radiation. In the foot, AVN commonly occurs in the talus; other sites include the metatarsals.

The bone experiences vascular occlusion and bone death followed by revascularization and repair. Plain films do not show the initial pathologic episode of bone death. The initial radiographic finding is a lucent line just beneath the cortex, the crescent sign, which is a subchondral fracture. If the disease is allowed to progress, the bone loses volume and appears more compact and dense. As the bone heals, osteosclerosis becomes more prominent, creating a "snowcapped" appearance.

Scintigraphy shows abnormally decreased focal tracer uptake in the early stages of the disease. As the bone regenerates, the bone scan gradually regains a normal appearance.[17] Some authors have found that MRI findings progress, correlating with the histologic and radiographic progression of ischemic necrosis.[13] At all stages and on both T1- and T2-weighted images, the area of necrosis is demarcated by a ring of intermediate signal intensity. The center of an early lesion (one without radiographic abnormalities) has high signal intensity and intermediate signal intensity on T1- and T2-weighted images, respectively. As the lesion becomes worse, consistent with hemorrhage in the

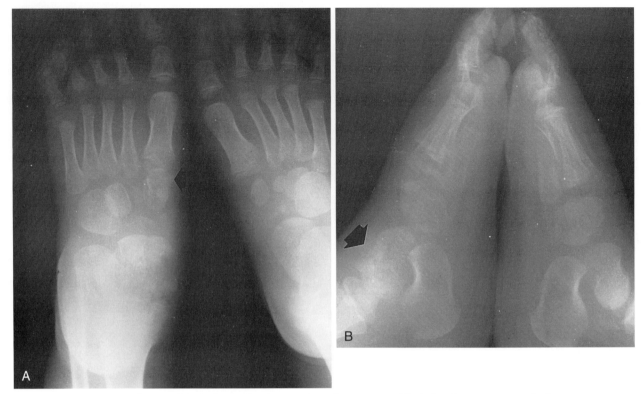

Figure 2–30. Dysplasia epiphysealis hemimelica (Trevor's disease). *A*, AP view of both feet shows asymmetrical enlargement of left medial cuneiform *(arrow)*. *B*, Lateral view of both feet shows irregular ossification of the left talus *(arrow)*.

center, the central signal characteristics change to high signal intensity on both T1- and T2-weighted images. Further deterioration with both edema and blood in the lesion (the crescent sign stage) causes the center to exhibit low signal intensity and high signal intensity on T1- and T2-weighted images, respectively. The formation of fibrosis results in low signal intensity on both sequences.[13]

Bone Infarcts

As with subchondral AVN, bone infarcts represent ischemic necrosis of bone followed by revascularization. Early radiographs do not show the initial bone necrosis. With revascularization comes deposition of new bone, which allows better visualization of the infarct. Radiographs may show a rim of sclerosis, usually in the metadiaphyseal region.

On T1-weighted images, MRI shows the rim of sclerosis as a dark peripheral band, with an inhomogeneous low signal intensity marrow in the center. Proton density images have central high signal intensity and a low signal intensity rim; T2-weighted images reveal a bright signal intensity serpentine rim with a heterogeneous central signal.[8]

The differential diagnosis for a metadiaphyseal infarct is an enchondroma. Enchondromas typically have a chondroid matrix with flecks of calcification and lack a sclerotic rim. MRI shows fat intensity within infarcts but not within enchondromas.

Sickle Cell Anemia

The abnormal hemoglobin S causes red blood cell deformity leading to vascular stasis and occlusion. Complications include osteopenia, bone infarcts, avascular necrosis, and osteomyelitis. Though *Staphylococcus aureus* causes most cases of osteomyelitis, people with sickle cell anemia have higher than normal rates of *Salmonella* osteomyelitis.

Bone infarcts can cause growth deformities, such as tibiotalar slant with the joint angulated inferiorly and medially. In addition, children with sickle cell disease may have infarcts in their hands and feet that differ from infarcts due to other causes. Known as the hand-foot syndrome or dactylitis, it affects infants and toddlers and encompasses the following signs: pain and soft tissue swelling of the hands and feet, patchy short tubular bone destruction, and pronounced periosteal reaction. The latter can render differentiation of osteomyelitis from bone infarct difficult.

Plain films help to diagnose infarcts and osteomyelitis (Fig. 2–31). Scintigraphy may help to differentiate infarction from infection. Some authors recommend scintigraphy using first gallium-67 and then technetium (Tc-MDP). Infarcts should show greater activity with technetium than with gallium, whereas infection should show the reverse. On MRI, patients with sickle cell anemia have decreased marrow signal intensity on T1- and T2-weighted images because of marrow hyperplasia. Infarcts cause dark signal intensity in the marrow on T1-weighted images; proton density-weighted images reveal central

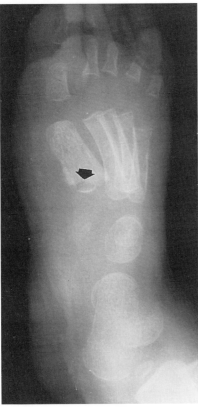

Figure 2–31. Sickle cell anemia. Dactylitis in a 16-month-old girl. Oblique view of the foot shows soft tissue swelling, osteolytic lesions, and periostitis involving predominantly the first metacarpal *(arrow)*.

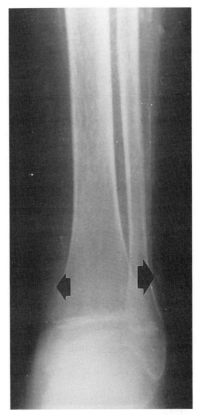

Figure 2–32. Dermatomyositis in an 11-year-old female. AP view of the lower leg shows extensive soft tissue calcifications *(arrows)*.

high signal intensity, and T2-weighted images show a high signal intensity rim with a heterogeneous signal in the center of the infarct.

Collagen Vascular Disorders

Collagen vascular disorders cause abnormalities in the soft tissues more commonly than in the bones. Dermatomyositis and polymyositis cause soft tissue calcifications in the subcutaneous and deeper soft tissues; rarely, patients develop flexion contractures (Figs. 2–32 and 2–33).

TRAUMA

1. Osseous injuries
2. Epiphyseal injuries
3. Dislocations
4. Open fractures
5. Soft tissue injuries
6. Osteochondral injuries
7. Reflex sympathetic dystrophy

Osseous Injuries

General Comments

Descriptions of pediatric fractures should include the number of fracture fragments, the orientation of the frac-

ture, and the type of cortical involvement. *Comminuted* fractures refer to fractures with more than two fragments. The fracture line can be oblique, spiral, transverse, or longitudinal. The *buckle* fracture causes lateral bulges along both sides of the bone; the *greenstick* fracture

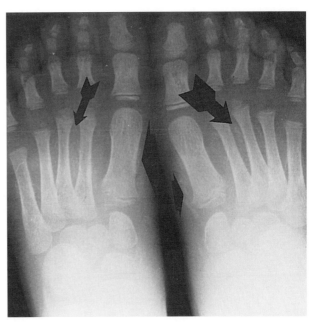

Figure 2–33. Dermatomyositis in a 3-year-old female. AP view of both feet shows bilateral symmetrical soft tissue calcifications *(arrows)*.

involves only one cortical aspect; the *bowing* fracture causes curvature but no distinct cortical disruption. Lastly, *compound* (or open) fractures extend to the skin, resulting in a higher risk of infection.[12]

Effusions commonly result from bony and ligamentous injuries, especially after trauma to the ankle. On a lateral film, an effusion creates a soft tissue density just anterior to the joint, beneath the tibia and anterior to the talus (Fig. 2–34).

Epiphyseal Injuries

Most injuries in children occur around the physis (growth plate). Salter and Harris described fractures across the unfused physis. Beginning along the growth plate itself (type 1 injury), the fracture extends first into the metaphysis (type 2), into the epiphysis (type 3), across both the epiphysis and the metaphysis (type 4), or results in impaction at the physis (type 5) (Figs. 2–35 to 2–37). The prognosis becomes worse with each successive type;

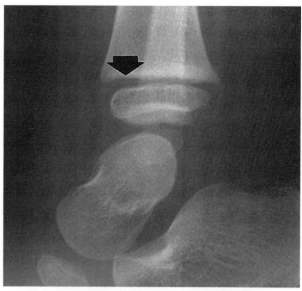

Figure 2–35. Salter-Harris I fracture of the distal tibia in a 4-year-old girl. Lateral view of the ankle shows widening of the distal tibial physis *(arrow)*.

type 4 and 5 injuries have poor prognoses because major injury to the growth plate often prevents normal growth. CT or MRI may be required to identify physeal tethering after such fractures.

Children commonly injure the distal tibia. Among epiphyseal injuries, the Salter-Harris type 2 injury is the most common (47%).[29] Fracture lines may be visible in only one plane or may become apparent only when compared to the noninjured extremity (especially in Salter-Harris type 1 fractures). Fractures may extend into a nonossified epiphysis. Differentiating Salter-Harris type 2 injuries from type 4 injuries in a child with a nonossified epiphysis may require MRI or arthrography.

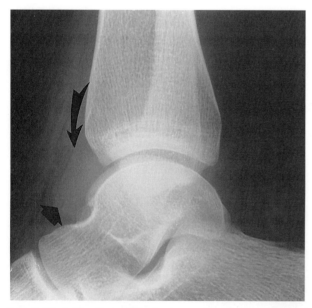

Figure 2–34. Ankle effusion following trauma. Lateral view of the ankle shows a well-defined soft tissue density anterior to the tibiotalar joint *(arrows)*.

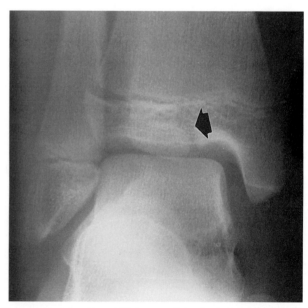

Figure 2–36. Salter-Harris III fracture of the distal tibia. AP view of the ankle shows a fracture extending from the medial tibial epiphysis to the physis *(arrow)*.

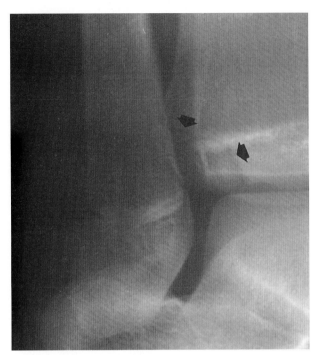

Figure 2–37. Salter-Harris IV fracture of the distal tibia in a 12-year-old female. Note the fracture extending from the epiphysis to the metaphysis *(arrows)*.

Outcome depends on the type of fracture, amount of displacement, presence of soft tissue injury, and the quality of postmanipulation reduction.[29] Salter-Harris type 3 to 5 injuries of the tibia often lead to secondary osteoarthritis because of articular disruption. Salter-Harris type 2 injuries of the tibia are unpredictable. Children with this type of injury should be imaged on a regular basis until either normal growth or skeletal maturity is documented. One should look carefully for a growth arrest line on each radiographic examination.[29]

Triplane Fracture

This fracture does not precisely fit the Salter-Harris classification but can be mistaken for a Salter-Harris type 2 injury. Called a triplane fracture because the fracture lines extend in three planes, the injury causes a horizontal fracture through the physis, a sagittal fracture through the epiphysis, and an oblique fracture through the posterior distal metaphysis. Plantar flexion with external rotation is the usual mechanism of injury. On radiographs, the fracture extends through the posterior distal metaphysis from the anterior-inferior margin to a posterior-superior position (seen best on the lateral or oblique view) (Fig. 2–38). The fracture may have two, three, or four fragments. It is important to differentiate fractures with two fragments from those with three. In the latter type, the entire epiphysis moves posteriorly, and more of the articular surface is disrupted. Thus, three-part fractures are more likely to require open reduction and internal fixation to reestablish the joint.[23]

CT scanning with three-dimensional reconstruction provides useful information for diagnosing the injury and determining therapy. After closed reduction has been performed, the child will not need invasive intervention if CT scans demonstrate a level articular surface and less than 2 mm of fracture fragment displacement.[23]

Various mechanisms of injury lead to predictable fracture patterns. Adduction of the foot results in Salter-Harris type 4 fracture or varus angulation (see Fig. 2–37). Abduction causes a Salter-Harris type 1 or 2 fracture of the distal tibia with or without fibular injury. Plantar flexion leads to a Salter-Harris type 2 fracture with posterior displacement of the distal tibial epiphysis and a separate metaphyseal fragment. External rotation and supination usually results in a Salter-Harris type 2 fracture with a posterior lateral fragment from the distal tibial metaphysis. Triplane or Tillaux fractures can also occur.

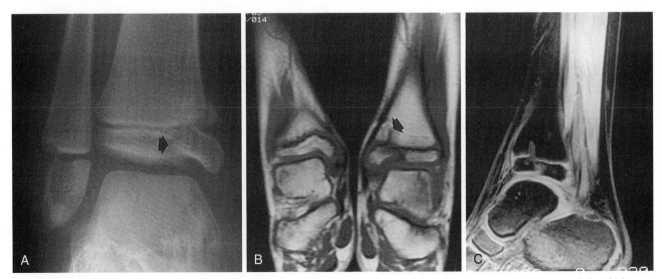

Figure 2–38. Triplane fracture of the distal tibia in a 7-year-old male. *A*, AP view of the ankle shows a vertical fracture of the tibial epiphysis *(arrow)* and widening of the medial portion of the physis. *B*, Coronal T1-weighted MR image shows the epiphyseal fracture extending to the metaphysis *(arrow)*. *C*, Sagittal SPGR (spoiled gradient recall echo sequence) MR image shows the fracture extending from the epiphysis to the metaphysis.

Juvenile Tillaux Fracture

This injury occurs only in children in whom the medial portion of the tibial physis is fused.[23] A Salter-Harris type 3 fracture, the vertical fracture line extends through the central or lateral distal tibial epiphysis, causing lateral physeal widening. Usually the medial physis, which has already closed, does not fracture. The lateral view is extremely important for diagnosing this injury.

As with the triplane fracture, CT scanning can determine the amount of fragment displacement (must be less than 2 mm) and the congruity of the articular surface (no step-off).

Calcaneal Injuries

Calcaneal fractures are common in falls from a height. Compression fracture of the calcaneus typically occurs. Boehler's angle, which is 20 to 40 degrees in a normal individual, is less than 20 degrees and sometimes less than 0 degrees after a severe fracture (Fig. 2–39). The same forces that break the heel can also cause vertebral body fractures, usually in the lumbar region, in 6% of pediatric cases (12% in adults). Thus, clinical and radiographic examination of the spine should be considered in any child with a calcaneal injury after a fall.

Other forms of calcaneal injuries in children under 14 years of age usually are extra-articular.[24] Children older than 14 years have fracture patterns similar to those seen in adults. Calcaneal fractures are easily overlooked; axial projections often help in identifying the fracture site. Avulsion fractures, along the anterior process of the calcaneus, occur after an adduction-inversion stress; oblique views may demonstrate the fracture fragment.[24]

CT is usually unnecessary but can determine the number of fragments, their location, and the integrity of the tibiotalar and calcaneocuboid joints. Most extra-articular fractures require only closed reduction.[24]

Tarsal Bone Fractures

These are uncommon (Fig. 2–40). See the later section on stress fractures for tarsal navicular stress fractures.

Talar Fractures

The type of fracture that occurs in the talus depends on the age of the child. Younger children usually have tonsillar fractures, whereas older children have linear neck fractures. Osteochondral fractures of the talar dome result from inversion injury (see later section, Osteochondral Injuries).

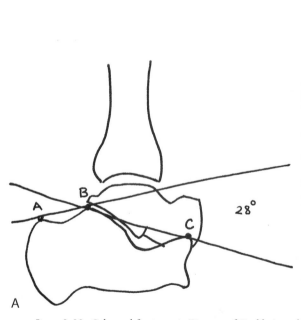

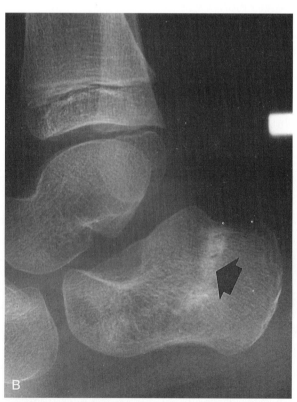

Figure 2–39. Calcaneal fracture. *A*, Diagram of Boehler's angle (the angle between lines A–B and B–C). The intact normal calcaneus has an angle of 20 to 40 degrees. Less than 20 degrees is abnormal and indicates the presence of an intra-articular fracture, even if the fracture line is not visible. *B*, Lateral view of the ankle showing a calcaneal compression fracture *(arrow)* in a 5-year-old boy following a fall from 5 feet. Boehler's angle is 38 degrees, indicating that the fracture is extra-articular.

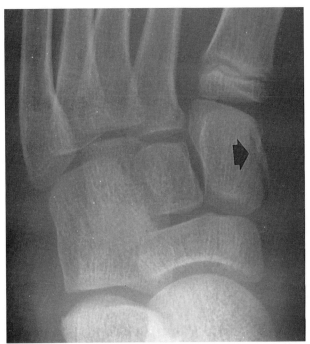

Figure 2–40. Medial cuneiform fracture. AP view of the foot in a child shows a longitudinal fracture *(arrow)* of the medial cuneiform.

Metatarsal and Phalangeal Fractures

Children may suffer torus or greenstick fractures of the phalanges (Fig. 2–41). When a child stubs his toe, a Salter-Harris type 1 or 2 injury to the epiphysis of the distal phalanx may result (Fig. 2–42). More important, in children the fracture is often open, since the growth plate

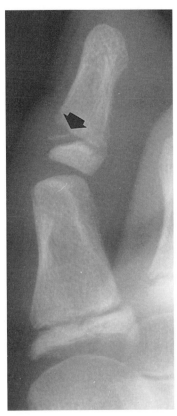

Figure 2–42. Distal phalanx fracture in a child who stubbed his toe. Oblique view of the great toe shows a fracture of the distal phalanx *(arrow)*.

and the nail bed are attached. Because the nail obscures the true nature of the fracture, the open wound is easily overlooked, and the injury can progress to cellulitis and osteomyelitis. Children require antibiotics prophylactically to prevent these complications.

Bunk Bed Fracture. In adolescents, a common fracture occurs at the base of the first metatarsal bone called a bunk bed fracture. This fracture results from a fall from a height. The trauma causes epiphyseal injury, which on radiographs can be subtle. The most common radiographic finding is irregularity and angulation along the medial proximal first metatarsal metaphysis.[24]

Fifth Metatarsal Avulsion Fracture. Often confused with the Jones fracture, the fracture line in the avulsion fracture exits through the cuboid-metatarsal joint. The physician should be sure not to confuse an avulsion fracture with a normal apophysis (Fig. 2–43). Both the avulsion fracture and the Jones fracture result from an inversion injury. Plain films usually are sufficient to diagnose the fracture, obviating the need for other radiologic procedures.[29]

Jones Fracture of the Fifth Metatarsal. This extra-articular fracture runs perpendicular to the long axis of the metatarsal bone and does not enter the cuboid-metatarsal joint (see Fig. 2–43). It occurs in the proximal portion of the bone after an inversion stress.[29]

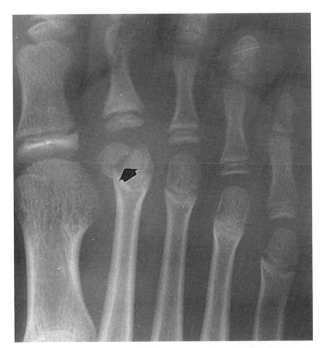

Figure 2–41. Second metatarsal fracture in a 12-year-old male. AP view of the forefoot shows a fracture in the head of the second metatarsal *(arrow)*.

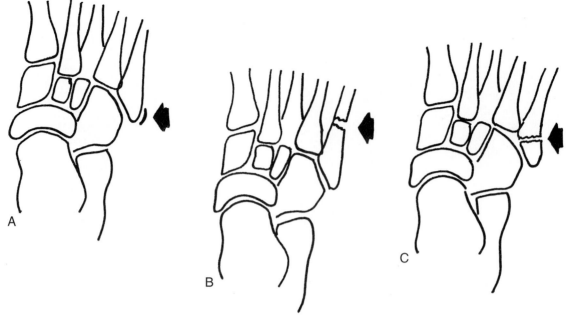

Figure 2–43. *A*, Apophysis of the fifth metatarsal. This curvilinear bone fragment should not be confused with a fracture. *B*, Jones' fracture of the fifth metatarsal shaft. Note that the fracture line is extra-articular and runs perpendicular to the long axis of the metatarsal. *C*, Avulsion fracture of the fifth metatarsal. The fracture line enters the metatarsal-cuboid joint.

Child Abuse

Multiple fractures in a child should always raise the suspicion of abuse. Metaphyseal fractures and periosteal new bone are the two most common manifestations of abuse. Hemorrhage between the periosteum and the bone leads to periosteal reaction. This finding, however, is nonspecific and can be seen with infection, blood dyscrasias, and various tumors. Metaphyseal corner fractures, on the other hand, are virtually pathognomonic for child abuse. The fracture extends across the physis, tearing a fragment off the metaphysis. Depending on the angle of the x-ray beam, the metaphyseal fragment may appear as a peripheral wedge fragment (corner fracture) or an arch of bone (bucket-handle fracture) (Fig. 2–44).

Thermal Injury

Frostbite, hot water exposure, and electrical injuries can all lead to severe injury of the pediatric foot. Extensive soft tissue injury is common; usually osseous injury of the phalanges occurs. Radiographs show osteopenia and eventual bone resorption. Thermal injury is included in the differential diagnosis of acro-osteolysis, which also includes, but is not limited to, neuropathic joints, Lesch-Nyhan syndrome, epidermolysis bullosa, and familial acro-osteolysis.

Bone Bruises

Trauma can cause occult bone injury not revealed by conventional radiographs. Bone bruises have a focal, nonlinear, dark signal intensity on T1-weighted images and intermediate to high signal intensity on T2-weighted images because of microfracture, hemorrhage, and edema. Stress fractures, on the other hand, have a more linear, nonfocal appearance and are eventually associated with positive radiographic findings.

Stress Fractures

Toddler's Fracture

The toddler's fracture, or spiral fracture of the distal tibia, is the most common bony injury in children 12 to 30 months of age. The fracture should be suspected in any afebrile child of this age who refuses to bear weight. The fracture occurs after a rotational stress to the tibia during a fall. AP and lateral radiographs are usually sufficient for diagnosis, but occasionally a 45-degree oblique view may be needed. If clinical suspicion remains high but plain radiographs are negative, a technetium bone scan should be considered.[12]

MRI can often locate early stress fractures with greater sensitivity and speed than conventional radiographs. MRI demonstrates an abnormal bone marrow signal (low on T1-weighted and high on T2-weighted images) at the site of stress fractures.

Calcaneal Stress Fracture

Much like the tibial stress fracture, the calcaneal stress fracture occurs in toddlers aged 20 to 40 months. This fracture is a less common but possible reason for a child's

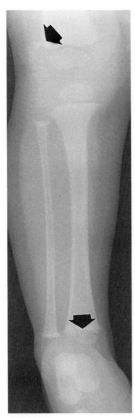

Figure 2–44. Child abuse and rickets in a 2-year-old boy. AP view of right leg shows corner fractures of the distal femoral metaphysis *(arrow)* consistent with child abuse. Note slight sclerosis and irregularity of the distal tibial metaphysis *(arrow)* consistent with rickets.

Table 2–4. **Indirect Findings Associated with Tarsal Navicular Fractures**

Sclerosis of proximal articular border of navicular
Short first metatarsal
Metatarsus adductus of 1st–4th rays
Metatarsal hyperostosis or stress fractures of the second, third, and/or fourth metatarsals
Talonavicular joint space narrowing (medial aspect)
Tarsal malalignment (seen on lateral radiograph)
Plantar displacement of the talus, navicular, and cuneiform
Talus and navicular lie dorsal to the cuneiforms

(anatomic AP films) provide the best opportunity for diagnosis. In dorsiflexion the dorsum of the navicular axis is placed parallel to the cassette and the tomographic plane.

Dislocations

Dislocations of the Ankle

Two forms of ankle dislocations may occur—posterior and anterior. Posterior dislocation of the ankle occurs rarely but accounts for the highest percentage of ankle dislocations. Severe plantar flexion with forward thrust of the leg causes anterior displacement of the tibia and fibula and posterior displacement of the talus and foot. Complications include fractures of either or both malleoli or of the posterior tibia. Both the dislocation and its complications are often visible on conventional radiographs.[3]

Anterior dislocation of the ankle is more rare than the posterior form. This type of dislocation results from forcible dorsiflexion, such as a fall onto a dorsiflexed foot. Radiographs demonstrate the forward displacement of the talus and posterior displacement of the tibia and fibula. In addition, they may reveal fracture of the malleoli or the anterior tibia.

Dislocation of the Talus

A severe inversion force can displace the talus out of the ankle mortise and lateral to the lateral malleolus. Such an injury is rare, and the wound is often open. In addition, the talar blood supply becomes disrupted, leading to avascular necrosis. Thus, dislocation of the talus is a surgical emergency. Radiographs demonstrate a rotated talus lying lateral and anterior to the lateral malleolus. The talus often rotates on the longitudinal axis so that the inferior articular surface faces posteriorly. Complications include osteomyelitis, soft tissue infection, arthritis, and avascular necrosis.[4]

Dislocation of the Calcaneus

This extremely rare injury occurs only after a severe twisting force. Radiographs show the calcaneus lying lateral to the rest of the foot. The remainder of the foot and its articulations often remain intact.[4]

refusal to walk or bear weight. Scintigraphy can locate the stress fracture site.[24]

Tarsal Navicular Stress Fracture

Athletes with navicular stress fractures often complain of soreness or cramping with exercise. The fracture afflicts men more often than women by a large margin and affects especially basketball players and runners. Bilateral fractures are unusual. Fractures may be complete or partial: partial fractures extend through the navicular dorsally for up to 5 mm, whereas the complete fracture lengthens to involve the entire bone, running from its dorsal to its plantar surfaces. The fracture lies in the sagittal plane, usually within the central third of the bone.

Radiographs in the AP, lateral, and oblique positions should be obtained. At times, coned-down views and magnification views may help. Incomplete fractures are difficult to visualize. Indirect findings that suggest the presence of a navicular stress fracture are listed in Table 2–4. Pavlov and colleagues found 100% diagnostic sensitivity using bone scintigraphy with ^{99m}Tc-MDP: all cases with stress fractures exhibited increased tracer uptake on both frontal and lateral views, and plantar views provided the best images for localizing the uptake to the tarsal navicular.[18]

Tomograms can also help to diagnose navicular fractures. Tomograms performed with the foot in dorsiflexion

Dislocation of the Cuneiform

This rare injury, resulting from a direct blow, causes subtle radiographic findings. The medial cuneiform and tarsal navicular overlap one another on the AP view. The medial cuneiform falls inferior (plantar) to the tarsal navicular on the lateral view. Often open reduction is required to reachieve stability.[4]

Dislocation of the Tarsal and Tarsal-Metatarsal Bones

Midtarsal joint dislocations are rare. In the most common form, the forefoot and midfoot move medially in relation to the talus and calcaneus. The cuboid often becomes fractured as the anterior tip of the calcaneus swings laterally. The tarsal bones lie superior to the hindfoot on the lateral view.

Direct mechanisms (a crush injury from a heavy weight) or indirect mechanisms (simultaneous abduction and plantar flexion while stepping in a hole or falling off a curb) can cause tarsal-metatarsal dislocations. A normal AP radiograph demonstrates perfect alignment between the medial margin of the second metatarsal shaft and the intermediate cuneiform. On the lateral view, the dorsal margins of the medial cuneiform and the metatarsal base should be equivalent. In patients with a dislocation, the AP or the lateral view shows abnormal alignment. Whether the first metatarsal bone follows the direction of the other metatarsal bones differentiates a convergent from a divergent dislocation.[4]

Dislocation of the Metatarsophalangeal Joints

These injuries are rare, have open wounds, and require immediate reduction. The first metatarsophalangeal joint is the most common site of injury. Typically, the lateral film in such cases shows dorsiflexion and dorsal displacement of the dislocated phalanx.[4]

Open Fractures

Any fracture that has pierced the skin is an open or compound fracture. The fragments need not protrude through the skin at the time of presentation to be called an open fracture. Radiographs and CT scans may show focal disruption of the soft tissues and overlying skin. MRI can definitively document the focal soft tissue abnormality. Nonetheless, diagnosis of a fracture as compound remains a clinical determination. The timing of treatment differs for compound and noncompound fractures. Compound fractures require meticulous debridement and use of antibiotics. Surgical fixation and primary closure are often delayed.[36]

Soft Tissue Injuries

Certain tendons, whether injured by fractures or lacerations, require prompt treatment to avoid deformity. Repair is important for injury to the Achilles, anterior tibial, and posterior tibial tendons but is contraindicated for injuries of the extensor hallucis longus tendon.[36] Peroneal tendon injury can occur during skiing.[29] Both CT and MRI can evaluate the integrity of tendons and help guide therapy.[36]

MRI can allow close examination of the soft tissue for focal thickening, irregularity, and discontinuity of ligaments and tendons. Complete tears of the Achilles tendon cause abrupt disruption of the normally dark tendon fibers on T2-weighted images as well as adjacent high signal material because of hemorrhage and edema.[8] Injury to other tendons causes an abnormally high signal intensity that is confined to the tendon on T2-weighted images; ligamentous injury may cause only disruption of the ligament without high signal to highlight the abnormality.[8] Differentiating partial tendon tears from focal tendinitis can be difficult, since both produce a bright signal within the tendon and tendon thickening on T2-weighted images. Bright signal around the tendon on T2-weighted images may indicate inflammation (tenosynovitis). It is important to recognize that some tendons have a small amount of fluid physiologically.[1]

Plantar Fasciitis

Plantar fasciitis causes focal or diffuse thickening of the plantar fascia. Conventional radiographs provide little assistance, but physical examination is usually sufficient to make the diagnosis. At times, MRI becomes necessary to exclude other diagnoses such as a soft tissue tumor. Some authors have found increased signal within the fascia on T1-weighted images.[8]

Sinus Tarsi Syndrome

This injury typically occurs after an inversion injury. MRI reveals abnormal bone marrow signal in the sinus tarsi (dark on T1-weighted images, bright on T2-weighted images) around the osteochondral injury. In addition, the cervical and talocalcaneal ligaments may lose their normal delineation because of inflammation. Some patients develop fibrosis that appears dark on T2-weighted images.[1]

Osteochondral Injuries

Osteochondritis Dissecans

This entity results from previous injury, usually involving foot inversion. In the foot and ankle, the talar dome is the most common site. The patient presents with pain and swelling. The abnormality has a four-stage classification system; higher stages indicate more damage and displacement. Stage I involves a focal trabecular compres-

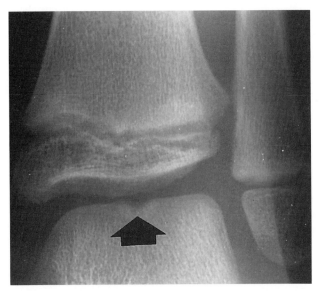

Figure 2–45. Osteochondral fracture (osteochondritis dissecans) in a 6-year-old boy. AP view of the ankle shows a small osteochondral fracture involving the middle third of the talar dome (*arrow*).

sion; stage II has an incompletely separated fragment (with a subchondral cyst the lesion is termed stage IIA). If the fragment is complete but nondisplaced, it is a stage III lesion, whereas an inverted or displaced fragment is a stage IV injury.[29] Conventional radiographs often reveal the lesion, showing a round or elliptical subchondral bone defect in the talar dome (Figs. 2–45 and 2–46). CT can help in staging the lesion and locating separated fragments.[29]

MRI can not only demonstrate the chondral and marrow extent of the lesion but can also delineate loose intra-articular bodies and the stability or instability of the

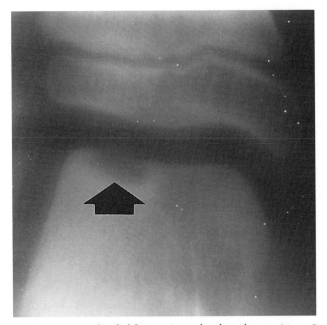

Figure 2–46. Osteochondral fracture (osteochondritis dissecans) in an 8-year-old boy. Coronal tomogram of the ankle shows an osteochondral lesion involving the lateral third of the talar dome (*arrow*).

lesion.[1] Thin sections with T1 and T2 weighting can document fluid within devitalized bone, whereas gradient echo images can identify intra-articular bodies that may be missed on other sequences.[26] In the dome of the talus, T1-weighted images show low signal intensity in the region of osteochondral injury; T2-weighted images have a variable signal intensity.[26] If conservative treatment (casting) is unsuccessful, MRI can help guide surgical therapy. MRI can also determine the integrity of the overlying cartilage: if this is disrupted, the patient will need curettage in addition to drilling of the lesion.[8]

Reflex Sympathetic Dystrophy

Patients with this idiopathic syndrome present with diffuse, nonanatomic pain, decreased function, and autonomic nerve dysfunction. Many experience relief of pain after lumbar sympathetic block.

Studying only adults, Holder and colleagues demonstrated the usefulness of three-phase bone scintigraphy in diagnosing reflex sympathetic dystrophy (RSD).[6] Delayed images invariably exhibited diffuse abnormal increased tracer uptake throughout the hindfoot, midfoot, and forefoot with marked periarticular accumulation of tracer. In addition, many had abnormal radionuclide angiograms (the tracer appeared in the blood vessels of the abnormal leg earlier than in the vessels of the normal leg) and abnormal blood-pool images (increased uptake throughout the foot). Holder and colleagues found 100% sensitivity and 80% specificity in three-phase bone scintigraphy. No one with RSD had a normal bone scan; nonetheless, many with conditions other than RSD (arthritis, infection, healing fractures, gout) also had abnormal bone scans.

Of note, several studies show that children with RSD are just as likely to have diffuse decreased radionuclide uptake as they are to have diffuse increased uptake.[11] Findings of decreased uptake may be more related to the stage of the illness than to the age of the patient.[6] In a small percentage of children the scintigram is normal despite significant clinical symptoms.[11] The scintigrams revert to normal after treatment in most children. Combining the clinical history with the scintigraphic findings often leads to the correct diagnosis.

ARTHRITIS

Juvenile Chronic Arthritis

Juvenile chronic arthritis (JCA) covers a spectrum of disease that can include systemic as well as skeletal abnormalities. The younger the age at onset, the less the illness resembles the adult form of rheumatoid arthritis. In general, younger children have monoarticular or pauciarticular involvement of the ankle, knee, or wrist. The older the child at age of onset, the more likely it is that he or she will have symmetrical polyarticular abnormalities. JCA causes hyperemia in the bone marrow, which in turn leads to premature physeal closure, short stature, and short tubular bones of the hands and feet.

Radiographs usually show periarticular osteoporosis,

joint effusions, and soft tissue edema. Periosteal reaction around the tubular bones of the hands and feet is common. Erosions and joint-space narrowing, characteristic of adult RA, rarely occur in children.

MRI can reveal abnormalities missed on conventional radiographs. Areas of synovial and cartilage inflammation become bright on T2 and enhance with gadolinium. MRI can show the extent of pannus and differentiate pannus from effusion.[1]

Hemophilia

In hemophilia, deficient clotting factors result in repeated hemorrhage into the joints, particularly the ankle, knee, and elbow. Acutely the child develops joint effusions; over time, synovitis, synovial thickening, and damage to the articular cartilage occur. Since hemophilia causes hyperemia, premature physeal fusion and diaphyseal undermodeling may result.

Depending on disease activity, conventional radiographs may show joint effusions acutely. In chronic cases, the radiographs reveal joint space narrowing, cartilage loss, subchondral cysts, and articular surface irregularity resulting from multiple episodes of bleeding (Fig. 2–47). MRI shows synovial hypertrophy as a lower than normal signal on both T1- and T2-weighted images.

A lytic expansile lesion along the bone (hemophilic pseudotumor) results from hemorrhage outside the joint capsule, typically in the calcaneus and the ilium but also in the tibia and small bones of the foot. Radiographs of this lesion typically show periosteal elevation, a soft tissue mass, and a lytic bone lesion.[9] MRI images differ depending on the age when the hemorrhage occurs but follow the usual signal characteristics of blood.[9]

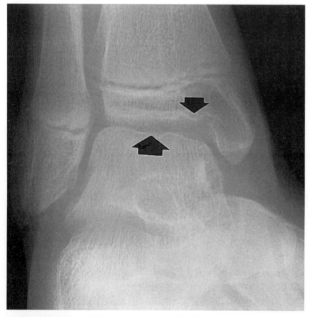

Figure 2–47. Hemophilia in a 12-year-old male. AP view of the ankle shows diffuse osteopenia as well as erosions of the articular surfaces *(arrows)* of the distal tibia and the talar dome.

Neuroarthropathy

A variety of disorders, including myelomeningoceles, congenital pain insensitivity, and Lesch-Nyhan syndrome, can lead to neuroarthropathy. Radiographs show the dreaded Ds: destruction, dislocation, distention of the joint, debris, disorganization, and eventually disappearance (of portions of bone, especially phalanges). In addition, bony sclerosis, subperiosteal hematomas, and physeal widening with metaphyseal fragmentation may be seen.

Most authors find that MRI of neuropathic joints shows decreased marrow signal on both T1- and T2-weighted images.[14] A few have found that acute spontaneous neuropathic fractures can exhibit a dark signal on T1-weighted images and a bright signal on T2-weighted images.[14] Both scintigraphy and MRI may help to distinguish infection from neuropathic arthropathy. Occasionally, biopsy is required for definitive diagnosis.

References

1. Aerts P, Disler DG: Abnormalities of the foot and ankle: MR imaging findings. AJR 1995; 165: 119–124.
2. Bresnahan PJ, Fung J: Magnetic resonance imaging of the foot and ankle in the pediatric patient. J Am Podiatr Assoc 1991; 81(3): 112–118.
3. Connolly JF: Injuries of the ankle: Sprains, dislocations, and fractures. *In* Connolly JF: Fractures and Dislocations—Closed Management. Philadelphia, W. B. Saunders, 1995, pp. 815–918.
4. Connolly JF: Fractures and fracture-dislocations of the bones of the foot. *In* Connolly JF: Fractures and Dislocations—Closed Management. Philadelphia, W. B. Saunders, 1995, pp. 919–1042.
5. Deutsch AL, Resnick D, Campbell G: Computed tomography and bone scintigraphy in the evaluation of tarsal coalition. Radiology 1982; 144: 137–140.
6. Holder LE, Cole LA, Myerson MS: Reflex sympathetic dystrophy in the foot: Clinical and scintigraphic criteria. Radiology 1992; 184: 531–535.
7. Fletcher B, Hanna SL, Fairclough DL, Gronemeyer SA: Pediatric musculoskeletal tumors: Use of dynamic, contrast-enhanced MR imaging to monitor response to chemotherapy. Radiology 1992; 184: 243–248.
8. Kier R, McCarthy S, Dietz MJ, Rudicel S: MR appearances of painful conditions of the ankle. Radiographics 1991; 11: 401–414.
9. Oestreich AE: Skeletal system. *In* Kirks DR (ed): Practical Pediatric Imaging. Diagnostic Radiology of Infants and Children, 2nd ed. Boston, Little, Brown, 1991, pp. 263–410.
10. Lateur LM, Van Hoe LR, Van Ghillewe KV, et al: Subtalar coalition: Diagnosis with the C sign on lateral radiographs of the ankle. Radiology 1994; 193: 847–851.
11. Laxer RM, Malleson PN, Morrison RT: Technetium 99m-methylene diphosphonate bone scans in children with reflex neurovascular dystrophy. J Pediatr 1985; 106: 437–440.
12. Mier RJ, Brower TD: Pediatric Orthopedics: A Guide for the Primary Care Physician. New York, Plenum Medical Book Co., 1994.
13. Mitchell DG, Rao VM, Dalinka MK, et al: Femoral head avascular necrosis: Correlation of MR imaging, radiographic staging, radionuclide imaging, and clinical findings. Radiology 1987; 162: 709–715.
14. Moore TE, Yuh WT, Kathol MH, et al: Abnormalities of the foot in patients with diabetes mellitus: Findings on MR imaging. AJR 1991; 157: 813–816.
15. Morrison WB, Schweitzer ME, Bock GW, et al: Diagnosis of osteomyelitis: Utility of fat-suppressed contrast-enhanced MR imaging. Radiology 1993; 189: 251–257.
16. Mott MP, Gebhardt MC: Pediatric bone tumors. Comprehens Ther 1993; 19(2): 73–81.

17. Ozonoff MB: Pediatric Orthopedic Radiology, 2nd ed. Philadelphia, W. B. Saunders, 1992.

18. Pavlov H, Torg JS, Freiberger RH: Tarsal navicular stress fractures: Radiographic evaluation. Radiology 1983; 148: 641–645.

19. Pineda C, Resnick D, Greenway G: Diagnosis of tarsal coalition with computed tomography. Clin Orth Rel Res 1986; 208: 282–288.

20. Resnick D, Niwayama G: Osteomyelitis, septic arthritis, and soft tissue infection: Mechanisms and situations. *In* Resnick D (ed): Diagnosis of Bone and Joint Disorders, 3rd ed. Vol. 4. Philadelphia, W. B. Saunders, 1995, pp. 2325–2418.

21. Resnick D, Niwayama G: Parathyroid disorders and renal osteodystrophy. *In* Resnick D (ed): Diagnosis of Bone and Joint Disorders, 3rd ed. Vol. 4. Philadelphia, W. B. Saunders, 1995, pp. 2012–2075.

22. Rogers LF: Introduction to skeletal radiology and bone growth. *In* Juhl JH, Crummy AB (eds): Paul and Juhl's Essentials of Radiologic Imaging, 6th ed. Philadelphia, J. B. Lippincott, 1993, pp. 21–31.

23. Rogers LF: The Ankle. *In* Rogers LF (ed): Radiology of Skeletal Trauma, 2nd ed. New York, Churchill Livingstone, 1992, pp. 1319–1428.

24. Rogers LF: The foot. *In* Rogers LF (ed): Radiology of Skeletal Trauma, 2nd ed. New York, Churchill Livingstone, 1992, pp. 1429–1521.

25. Sartoris DJ: Radiological review: Radiography of articular disorders in the foot. J Foot Ankle Surg 1994; 33(5): 518–525.

26. Sartoris DJ, Resnick D: Magnetic resonance imaging of pediatric foot and ankle disorders. J Foot Surg 1990; 29: 489–494.

27. Sartoris DJ, Resnick DL: Tarsal coalition. Arthr Rheum 1985; 28(3): 331–338.

28. Shapeero LG, Couanet D, Vanel D, et al: Bone metastases as the presenting manifestation of rhabdomyosarcoma in childhood. Skel Radiol 1993; 22(6): 433–438.

29. Sullivan JA: Ankle and foot injuries in the pediatric athlete. Instr Course Lect (IFC), 1993, 42: 545–551.

30. Wechsler RJ, Karasick D, Schweitzer ME: Computed tomography of talocalcaneal coalition: Imaging techniques. Skel Radiol 1992; 21: 353–358.

31. Wechsler RJ, Schweitzer ME, Deely DM, et al: Tarsal coalition: Depiction and characterization with CT and MR imaging. Radiology 1994; 193: 447–452.

32. Wenger DR, Leach J: Foot deformities in infants and children. Pediatr Clin North Am 1986; 33(6): 1411–1427.

33. Widhe T, Aaro S, Elmstedt E: Foot deformities in the newborn—incidence and prognosis. Acta Orthoped Scand 1988; 59(2): 176–179.

34. Yao DC, Sartoris DJ: Musculoskeletal tuberculosis. Radiol Clin North Am 1995; 33(4): 679–689.

35. Yeager KK, Mitchell M, Sartoris DJ: Diagnostic imaging approach to bone tumors of the foot. J Foot Surg 1991; 30(2): 197–208.

36. Rockwood CA Jr, Green DP: Fractures. Philadelphia, J. B. Lippincott, 1975.

37. Goldman AB: Heritable disease of connective tissue. *In* Resnick D (ed): Diagnosis of Bone and Joint Disorders, 3rd ed. Philadelphia, W. B. Saunders, 1995, pp. 4122–4129.

3

Management of the Pediatric Patient

Kevin D. Roberts, D.P.M., R.Ph.

Pediatrics is a specialized branch of podiatric surgery dealing with the study and the treatment of the foot and ankle from birth to adolescence. As this population continues to grow in today's podiatric practice, certain guidelines for the preoperative, intraoperative and postoperative management of these patients should be addressed. It is not in the scope of this paper to cover every detail of the management of the pediatric surgical patient but instead to highlight some considerations in such management.

The pediatric population differs greatly from its adult counterpart and offers many new challenges. To complicate the issue further, the pediatric population itself is made up of many different subgroups: (1) premature infants, less than 38 weeks of gestation; (2) neonates, birth to 1 month old; (3) infants, 1 to 24 months old; (4) small children, 1 to 5 years old; (5) older children, 6 to 12 years old; and (6) adolescents, 13 to 18 years old. As can be easily surmised, not only do these subgroups differ chronologically, they also differ physiologically, psychologically, and cognitively. Owing to these differences, patients in each subgroup present their own special challenges when they become surgical candidates.

PREOPERATIVE PERIOD

The most difficult person to deal with in this period is the parent. The thought of surgery can be as overwhelming to the parent as it is to the child. It is important to remember that the parents are making difficult decisions about one of their most cherished gifts. Most parents realize that this decision could affect their child for the rest of his or her life.

The responsibility of decision making may cause anxiety in the parents that will be perceived by the child as fear. Therefore, it is very important for the physician to spend an adequate amount of time with the parents discussing the surgery and any anticipated complications. All questions should be answered honestly (e.g., Yes, there will be some pain, but medication will be given for this, and the pain will decrease greatly after several days). This honesty, will gain the trust of the parents and greatly decrease their anxiety when the child complains of pain

postoperatively. The surgery or hospital stay should be explained to the child after the decision has been made by the parents and all questions and concerns have been addressed. The explanation should include both cognitive information (what will happen) and sensory information (how it will feel) in easy-to-understand terms that the child can relate to. The explanation given to children in each subgroup will vary.

The small child, aged 1 to 5 years, who has a vivid imagination may believe that the surgery is a punishment for something that he has done wrong. In this case, the child must be informed that the procedure is intended to help him or her, not to punish him. Terms such as "going to sleep" may be easily understood by the adolescent but can be misinterpreted by the small child. He should be reassured that he will wake up (yes, you will go to sleep, but then you will wake up, and the surgery will be all done).

Older children, aged 6 to 12 years, can be very curious about what is going on around them. This energy can be directed into a positive experience by letting them try out anesthesia masks, work blood pressure cuffs, and wear surgical attire before the surgery. This will help to acclimate them to the equipment used on the day of surgery and will therefore decrease their anxiety level.

Adolescents, 12 to 18 years old, should be treated like adults, openly and honestly. Self-esteem is important in this age group. They usually state that they "don't want to be treated like a child."

Several institutions have adopted programs in which children and parents can tour the hospital and be introduced to the medical team before the hospital stay begins. Various other methods have been used to provide useful information to children about surgery or the hospital stay including coloring books and playing with dolls. Most important, the child's feelings and fears should be discussed with both the physician and the parents before the surgical procedure is performed.

Both small and older children can experience a great amount of anxiety if they are separated from their parents. The parent or parents should be present at the time of induction of anesthesia as well as in the recovery room if this is allowed by the institution to decrease separation anxiety. Security blankets and favorite dolls are a comfort

SMA7

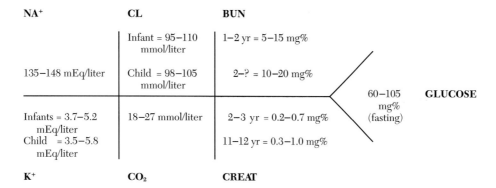

NA+	CL	BUN		
	Infant = 95–110 mmol/liter	1–2 yr = 5–15 mg%		
135–148 mEq/liter	Child = 98–105 mmol/liter	2–? = 10–20 mg%		GLUCOSE
			60–105 mg% (fasting)	
Infants = 3.7–5.2 mEq/liter	18–27 mmol/liter	2–3 yr = 0.2–0.7 mg%		
Child = 3.5–5.8 mEq/liter		11–12 yr = 0.3–1.0 mg%		
K+	CO₂	CREAT		

to some children and should be present both before and after the surgical procedure to provide reassurance. Whenever it is possible to do safely, the surgical procedure should be performed as an outpatient procedure because children usually recover faster in familiar surroundings such as home.

With the psychologic and cognitive issues addressed, the physician should carefully screen the child's physiologic health. This screening procedure should include a thorough podiatric history and physical examination. The physician should also discuss the patient's history and treatment plan with the treating pediatrician before performing the history and physical examination; this discussion will offer important insights into the patient's preoperative, intraoperative, and postoperative care.

As with all preoperative patients, laboratory tests are a must. Routine lab work should include a complete blood count (CBC) with differential, erythrocyte sedimentation rate (ESR), prothrombin time (PT), partial thromboplastin time (PTT), urinalysis with microbiology, and an SMA 7 panel. Some pediatric lab values can vary outside the usual norm of adults (e.g., a normal CBC in a 3-month-old child ranges from 6000 to 18,000 with a greater percentage of lymphocytes compared to polymorphonuclear leukocytes). A knowledge of these different lab values is necessary to adequately assess the preoperative pediatric patient. Preoperative laboratory evaluation is individualized for each patient. For example, in young black children a sickle cell screen should be performed, and a screen for human chorionic gonadotropin (hCG) should be performed in female patients who have reached puberty.

On admission to the hospital or outpatient center, the history and physical findings as well as the preoperative lab work should be reviewed for completeness and correctness. Vital signs (blood pressure, temperature, pulse,

Partial thromboplastin time	42–54 sec
Prothrombin time	11–15 sec
Sedimentation rate (micro)	<2 yr: 1–5 mm/hr
	>2 yr: 1–8 mm/hr

CBC

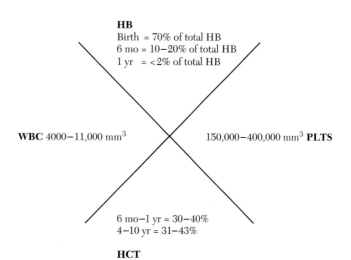

HB
Birth = 70% of total HB
6 mo = 10–20% of total HB
1 yr = <2% of total HB

WBC 4000–11,000 mm³   150,000–400,000 mm³ **PLTS**

6 mo–1 yr = 30–40%
4–10 yr = 31–43%

HCT

and respirations) should be taken and recorded. Once again, the values for children usually differ from those seen in adults. Some of these differences include higher pulse and respiratory rates and a lower systolic blood pressure. It is recommended that children 3 years old or younger have their temperature taken rectally. Rectal temperatures may run 1 degree higher than oral temperatures, and axillary temperatures may be 1 degree less. Some auditory temperature monitoring devices are available, but these are usually too large to fit the small external canal of a child to give a reliable reading. The child's height and weight are essential for his or her management and should be documented.

Preoperative orders in children do not follow the standard NPO orders after midnight as in adults. Food solids and milk should be discontinued 12 hours preoperatively, but fluids should be maintained as long as possible. Children have an increased metabolic requirement. An infant is usually fed every 4 hours. If feedings are decreased, the baby becomes hungry and restless, and his or her stores of glycogen become depleted. Infant feedings should not be discontinued any longer than necessary. The last bottle for an infant 6 months or younger should be given approximately 4 hours before surgery and should consist of plain or sweetened water. Children 6 months to 3 years old should be hydrated up to 6 hours preoperatively and those over 3 up until 8 hours preoperatively. These recommendations vary from institution to institution and should be discussed with the anesthesia department to determine their procedures and policy.

Preoperative Medications

Physicians should have an increased awareness of the unique drug-related considerations that apply to prescribing medications for pediatric patients. Neonates, infants, and children have special pharmacokinetic and pharmacodynamic parameters that differ as changes in their body organ functions occur. These parameters include drug absorption, distribution, metabolism, excretion, sensitivity, and dosing. Drug absorption is defined as the uptake of a drug into or across tissues.

Route

1. The oral route is most commonly used, but it can differ greatly in this population, especially in neonates and infants. Some of the differences in oral absorption are related to faster transit times in the gut, decreased gastric acid production, and lack of hydrolytic enzymes. Therefore, alterations in the amount, interval, and route of the drug may be needed.
2. The rectal route is used more often in children than in adults. There is no difference in absorption of medications given rectally in children compared with adults. This may be a good alternative route to use in children who have problems taking oral medications.
3. The parenteral route is commonly used in hospitalized pediatric patients. The intravenous (IV) route offers

100% bioavailability, and dosing by this route is reliable. This is not the case with the intramuscular (IM) route in neonates and infants. Because they have a smaller muscle mass and a smaller blood supply, the rate of drug absorption can be erratic and slower. Therefore, the IV route is preferred to intramuscular administration when possible.[11-13]

Metabolism

Drug distribution in pediatric patients is governed by a number of age-dependent factors. The main one is the change in body composition as the child grows and matures. Since most drugs are distributed by plasma protein in the aqueous portion of the body, changes in these components dramatically alter the distribution of drugs. Body weight in the neonate is approximately 75% water, whereas in the adult it is 60% water. The larger percentage of water increases the volume of distribution. Neonates and infants also have a decreased level of plasma proteins, which can cause an increase in the amount of unbound or pharmacologically active drug, leading to increased pharmacologic or toxic effects.

Drug metabolism takes place in many organs and tissues of the body (lungs, kidneys, blood, gastrointestinal (GI) tract, and liver). Active lipid-soluble drugs are converted to inactive water-soluble metabolites primarily in the liver. A number of hepatic metabolic pathways in the liver mature at different rates. Most of these pathways reach the adult level by age 4.

Elimination of drugs from the body is performed by a number of organs and tissues including the lungs, GI tract, sweat glands, and kidneys. The kidneys are primarily responsible for eliminating drugs in the pediatric patient. As with other organs, kidney function is age dependent. The normal developing kidney reaches the adult level of function by about 7 months of age.

Neonates and infants, due to their developing systems, can be especially sensitive to some drugs. This is very important when one is prescribing medications that are active in the central nervous system. The central nervous system matures slowly and does not reach adult levels until about age 8. Therefore, drugs like morphine and chloral hydrate may have an increased depressant effect in the immature central nervous system (CNS).

The challenge of dosing in pediatric patients can now be easily appreciated. Many formulas have been developed to help calculate pediatric doses. These formulas offer a quick reference for dosing pediatric medications, but the child's body surface area should be used for a more accurate dose. These calculations or nomograms take the child's height and weight into account, giving a dose in milligrams per meter squared,

Clark's Weight Rule (for patients over 2 years):

$$\frac{\text{Weight in lb}}{150} \times \text{adult dose} = \text{child dose}$$

Young's Rule (for patients over 2 years):

$$\frac{\text{Age in years}}{\text{Age in years} + 12} \times \text{adult dose} = \text{child dose}$$

Fried's Rule (for patients under 2 years):

$$\frac{\text{Age in months}}{150} \times \text{adult dose} = \text{infant dose}$$

which is more accurate than the age-dependent calculations referred to earlier.

Preoperative Analgesia

Several medications can be used alone or in combination to provide preoperative analgesia and sedation. Although none are perfect, many have been used successfully.

Barbiturates. Barbiturates produce sedation by depressing the CNS. They offer no analgesic effect and in fact may increase the patient's sensitivity to pain. Therefore, barbiturates can be used for nonpainful procedures (i.e., magnetic resonance imaging [MRI]) but should not be used alone before painful surgical procedures.

Dose (e.g., pentobarbital)
- Oral: 2–6 mg/kg per day (maximum 100 mg per day)
- Rectal: Age 2 months to 1 year (10 to 20 lb)— 30 mg
                   Age 1 to 4 years (20 to 40 lb)— 30 or 60 mg
                   Age 5 to 12 years (40 to 80 lb)— 60 mg
                   Age 12 to 14 years (80 to 110 lb)— 60 or 100 mg
- Intramuscular: 2–6 mg/kg but no more than 100 mg in any one dose. Usual dose is between 25 and 80 mg

Benzodiazepines. Benzodiazepines are sedative-hypnotic drugs that offer the added benefits of muscle relaxation and an amnesia effect. Again, this group of drugs offers no analgesic effect and can heighten the patient's response to pain.

Dose (e.g., diazepam)
- Oral: Age older than 6 months—0.04–0.2 mg/kg
- Parenteral: 0.04–0.2 mg/kg dose every 2 to 3 hours, to a maximum of 0.6 mg/kg an 8-hour period

Chloral Hydrate. Chloral hydrate (Roxane Laboratories Inc., Columbus, OH 43228) is a nonbarbiturate that is frequently used for preoperative sedation. Chloral hydrate is a prodrug that depends on conversion by the liver to its active metabolite trichloroethanol. The CNS depression that results is similar to that produced by barbiturates. Oral use of chloral hydrate is frequently associated with problems such as its bad taste and GI upset. These problems can be overcome by using the suppository formulation.

Dose
- Oral or rectal: 25 mg/kg per day up to 500 mg in a single dose.

Narcotic Agents. Narcotic agents can produce analgesia and sedation. The analgesic dose is lower than that needed for sedation, and since narcotics produce dose-related respiratory depression, they are very seldom used alone for preoperative sedation.

Dose
- Meperidine: Intramuscular or subcutaneous—1–2 mg/kg
- DPT (Demerol/Phenergan/Thorazine):
  Given in a single IM injection—1 mg/kg Demerol; 0.5–1.0 mg/kg Phenergan; 0.5 mg/kg of Thorazine

DPT* is probably the most widely used combination of sedative drugs in the pediatric population. The antihistamine Phenergan (promethazine) is used to potentiate the effect of the narcotic Demerol (meperidine), allowing use of a lower dose of the narcotic. The antipsychotic Thorazine (chlorpromazine) is added to relieve the restlessness and apprehension that are often experienced prior to surgery. Thorazine also combats the nausea and vomiting induced by the use of narcotics.

Atropine, Scopolamine, Hyoscyamine, and Glycopyrrolate. Atropine, scopolamine, hyoscyamine, and glycopyrrolate are anticholinergics that can be used in combination to help decrease secretions as well as block cardiac vagal inhibitory reflexes during induction of anesthesia and intubation.

Knowledge of a drug's onset and duration is important when ordering a preoperative medication. The patient should arrive in the operating room drowsy but cooperative. Proper administration of the preoperative medication should be reviewed with the parents or caretaker if they are responsible for giving it. Whenever possible, the medication should be administered by medical personnel in a controlled environment (e.g., a nurse in a preoperative holding area).

INTRAOPERATIVE PERIOD

The anesthesiologist is an important member of the surgical team. He or she monitors many parameters during the procedure. It is the responsibility of the surgeon to know these parameters and aid in decreasing fluctuations in them. Fluid loss is one of these parameters. Although it usually is not a problem in podiatric procedures, the surgeon should be aware of it, especially when performing surgery on neonates and infants, who have small reserves. Replacement is a must with even a small loss. Lactated Ringer's solution or whole blood may be used for this purpose.

*DPT comprises Demerol (Sonofi Winthrop Pharmaceuticals, New York, NY 10016; Phenergan (Wyeth-Ayerst Laboratories; Philadelphia, PA 19101; and Thorazine (SmithKline Beecham Pharmaceuticals, Philadelphia, PA 19101.)

General anesthesia is the preferred method of anesthetizing the pediatric patient whenever possible. It decreases the anxiety of the child to know that he or she will receive an injection to numb the area, and, in fact, most children prefer to go to sleep during the procedure.[2–5]

Hypothermia

The risk of hypothermia is a concern with the use of general anesthesia and is exaggerated in neonates and infants because of their immature temperature-regulating system. Also, they have a high ratio of surface area to body and are unable to shiver, which further decreases their ability to maintain body temperature. Warm blankets and warming devices such as the Bair hugger should be employed. In some cases, the temperature of the operating room suite can be raised to minimize loss of body heat by the patient.[1]

Tourniquet size must be scaled down and the pressure adjusted to approximately 100 mm of mercury above the systolic blood pressure. Timing of the thigh tourniquet is recommended to last approximately 1 hour in a pediatric patient instead of the 1 to 2 hours recommended for an adult.

Intraoperative Blocks

Intraoperative blocks can be employed to help decrease the anesthetic requirements during the procedure as well as to speed emergence from the anesthetic. They can also offer great postoperative pain control, thereby decreasing the need for opiates in the postoperative period. Great care should be taken to avoid toxic doses of local anesthetics in this population. Diluted solutions should be used in most cases. Local anesthetics can be diluted with preservative-free normal saline to the desired concentration. Bupivacaine is especially useful postoperatively because of its long-acting blockade of pain. Use of it in the pediatric population is controversial and, according to the package insert, it should not be used in children under the age of 12 because of lack of clinical experience. However, a number of institutions have employed bupivacaine in infants with no deleterious effects.

POSTOPERATIVE PERIOD

Many of the parameters that are monitored intraoperatively should be monitored postoperatively as well, including oxygenation of blood and cardiac electrical activity. Vital signs should also be taken according to the protocol of the institution. If the infant or neonate received intravenous therapy during the procedure, his or her weight should be recorded and compared with preoperative values.

Restoration of respiratory function is important in the pediatric patient postoperatively. Atelectasis or lung collapse is frequently due to an obstruction of the bronchus by a mucus plug. This occurs postoperatively when anesthesia has stimulated an increase in bronchial secretions.

Postoperative use of analgesic medications may lead to shallow breathing and discourages the patient from coughing to clear these secretions. Therefore, infants and neonates should sleep propped on one side with pillows, and the side should be switched every several hours to allow aeration of both lungs.

To clear any mucus that has formed, infants should be awakened every 4 hours and forced to cry. Young children and older children should cough or blow up balloons when available. Voldyne incentive spirometry can be used with adolescent patients. The most common cause of death in infants undergoing surgery is aspiration. When these children are fed, the head of the bed should be elevated, and suction equipment always should be nearby.

The greatest challenge postoperatively is adequate and proper management of the patient's pain. This challenge is even greater in pediatric patients, in whom little research has been done, and few clinical trials of controlling postoperative pain have been performed. This situation has led to a great many misconceptions about the control of pain in this population. One of these misconceptions is that the pediatric patient does not feel the same amount of pain postoperatively as the adult patient. There is good evidence now that children are anatomically and neurochemically capable of experiencing pain at the time of birth and respond to painful stimuli in the same way as adults. The World Health Organization recommends treating pain by a three-step method.[6]

1. Mild pain can be treated with nonopioids.
2. Moderate pain should be treated with weak opiates and nonopiates in combination.
3. Severe pain is treated with strong opiates and nonopiates in combination.

Continuous administration of analgesics is superior to the prn administration most commonly used with these medications. The latter often leaves patients with prolonged periods of inadequate analgesia and requires larger doses to rescue them from painful experiences.[8–10]

Acetaminophen

The most commonly used analgesic for mild pain in pediatric patients is acetaminophen. Its exact mechanism of action in causing the analgesic effect is unclear, but it is thought that the drug inhibits the generation of afferent pain signals. Acetaminophen also has an antipyretic effect through its direct action on the hypothalamic regulating center. This direct action increases the dissipation of body heat by increasing vasodilatation and sweating. Acetaminophen has very little effect on prostaglandin synthesis peripherally and therefore has very little anti-inflammatory effect. Acetaminophen also offers an advantage over nonsteroidal anti-inflammatory drugs and aspirin in that it does not inhibit platelet aggregation or produce GI bleeding. The availability of various dose forms also offers advantages in administering the medication. These dose forms include suppositories, chewable tablets, granules, tablets, capsules, and elixir.

Dose:
• 10–15 mg/kg per dose every 4 to 6 hours

Aspirin

Aspirin, a medication that was formerly extensively used in this population, has fallen from grace because of its association with Reyes' syndrome.

Nonsteroidal Anti-Inflammatory Drugs

Recently there has been an increased use of nonsteroidal anti-inflammatory drugs (NSAIDs) in the pediatric population. This usage was further augmented by the formulation and release of an over-the-counter ibuprofen suspension. NSAIDs can be especially useful in podiatric postoperative patients in whom pain originates from the inflammatory response to bone and joint manipulation. To date three NSAIDs are recognized by the Food and Drug Administration (FDA) for use in children. They are ibuprofen administered in children 12 months old and older, tolmetin, and naproxen, administered in children aged 2 years old and older. Ibuprofen and naproxen offer the added benefit of the availability of suspension forms. The suspension form of ibuprofen is formulated to have 100 mg of drug per 5 mL (a teaspoon). The suspension of naproxen is formulated to have 125 mg of drug per 5 mL. The recommended dose of ibuprofen for children is between 20 and 40 mg/kg per day divided into three or four doses. Although NSAIDs have not been implicated in Reye's syndrome, experimental studies in animals have suggested that ibuprofen coupled with influenza B viral infection in a patient ingesting a diet free of arginine may cause significant hepatic disruption and increase mortality. Further investigation is needed, and the cautious use of these medications postoperatively in the pediatric population cannot be overstressed. Unfortunately, these drugs as a class have some of the same side effects as aspirin. Most important in postoperative patients are GI irritation and the inhibitory effect on platelet aggregation. For these reasons, it is recommended to delay starting these medications until approximately 24 hours after the surgical procedure has been performed. This delay ensures that adequate clotting has occurred at the surgical site and that the patient is tolerating oral feedings. As with all oral NSAIDs, the drugs should be given on a full stomach to help decrease GI side effects.

Dose
- Naproxen suspension: Approximately 10 mg/kg per day divided into two equal doses

Codeine

Codeine, a weak opiate, is probably the most commonly used medication for the treatment of moderate pain in pediatric patients, both alone and in combination with other drugs. Codeine acts like morphine in its antagonist activity at three of the five known opiate receptors. Since codeine has a ceiling effect, it is most often used in combination with other medications to reach a higher analgesic effect. The most commonly used combination is codeine and acetaminophen. When codeine is used as a single agent in children over 1 year of age, it may be administered as a subcutaneous injection, an intramuscular injection, or orally. The elixir formulation of acetaminophen and codeine is the form most commonly used in children. This formulation includes 12 mg of codeine phosphate and 120 mg of acetaminophen per 5 mL (a teaspoon). The dose of this combination should be based on the codeine content. The dosing criteria shown below can be used when administering the elixir form of acetaminophen with codeine.

Dose
- Codeine: 0.5 mg/kg or 15 m² of body surface area every 4 to 6 hours

Narcotic Agonists (Morphine and Meperidine)

Narcotic agonists are the mainstay of treatment of severe postoperative pain. Their analgesic activity is related to the binding of these agents to opiate receptors in the CNS, thereby altering the central release of neurotransmitters from afferent nerves that have been activated by painful stimuli. Unfortunately, their greater analgesic effects are accompanied by a variety of secondary pharmacologic effects. These side effects can vary from being a nuisance in postoperative patients to effects that can be fatal. They include but are not limited to drowsiness, nausea, vomiting, respiratory depression, orthostatic hypotension, constipation, and urinary retention. A number of these narcotic agonists are available for use in the postoperative patient. Morphine and meperidine are most commonly used in pediatric patients.

Morphine should be used cautiously in patients 3 months old and younger because of the immaturity of the blood–brain barrier in these infants. Morphine, due to its low lipid solubility, usually has a slower onset and a longer duration of action, but when administered to these very young infants it can reach higher levels more quickly, thereby causing an increase in respiratory depression. Meperidine, which is more lipid soluble, is usually more reliable in these young infants. Meperidine also offers an advantage over morphine in that it causes less intestinal muscle spasm and constipation in an equal analgesic dose.

In a number of patients with preexisting disease extreme caution should be used when prescribing narcotic agonists. These include asthmatic patients, who may already have a decreased respiratory reserve. Also, patients with preexisting seizure disorders must be monitored closely for opiate-induced seizure activity. Special care should be taken when dealing with a patient with renal dysfunction who needs meperidine because the active metabolite normeperidine may accumulate, resulting in increased CNS adverse effects.

The use of the piperazine antihistamine hydroxyzine can help to potentiate the actions of the narcotic agonist. When these drugs are used in combination, it is recommended that the narcotic agonist dose be decreased by 50%. The only parenteral route acceptable for the use of hydroxyzine is the IM route. Tissue necrosis and hemolysis have been associated with the subcutaneous and IV routes. Meperidine has been formulated with a number of other drugs to take advantage of each medication's ability to alleviate pain. Most notable of these other medications are acetaminophen and promethazine. Morphine formulations include injectables, soluble tablets, tablets, sustained controlled-release tablets, solutions, and rectal suppositories. As can be seen, a number of different routes can be used to administer morphine in postoperative patients. When administering morphine orally, it should be remembered that it is approximately a third to a sixth as effective as the parenteral route because of the first-pass effect.

Dose
- Morphine: Starting dose for postoperative pain in infants older than 3 months of age—0.3 mg/kg every 4 hours
  Intramuscular dose—0.15 mg/kg every 3 to 4 hours
- Meperidine: Oral and parenteral dosage is approximately the same, starting at 1 to 1.5 mg/kg every 3 to 4 hours

Antibiotics

When prophylactic antibiotics are used, administration should begin about 30 minutes before the incision is made, with the intent of achieving peak concentrations of the drug at this time. In most instances, IV administration is preferred for major procedures. The intent is to maintain adequate plasma and tissue concentrations of the drugs until the incision is closed. With prolonged procedures lasting 2 to 3 hours, an additional dose may be required. Drugs administered postoperatively for prophylaxis do not reduce the infection rate.

The selection of antibiotics for prophylaxis is based on the procedure, the expected contaminating organisms, and the safety of the drugs. Because of the vast array of antibiotics now available, more than one may qualify well for use. Some suggestions for preventing infection in a clean-contaminated compound fracture are cefazolin, nafcillin, and vancomycin.[7]

SUMMARY

The pediatric surgical patient is not merely a miniature adult. Many aspects of the preoperative, intraoperative, and postoperative care of these patients must be addressed before the patient is even considered a surgical candidate. This chapter has highlighted only a few of these considerations. A working knowledge of the psychologic, physiologic, and cognitive parameters of each age group is needed before treatment can be initiated. Children are truly special patients, and their management should be approached accordingly.

References

1. Goudsouzian NG, Morris RH, Ryan JF: The effects of a warming blanket on the maintenance of body temperature in anesthetized infants and children. Anesthesiology 1973; 39:351–353.
2. Ararnoff P, Woody PD: Preparation of children for hospitalization in acute care hospitals in the United States. Pediatrics 1981; 68:361–368.
3. Egbert LD: The value of the preop visit by an anesthetist. JAMA 1962; 185:553–555.
4. Wood RA: Value of the chest x-ray as a screening test for elective surgery in children. Pediatrics 1981; 67:447–452.
5. Steward DJ: Outpatient pediatric anesthesia. Anesthesiology 1975; 43:268–276.
6. Soumerai SB: Drug prescribing in pediatrics: Challenges for quality improvement. Pediatrics 1990; 86:782–784.
7. Hoekelman RA: Choosing the right antibiotic. Pediatr Ann 1993; 22:155–156.
8. Weisman SJ: The management of pain in children. Pediatr Rev 1991; 12:237–243.
9. Bede CB: Pediatric postoperative pain management. Pediatr Clin North Am 1989; 36:921–938.
10. Zeltzer LK: The management of pain associated with pediatric procedures. Pediatr Clin North Am 1989; 36:941–961.
11. McLeod HL: Pediatric pharmacokinetics and therapeutic drug monitoring. Pediatr Rev 1992; 13:413–421.
12. Berlin CM: Advances in pediatric pharmacology and toxicology. Adv Pediatr 1993; 40:405–431.
13. Walson PD: Principles of drug prescribing in infants and children. A practical guide. Drugs 1993; 46:281–288.

4

Pediatric Anesthesia

John G. Goode M.D., D.A.B.P.M.

Because children are not just small adults but differ physiologically, pharmacologically, and psychologically from adults, the provision of safe pediatric anesthesia requires special knowledge and understanding. Although Patel and Hannallah[1] have demonstrated the safety of pediatric ambulatory surgery, the risk of a major or minor adverse event during pediatric anesthesia may be as high as 35% compared with 17% during adult anesthesia.[2] Furthermore, the risk of cardiac arrest for infants younger than 1 year of age has been reported to be 19 per 10,000 anesthetics compared with 7 per 10,000 anesthetics for adults.[3] Routine techniques that may be appropriate for adult anesthesia are not always appropriate for pediatric anesthesia. Instead, the anesthesiologist must design a technique that is best for each individual child.

EQUIPMENT

A hospital that performs primarily adult surgery should have a pediatric cart or box that contains all necessary equipment. Minimal equipment is listed in Table 4–1.

PHYSIOLOGIC DIFFERENCES

The body surface-to-volume ratio is 70 times higher for neonates than for adults.[4] Children, and especially neonates, are thereby prone to heat loss with resultant hypothermia. Oxygen consumption for the infant is about twice that of the adult per unit weight.[5] Furthermore, the child's airway is more prone to obstruction because of the relatively large tongue and anterior larynx.[6] The possibility of airway obstruction in conjunction with increased oxygen consumption explains the decreased margin of respiratory reserve during pediatric anesthesia. Next, the incidence of malignant hyperthermia has been reported to be as high as 1 in every 14,000 pediatric anesthetics[7] compared with an overall incidence of 1 in 250,000 anesthetics.[8] The clinical picture of malignant hyperthermia includes increased CO_2 production, muscle rigidity, acidosis, tachycardia, and increased temperature. Temperature elevation may be a late manifestation. With early diagnosis and specific therapy, the mortality rate has fallen from 70% to 10%.[8] A study by Dubrow and colleagues[9] demonstrated that patients at risk for malignant hyperthermia can be anesthetized safely with carefully selected general anesthesia. Both succinylcholine and potent inhalational anesthetics must be avoided because they are triggering agents. The muscle relaxant succinylcholine, which is routinely used for adult anesthesia, should be used only selectively in pediatric anesthesia. Succinylcholine has been reported to cause hyperkalemic cardiac arrest in asymptomatic pediatric patients with subclinical myopathy.[10]

PHARMACOLOGIC DIFFERENCES

The uptake of the inhalational anesthetics (halothane, isoflurane, sevoflurane) is more rapid in children because of their faster respiratory rate and higher cardiac index. This explains why it is relatively easy to give an overdose to young children. Body composition also changes from infancy to adulthood. The percentage of total body water decreases as fat and muscle mass increase.[11] The changes in body composition explain why an initial drug dose requirement for a water-soluble drug (succinylcholine) may be higher in a young child and why some drugs that redistribute into fat (thiopental) and muscle (fentanyl) may have longer clinical effects.[12] As opposed to adult anesthesia, pediatric drugs are given according to weight in kilograms. Table 4–2 lists the resuscitation doses and miscellaneous doses.

PSYCHOLOGIC DIFFERENCES

Prolonged hospitalization and major surgery can result in psychologic trauma in children.[13] In comparison, day

Table 4–1. **Pediatric Surgical Equipment**

Airway equipment
  Laryngoscope handles and blades (MAC + Miller, sizes 1 and 2)
  Endotracheal tubes (2.5 through 6.0 uncuffed, 5 and 6 cuffed)
  Airways (assorted sizes)
  Suction catheters (12 Fr, 10 Fr, 8 Fr, 6 Fr)
  Stylettes (pediatric)
  Masks (assorted sizes)
Monitoring equipment
  Pediatric blood pressure cuffs
  Esophageal or rectal temperature probes
  Pediatric oximeter probes
Warming blankets or Bair Huggers
Pediatric ventilator for anesthesia machine
Pediatric IVs and Soluset administration sets

Table 4–2. **Resuscitation and Other Drug Doses**

Resuscitation Drug Doses	Concentration	Dose for Selected Ages		
		1 yr (10 kg)	*6 yr (20 kg)*	*9 yr (30 kg)*
Atropine	0.02 mg/kg (IV) (max = 0.4 mg)	0.1 mg/mL (0.01%)	0.2 mg (0.2 mL)	0.4 mg (0.4 mL)	0.4 mg (0.4mL)
Calcium gluconate	30 mg/kg (IV)	100 mg/mL (10%)	300 mg (3 mL)	600 mg (6 mL)	900 mg (9 mL)
chloride	10 mg/kg (IV)	100 mg/mL (10%)	100 mg (1 mL)	200 mg (2 mL)	300 mg (3 mL)
Dextrose (50%)	1 mL/kg (IV)	0.5 mg/mL (50%)	10 mL	20 mL	30 mL
Epinephrine	10 μg/kg (IV)	1:10,000 (100 μg/mL)	100 μg (1 mL)	200 μg (2 mL)	300 μg (3 mL)
Lidocaine	1 mg/kg (IV)	20 mg/mL (2%)	10 mg (0.5 mL)	20 mg (1 mL)	30 mg (1.5 mL)
Sodium bicarbonate	1–2 mEq/kg (IV)	1 mEq/mL	15 mEq (15 mL)	30 mEq (30 mL)	45 mEq (45 mL)
Defibrillation dose	2 watts (second/kg)	**Epinephrine:**	If the pulseless child fails to respond to above epinephrine doses, consider giving 0.1 mg/kg (100 μg/kg) as 0.1 mL/kg of 1:1000 epinephrine.		

Miscellaneous Drug Doses	
Decadron	1 mg/kg (IV)
Droperidol	25–75 μg/kg (IV)
Fentanyl	1 μg/kg (IV)
Hydrocortisone	2 mg/kg (IV)
Ketamine (induction)	4 mg/kg (IM) or 1 mg/kg (IV)
Lasix	1 mg/kg (IV)
Midazolam (premed)	0.5 mg/kg max = 1.5 mg (PO)
Morphine	0.05–0.1 mg/kg (IV)
Narcan	5–10 μg/kg (IV)
Neostigmine (reversal)	0.07 mg/kg (IV)
Epinephrine	0.2–0.5 mL in 3 mL normal saline Nebulization
Valium (status)	0.2 mg/kg (IV)

surgery appears to cause minimal problems.[14] Eckenhoff[15] observed that 17% of children had postoperative personality changes that were thought to be related to their hospital/surgical experiences and that the incidence of changes was inversely related to the child's age. Parental reactions are very important, since anxiety is readily communicated to the child and affects his or her behavior.[16] To reduce the overall stress of surgery, the following guidelines should be followed:

1. Be completely honest with parents and the patient.
2. Encourage parents to bring children's security objects (blankets, stuffed animals) to the hospital.
3. Minimize the separation time preoperatively as well as postoperatively.
4. Recommend reading materials such as *A Visit to Sesame Street Hospital*,[17] *Going to the Hospital*,[18] and *When Your Child Needs Anesthesia*.[19]
5. Establish and encourage hospital tours for children with their parents.

PREOPERATIVE CONSIDERATIONS

The American Society of Anesthesiologists (ASA) has developed a physical status (PS) rating that can be applied to all preoperative patients.[20] There are five classes as follows:

    I. Healthy patients
    II. Patients with mild systemic disease
    III. Patients with severe systemic disease
    IV. Patients with life-threatening disease

    V. Moribund patients.

The PS I through III patients should be considered for outpatient surgery; PS III patients should have a written statement from the primary care physician as well as a preoperative anesthetic consultation to determine if outpatient surgery is appropriate.[21] Patients who require postoperative parenteral analgesics should not undergo outpatient surgery. Furthermore, premature infants should not undergo outpatient surgery unless their *postconceptual age* is greater than 60 weeks, since they are at risk for postoperative apnea.[22]

It is probably prudent to postpone elective surgery for the child with an upper respiratory tract infection. Although Tate and Knight[23] concluded that there was no increase in complications, two other studies demonstrated more respiratory problems intraoperatively or postoperatively in this subset of patients.[24, 25]

The guidelines for preoperative fasting have of late been liberalized. Several studies have shown that it is safe to give clear liquids up to 2 to 3 hours before induction of anesthesia.[26–28] Solid food should probably still be restricted for 6 to 8 hours before induction.

Premedication is often administered prior to induction of anesthesia. The purpose of premedication is to allay anxiety and to decrease secretions and vagal responsiveness.[29] Nicholson and colleagues[30] have demonstrated that oral premedication can be as effective as intramuscular premedication. Intranasal[31] and rectal[32] routes have also been shown to be effective. One study has shown that a premedication of midazolam (0.5 to .75 mg/kg with max = 18 mg), atropine (.03 mg/kg), and apple juice (5 mL) given

30 minutes prior to entering the operating room increased sedation, decreased separation anxiety, and improved the quality of an inhalational anesthetic.[33]

INTRAOPERATIVE CONSIDERATIONS

Anesthesia for pediatric podiatric surgery consists of one of the following options:

1. Monitored anesthesia care (MAC) (conscious sedation with a peripheral anesthetic block, i.e., popliteal fossa, ankle, or more peripheral)
2. General anesthesia (GA)
3. Neuraxial anesthetic (spinal, lumbar, or caudal epidural block)
4. Combined anesthesia (GA with peripheral or neuraxial block).

The goal of conscious sedation is to produce a comfortable, cooperative, amnesic patient who has an elevated pain threshold, but who is still conscious and able to protect his or her airway. A combination of three rapid but short-acting agents, such as fentanyl, midazolam, and propofol, is very satisfactory. In comparison, Harris and others have described the use of nitrous oxide and diazepam for conscious sedation.[34] After an appropriate level of sedation has been reached, the block can be performed by the surgeon or anesthesiologist. This type of anesthesia is not appropriate for patients who would be uncooperative or impossible to communicate with such as very young children.

Because the volume of distribution of local anesthetics is greater in children than adults, the dose in mg/kg tolerated by children is probably greater than the dose tolerated by adults. Doses of bupivacaine up to 3 mg/kg and lidocaine up to 10 mg/kg have been associated with safe plasma levels.[35–37] Accepted pediatric doses of local anesthetics are listed in Table 4–3.

A pediatric ankle block is performed in a manner similar to an adult block, but care is taken not to exceed the recommended upper doses. The popliteal fossa block is performed with the patient in the prone position. It provides anesthesia below the knee except to the saphenous nerve, which must be blocked separately. With the aid of a low-output peripheral nerve stimulator, Singelyn and others have described popliteal fossa block for surgery below the knee in 507 patients from 6 to 87 years old.[39] Only 3% required general anesthesia. A Teflon-insulated needle was placed in the midline 10 cm above the popliteal skin crease and advanced until a motor response was seen with an output less than 1 mA. Subsequently, a 30-mL dose of either 1% mepivacaine plus

1:200,000 epinephrine or 0.5% bupivacaine plus 1:200,000 epinephrine was injected.

General anesthesia alone or in conjunction with regional anesthesia or neuraxial block is most appropriate for young children undergoing podiatric surgery. If the child receives heavy premedication and comes to the operating room sleeping, the mask with anesthetic gas can be applied lightly so that the child is anesthetized without waking up (steal induction). Because it is not irritating to the airway, halothane is often used for inhalational induction. Sevoflurane is a newer inhalational agent that is theoretically better than halothane because it provides more rapid inductions and emergences. It remains to be seen whether sevoflurane will replace halothane in pediatric anesthesia. Sevoflurane is definitely more expensive and has been associated with emergence delirium.

Many children who come to the operating room awake will accept a mask especially if it is flavored with a familiar and pleasant scent. A variety of flavored scents (root beer, cherry, and so forth) are available (Loran Oils, Inc., Lansing, Michigan). There are several other options for the uncooperative child. For the younger child, rectal methohexital produces sleep within 4 to 13 minutes while the patient is still in his or her parent's arms.[40] Low-dose intramuscular ketamine also facilitates an inhalational induction.[41] Patel and Hannallah[1] reported the use of intravenous induction if the child does not readily accept the mask.

Neuraxial blocks (spinal anesthesia, lumbar or caudal epidural anesthesia) should be considered for pediatric podiatric surgery unless they are contraindicated because of coagulopathy, local infection, or patient/family refusal. Unless the patient is older, these blocks are performed after induction of general anesthesia. This combined technique reduces the requirement for general anesthesia agents and provides postoperative analgesia. Theoretically, any neuraxial block (or even peripheral block) that is performed preoperatively, with or without general anesthesia, may reduce postoperative pain through the provision of "preemptive" analgesia. Preemptive analgesia occurs when pain pathways are blocked preoperatively such that spinal cord pain circuits are not activated.

In a randomized study, Payne and colleagues[42] described the benefits of caudal anesthesia with 0.7 mL/kg of 0.25% bupivacaine (versus no caudal anesthesia) after induction of anesthesia and before incision in 100 pediatric patients (1 to 15 years of age) who were undergoing orthopedic surgery to the lower limbs.[42] The caudal block had a duration effect of 5 to 6 hours and provided better analgesia in the recovery room. Although McGowan[43] reported serious complications (cardiac arrests and

Table 4–3. **Pediatric Doses of Local Anesthesia**

Local Anesthetic	Usual Concentration	Usual Doses (mg/kg)	Max Doses Without Epinephrine (mg/kg)	Max Doses With Epinephrine (mg/kg)	Duration of Effects (Hours)
Lidocaine	0.5–2%	5	7.5	10	0.75–2
Mepivacaine	0.5–1.5%	5–7	8	10	1–1.25
Bupivacaine	0.15–0.5%	2	2.5	3	2.5–6

deaths) after caudal blocks, Broadman and colleagues[44] describe no toxic reactions or complications in 1154 caudal blocks. Dalens and Hasnaoui[45] reported that a number of their patients who accepted caudal blocks as the sole anesthetic agent were unable psychologically to tolerate the surgical procedure even though they were able to tolerate the block.[45]

POSTOPERATIVE CONSIDERATIONS

Recovery from anesthesia requires careful attention to the respiratory, circulatory, and central nervous systems. Postoperative pain must be anticipated and treated aggressively. Intraoperative peripheral blocks and neuraxial blocks reduce the need for postoperative analgesics. Intraoperative local anesthetic infiltration also promotes analgesia.[46] For inpatients, epidural catheters can be placed for postoperative analgesia. Low doses of narcotics and local anesthetics should be given. Caudal morphine can produce postoperative analgesia for more than 8 hours in most children.[47] However, caudal narcotics should be given only to inpatients, since this approach can be associated with several complications, including delayed respiratory depression. Intravenous patient controlled analgesia (PCA) has been used widely for children over 6 years of age.[48]

Nonsteroidal anti-inflammatory drugs should be considered for outpatients as well as inpatients. These drugs have an opioid-sparing effect. Furthermore, Splinter and colleagues[49] have shown that intravenous ketorolac to supplement local anesthesia infiltration after hernia repair is superior to caudal analgesia.

Protracted vomiting was the most common cause for unanticipated admission of ambulatory pediatric patients in a study of 10,000 patients by Patel and Hannallah.[1] Intraoperative administration of droperidol may reduce the incidence of postoperative nausea and vomiting.[50] Ondansetron has also been found to be useful to both prevent and treat postoperative nausea and vomiting. Davis and colleagues[51] have shown that compared with droperidol and placebo, ondansetron reduced the 24-hour incidence of emesis in ambulatory pediatric patients after dental surgery. Furthermore, the length of hospital stay was significantly prolonged after droperidol as compared with ondansetron.

SUMMARY

Pediatric podiatric anesthesia requires special attention to the physiologic, pharmacologic, and psychologic factors of children. All children cannot be approached in an established, routine manner—the anesthesiologist must individualize his or her approach. Careful attention to detail can provide a minimally traumatic experience for the child and the family as well as a satisfying experience for the perioperative care team. Table 4–4 provides some guidelines for choice of anesthesia.

Table 4–4. Choice of Anesthesia

	Age < 6–8 yr		Age > 6–8 yr	
	Out-patient	In-patient	Out-patient	In-patient
MAC (sedation with peripheral block)			+	
GA (alone)	+	+	+	+
Neuraxial block (without GA)			+	+
Combined (GA with peripheral or neuraxial block)	+	+	+	+
Postoperative analgesia with catheter technique, caudal morphine, or PCA		+		+

References

1. Patel RT, Hannallah RS: Anesthetic complications following pediatric ambulatory surgery: a 3-year study. Anesthesiology 1988; 69:1009–1012.
2. Cohen MM, Cameron CB, Duncan PG: Pediatric anesthesia morbidity and mortality in the perioperative period. Anesth Analg 1990; 70:160–167.
3. Tiret L, Nivoche Y, Hatton F, Desmonts JM, Vourc'h G: Complications related to anesthesia in infants and children. Br J Anaesth 1988; 61:263–269.
4. Gregory GA: Pediatric anesthesia. In Miller RD (ed): Anesthesia. New York, Churchill Livingstone, 1986, p. 1755.
5. Cross KW, Flynn DM, Hill JR: Oxygen consumption in normal newborn infants during moderate hypoxia in warm and cool environments. Pediatrics 1966; 37:565–576.
6. Coté CJ, Todres ID: The pediatric airway. In Ryan JF, Todres ID, Coté C, Goudsouzian NG (eds): A Practice of Anesthesia for Infants and Children. Boston, Grune & Stratton, 1986, p. 37.
7. Britt BA, Kalow W: Malignant hyperthermia, a statistical review. Can Anaesth Soc J 1970; 3(17):293–315.
8. Mott JM, Schulman SR, Gronert GA: Malignant hyperthermia. Curr Rev Clin Anesth 1989; 9:187–191.
9. Dubrow TJ, Wachym PA, Abdul-Rasool IH, Moore TC: Malignant hyperthermia: Experience in the postoperative management of eight children. J Pediatr Surg 1989; 24:183–185.
10. Rosenberg H, Gonert GA: Intractable cardiac arrest in children given succinylcholine. Anesthesiology 1992; 77:1054.
11. Friis-Hansen B: Body composition during growth. In vivo measurements and biochemical data correlated to differential anatomical growth. Pediatrics 1971; 47:264.
12. Cote CJ, Pediatric anesthesia. In Miller RD (ed): Anesthesia. New York, Churchill Livingstone, 1994, p. 2102.
13. Vernon DTA, Schulman JL, Foley JM: Changes in children's behavior after hospitalization. Am J Dis Child 1966; 111:581–593.
14. Steward DJ: Experiences with an out-patient anesthesia service for children. Anesth Analg 1973; 52:877–880.
15. Eckenhoff JE: Relationship of anesthesia to postoperative personality changes in children. Am J Dis Child 1953; 86:587–591.
16. Steward DJ: Psychological preparation and premedication. In Gregory GA (ed): Pediatric Anesthesia. New York, Churchill Livingstone, 1983, p. 424.
17. Hautzig D: A Visit to the Sesame Street Hospital. New York, Random House, 1985.
18. Rogers F: Going to the Hospital. New York, Putnam, 1988.
19. American Society of Anesthesiologists: When Your Child Needs Anesthesia. Park Ridge, IL, American Society of Anesthesiologists, 1994.
20. Schneider AJL: Assessment of risk factors and surgical outcome. Surg Clin North Am 1983; 63:1113–1126.
21. Epstein BS, Hannallah RS: Anesthetic considerations for pediatric ambulatory surgery. Curr Rev Clin Anesth 1988; 8:146–151.
22. Kurth CD, Spitzer AR, Broennie AM, Downes JJ: Postoperative apnea in preterm infants. Anesthesiology 1987; 66:483.

23. Tait AR, Knight PR: Intraoperative respiratory complications in patients with upper respiratory tract infections. Can J Anaesth 1987; 34:300–303.

24. Cohen MM, Cameron CB: Should you cancel the operation for a childhood URI? Anesth Analg 1990; 70:S63.

25. Desoto H, Patel RI, Soliman IE, Hannallah RS: Changes in oxygen saturation following general anesthesia in children with upper respiratory infection signs and symptoms undergoing otolaryngological procedures. Anesthesiology 1988; 68:276–279.

26. Splinter, WM, Schaefer JD: Ingestion of clear fluids is safe for adolescents up to 3 hours before anesthesia. Br J Anaesth 1991; 66:48.

27. Splinter WM, Schaefer JD: Unlimited clear fluid ingestion two hours before surgery in children does not affect volume or pH or stomach contents. Anaesth Intensive Care 1990; 18:522.

28. Schreiner MS, Triebwasser A, Keon TP: Ingestion of liquids compared with preoperative fasting in pediatric outpatients. Anesthesiology 1990; 72:589.

29. Gregory GA: Pediatric anesthesia. *In* Miller RD (ed): Anesthesia. New York, Churchill Livingstone, 1986, p. 1771.

30. Nicholson SC, Betts EK, Jobes DR, Christianson LA, Walters JW, Mayes KR, Korevaar WC: Comparison of oral and intramuscular preanesthetic medication for pediatric inpatient surgery. Anesthesiology 1989; 71:8–10.

31. Slover R, Dedo W, Schlesinger T, Mattison R: Use of intranasal midazolam in preschool children. Anesth Analg 1990; 70:S377.

32. Saint-Maurice C, Meistelman C, Rey E, Esteve C, DeLauture D, Olive G: The pharmacokinetics of rectal midazolam for premedication in children. Anesthesiology 1986; 65:536–538.

33. Feld LH, Negus JB, White PF: Oral midazolam preanesthetic medication in pediatric outpatients. Anesthesiology 1990; 73:831–834.

34. Harris WC, Alpert WJ, Gill JJ, Marcinko DE: Nitrous oxide and Valium use in podiatric surgery for production of conscious sedation. J Am Podiatr Assoc 1982; 72:505–510.

35. Bruguerolle B, Giaufre E, Morisson Lacombe G, Rousset Rouviere B, Arnaud C: Bupivacaine free plasma levels in children after caudal anaesthesia: Influence of pretreatment with diazepam. Fundam Clin Pharmacol 1990; 4:159–161.

36. Mobley KA, Wandless JG, Fell D: Serum bupivacaine concentrations following wound infiltration in children undergoing inguinal herniotomy. Anaesthesia 1991; 46:500–501.

37. Stow PJ, Scott A, Phillips A, White JB: Plasma bupivacaine concentrations during caudal analgesia and ilioinguinal-iliohypogastric nerve block in children. Anaesthesia 1988; 43:650–653.

38. Dalens BJ: Regional anesthesia in children. *In* Miller RD (ed): Anesthesia. New York, Churchill Livingstone, 1994, p. 1570.

39. Singelyn FJ, Gowerneur JA, Gribomont BF: Popliteal sciatic nerve block aided by a nerve stimulator. A reliable technique for foot and ankle surgery. Reg Anesth 1991; 16:278.

40. Kestin IG, Mcllvaine WB, Lockhart CH, Kestin KJ, Jones MA: Rectal methohexital for induction of anesthesia in children with and without rectal aspiration after sleep. Anesth Analg 1988; 67:1102–1104.

41. Hannallah RS, Patel RI: Low-dose intramuscular ketamine for anesthesia preinduction in young children undergoing brief outpatient procedures. Anesthesiology 1989; 70:598–600.

42. Payne KA, Hendrix MRG, Wade WJ: Caudal bupivacaine for postoperative analgesia in pediatric lower limb surgery. J Pediatr Surg 1993; 28:155–157.

43. McGowan RG: Caudal analgesia in children: Five-hundred cases for procedures below the diaphragm. Anesthesia 1982; 37:806–818.

44. Broadman LM, Hannallah RS, Norden JM, et al: "Kiddie caudals": Experience with 1154 consecutive cases without complications. Anesth Analg 1987; 66:S18.

45. Dalens B, Hasnaoui A: Caudal anesthesia in pediatric surgery. Anesth Analg 1989; 68:83–89.

46. Bourne MH, Johnson KA: Postoperative pain relief using local anesthetic instillation. Foot Ankle 1988; 8:350–351.

47. Krane EJ, Tyler DC, Jacobson LE: The dose response of caudal morphine in children. Anesthesiology 1989; 71:48–52.

48. Berde CB: Acute postoperative pain management in children Refresher Course #225. American Society of Anesthesiology Annual Meeting, 1995.

49. Splinter WM, Reid CW, Roberts DJ, Bass J: Reducing pain after inguinal hernia repair in children. Anesthesiology 1997; 87:542–546.

50. Abramowitz MD, Oh TH, Epstein BS, et al: The antiemetic effect of droperidol following outpatient strabismus surgery in children. Anesthesiology 1983; 59:579–583.

51. Davis PJ, McGowan FX, Landsman I, et al: Effect of antiemetic therapy on recovery and hospital discharge time. A double-blind assessment of ondansetron, droperidol, and placebo in pediatric patients undergoing ambulatory surgery. Anesthesiology 1995; 83:956–960.

5

Neuromuscular Disorders and Reflexes

Jeanean Willis, D.P.M., and Richard M. Jay, D.P.M.

A number of neurologic disorders produce clinical symptoms in the lower extremity in the pediatric population. Disorders that affect gait, posture, and coordination may be diagnosed by the podiatric physician. Examples of some of the more common disorders of the lower extremity that should be recognized by a specialist are chronic motor disorders classified under the term cerebral palsy and neuromuscular disorders such as Charcot-Marie-Tooth disease, myotonia congenita, and the muscular dystrophies.

NEUROMUSCULAR DISORDERS[1–8]

Neuromuscular disorders in children comprise a group of diseases that cause dysfunction of the lower motor neuron. The components of a lower motor neuron include the anterior horn cell (gray matter in the spinal cord), the axon, the neuromuscular junction, and the muscle fibers innervated by the axon.

Hallmarks of these disorders include muscle weakness, decreased muscle tone, hyporeflexia or areflexia, muscle atrophy, and fasciculations. Weakness can present intermittently, progressively, acutely, or chronically. Generally, proximal muscle weakness is associated with a primary muscle disease, and distal weakness is seen in neurogenic disorders or peripheral neuropathy. However, there are many exceptions to this rule. Intermittent weakness implies a toxic or a myasthenic syndrome. Examples of myasthenic disorders include myasthenia gravis, botulism, and organophosphate poisoning.

Myasthenia Gravis

This nonhereditary, autoimmune disease of the neuromuscular junction is the disease that most commonly affects neuromuscular transmission. The symptoms result from an attack by antibodies on the acetylcholine receptors. This disease affects voluntary skeletal muscles and causes weakness and fatigability. Generally, the ocular and bulbar muscles are affected most prominently. Girls are affected more often than boys. The course varies in presentation and can be focal or generalized and progressive

or relapsing. The clinician should be aware of skeletal weakness, diplopia, bilateral lid ptosis, and changes in facial expression and quality of voice. The physician can quickly test whether the patient can sustain a gaze for a minute or two. This disorder can affect all age groups; however, it is rare for involvement to occur before the age of 2. The disease is initially treated with anticholinesterases.

Myotonia Congenita

Myotonia congenita is a hereditary neuromuscular condition that is less common than myasthenia gravis. It is characterized by increased muscle tone and becomes worse in cold temperatures. The disease begins before 6 years of age. Infants walk later than expected and appear to be very muscular. Parents may state that the patient has to "warm up" or stretch before moving. The muscles of the hands, tongue, and orbicularis oculi are most commonly affected.

The most common diseases affecting the peripheral nerve or nerve root in children are Charcot-Marie-Tooth disease, a hereditary myopathy, and Friedreich's ataxia, a hereditary ataxia.

Charcot-Marie-Tooth Disease

Charcot-Marie-Tooth disease is also known as peroneal muscular atrophy and is inherited as an autosomal dominant trait. This disease has been classified into two types. The first type usually begins in the first or second decade of life and is characterized by a foot drop and steppage gait. Distal muscle weakness produces a stork-like appearance of the legs. Scoliosis and cavus feet are also common. Peroneal weakness is manifested by difficulty in walking, running, and climbing stairs. The steppage gait is due to prominent weakness in the anterior and peroneal muscles of the leg. The peripheral nerves are often palpable. Tremor is prominent in some patients. If tremor is present, the disease is termed Roussy-Levy syndrome. There is minimal sensory loss in the first stage of the disease, but as it progresses, diminished sensation occurs in a stocking-glove distribution. Achilles reflexes are diminished or absent.

In type II Charcot-Marie-Tooth syndrome, symptoms usually appear in adulthood; however, foot deformities are present in childhood. This disease is similar to type I disease but is less severe, and the nerves are not usually palpable.

Friedreich's Ataxia

Friedreich's ataxia is also an inherited neuromuscular disease. The cause is degeneration of the dorsal portion of the spinal cord and cerebellum. The nerve roots are also sometimes affected. Clinically, the disease is characterized by ataxia of the limbs, weakness, loss of proprioception in the limbs, loss of tendon reflexes, and a positive Babinski's response. Friedreich's ataxia is slightly more common in boys than in girls and usually occurs between the ages of 7 and 13. Ataxia of gait is the most common symptom and is usually the first symptom to appear. Commonly, these children are slow to begin walking, move awkwardly, and have a loss of agility. Clubfoot and kyphoscoliosis are characteristic deformities. The foot deformity is present in 75% of cases and can present at any time during the course of the disease. Kyphoscoliosis develops late in the disease and is present in 80% of patients. It is important to realize that less severe disease or variations of Friedreich's ataxia exist in which the patient may have only a few symptoms. These patients usually go on to lead normal healthy lives.

Muscular Dystrophy

Also under the category of neuromuscular diseases are the muscular dystrophies classified as hereditary myopathies. The muscular dystrophies are divided into Duchenne's muscular dystrophy, myotonic muscular dystrophy, and fascioscapulohumeral muscular dystrophy. The term limb-girdle muscular dystropy is also common; however, it is typically used as a general term when manifestations of the disease do not fit within the typical classification. The muscular dystrophies are a group of inherited disorders that cause degeneration of skeletal muscle.

Duchenne's muscular dystrophy is the most common of the hereditary myopathies. It is an X-linked recessive disease that affects boys almost exclusively. Not apparent early in infancy, the symptoms usually appear after the age of 3. There is usually a history of late walking, clumsiness, problems with climbing stairs or getting up from a chair and difficulty in riding a tricycle. The patient "climbs" up his legs to get from a sitting position to a standing position; this is called Gowers' sign. The calves are hypertrophic, and lordosis is common. Toe-walking and a waddling gait are early manifestations. Most boys cannot walk by the age of 11. If a child can walk at 12 years of age, the disease is called Becker's dystrophy.

Typically the dystrophy is limited to the muscles of the trunk and limbs. Pseudohypertrophy usually occurs in the gastrocnemius, deltoids, and triceps. There is symmetry of both sides of the body. Although no cerebral involvement has been discovered, a slight mental retardation appears to be associated with this disorder.

On physical examination, sensation is normal. Reflexes may be absent or present even in wasted muscles. The knee jerk usually disappears before the ankle jerk; however, contractures at the ankle may impede an accurate assessment of the reflexes. Diagnosis can be confirmed by the pressure of elevated levels of creatine kinase and other enzymes and by muscle biopsy.

CEREBRAL PALSY

Insults to the brain can cause dysfunction in various areas of the brain. If there is primarily motor involvement, it is assumed that the motor areas of the brain are involved, and the disorder is termed cerebral palsy. If the areas of the brain that control learning and reasoning are involved, the disorder is called mental retardation. If a child's concentrating ability and attention span are diminished, the disorder is termed attention deficit disorder or minimal brain dysfunction.

Cerebral palsy (CP) is a catch-all term for chronic motor disorders and encompasses many different conditions. Certain criteria must be met for a condition to be categorized as cerebral palsy. The pathology must occur in the brain and involve the motor system, the disorder cannot be progressive, and the pathology must have occurred before birth, perinatally, or during the first few years of life.

The etiology of CP is not completely known; however, low birth weight is the single factor most frequently associated with the pathology. All complications of pregnancy that predispose the neonate to hypoxia and intracranial bleeding along with toxins, threats of miscarriage, metabolic disorders, and maternal diseases contribute to the development of CP.

Although CP is not progressive, the patient's clinical symptoms may change. For example, children with spasticity may develop fixed deformities if the spasticity is untreated, and if the child gains too much weight, walking may be reduced owing to the increased effort or energy required. Diagnosis can be made by noting the clinical manifestations in infancy and by detecting abnormal posturing and asymmetry of the limbs in appearance and movement.

There are three major types of cerebral palsy: spastic, dyskinetic, and ataxic. Spastic cerebral palsy is the most common form of CP. Commonly, the limbs on one side are smaller and thinner than those on the other side. There is increased tone of the flexors of the hip, arms, adductors, knee flexors, and plantar extensors. Running exaggerates the characteristic gait. The reflexes on the affected side are increased, and ankle clonus may be present. A positive Babinski's reflex is usually present in postnatal cases. Treatment of spastic CP includes physical therapy, orthoses, speech and occupational therapy, and possibly surgical intervention if conservative measures have failed.

Children with dyskinetic cerebral palsy have involuntary abnormal movements termed chorea. This diagnosis is hard to make in infants, but as the patient matures the movements become much more noticeable. Due to the continuous movement, especially in the neck and shoulders, hypertrophy of the muscles in constant use occurs.

Ataxia exists in less than 5% of chilren with CP, and the etiology is not understood. Most children learn to compensate for this movement disorder.

THE REFLEXES

During child development there are a number of reflexes that should be tested routinely. Normal or abnormal responses may be an important clue to proper neurologic development in the child. For most of these responses there is a particular period during development in which a positive or negative response is deemed appropriate (Table 5–1). The following is an outline of specific reflexes, the tests used for them, and the responses that can be expected during development.

Plantar Grasp Reflex

Tonic flexion and adduction of the toes occurs on light digital pressure on the plantar surface of the foot. This reflex is present in the newborn and disappears by the end of the first year but may persist in children with birth injuries and retarded development.

Steppage Reflex

In eliciting this reaction, the infant is supported upright from the waist. The anterior aspect of the distal tibia or dorsum of the foot is then brought against the edge of the table. The infant will flex the hip and knee spontaneously, dorsiflex the ankle, and place the foot on the table, extending the lower extremity on active or passive contact of the sole with the table. Normally, this reaction is fully present at birth in full-term infants. Its absence suggests brain damage. To obtain the walking reaction, the infant is held upright with the soles of the feet pressing the table and is then gently moved forward. This initiates reciprocal flexion and extension of the lower extremities, which simulates walking.

Crossed Extension Reflex

When one lower extremity is held extended by the examiner at the knee and firm pressure is applied to its sole by running or stroking with the hand, the opposite free leg flexes, adducts, and then extends. This stimulation of the sole of the foot causes flexion movements of the ipsilateral extremity away from the stimulus and extensor movement of the contralateral extremity toward it. This reflex is not normally obtained after the first month. Its persistence indicates a partial spinal lesion.

Withdrawal Reflex

A pinprick is applied to the sole of the foot, causing dorsiflexion at the ankle and flexion of the knee and hip, which draws the extremity away from the noxious stimulus. This reflex is absent or weak in children born with myelomeningocele or other intraspinal lesions.

Table 5–1. **Important Landmarks in Development**

Birth to 1 month	Tonic neck reflexes	13 to 15 months	Walks independently
	Moro's reflex		Climbs stairs if one hand is held
	Sucking and rooting reflexes		Vocabulary of three to six words
	Grasping reflex	16 to 18 months	Begins to run
	Crossed extension reflex (reciprocal kick reflex)		Climbs chairs and beds
	Acoustic blink reflex		Vocabulary of six words or more
	Support reaction		Shows hand dominance
	Extensor thrust		Feeds self
	Neck righting reflex	19 to 21 months	Climbs stairs holding rail
2 months	May begin to smile		Runs well
	Begins to vocalize single vowel sounds		Walks backward
3 months	Babinski's response is positive		Begins to combine words
	Chuckles		Vocabulary of 12 words or more
	Picks up objects	22 to 24 months	Walks alone up and down stairs
4 months	Steppage reflex		Attempts to climb fences
	Brings objects toward mouth		Speaks in sentences
	Laughs		Gains voluntary control of bladder and bowel
	Supports a fraction of his weight		Can turn pages singly
5 to 6 months	Rolls from supine to prone position	3 years	Walks upstairs alternating feet
	Babbles		Stands on one foot
7 to 8 months	Begins to creep		Feeds self
	Sits independently		Puts on own shoes
	Monosyllables "ma," "ba," clearly pronounced		Comprehends questions and answers
9 to 10 months	Pulls self up to standing position	4 years	Walks downstairs one foot to a step
	Polysyllables "ma-ma," "da-da"		Washes and dries hands, brushes teeth
	Landau's reaction well developed	5 years	Skips on one foot
	Parachute reaction well developed		Recognizes colors
11 to 12 months	Walks if led		May print a few letters
	Stands momentarily alone		Has a considerable vocabulary
	Vocabulary of one to three words		Knows some of the alphabet
	Understands simple requests and gestures		

Extensor Thrust

When pressure is applied to the sole of the foot with the lower extremity in a flexed position, the infant suddenly extends the entire leg. This response is normal up to 2 months of age; persistence indicates brain damage or delayed maturation of the CNS.

Babinski's Reflex

This reflex is tested for by running the examiner's thumbnail along the lateral side of the heel toward the fifth toe and then across the ball of the foot to the great toe. An extensor plantar (or positive Babinski's) response is generally present in infants from 3 to 12 months of age. This response becomes flexor after 1 year of age. Persistence of a positive Babinski's reflex is indicative of corticospinal tract dysfunction.

Moro's Reflex

The patient is placed supine with both upper and lower extremities extended. The response can be elicited by a variety of stimuli that have in common sudden extension of the neck. The reflex consists of abduction and extension of all four extremities and extension of the spine, with extension and fanning of the digits. This phase is followed in turn by flexion and adduction of the extremities as if in an embrace. The reflex is present during the first 3 months of life and then gradually disappears by 4 to 6 months, probably with the development of myelinization.

Startle Reflex

This reflex is elicited by a sudden loud noise or by tapping the sternum. The elbows are then flexed (not extended, as in the Moro reflex), and the hands remain closed.

Hand-Grasp Reflex

If the examiner's finger or some other thin object is introduced into the palm from the ulnar side, flexor tonus is enhanced, and the fingers flex and grip the object. If the examiner then pulls the object being grasped, the flexor tone is increased synergistically, making his grip so strong that he can often be suspended by the object he is grasping. The hand will open on tactile stimulation over the dorsum and thus should not be touched during the test. This reflex is present in the newborn and very young infant and disappears at the age of 2 to 4 months. Its persistence after 4 months of age may indicate cerebral palsy.

Tonic Neck Reflexes

Tonic neck reflexes are both symmetrical and asymmetrical. To elicit the asymmetrical reflex, the infant is placed in the supine position, and the head is rotated without flexion to one side, kept rotated for 5 to 10 seconds, and then rotated to the other side. In a positive response, the arm on the side toward which the chin is rotated becomes rigid and goes into extension and the leg may go into extension as well. On the occiput side the arm goes into flexion and the leg may also flex. This reflex usually disappears by the age of 4 to 6 months. In states such as severe cerebral palsy, this reflex persists and may even increase.

The symmetrical tonic neck reflex is tested by having the patient rest in the prone position over the examiner's knee. When the head and neck are extended, the arms extend also and the legs go into flexion, whereas when the neck is flexed, the arms flex and the legs go into extension. This reflex is normally present by 6 months of age. There is no absolute time for its disappearance.

Neck Righting Reflex

To obtain this reflex, the child is placed supine with the head in midposition and all four limbs fully extended. The head is rotated to one side, and this position is held for 10 seconds. When the reflex is present, the body rotates as a whole in the same direction as the head. This reflex is normally present between birth and 6 months of age. If it is absent after the first month, delayed maturation is indicated.

Landau's Reflex

The child is held in the air in the prone position with the examiner's hand supporting him under the abdomen. The child's body should be parallel to the floor. The examiner should note whether the neck, spine, and hips assume a hyperextended position or whether they hang lifelessly. The head is first flexed and then extended, and the respective positions of the extremities and trunk are noted. The Landau reflex is positive when, on passive flexion of the head with the body in an extended position, the trunk, arms, and legs go into flexion; when the head is extended, the limbs and body are brought into an extended position. This reflex is positive normally from 6 months to 2 1/2 years of age. If elicited beyond 2 1/2 years of age, delayed reflex maturation is suggested.

Parachute Reaction

The patient is suspended in the air by the waist in the prone position, and the head is moved suddenly toward the floor. In a positive response, the child immediately extends his arms and wrists to protect his head, as if to break the force of the fall. The parachute reaction begins at about 6 months of age and persists throughout life.

Acoustic Blink Reflex

This response is very easily elicited in the newborn child by a loud hand clap. In response to this stimulus the infant blinks his eyes. This reflex is present from birth to approximately 4 months of age. After 4 months of age this reflex is replaced by the startle reflex.

Many other reflexes can be tested, but such specific testing is usually reserved for patients in whom some type of neurologic disorder is suspected.

Positive Support Response or Leg Straightening Reflex

The patient is held in a standing position, and the soles of the feet are pressed to the ground or table several times. When the support response is positive, the lower extremities and trunk go into extension when the feet contact the ground. The legs thereby serve as strong supporting pillars for weight bearing. This response is normal up to 4 months of age. If it persists, reciprocal leg movements cannot occur, and the infant is able to neither stand nor walk.

Body Righting Reflex

To elicit this reflex, the same test position and stimulus are used as for the support response, but on rotation of the head, the body, instead of rotating as a whole, rotates cephalocaudally in segments (i.e., the head turns first, then the shoulders and trunk, and finally the pelvis). This reflex appears at 6 months of age.

Galant's Reflex or Trunk Incurvation

With the infant in the prone position, the lateral aspect of the back in the lumbar region is stimulated with the index finger. When the reflex is present, the trunk flexes toward the side of the stimulus.

Oral Reflexes

The following reflexes are present in all full-term newborns. Their absence is indicative of severe developmental defect or marked prematurity. The sucking reflex is induced by introducing a nipple or a finger into the mouth. The rooting or search reflex enables the infant to find the nipple without being directed to it. When areas of the infant's mouth are stimulated, the lip retracts and the tongue moves toward the area of stimulus. When the stimulus is moved to the cheek or chin, the neck is either flexed or rotated to follow the stimulus.

Tilting Reactions

Tilting reactions are tests for maturation and equilibrium. The center of gravity is changed in various postures of the body, and protective adoptive responses are observed. There are several levels of performance, all of which test the patient's ability to maintain his or her center of gravity and thus equilibrium (or balance). These responses appear at about 6 to 7 months and persist throughout life.

References

1. Armstrong R, Appel S: Neuromuscular Disorders. Current Neurology, Vol. 3. New York, John Wiley and Sons, 1981.
2. Bray P: Neurology in Pediatrics. Chicago, Year Book, 1969.
3. Dodge P, Gamstrop I, Byers R: Myotonic dysrophy in infancy and childhood. Pediatrics 1965; (35: 3–19.)
4. Fishman M: Pediatric Neurology. Orlando, Grune & Stratton, 1986.
5. Lansky L: Pediatric Neurology: A Practitioner's Guide. Flushing, NY, Medical Examination Publishing Co., 1975.
6. Moosa A: Muscular dystrophy in childhood. Develop Med Child Neurol 1974; 16:97–111.
7. Quinn N, Jenner P: Disorders of Movement: Clinical, Pharmacological and Physiological Aspects. San Diego, Academic Press, 1989.
8. Swaiman KF, Wright FS: Neuromuscular Diseases of Infancy and Childhood, Springfield, IL, Charles C Thomas, 1970.

Two

Forefoot

6

Metatarsus Adductus

Richard M. Jay, D.P.M.

Metatarsus adductus is a congenital transverse plane deformity that occurs at Lisfranc's tarsometatarsal articulation. Clinically the forepart of the foot is adducted. The incidence is 3 in 1000[1] (Fig. 6–1). Adduction of the foot may be associated with internal tibial torsion and is also seen as a residual component of clubfoot. As such, treatment must address the rearfoot as well as the forefoot.

ETIOLOGY

The etiology of metatarsus adductus is not fully understood at this point, but there are a few theories. It is possibly due to excessive pressure, which is characteristically present in the uterus with the firstborn, or the uterus may just be generally constrictive regardless of the number of children. It is also possible that malposition of the fetus or lack of ontogeny has a deforming effect on the metatarsals. Whether because of the malposition of the fetus or the number of fetuses present in the uterus, it is still a fight for space because the fetus is packed into the tight compressive uterus. Due to the internal torque and flexion of the leg segment, the feet wrap around the buttocks. The increase in size of the fetus along with the strong uterine musculature prevent the foot and leg from going through the external abducting torque that normally occurs.

With malposition, specific muscles gain a mechanical advantage. For example, the abductor hallucis may become overactive, causing the hallux and the first ray to adduct, thus creating a metatarsus adductus (metadductus) deformity. The abductor hallucis muscle and tendon lie on the medial side of the foot. They arise from the medial aspect on the calcaneal tuberosity, the flexor retinaculum, and the aponeurosis distally. The muscle travels along the medial border of the plantar aspect of the foot, and the tendon eventually inserts into the base of the proximal phalanx along with the medial head of the flexor hallucis brevis. The abductor hallucis tendon abducts the great toe on the metatarsal phalangeal joint as well as flexing the joint. In a malposition of the metatarsal that is adducted, the muscle tendon apparatus of the abductor lies even more medially, creating an even greater effect of abduction on the great toe. The muscle tendon apparatus may become overactive due to this shortened position rather than from a neurologic dysfunction. If the peroneal muscles are weak, the tibialis anterior and tibialis posterior muscles gain a mechanical advantage that causes the forefoot to supinate and adduct.

CLINICAL SIGNS

The diagnosis of metadductus is made predominantly on clinical grounds. The following five clinically diagnostic criteria can be observed in weight-bearing and non-weight-bearing positions.

1. The foot maintains an inward position when the lateral border is stroked; it may twist outward for a moment but then returns to the original adducted position.
2. The foot develops a medial concave border and a lateral convex border with a prominent base of the fifth metatarsal. The prominence of the fifth metatarsal

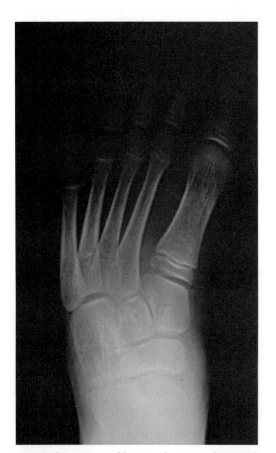

Figure 6–1. Total metatarsus adductus with rectus right toe in line with first metatarsal.

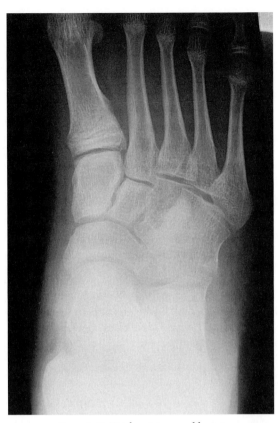

Figure 6–2. Total metatarsus adductus.

base becomes more evident after the foot loses some of its fat and the fifth metatarsal base becomes ossified. A **C**-shaped foot is observed from the plantar aspect.

3. The metadductus foot may appear to have a high arch. In the infant the foot looks as if it were in a cavus position.

4. One can observe a marked separation of the great toe from the lesser toes. The great toe can remain in this adducted position, yielding a hallux varus and a high first metatarsal adductus angle. In the presence of a tight tendoachilles, the foot pronates. Eventually the adducted hallux will drift laterally as the first ray and metatarsal phalangeal joint compensate by dorsiflexing. The first metatarsal phalangeal joint loses its stability, and a hallux valgus deformity develops.

5. The metatarsus adductus foot should be viewed plantarly in a nonweight-bearing attitude, two imaginary lines should be constructed. One line should bisect the heel longitudinally, and the other should bisect the forefoot area longitudinally. In a metadductus foot these two lines intersect, creating an angle of greater than 25 degrees.

There are three types of metadductus. Each is a separate entity. However, depending on the degree of severity and the treatment provided, each can progress to the severe pronated form, the so-called **Z** foot.

1. *Total metadductus*. Metatarsals 1 through 5 are adducted relative to the lesser tarsus with a mild to moderate degree of pronation at the subtalar and midtarsal joints. The great toe and the lesser digits are

also adducted. At times the great toe is in valgus if the degree of pronation is high, but this does not usually occur until the child is at least 5 to 6 years old (Fig. 6–2).

2. *Atavistic form, or metatarsus primus adductus*. The first ray is adducted so that the intermetatarsal angle is increased above 15 degrees. The hallux assumes an adducted attitude, since it stays in line with the metatarsal. This adducted position is maintained by the abductor hallucis, the insertion of which is in the medial base of the proximal phalanx. The lesser metatarsals remain normal or slightly adducted (Figs. 6–3 and 6–4).

3. *Serpentine, skew, or* **Z**-*shaped foot*. This is a severe metadductus of all five metatarsals. Compensation occurs through an increased amount of subtalar and midtarsal joint pronation. The hallux has an abducto-valgus deformity due to the pronatory effect of the rearfoot; an uncontrolled, longstanding total metadductus can develop into this type of metadductus deformity. The clinical appearance of this foot is not typical of the adducted foot. The foot is flat and rectus due to the pronatory compensation (Fig. 6–5).

RADIOGRAPHIC INTERPRETATION

Proper evaluation of metatarsus adductus deformity requires weight-bearing angle and base-of-gait films, including dorsoplantar and lateral views of the foot and anteroposterior (AP) views of the ankles. The radiograph, however, is not a necessary diagnostic tool. The clinical appearance makes the diagnosis, and radiographs are used to assess the deformity. The dorsoplantar view allows measurement of the adductus deformity through the metadductus angle and localization of the deformity at either

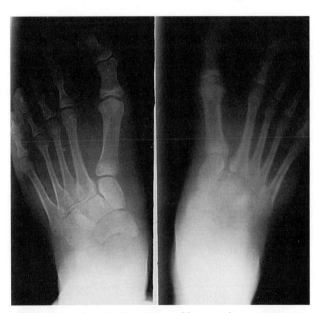

Figure 6–3. Left foot. Total metatarsus adductus with metatarsus primus adductus. First ray equals 15 degrees of adduction to an already adducted metatarsal. Hallux position is rectus; however, as seen by the interphalangeal joint and joint adaptation, a lateral drift is noted.

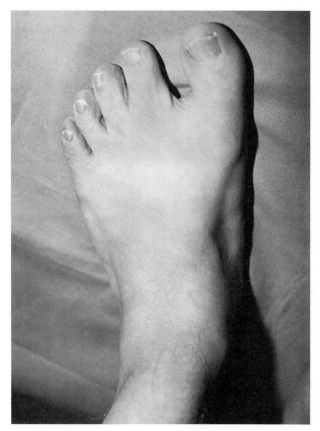

Figure 6–4. Hallux varus with increase in metatarsus primus adductus.

the tarsometatarsal joint, the midtarsal joint, or both. Therefore, radiographs help in establishing a value system for the deformity. The severity of the deformity can be assessed and an appropriate surgical or nonsurgical approach can be determined from radiographic evaluation.

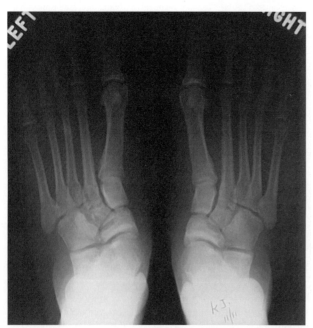

Figure 6–5. Z-type metatarsus adductus with beginning of juvenile hallux valgus. Talus is adducting in relation to calcaneus.

Postoperative or postcasting monitoring can also be accomplished through the use of radiographs.

The metatarsus adductus angle is the relationship between the line representing the bisection of the second metatarsal and the line representing the lesser tarsus abductus angle. A normal metatarsus adductus angle is approximately 22 degrees. A significant metatarsus adductus angle is greater than 25 to 30 degrees with a normal midtarsal joint position.[2] Since the foot of the infant is not osseously mature, the lesser tarsus cannot be identified accurately. The spaces between the points of identification are too wide at the articular margins of the medial aspect of the first metatarsal and cuneiform, navicular, and talus, the lateral aspect of the calcaneus and cuboid, the fifth metatarsal, and the cuboid (Figs. 6–6 and 6–7).

An alternative method can be employed; however, the following method is not as accurate as a full bisection of the lesser tarsus. In the older child, metatarsus adductus can be ruled out by bisecting the middle cuneiform and the second metatarsal. The angle formed between these bones approximates the lesser tarsus metatarsus adductus angle (Fig. 6–8). This measurement, however, cannot be used in infants because the middle cuneiform is not fully developed and thus cannot be bisected accurately. Ossification begins at 28 months in males and 21 months in females.[6]

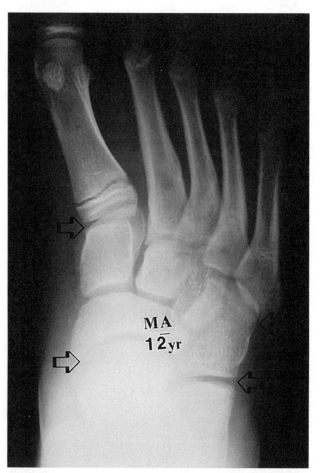

Figure 6–6. Arrows show the notable portions that are used to measure the lesser tarsus for metatarsus adductus. The infant will not have these well-demarcated landmarks.

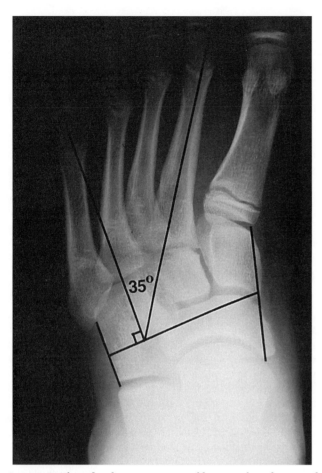

Figure 6–7. Thirty-five degree metatarsus adductus angle as determined by bisecting the second ray and comparing this result with the perpendicular of the bisection of the lesser tarsus.

Radiographically, on the anteroposterior view, the metatarsal position must be noted. Are metatarsals 1 through 5 adducted as a group, or is the first metatarsal adducted individually? The first metatarsal adducted alone is an atavistic type of metatarsus adductus. The hallux is directly in line with the first metatarsal in the atavistic form and can result in a hallux varus deformity. If left untreated, this type of early metatarsus primus adductus angle can result in a compensated juvenile hallux valgus deformity (Fig. 6–9). This is a direct result of midtarsal and subtalar joint pronation. Without subtalar and midtarsal joint pronation, the adductor hallucis muscle will maintain the hallux in a varus position with a resultant hallux varus. The base of the proximal phalanx ossifies at 30 months in males and at 20 months in females.[6] In the presence of continued tension at the epiphysis, the varus deformity results secondary to Wolff's law.

Juvenile hallux valgus is an avoidable complication that is all too often neglected during the early stages. It is not until the deformity progresses that attention is finally given to this controllable and reducible problem. As the first metatarsal drifts medially secondary to the retrograde force of the abducting proximal phalanx, an increase in compression arises on the medial physis; the lateral portion of the physis is pulled open with the increase in tension. Tension at the physis induces lateral metatarsal growth, while compression on the opposite side of the physis reduces medial growth. The result is an increase in the intermetatarsal angle (see Chapter 11).

Early intervention reduces the medial compressive force and lateral tension. The forces can be converted to a tension force on the medial side and to a compressive force on the lateral side. Reversing the forces on the physis eliminates the possibility of recurrence. Simple bunion procedures in children with high intermetatarsal angles are contraindicated because they do not address the deforming forces mentioned earlier (see Chapter 17). The newly distributed forces are exerted after intermetatarsal reducing angle procedures have been performed. These redistributed forces, along with alignment of the new bone, permit growth in the proper rectus direction. Control of the subtalar and midtarsal joints in a neutral position is imperative to ensure that this growth pattern is maintained.

The position of the navicular on the talar head should be considered when determining whether to pursue a surgical or a conservative approach. A laterally positioned navicular indicates subtalar pronation, while a medially positioned navicular on the talar head is seen with talipes equinovarus and cavus foot deformities. This type of supinated position must be addressed separately and is usually seen with a forefoot adductus deformity. Radiographs are

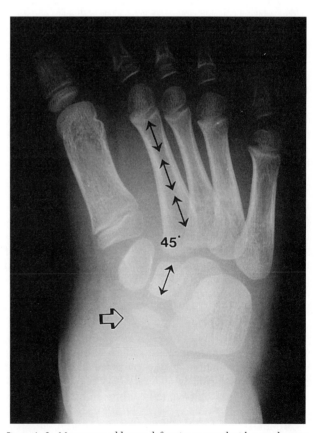

Figure 6–8. Metatarsus adductus deformity as noted with a crude angular measurement utilizing the middle cuneiform. The middle cuneiform is bisected, and the longitudinal bisection of the second ray is measured and compared with this cuneiform. The navicular is noted to be lateral to the talar head as seen in metatarsus adductus.

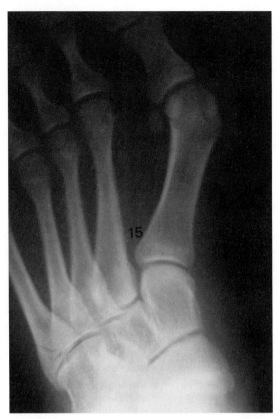

Figure 6–9. Metatarsus adductus with 15-degree intermetatarsal angle yielding a high metatarsus primus adductus along with a juvenile hallux valgus deformity.

used to assess the navicular position on the talar head. When reducing the metatarsus adductus angle with transverse plane abduction, an abductory force may be exerted at the Choparts articulation. If a lateral deviation of the navicular occurs during this cast reduction, cast therapy should cease. In the presence of continued transverse force and midtarsal joint abduction, the result will be a rectus foot at the expense of a pronated flatfoot.

The calcaneal cuboid relationship is studied to determine the presence or absence of forefoot adductus. Forefoot adductus is a soft tissue deformity produced by midtarsal joint supination around the oblique axis, resulting in plantar flexion, adduction, and inversion of the forefoot. Forefoot adductus is evident with an adducted position of the cuboid on the calcaneus. On radiographs of an adducted forefoot, a line from the calcaneus through the lateral surface of the cuboid deviates in the direction of adduction. Normally, these two lines do not converge. An adducting line demonstrates oblique axis supination, whereas an abducting line indicates midtarsal joint oblique axis pronation. In the presence of abduction of the cuboid (midtarsal joint pronation), a metatarsus adductus deformity will have to be addressed more radically and aggressively.

Metatarsus adductus is frequent in children, and it is of interest to examine whether it will correct spontaneously or whether early treatment is necessary. A study[1] was performed on 84 patients with metatarsus adductus, 50 boys and 34 girls (124 feet). The age spread was 5-1/2 months to 2-1/2 years. Weight-bearing AP and lateral radiographs were taken. It was found that more than 43% of the children with a simple metatarsus adductus required no treatment; their midfoot and hindfoot were in normal alignment. Fourteen percent of children with a metatarsus adductus in whom the midfoot was laterally translated required no treatment.

The remaining children with a severe complex rearfoot deformity and an adducted deformity of the forefoot required cast treatment twice as long as the 43% with simple metatarsus adductus. When a severe breakdown at the midtarsal or subtalar region is present, the foot requires more aggressive therapy. Prolonged cast therapy with the possibility of surgical intervention and rearfoot stabilization with or without tendoachilles lengthening must be considered.

CASTING TECHNIQUE

Application of the cast prior to the age of ambulation is preferred because the metatarsal bases are cartilaginous. Weight bearing puts pronatory forces at the Lisfrancs, midtarsal, and subtalar joints. I personally refrain from casting within 2 months after the age of ambulation. If it is necessary to apply a cast after the child has begun to ambulate, care must be taken. The foot is maturing and the bases of the metatarsals are becoming more rigid.[3] Once the bases of the metatarsals become mature, the results obtained with casting are reduced. If a transverse force from the cast is applied to this weight-bearing foot, the more proximal articulations of the midtarsal and subtalar joints will be affected. The entire foot will abduct with the exception of the originally deformed adducted metatarsals, and the result will be a maximally pronated, iatrogenically induced flatfoot.

Prior to the application of the cast, the foot is prepared for the correction by manipulating it for approximately 5 to 10 minutes. The initial reduction is more successful with this preparation because it relaxes the child and seems to loosen the ligaments. Once the child's foot is relaxed, the heel is placed between the clinician's thumb and index finger and locked to prevent motion. With the opposite hand, the clinician grasps the forefoot and applies an abductory force. He or she should be sure that the abductory force is applied at the first metatarsal head, with counterpressure applied on the base of the fifth metatarsal. This transverse force is applied to the point of resistance for approximately 15 seconds and then released. This maneuver is repeated for 5 to 10 minutes. Eventually the stiff deformity becomes easily reducible. At this point the cast can be applied (Table 6–1). If the deformity in the foot is still stiff or the infant is unmanageable, the parents should continue this manipulation for another week. Prior to cast application one should make sure that the parents do not allow the heel to evert and unlock because this will force the foot into a pronated position.

ABDUCTORY CASTING

As stated previously, the reduction must be precise; plaster cast material is recommended for use in the re-

Table 6–1. **Metatarsus Adductus—Cast Treatment**

1. Cast before age of ambulation.
2. Apply two layers of 2-inch Webril, cover distally past toes and proximally to below the knee joint.
3. Apply plaster of Paris using 3-inch rolls.
4. Rub and mold the cast until it becomes semirigid.
5. Hold the heel in neutral to slightly inverted position.
6. Extend the hold on the heel to include the lateral fifth metatarsal cuboid articulation to act as counterpressure.
7. Grasp forefoot or apply pressure directly to the medial side of the first metatarsal head with the opposite hand.
8. Abduct the forefoot while stabilizing the fifth metatarsal base–cuboid articulation and the rearfoot inverted position.
9. Rub and smooth the plaster during this reduction.
10. Let the plaster set.
11. Change the cast and repeat the above procedure every 1 to 2 weeks until reduction is accomplished.

duction rather than flexible fiberglass because plaster is easily molded. After applying the stockinette and two layers of 2-inch Webril (Johnson and Johnson Orthopedics, Raynham, MA) past the ends of the toes and snugly around the foot and leg, the plaster is rolled on rapidly. The 3-inch wide plaster is also applied through to the tips of the toes from a point just proximal to the knee joint. This incorporates the toes in the reduction of Lisfranc's articulation and decreases the possibility that a hallux varus and adducted digits will remain after the cast is removed. When applying the cast, folded tabs are placed at the end of the roll to allow for easy removal after soaking.

While the plaster is setting, the hands are positioned around the foot to reduce the deformity. The heel is secured in one hand in a neutral to inverted attitude with respect to the leg. To prevent breakdown of the midtarsal and subtalar joints, the rearfoot is maintained in this neutral or slightly inverted position. One should make sure that the fifth metatarsal-cuboid joint is stabilized with the same hand as it extends distally on the lateral border of the foot; this is simply performed with the thumb and index finger.

It has been reported that counterpressure on the first metatarsal head is enough to reduce the metatarsus adductus deformity.[7] When three points of pressure are applied—at the medial heel, the lateral fifth metatarsal base, and the medial first metatarsal head—the correction does occur. However, when the intermetatarsal angle is increased along with adduction of the lesser metatarsals, simply applying a transverse force on the first metatarsal addresses only the metatarsal primus adductus deformity. Correction is gained, but not enough to reduce or abduct the remaining lesser metatarsals. To completely reduce the metatarsus adductus deformity, the metatarsals must be adducted as a unit. This is accomplished by placing the child's first metatarsal head in the sulcus of the hand, between the index finger and thumb. The remaining metatarsals are then grasped by the thumb and index finger. In this way, an abductory force is applied on the forefoot while stabilizing the rearfoot and applying counterpressure on the fifth metatarsal base. This provides reduction of the first metatarsal head and a sequential abductory reduction of the lesser metatarsals. The

fingers and hands should be continually smoothing the plaster while maintaining the correction; this will eliminate pressure point marks on the cast. After a few weeks of casting, it is a good idea to take an x-ray film of the foot to determine the position of the cuboid relative to the calcaneus. This is important in studying the integrity of the calcaneocuboid angle and preventing pronation at the midtarsal joint. The cast is removed and reapplied at weekly intervals.

It is advisable to start manipulative casting before the age of ambulation. At the age of 12 to 13 months the malleable foot starts to mature and becomes resistant to casting. The bases of the metatarsals calcify with age. With the addition of weight-bearing forces, which increase the chance of pronation, casting of metadductus after the age of ambulation increases the potential risks of inducing a permanent flatfoot. Since the bases of the metatarsals are starting to mature and square off, transverse motion in the direction of abduction will be transferred more proximally to the midtarsal and subtalar joints. The result will be a serpentine deformity. To ensure that the physician does not induce this pronated flatfoot position while casting a child, holding the rearfoot in a neutral to slightly inverted position is recommended. This is accomplished by grasping the heel in a slightly inverted position relative to the leg. As the rearfoot is stabilized and locked, the lateral border is also stabilized by applying pressure on the base of the fifth metatarsal cuboid area. It is at this point that the forefoot is abducted.

One method of doing this is to grasp the entire forefoot with the opposite hand and allow the first metatarsal head to rest in the sulcus of the hand between the thumb and index finger. While applying a grasping force on the forefoot, the entire hand is shifted laterally, thus applying an abductory transverse plane position. An alternative method is to use the thumb of the opposite hand to press on the metatarsal head, driving this first metatarsal in an abductory position on the transverse plane. The rearfoot must remain inverted as an abductory force is applied to the metatarsals. If the rearfoot is everted, the abductory force will result in midtarsal joint pronation.

Plaster of Paris is recommended while the cast is manipulated and molded. Using plaster of Paris, the foot can be molded into the exact position needed to reduce the adductory force of the metatarsals while maintaining the rearfoot in a neutral position. Either 2-inch or 3-inch plaster can be used after Webril is applied to the foot extending over the toes and proximally below the knee. The plaster of Paris is then rolled in a continuous manner. Try to keep the plaster wet enough so that it can be easily molded. I have found that 3-inch plaster is easier to work with when trying to manipulate the foot at the same time. Once the complete roll is placed about the foot, the plaster of Paris on the foot is rubbed continuously. This rubbing continues until the cast just about sets.

Once the plaster begins to harden, the technique described earlier of holding the rearfoot in position and reducing the metatarsus adductus is begun. Enough force is applied to reduce the deformity. Excessive pressure is limited to avoid hurting the child and to prevent midtarsal and subtalar joint breakdown. The plastered foot is held in position until the plaster has completely set. One should be sure when applying the plaster and Webril that it extends distally over the toes to capture the adduction deformity in the digits as well. If the cast is proximal to the metatarsophalangeal joints, the metatarsals may be well reduced, but the digits will still lie in an adducted position.

The cast is kept in position for 1 to 2 weeks. It is changed every week, and a new cast is applied in the same manner until the metatarsus adduction is completely reduced. Depending on the resistance of the metatarsus adductus deformity, casting may last for 3 weeks to 3 months.

Removing the cast can be a difficult chore for both the physician and the parent. I have found that use of a cast cutter can be traumatic not only for the child but also for the family. The cast cutter with its vacuum noise and saw blade is very frightening. For this reason, I elect to have the parents participate in the treatment by removing the cast themselves. I advise them to allow approximately 1 hour to remove the cast. They can place the child in a warm tub or basin and let the cast soak for about a half hour. A cap full of vinegar added to the water aids in the breakdown of the cast. Using the heels of both hands on the cast will help to crack the cast and allow more absorption of water to soften the cast itself. I have also found that use of a thickened tab of plaster at the end of the roll when it is applied to the leg facilitates removal. Once this end softens up, the parent can simply unravel it without any difficulty. The cast should be removed just prior to the office appointment. The family should avoid using sharp utensils when unraveling the softened cast.

MODIFIED FURLONG PROCEDURE

A short leg cast is applied to the foot as described earlier. The cast is then modified in such a way that only the forefoot can abduct at the Lisfranc articulation while the rearfoot is held locked in an inverted stable neutral position; a wedge is cut out of the dorsolateral aspect of the cast and removed. A triangular window is created that allows the forefoot to escape laterally. A wedge-shaped felt piece is then placed between the great toe joint and the medial aspect of the cast. The foot is subsequently wrapped in elastic wrap to avoid window edema. Each week the wedge of felt is increased in size and is placed back in the medial aspect of the cast. This wedge creates an abductory force around the Lisfranc articulation. Caution must be exercised when attempting this procedure because as the forefoot abducts, it has a tendency to abduct at the midtarsal joint rather than at the Lisfranc articulation. It is imperative for the rearfoot to be locked and stabilized in a neutral position to prevent midtarsal and subtalar joint breakdown. The cast should be well molded and conform to the heel, thus preventing rearfoot motion when the forefoot starts to abduct. It is also important to cut the cast so that the dorsolateral piece that is removed extends no further proximally than the fifth metatarsal base. Casting is continued until the desired degree of abduction is attained. Final position is

maintained in a below-the-knee closed cast for 2 weeks[4] (Fig. 6–10).

AFTER-CAST MAINTENANCE AND ALTERNATIVES TO CASTING

After the deformity has been reduced with casting, the correction must be maintained. The question then arises as to how long the position must be maintained. If casting is performed prior to the age of ambulation, it is not uncommon for casting to last between 3 weeks and 3 months. The Ganley splint (J. Ganley, Norristown, PA) or any adjunct splinting is used for an additional 3 to 6 months.

Ganley Splint

Application of the Ganley splint is descibed under calcaneovalgus except for the shape of the longitudinal bar. This bar is bent with bending irons to create an abducted forefoot position. The rearfoot is still maintained in approximately 5 degrees of varus. If medial tibial torsion is present, the transverse bar is also abducted on the transverse plane. When the splint is used in the treatment of metatarsus adductus, the torsion bar is bent to allow the foot to be externally or laterally rotated with reference to the leg. In metatarsus adductus a concomitant internal tibial torsion is commonly present, and external rotation of this bar maintains an abductory position rather than allowing the foot to rotate inward. The shank bar is bent outward to allow the forefoot to abduct on

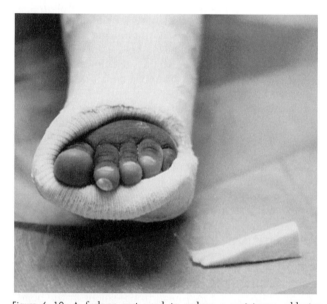

Figure 6–10. A furlong cast used to reduce a metatarsus adductus deformity. The wedge is placed in the medial aspect of the cast, forcing the first metatarsal laterally. The cast is cut out on the lateral and dorsal surface to allow transverse plane motion while securing the rearfoot in a mild varus attitude. The wedge is placed with the apex pointing proximally into the cast. This wedge is changed weekly and is gradually increased in size. In time, the adduction component of the metatarsals will be reduced. Care must be taken to secure the rearfoot in a neutral position.

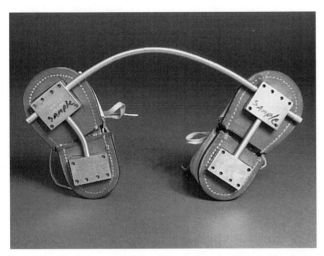

Figure 6–11. Ganley splint. The right foot is positioned to reduce a metatarsus adductus deformity. Both shoes are split in the center. The longitudinal bar of the right shoe has been bent in an abducted position to correct for the transverse plane of the metatarsus adductus. The rearfoot of the right foot is inverted in relationship to the forefoot to prevent pronation. The transverse bar connecting the two shoes is bent to allow abduction and maintain the external axial position.

the rearfoot, and at the same time the heel plate is placed in varus. It is important to maintain rearfoot inversion with the abduction of this shank to prevent severe pronatory changes that can be driven through the entire rearfoot and midfoot joints (Fig. 6–11).

Bebax

An alternative to casting is available in the Bebax shoe (made by Inter Axial France, Sallanches, France). This device is designed for infants who do not yet walk. It works on the same principle as casting. The device can also be used after casting, but if the child is ambulatory it must be used only during nap and sleep time. When stimulating the cast, the shoe should be worn at all times. The shoe itself should be snug on the foot and is worn over a sock. Various sizes are available and may be changed as the child grows.

The Bebax shoe is used as an adjunct to casting for children with metatarsus adductus, talipes equinovarus, and calcaneovalgus. The shoe allows triplanar changes in position through the universal joints placed underneath the forefoot and rearfoot shoe compartments. The position is determined by the diagnosis, and the deformity is manipulated in the same way as it is during cast correction. The heel seat should be snug as well as the forefoot strap. The heel segment is held in varus, and the forefoot section is abducted.

In the treatment of metatarsus adductus, the Bebax shoe maintains and reduces the deformity nicely. A central longitudinal bar connects the segmented forefoot and rearfoot by universal joints. The child's foot is placed in the Bebax device, and the straps are applied firmly around the ankle and forefoot. The plantar universal joints are loosened with an Allen wrench, and the foot is positioned. The heel is held in slight inversion (3 to 5 degrees) to

the forefoot, and the fore part of the foot is abducted on the transverse plane. In the final position of the first ray should appear slightly plantar-flexed to the rearfoot. When the desired position is attained, the plantar universal joints are tightened. The child wears the Bebax shoe continually. Every week the forefoot is readjusted by abduction (Fig. 6–12).

Ipos

Another device, the Ipos (Ipos USA, Niagara Falls, NY), is similar in purpose to the Bebax and may be used as a primary device or as an adjunct to casting. The Ipos, however, offers no rearfoot locking mechanism and provides only transverse torque on the forefoot. Because there is no locking mechanism or ability to invert the rearfoot with the IPOS shoe, it is necessary to make sure that the foot fits tightly into the heel cup of the shoe. If it is too loose, the foot will have a tendency to pronate when the forefoot is abducted. The shoe is offered in various sizes and also has a selection of rubber elastic rings that apply the transverse abductory force. In severely rigid or resistant deformities, a tighter band can be used to abduct the foot at Lisfranc's articulation (Fig. 6–13).

Wheaton Brace

This relatively expensive device is an orthosis made of polypropylene. The device is intended to serve as an

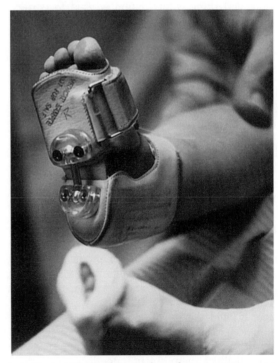

Figure 6–12. A child placed in a Bebax splint to maintain metatarsus adductus. Note that the longitudinal footplate is inverted in the rearfoot, and the forefoot is abducted in relation to the rearfoot. This shoe may be used after casting or in lieu of casting.

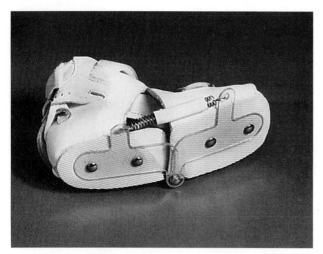

Figure 6–13. IPOS. The shoe is split in the center with a lateral spring that yields varying degrees of tension. By increasing the tension on this lateral spring, the force in the transverse plane motion is increased, thereby reducing a metatarsus adductus deformity. There is no control of the rearfoot position, and the shoe must be firmly fitted to the heel of the child's foot.

alternative to serial casting but may be better used as an adjunct to casting. Serial casting has the advantage of providing correction in an exact mold and position of the foot. Since the Wheaton brace (Wheaton Brace Co., Carol Stream, IL) is manufactured, it inherently does not mold to the exact shape of the foot. Although three-point pressures and counterpressures are applied, they may not be in the desired position on each individual's foot. Using either a heat gun or a hot water bath, the brace is molded to the inner border of the foot in the overcorrected position, and three-point fixation is used to correct the deformity as described earlier in this chapter. When the brace is malleable after heating, the rearfoot is held by the heel portion of the orthosis to prevent rearfoot pronation while an abductory force is exerted on the forefoot. The amount of correction obtained can be altered by abducting the forefoot and adjusting the tightness of the straps. The rearfoot position must be inverted to prevent pronatory changes within the foot. The brace is kept on the child continually and should be evaluated weekly and abducted if necessary (Fig. 6–14).

Orthotic Device Control (DSIS)

The ambulating child who presents with compensated metatarsus adductus needs an orthosis. The compensated metatarsus adductus foot is flat or pronated; an orthotic supinates the foot while at the same time visually increasing the apparent toe-in position. A device that controls rearfoot pronation and prevents transverse drift of the forefoot is needed.

Addressing the deformity at the earliest age is paramount. Because this is not always possible, the physician should still attack the problem immediately with the most aggressive form of conservative therapy. Cast treatment is optimal but is not possible in children who have begun to walk. I have developed a technique for these early

ambulators that incorporates cast therapy and orthotic control together. This is accomplished by using a neutral position cast constructed in the usual manner. As the plaster is starting to set, and as the rearfoot is held in a neutral position, the forefoot is abducted. The method is similar to that used for cast reduction for metadductus in the infant. The rearfoot is locked in the neutral position while the lateral column at the fifth metatarsal base–cuboid area is stabilized. The transverse abducting force is applied to the first metatarsal head. The laboratory can press a Dynamic Stabilizing Innersole System (DSIS) (Longer Laboratories, Deer Park, NY) from this cast. The DSIS has a deep shelled heel seat with high medial and lateral flanges that extend just proximal to the first and fifth metatarsal heads. The DSIS now has an imprinted foot in a corrected rectus position with a neutral rearfoot. When the child's adducted foot is placed in this device, it is forced into an abducted position. With weight bearing, the rearfoot is still held in varus to prevent the pronated skewfoot deformity (Fig. 6–15).

The child who presents with a complicated and compensated metatarsus adductus deformity who is over the recommended age of casting (usually considered to be the age at which the child starts to ambulate fully without assistance) needs some control for the foot. This is not to say that orthotic control is going to reduce the foot defor-

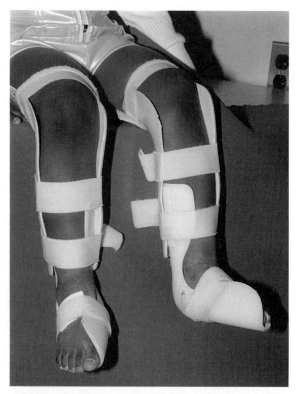

Figure 6–14. Wheaton brace. This brace is designed to maintain and correct for a transverse plane deformity in the foot as in metadductus and internal or external tibial torsion. The two components are held together in the calf region by Velcro straps. Rotating the lower tibial segment on the upper thigh segment drives externally the leg on the thigh. The forefoot can be held in abduction, and the rearfoot can be held in inversion by the moldable rearfoot component. The splint is placed on the child in a nonirritating fashion and can be molded with either a heat gun or hot water before it is applied.

mity, but it will prevent the foot from pronating. A visual toe-in is noted as the orthotic supinates the foot. Because the foot is maturing and the protective fat about the foot is decreasing, a device has to be constructed that will control rearfoot pronation and also prevent the transverse drift of the forefoot that is commonly seen in children with the compensated metadductus deformity.

It was mentioned that when controlling a metadductus foot with an orthosis the result will be control but a toe-in will appear. This is due to the supinatory effect on the rearfoot. Imagine a concomitant internal axial deviation (internal tibial torsion, internal femoral position) occurring at the same time as a metadductus. The result would be a severely internally positioned foot that is controlled and protected against the pronatory effects. It is imperative to explain the purpose of the orthosis and its visual effect to the parents prior to dispensing the device.

The major complication occurs when the deformity is unchecked and a surgical procedure is performed to reduce the adducted metatarsals. The result is a complete breakdown of the midtarsal joint secondary to the transverse plane deformity in the axial segment. This complication is avoidable even when the adductus angle is greater than 35 degrees and the child presents with severe tripping owing to the foot, leg, or femoral deformity. This condition must be controlled after surgery to prevent a transverse midtarsal break. A deep-seated, neutral position, posted orthosis, which is cut out proximal to the fifth metatarsal base, is recommended.

The child with a metatarsus adductus is prone to Iselin's apophysitis because of an increase in pressure and irritation on the lateral prominence of the fifth metatarsal. This pressure can be decreased by using a rigid molded acrylic orthosis. This orthosis is a modified version of a Roberts plate; the flanges are kept low, but it has a deep heel seat. The lateral flange is cut proximal to the fifth metatarsal base. Thus, the orthotic device controls pronation and removes direct pressure on the fifth metatarsal base. With a healthy fat pad in younger patients, this cut out portion is not necessary; the flange should be extended distally, just proximal to the fifth metatarsal head.[5]

Reverse-last shoes are contraindicated because they pronate the foot maximally at the midtarsal and subtalar joints. In the toddler, a straight-last shoe with a scaphoid pad can be used before an orthosis is constructed. The straight-last shoe maintains the foot in a rectus position

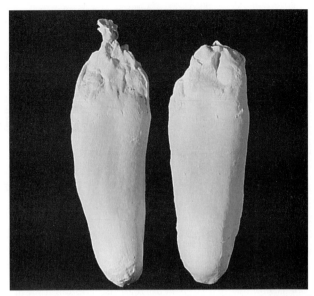

Figure 6–15. Neutral position cast. Cast on the left demonstrates adducted metatarsal position with prominent fifth metatarsal base. Right neutral position cast is taken with the foot reduced manually. A positive impression will be made from these neutral position casts, and the DSIS will be pressed to this impression of the reduced metatarsus adductus deformity. The foot will function with the orthotic in a corrected position and the foot rectus.

while the scaphoid pad prevents some degree of midtarsal joint abduction.

References

1. Wynne-Davis R: Family studies and the cause of congenital clubfoot. J Bone Joint Surg 1954; 46B:445.
2. Sgarlato TE: A Compendium of Podiatric Biomechanics. San Francisco, California College of Podiatric Medicine, 1971, pp. 31.
3. Jay RM, Johnson M: Recurrent metatarsus adductus. Curr Podiatr 1984; 33:12.
4. Bestard EA: A modified Furlong procedure for the correction of metatarsus adductus. Contemp Orthop 1984; 8:19–23.
5. Schwartz B, Jay RM, Schoenhaus HD: Apophysitis of the fifth metatarsal base: Iselin's disease. JAPMA 1991; 81:128–130.
6. Hoerr NL, Pyle SI, Francis CC: Radiographic Atlas of Skeletal Development of the Foot and Ankle. Springfield, IL, Charles C Thomas, 1962
7. Kite JH.: Congenital metatarsus varus. J Bone Joint Surg 1967; 49A:388–397.

7

Surgery for Metatarsus Adductus

Richard M. Jay, D.P.M.

The decision to perform surgery on the metadductus foot is *not* made for cosmetic reasons. The child should present with difficulty in finding comfortable foot gear, tripping, or pain at the various pressure points of the foot (e.g., first metatarsal head, fifth metatarsal base). To determine the surgical procedure, one examines the metatarsal bases to evaluate the progression of development. During the developmental years, the bases appear rounded at the cartilaginous junction. However, the cartilaginous base is actually squared off at Lisfranc's articulation. The rounded base is only a radiographic appearance, and eventually the cartilaginous base ossifies and then appears squared off.

CRESCENTIC OSTEOTOMY

If the metatarsus adductus deformity is considered a transverse plane osseous deformity, the deformity must be addressed at the bases of the metatarsals. The adducted position (greater than 25 degrees deviation) occurs through the midline of the body of the second metatarsal in reference to the perpendicular to the bisection of the lesser tarsus. When the deformity is resistant or the metatarsals are mature, surgical intervention with a base wedge osteotomy is indicated. The procedure, described in 1966 by Steytler and Van Der Welt,[1] uses osteotomies with connecting drill holes in a wide **V** design. The metatarsals are then shifted into an abducted position. The procedure was later modified into a crescentic osteotomy, which allowed rotation at the crescentic cut. This allowed the metatarsals to abduct on the transverse plane on a single axis with maximal bone contact.[2]

The advent of the crescentic blade permitted performance of an osteotomy that alleviated the usual problems associated with closing wedge osteotomies. The crescentic osteotomy is an acceptable procedure for simultaneously reducing the adducted metatarsal and maintaining the metatarsal length. The standard surgical technique for performing the crescentic osteotomy is relatively simple. Appropriate soft tissue dissection and preservation of the vital structures are much more tedious than performance of the actual osteotomy itself. An inherent weakness of the osteotomy is the position of the cut; the cut is unstable

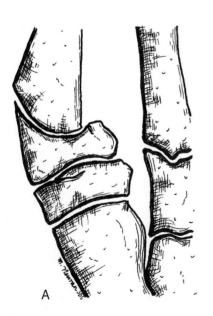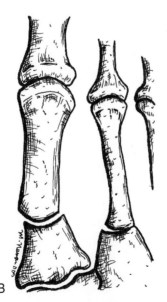

Figure 7–1. *A*, Crescentic osteotomy approximately 1 cm distal to the epiphysis. The crescentic cut is offset medially to allow a buttress effect, which prevents the drift of the first metatarsal medially. In addition, it allows a greater amount of bone contact. *B*, Centrally placed crescentic osteotomy loses bone contact as it loses the buttress effect and allows possible slipping of first metatarsal medially.

A   B

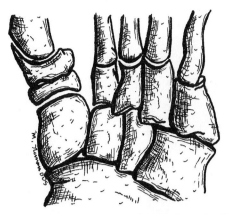

Figure 7–2. Crescentic osteotomies one through five with offset medial cut mode on first metatarsal. Remaining metatarsals can be centrally placed. In the final reduction one should attempt to keep the bases in contact with the shaft.

on the frontal plane. Translation of the entire metatarsal can occur at the osteotomy site in the direction of dorsiflexion or plantar flexion. A similar drift of the metatarsal can cause the entire base to shift medially or laterally.

Modification of the crescentic osteotomy of the base is done very simply to prevent drift and translation. The osteotomy is modified by making the cut with the crescentic blade angulated and rotated medially (Fig. 7–1). The apex of the blade is positioned laterally off center to the metatarsal base. One of the most important effects of the angulated crescentic osteotomy is the intrinsic bolstering that is produced by the high medial lip on the medial side of the base. This lip of bone acts as a significant counterforce to any medially directed forces at the osteotomy site.[3] Tachdijian believes that this bolstering effect is useful in the correction of metatarsus adductus.[4] A shelf

of bone protrudes medially into the adjacent soft tissue at the proximal cut in the shaft after the metatarsal has been manipulated into an abducted position. Manual displacement reduces the adductus angle of the metatarsal and maintains more bone-to-bone contact than does the conventional transversely placed crescentic osteotomy. Since the angulated cut is made with the medial surface higher than the lateral surface, the metatarsal is also effectively lengthened when the shaft is abducted. The rotation takes place in an arc so that loss of bone length secondary to the width of the osteotomy blade is prevented; length is gained because of the geometry of the cut (Figs. 7–2 and 7–3).

Healing potential is markedly increased when the osteotomy is performed in the proximal region of the metatarsal (Fig. 7–4). If the osteotomy is performed too distally, in the presence of more cortical bone and less cancellous bone, increased callus formation could result (Figs. 7–5 and 7–6). In addition, this procedure could initiate a vascular insult in the vulnerable diaphyseal blood supply, leading to a delay in healing with the potential of nonunion.[5]

The proximal aspect of the first metatarsal base is meticulously dissected because the epiphysis is approximately 1 cm from the metatarsal-cuneiform joint. The osteotomy is made another 1 to 1.5 cm proximal to the epiphysis. The epiphysis can be identified in the young child by its pale blue color in contrast to the white bone. The periosteum is reflected carefully off all the metatarsal bases and closed after the osteotomies have been made; this minimizes large bone callus and possible intermetatarsal bone fusion. All osteotomies are made in the proximal segment to maximize reduction and increase the healing potential of the metatarsal (Fig. 7–7).

Two methods of fixation are commonly employed when

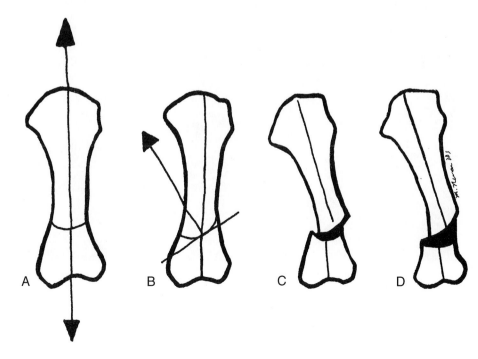

Figure 7–3. A, Longitudinal axis of first metatarsal with crescentic cut. B, Crescentic cut offset medially, thus increasing height on medial surface of metatarsal. C and D, Standard central crescentic cut and three-dimensional medially placed crescentic cut. Note the increase in bone contact surface area.

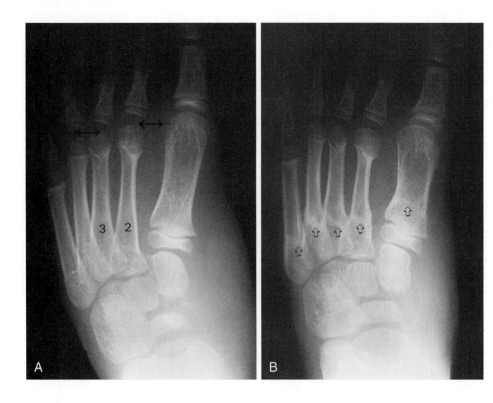

Figure 7–4. *A* and *B*, Preoperative and postoperative views of metatarsus adductus. Note crescentic line that is present 1 year postoperatively.

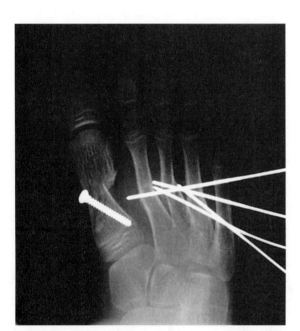

Figure 7–5. A Lepird procedure performed on the right foot. The first metatarsal is nicely reduced with a closing base wedge osteotomy. The remaining metatarsals, however, were cut midshaft to allow rotation. However, the angular cut was not made parallel to the ground but rather angulated in the metatarsal at midshaft level.

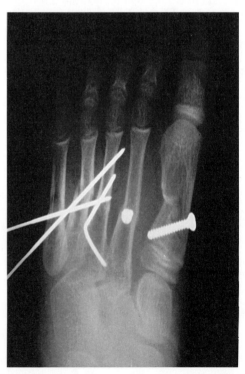

Figure 7–6. A Lepird procedure performed on the left foot. The first metatarsal is nicely reduced with a closing base wedge osteotomy. As in Figure 7–5, the remaining metatarsals were cut midshaft to allow rotation, and the angular cut was angulated in the metatarsal at midshaft level rather than made parallel to the ground.

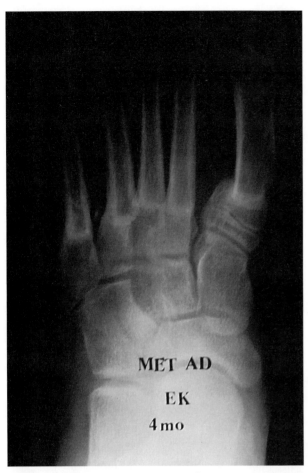

Figure 7–7. Four-month postoperative view of crescentic osteotomy performed for metatarsus adductus.

performing crescentic osteotomies on the metatarsals—transverse pin fixation and cross-pinning of the first and fifth metatarsals (Figs. 7–8 through 7–12). Care must be taken to avoid the distal growth plates of metatarsals 2 through 5. If one enters from the lateral side of the fifth metatarsal and the pin is placed just proximal to the neck, one avoids damaging the plates because the fifth growth plate is the most proximal one. Another advantage of the lateral entrance is the ease with which the pin can be guided from the thin fifth metatarsal to the thicker first metatarsal shaft. A large (.062) Kirshner wire (Micro-Aire, Valencia, CA) is placed across the metatarsals distally and then secured in a plaster cast that maintains alignment. This provides adequate maintenance of the fracture sites, but if the proper sequence of pin fixation is not followed, complications such as delayed union, malunion, or nonunion may result.[5, 6]

The forefoot must be abducted before the pin is inserted. One should make sure that metatarsal bases 1 through 5 are in good rotated contact at the osteotomy sites. The forefoot is stabilized in the corrected position, and pinning is begun. If the pin is passed through all the metatarsals before the forefoot is abducted, subluxation with loss of contact occurs. When abduction occurs, the forefoot will move as a unit and pivot on the fifth metatarsal base while lifting off and losing contact with the first metatarsal base osteotomy cut.

An alternative method of fixation of the metatarsals is to use two .062 Kirshner wires, one fixing the first metatarsal to the middle cuneiform and the other fixing the fifth metatarsal to the medial portion of the cuboid. Proper alignment and reduction of the metatarsal bases is most important. The buttress effect helps in achieving some stabilization; however, the pins are only maintaining the first and fifth metatarsals. For this reason, good visualization of the osteotomy sites is mandatory. The child's foot has amazing healing properties, and metatarsals 2 to 4 usually align themselves well without too much effort in fixation; however, this phenomenon does not override the need for proper positioning and fixation. Once the pins are in place and the incisions are closed, a well-molded cast is applied. The foot is immobilized for at least 6 weeks.

HEYMEN-HERNDON-STRONG TARSOMETATARSAL CAPSULOTOMY

The Heymen-Herndon-Strong (HHS) procedure is indicated in the reduction of flexible metatarsus adductus. Flexibility is determined by the degree of reducibility seen on manipulation. Since this is truly a soft tissue deformity of adduction at the Lisfranc articulation, the procedure should be performed by releasing the liga-

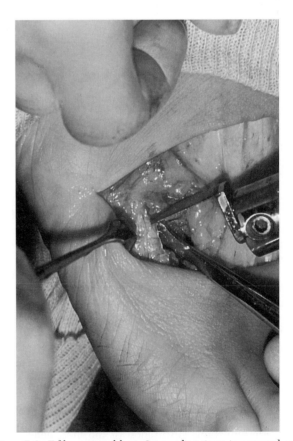

Figure 7–8. Fifth metatarsal base. Surrounding tissue is protected, and a crescentic blade is used to create the osteotomy. The periosteum is dissected. The incision can be transverse or individual incisions can be made over metatarsals one, two, and three and between metatarsals four and five.

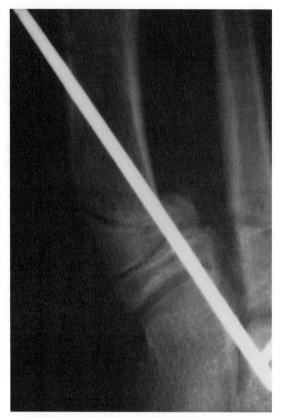

Figure 7–9. Buttress effect of medially placed crescentic osteotomy along longitudinal axis of first metatarsal. First metatarsal is stabilized with a smooth **K**-wire. Note the amount of bone contact on the medial aspect of the first metatarsal base.

ments by the age of 5 to 6 years. This procedure is reserved for children who demonstrate no osseous adduction of the metatarsals.

Exposure is gained by making three longitudinal incisions on the dorsum over the foot. The first incision is made over the base of the first metatarsal. The second and third incisions are made between the second and third metatarsals, and between the fourth and fifth metatarsals, respectively. Both of these incisions are located at the bases. The incisions are long enough to expose Lisfranc's articulation. Using a No. 64 miniblade, the ligaments surrounding each of the metatarsal bases are incised except the lateral interosseous ligaments. These ligaments maintain the stability of the joints being released and act as a stabilizing pivot point. Very careful dissection is needed because damage to the soft surrounding cartilaginous bases can leave small fragments that may eventually fuse to the other adjacent joints. When sectioning the first metatarsal base ligaments, an exact knowledge of their location is imperative. The epiphysis is located proximally on the shaft and may be mistaken for the metatarsal-cuneiform joint.

After complete release of all the joints, the foot is now ready for reduction. Pin fixation of the first metatarsal-cuneiform and the fifth metatarsal-cuboid joints can be used to stabilize the foot after forefoot abduction. The joints can also be stabilized with the application of a well-molded abducted cast. The adduction should be re-

duced in the same manner as that described earlier in Chapter 6.

The cast is changed every 2 weeks and mild abduction is applied to the forefoot while the rearfoot is stabilized in a neutral position. The cast is used for a minimum of 6 weeks. Overcorrection should Lisfranc's joint can dislocate. If a dorsal force is used on the metatarsals, the result is dorsal dislocation. One major complication of this procedure is damage to the articular surfaces. If this occurs, degenerative changes result, and fusion is likely to develop.

In a study performed at the Gillette Children's Hospital in St. Paul, Minnesota, 37 children (56 feet) with metatarsus adductus opted for a capsulotomy procedure as described earlier after experiencing failed conservative treatment. Tarsometatarsal capsulotomy release failed in 41% of cases, with no true overcorrection. This raises the question of whether this procedure deals with the actual pathology present. Pain was noted frequently postoperatively, and radiographically the outcome yielded fusion of the metatarsal joint bases and degenerative joint changes in the late stages. These occurred independently of whether the surgical procedure was performed in a younger child or older child. The high failure rate in this study of capsule releases of the metatarsal bases shows that care must be taken in the release of these cartilaginous surfaces.[7]

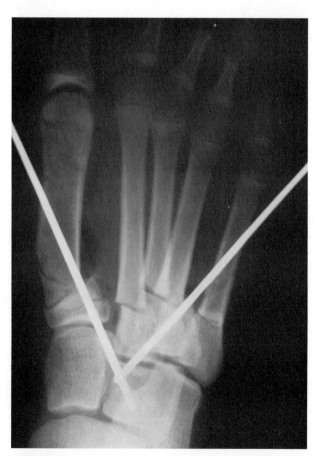

Figure 7–10. Crescentic osteotomies of bases of metatarsals for correction of metatarsus adductus. Cross **K**-wire fixation of metatarsals one and five is shown.

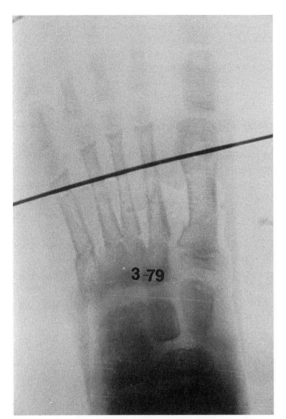

Figure 7–11. Transverse pin fixation of metatarsals one through five with a smooth K-wire. Crescentic osteotomies were performed to reduce metatarsus adductus. The osteotomy sites are lined up prior to reduction, and reduction of the metatarsus adductus deformity is made prior to insertion of the K-wire. If the K-wire is placed through the metatarsal shafts before reduction, the entire medial column will lift with loss of bone contact.

OPEN WEDGE OSTEOTOMY OF THE FIRST CUNEIFORM AND CLOSING WEDGE OSTEOTOMY OF THE CUBOID

Development of the crescentic osteotomy for the correction of metatarsus adductus resulted from an inability to apply closing and opening wedge osteotomies to all cases of pathologically increased intermetatarsal angles. Specifically, the opening wedge osteotomy was an acceptable procedure when the first metatarsal was not too short or when the second metatarsal was not too long. Either of these situations assumes an absolute or relative shortening of the first metatarsal, which could only be accentuated by using a closing wedge osteotomy at the base of the metatarsal. When an absolute or relative shortening of the first metatarsal is a consideration, the opening wedge osteotomy can reduce the intermetatarsal angle while simultaneously preserving a functionally acceptable metatarsal length. In fact, the opening wedge osteotomy was developed for the specific purpose of increasing the length of an absolute or relatively shortened first metatarsal. The opening wedge osteotomy must be grafted with approximately 6 to 10 mm of bone. It is preferable to use a combination of cancellous bone to

provide good osteogenesis and cortical bone to provide a strong strut to prevent collapse at the osteotomy site.

The opening wedge cuneiform osteotomy with the insertion of a bone graft and the closing wedge osteotomy of the cuboid address the adductus deformity proximal to Lisfranc's articulation and can provide a greater amount of correction on the transverse plane. Since the medial column increases in length and the lateral column shortens, the risk of midtarsal joint pronation increases. Lateral cuboid stability must be ensured to prevent the first ray from elevating secondary to the weakened pull of the peroneus longus. Adjunct procedures are usually indicated with this procedure. With an equinus foot, the tendoachilles or gastrocnemius may have to be lengthened. If the procedure is done on a skew foot with severe rearfoot pronation, the lateral column must be preserved with an Evans calcaneal osteotomy. With any sag of the sagittal plane, one must consider an arthroereisis procedure.[8]

In a study performed at Indiana University in Indianapolis, resistant metatarsus adductus deformities were studied. It was noted that a severe first metatarsal–cuneiform joint adductus angle was present. Opening wedge osteotomy of the medial cuneiform was selected to correct this angulation. All records and radiographs of 32 feet in 22 patients who underwent an opening wedge medial cuneiform osteotomy with two to four metatarsal osteotomies were reviewed. The mean age at the time of osteotomy surgery was 11 years (range, 3.5 to 21 years) and the average period of follow-up was 2 years (range, 1 to 5.5 years). At follow-up, patients and parents were asked about the appearance of the foot, shoe fit, pain, and level of activity. The adduction deformity and the

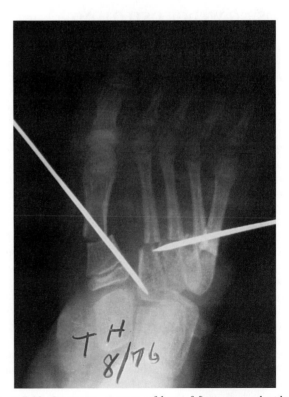

Figure 7–12. Crescentic osteotomy of base of first metatarsal without buttress. Minimal bone contact to remaining metatarsals causes loss of stability.

obliquity of the first metatarsal-cuneiform joint were measured on standing AP and lateral radiographs.

All patients and parents rated the foot as good or excellent in appearance; shoe fitting was easy; and none had pain or limited activity postoperatively. Radiographically, correction of the adduction deformity was 13 degrees (64%) as measured by the talar-first metatarsal angle. The remaining adduction deformity was 0 degree in 13 feet, 1 to 10 degrees in 6 feet, 11 to 20 degrees in 8 feet, and greater than 20 degrees in 5 feet. The average amount of correction of the first metatarsal–cuneiform angle was 10 degrees or 71%. Patients with greater adduction deformities preoperatively had larger adduction deformities postoperatively. This suggests that there is a limit to the amount of correction possible with this procedure. No wound or pin tract problems, nonunions, or osteomyelitis occurred in this series.

The preliminary report suggests that the first cuneiform opening wedge osteotomy addresses the region of deformity in resistant metatarsus adductus and that it is safe and effective. It reduces the obliquity of the first metatarsal–cuneiform joint, which should prevent recurrent deformity. In addition, it avoids the tarso-metatarsal joints, which if damaged can lead to degenerative joint disease, and it also avoids the first metatarsal growth plate, which if damaged can lead to a growth arrest and shortened first metatarsal. If the adduction deformity is severe (greater than 25 degrees), full radiographic evidence of correction of the deformity should not be anticipated even though the patient and the parents may be satisfied with the appearance of the foot.[9]

CLOSING WEDGE OSTEOTOMY

In the child older than 6 years with adduction of the metatarsals osteotomy of the metatarsals can be performed in a manner similar to the crescentic procedure in technique and indications. Care must be taken with regard to the first metatarsal epiphysis. Periosteal dissection and closure must be meticulous to avoid unwanted bone growth and fusion of the metatarsal base to adjacent structures.

The osteotomy is made with the apex of the wedge located at the proximal-medial aspect of each metatarsal, distal to the articular facets of metatarsals 1 through 5. The cut on the first metatarsal is made 1 to 1.5 cm distal to the epiphysis. Various types of surgical fixation can be used after the resected wedge is removed. Fixation of the first and fifth metatarsals provide a good buttress effect in stabilizing the central metatarsals. Various techniques employed to fix the osteotomy include Kirschner wire fixation (which provides uniplanar stability at the osteotomy site), internal monofilament wire fixation along the lateral aspect to close down the osteotomy site (but only when the medial cortex is still intact), and screw fixation. A large base is necessary for screw fixation to allow the insertion of the 2.7-mm cortical screw. The technique for entering the central metatarsals for screw fixation is somewhat difficult due to the position of the adjacent metatarsal. Because the metatarsals are small and close together, it is tempting to perform the osteotomy distally, but the cut must be made as far proximal as possible to ensure bone healing.

Postoperatively the foot is immobilized in a below-the-knee cast. The cast is changed at the time of incision inspection and suture removal. Mild adduction is held to the forefoot, and a neutral to inverted heel position is maintained with cast changes.

LEPIRD PROCEDURE

The osseous Lepird procedure[10] is indicated in children between the ages of 6 and 16 years. Three linear dorsal incisions expose all the metatarsal bases and shafts. The first incision is located over the base and proximal shaft of the first metatarsal. The second incision is made between the bases and shafts of metatarsals 2 and 3. The third incision is like the second incision but is located between the fourth and fifth metatarsals. Identification of neurovascular structures is made to minimize any trauma to these structures. Closing base wedge osteotomies are performed on metatarsals 1 and 5 in standard fashion (as described earlier). Osteotomies are now made in metatarsals 2, 3, and 4. The cuts are made from the distal dorsal cortex through the proximal plantar cortex. These are diagonal cuts through the metatarsal. The first and fifth metatarsals are closed and fixed from the medial and lateral surfaces. Metatarsals 2, 3, and 4 can now rotate on the diagonal plane and are fixed from dorsal to plantar with a single 2.7-mm cortical screw. The first and fifth metatarsal closing base wedge osteotomies must have a strong medial hinge. Their fixation is accomplished using 2.7-mm cortical screws. These two osteotomies act as a buttress for the central metatarsals because they are unstable on the transverse plane.

The procedure in theory is excellent; however, in actuality if the procedure is to be successful the osteotomies of metatarsals 2, 3, and 4 must be parallel to the supporting surface. Since the lesser metatarsal declination angle is approximately 20 degrees, the parallel cut would extend nearly to the metatarsal head distally and to the metatarsal base proximally. This would require excessive dissection in the child's foot. To localize the osteotomy in the proximal segment of the metatarsal, the metatarsal declination angle would have to be as high as 45 degrees, a rare finding. A common error of this procedure is making the osteotomy too perpendicular to the ground axis rather than parallel to it. The axis of rotation with this cut is not on the transverse plane but rather on the long axis of the metatarsal. This procedure results in more of a frontal plane change in the metatarsal than a reduction in the transverse plane.

THOMSON PROCEDURE

This soft tissue release procedure is indicated for the flexible atavistic form of metatarsus adductus with a hallux varus deformity secondary to a hyperactive abductor hallucis muscle. An incision is made on the medial side of the first metatarsal phalangeal joint. The abductor hallucis muscle and tendon are identified. Depending on the tightness of this myotendinous structure, the tendon can be lengthened or a segment of tendon and muscle belly can be transected and removed. The medial capsule of the first metatarsal phalangeal joint may have to be incised, depending on the varus deformity.

Caution is needed at this point because a hallux valgus can result. If the forefoot adduction is not addressed and the rearfoot pronates, hallux valgus is very likely to occur. This procedure is not indicated in lieu of a complete metatarsus adductus release or osseous correction.

Postoperatively the hallux is maintained in a rectus position by either splinting or pin fixation through the great toe. I have found that a Betadine-impregnated gauze shell serves the purpose of maintenance quite well. The splint is kept in place for 3 weeks.

References

1. Steytler JCS, Van Der Walt ID: Correction of resistant adduction of the forefoot in congenital clubfoot and congenital metatarsus varus by metatarsal osteotomy. Br J Surg 1966; 53:558.

2. Berman A, Gartland JJ: Metatarsal osteotomy for the correction of adduction of the forepart of the foot in children. J Bone Joint Surg 1971; 53A:498.

3. Jay RM, Schoenhaus HD, Donohue CM: A modified crescentic osteotomy in children. J Foot Surg 1990; 29:417–420.

4. Tachdijian MO: Pediatric Orthopedics. Philadelphia, W.B. Saunders, 1972, p. 1340.

5. Jaworek TE: The intrinsic vascular supply to the first metatarsal. J Am Pediatr Med Assoc 1973; 63:555–563.

6. Turek SL: Orthopedics: Principles and Their Application. Philadelphia, J.B. Lippincott, 1977.

7. Stark JG, Johanson JJ, Winter RB: The Heyman-Herndon-Strong tarsometatarsal capsulotomy for metatarsus adductus. J Pediatr Orthoped 1987; 7:305–310.

8. Berg EE: A reappraisal of metatarsus adductus and skewfoot. J Bone Joint Surg 1986; 68A:1185–1196.

9 Kling TF, Schmidt T. L, Conklin MJ: Open wedge osteotomy of the first cuneiform for metatarsus adductus. J Bone Joint Surg. 1991; 15(2):331.

10. McGlamry ED: Comprehensive Textbook of Foot Surgery. Baltimore, Williams & Wilkins, 1987.

8

Medial Column Soft Tissue Release for Metatarsus Adductus Correction

Bruce D. Harley, D.P.M.

Metatarsus adductus is a transverse plane deformity in which the forefoot is in an adducted position relative to the lesser tarsals.[1, 4, 10, 12, 14] Frontal plane deformity[7] may also be seen but is usually found in individuals approaching osseous maturity. Hallux adductus is often associated with metatarsus adductus deformity in pediatric patients.[2, 3] Hallux adductus tends to reduce with shoe wear.

Metatarsus adductus deformity occurs at the tarsometatarsal joint.[1, 10, 12, 13, 14] The osseous deformity has generally been considered to be in the metatarsus segment, but some recent authors have proposed that the level of deformity is in the lesser tarsus.[10, 13, 14, 16] The regions of articular deformity are of prime importance when one is contemplating correction by soft tissue release.

CLINICAL PRESENTATION

Metatarsus adductus generally presents as a C-shaped foot with a convex lateral border and a concave medial border.[1, 4, 9, 10, 14, 15] The medial metatarsals are usually adducted to a greater degree than the lateral column. The base of the fifth metatarsal is often more prominent than usual.

Evaluation should include open and closed kinetic chain examination to ensure accurate diagnosis of all components of the foot deformity. Children often have a concomitant hallux adductus deformity and a contracted abductor hallucis.[2, 3] Proximal compensations such as subtalar and midtarsal joint pronation are less common in children. For this reason, young patients often present with uncompensated conditions that become manifest as tripping and stumbling.

RADIOGRAPHIC EXAMINATION

Metatarsus adductus is visible on a weight-bearing anteroposterior (AP) projection. A metatarsus adductus condition is diagnosed by the presence of a metatarsus adductus angle of greater than 15 degrees. This measurement assesses the position of the metatarsus relative to the lesser tarsus.

TREATMENT OF METATARSUS ADDUCTUS

Selection of the most appropriate treatment for metatarsus adductus must be based on the amount of clinical deformity, the impact of the deformity on the gait pattern, and the age of the individual. Treatment of infants with metatarsus adductus should be initiated at the time of diagnosis because of the malleable nature of the deformity. Corrective casting should be attempted in children less than 36 months of age, which leads to good results generally especially in those 16 to 18 months.[1, 10, 13, 14]

The transverse plane correction should be obtained entirely at the tarsometatarsal joint. Care should be taken to ensure that the midtarsal joint is not laterally subluxed in a pronatory direction during the casting regimen.

Casting is used as an initial treatment to obtain correction. Splint and shoe therapy is used for follow-up maintenance. The casting technique is initiated by manual supination of the subtalar and oblique midtarsal joint axes, which prevents pronatory oblique midtarsal axis subluxation during the abductory maneuver. Supination of the subtalar joint locks up the oblique midtarsal joint in a supinatory direction. Three-point manipulation is performed with a laterally directed force applied to the medial side of the supinated heel and to the forefoot. A medially directed force is applied to the lateral surface of the cuboid and the fifth metatarsal base.

The manipulative force should be gentle, and the correction should be obtained gradually. The urge to obtain correction rapidly should be avoided because subluxation of the midtarsal joint often occurs in such cases. The cast padding is kept to a minimum because excess padding decreases the ability of the cast to maintain the corrected position.

When hallux adductus is present along with metatarsus adductus, the abductor hallucis is generally a deforming force.[2, 3] In this condition, the corrective cast is extended distally to allow abduction of the hallux. This technique stretches the abductor hallucis muscle–tendon complex, allowing simultaneous correction of both deformities.

Straight-last shoes and splints are used to maintain the correction achieved by casting. Orthotic therapy is useful as an antipronation device but does not correct the metatarsus adductus condition.

Medial column soft tissue release of the first metatarsocuneiform and the naviculocuneiform joints is indicated when conservative therapy fails to provide correction in patients less than 36 months of age. Because I believe that both articulations contribute to the adductus deformity, release the ligaments at both levels. The first metatarsophalangeal joint (MPJ) is released, and an abductor hallucis tendon Z-lengthening procedure is performed when hallux adductus is present. A corrective cast is applied at the completion of surgery. Soft tissue techniques involving both the medial and lateral columns have been advocated by various authors for correction of the immature skeleton.[1, 4, 7, 14]

Technique

An incision is placed along the osseous structures of the medial column. The incision extends from the navicular tuberosity to the midshaft of the first metatarsal, and to the midshaft of the proximal phalanx when hallux adductus is present. The incision is deepened through skin and superficial fascial tissue to the deep fascial layer. The abductor hallucis muscle belly is bluntly dissected

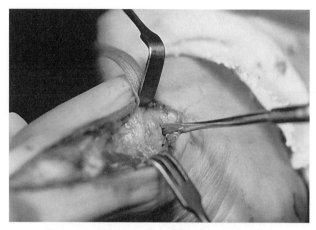

Figure 8–2. The naviculocuneiform joint is identified.

away from the osseous structures to allow complete visualization of the articulations.

The tibialis anterior tendon is identified and separated from the surrounding tissue (Fig. 8–1). It is mobilized and retracted with umbilical tape or a Penrose drain. The tendon is retracted away from the joints while ligamentous releases are performed. The tibialis anterior tendon should not be released for correction of transverse plane deformities because it controls the sagittal and frontal plane positions of the forefoot but does not affect the transverse plane position.

The medial column articulations are identified using a Freer elevator and manipulation of the first ray (Figs. 8–2 and 8–3). Extreme care is taken to find the joint before dividing the ligaments because of the delicate nature of these small immature osseous structures.

The joints are entered using a very delicate scissors technique. Blunt-blunt curved iris scissors are preferred because they generally do not damage the articular cartilage. Scalpel blades should be avoided because of their potential for cartilage violation.

The first metatarsocuneiform joint is released initially, followed by release of the naviculocuneiform articulation. The joints are entered tentatively while the first ray is manipulated to stretch and apply tension on the ligaments

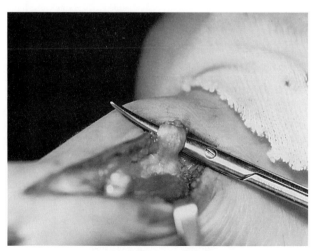

Figure 8–1. The tibialis anterior tendon is identified and preserved.

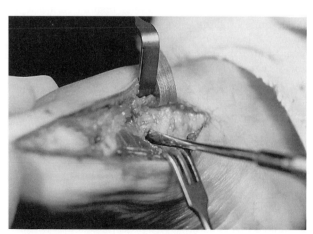

Figure 8–3. The first metatarsocuneiform joint is identified.

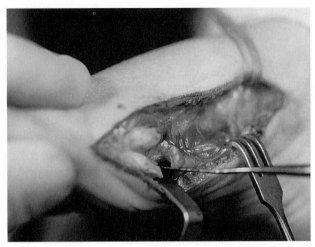

Figure 8–4. The abductor hallucis tendon and first metatarsophalangeal joint are released.

being severed. After entering the joint, the scissors are rotated to release the medial, dorsal, and plantar ligaments. Care is taken when dividing the dorsal ligaments to avoid damage to the dorsalis pedis artery and deep peroneal nerve.

After the ligaments have been released, lateral pressure is applied to the forefoot to ascertain the resistance to abduction and the effectiveness of the procedure. The contribution of the abductor hallucis and first MPJ is gauged. A first MPJ release is performed as necessary to allow complete reduction of the metatarsus adductus deformity (Fig. 8–4). This involves a Z-lengthening of the abductor hallucis tendon using a scalpel and a frontal plane first MPJ release using scissors.

Reduction is reassessed after the first MPJ release. When further correction is needed, a dorsal linear incision is placed over the second and third MPJs, and a soft tissue release of the Heyman-Herndon-Strong[4] type is performed. I have never had to make this second incision on individuals under the age of 3.

When the foot can be easily manipulated into a rectus position the wound is closed. Closure consists of coaptation of the subcutaneous and skin layers. The ligamentous releases are not repaired. A sterile dressing and corrective cast are applied.

Serial casting is performed in a manner identical to that described for the preoperative technique. The duration of the postoperative casting period has been 4 to 6 weeks in my experience. Maintenance therapy is achieved with straight-last shoes. The foot is kept non-weight-bearing for 2 to 3 weeks.

I have performed 12 medial column releases for metatarsus adductus in children under 3 years of age. Correction has been complete in 11 cases. One patient with bilateral deformity had approximately a 60% reduction on one side. Four of the cases were performed in conjunction with the STA-Peg procedure. All 12 patients are asymptomatic and are able to engage in all activities without restrictions.

The soft tissue release may be performed bilaterally at the same surgical setting. The procedure is less invasive

and creates less disability than the osseous techniques used in older age groups (ages 5 to 16).

In my opinion, correction of metatarsus adductus in infants by the soft tissue technique is preferable to subjecting adolescents to the long recovery periods required for osseous procedures.[10] An aggressive conservative and surgical regimen is recommended in infants to avoid the more debilitating operations needed in the more mature skeleton.

SUMMARY

A brief review of metatarsus adductus deformity has been presented, including clinical and radiographic findings. An aggressive approach to both serial casting and surgical therapy is recommended to avoid the need for osseous surgery in adolescence or adulthood. A medial column soft tissue release technique is presented for use in infants up to age 3. Manipulative casting is used to obtain the correction after ligamentous release has been performed.

References

1. Yu GV, Wallace GF: Metatarsus adductus. *In* McGlamry ED (ed): Textbook of Foot Surgery, Vol. 2. Baltimore, Williams & Wilkins, 1987, pp. 327–351.
2. Thompson SA: Hallux varus and metatarsus varus. Clin Orthop 1960; 16:109.
3. Lichblau S: Section of the abductor hallucis tendon for correction of metatarsus varus deformity. Clin Orthop 1975; 110:227.
4. Heyman CH, Herndon CH, Strong JM: Mobilization of the tarsometatarsal and intertarsal joints for the correction of resistant adduction of the forefoot of the foot in congenital clubfoot or congenital metatarsus varus. J Bone Joint Surg 1958; 40A:299–310.
5. Peabody CW, Muro F: Congenital metatarsus varus. J Bone Joint Surg 1933; 15:171–189.
6. McCormick D, Blount WP: Metatarsus adductovarus. JAMA 1949; 141:449.
7. Fowler B, Brooks AL, Parrish TF: The cavovarus foot. J Bone Joint Surg 1959; 41A:747–752.
8. Steytler JCS, Van Der Walt ID: Correction of resistant adduction of the forefoot in congenital clubfoot and congenital metatarsus varus by metatarsal osteotomy. Br J Surg 1966; 53:558–560.
9. Berman A, Gartland JJ: Metatarsal osteotomy for the correction of adduction of the fore part of the foot in children. J Bone Joint Surg 1971; 53A:498–506.
10. Ganley JV, Ganley TJ, Castellano BA: Metatarsus adductus: neonatal management. *In* McGlamry ED (ed): Reconstructive Surgery of the Foot and Leg. Tucker, GA, Doctors Hospital Podiatry Institute Publications, 1989, pp. 219–229.
11. Hara B, Beck CJ, Woo RA: First cuneiform closing abductory osteotomy for reduction of metatarsus primus adductus. J Foot Ankle Surg 1992; 31(5):434–439.
12. Benard MA: Treatment of skewfoot by multiple lesser tarsal osteotomies and calcaneal osteotomy. J Foot Ankle Surg 1990; 29(5):504–509.
13. Brody PJ, Grumbine N: Peroneus tertius reconstruction for flexible claw toes. J Foot Surg 1994; 23(5):357–361.
14. Ganley JV, Ganley TJ: Metatarsus adductus deformity. *In* McGlamry ED, Banks AS (eds): Comprehensive Textbook of Foot Surgery, 2nd ed, Vol. 1. Baltimore, Williams & Wilkins, 1992, pp. 829–852.
15. Tachdjian MO: Pediatric Orthopedics, Vol. 2. Philadelphia, W.B. Saunders, 1972.
16. Harley BD, Fritzhand AJ, Little JM, Little ER, Nunan P J: Abductory midfoot osteotomy procedure for metatarsus adductus. J Foot Surg 1995; 34(2):153–162.

9

Abductory Midfoot Osteotomy for Metatarsus Adductus

Bruce D. Harley, D.P.M.

Metatarsus adductus is a transverse plane deformity in which the metatarsus is adducted relative to the longitudinal axis of the lesser tarsus. The deformity is believed to be located in the tarsometatarsal joint region. Traditionally, this deformity has been surgically corrected in the metatarsal base region. More recently, it has been corrected in the lesser tarsus.

Osseous surgery has been advocated for moderate to severe degrees of this condition in individuals 8 years and older. Prior to this age conservative treatment and soft tissue procedures are indicated. The metatarsal base techniques have been described by Berman and Gartland[16] and by Lepird. The geometric concept involves achieving a transverse plane angulational correction by performing an abductory metatarsal base osteotomy. The osteotomy may be a frontal plane or oblique wedge procedure, an arcuate procedure, or a transverse plane rotational osteotomy. All of these techniques have achieved some degree of success. Common complications include (1) undercorrection because of the relatively short lever arm of correction, (2) plantar forefoot lesions due to the difficulty of keeping all metatarsals on the same weight-bearing plane, (3) nonunion, resulting from the instability of the osteotomy, and (4) technical difficulty in performing the procedure (Lepird procedure).

Ganley and colleagues stated that the metatarsus adductus deformity is the lesser tarsal region rather than in the metatarsal bases.[11] Their study found that the shape of the individual metatarsal bases is normal in metatarsus adductus conditions. They concluded that the deformity is within the lesser tarsus and advocated surgical correction at the apex of the deformity within the lesser tarsals. Their initial article described an opening cuneiform osteotomy technique in the medial column. Ganley's follow-up textbook chapter discussed a technique involving an opening osteotomy of the first cuneiform and a closing osteotomy of the cuboid.[20]

Grumbine advocated a closing osteotomy of the lateral column in the lesser tarsal region.[19] His technique involved osteotomy of the cuboid and of the third and second cuneiforms. He reported very good correction and a very small incidence of complications in a relatively large series. His procedure was often performed in conjunction with flatfoot correction, and fixation was generally achieved by Steinmann pins or Kirschner wires.

I have been performing the abductory midfoot osteotomy for metatarsus adductus correction since 1991.

PRINCIPLES

1. The osteotomy is performed at the apex of the adductus deformity.
2. According to the central axis concept the combination of a closing wedge osteotomy of the lateral column and an opening wedge osteotomy of the medial column increases the angular correction by a factor of 2 compared with either the closing or opening technique used alone.
3. I believe that the deformity is more severe in the medial column. The angle of the medial opening wedge is generally slightly larger than that of the lateral closing wedge.
4. Lengthening of the medial column and shortening of the lateral column is achieved.
5. The lever arm of correction is greater than with the metatarsal base osteotomy technique. This is the distance from the osteotomy to the metatarsal heads.

TECHNIQUE

The medial incision is placed over the extensor hallucis longus tendon and is centered over the first cuneiform. The skin and superficial fascia are incised, and superficial bleeders are ligated. Ligation is preferred over electrocoagulation because of the proximity of the medial marginal vein.

The extensor hallucis longus tendon is retracted laterally, and the neurovascular bundle just lateral to the tendon is protected. The capsuloperiosteal layer is incised in a linear fashion just medial to the extensor hallucis longus tendon. Subperiosteal dissection technique is used to expose the cortical bone. Use of a No. 15 blade is preferred to periosteal elevators because of the uneven osseous surface in this region. Very delicate dissection should be used in children because of the soft nature of the bone in such patients.

The lateral incision is placed along the lateral border of the extensor digitorum brevis and centered over the cuboid. Dissection is carried through the skin and the superficial fascial and capsuloperiosteal layers to the cortical tissue. The foot is dorsiflexed to reduce tension on the dorsal soft tissue structures, and subcapsuloperiosteal dissection unites the medial and lateral incisions. Medial and lateral dissection exposes the entire lesser tarsus.

The articulations of the midfoot region are carefully identified, including midtarsal, lesser tarsal, and tarsometatarsal joints. The position and orientation of the various articulations are noted. A malleable retractor is generally used to protect the isthmus of soft tissue between the two incisions. A 0.045 K-wire or blunt electrocoagulation tip can be inserted manually in the second intercuneiform joint as an osteotomy guide.

Templates provide the surgeon with an idea of the size of the wedge to be resected. The lateral wedge is generally oriented in a somewhat oblique fashion, extending from a central position on the lateral surface of the cuboid to the proposed apex at the second intercuneiform joint. The advantage of accurate preoperative planning is that a definitively performed wedge preserves a component of the cuboid for autogenous grafting to the medial cuneiform.

The medial osteotomy is oriented from a central position on the medial aspect of the first cuneiform to the proposed apex at the second intercuneiform joint. The second cuneiform should be divided into equal anterior and posterior halves. The tarsometatarsal, midtarsal, and naviculocuneiform joints are carefully avoided. The lateral

column osteotomy is closed and reciprocally planed to obtain flush osseous apposition. Extreme care is taken to maintain the alignment of each of the intertarsal articulations.

The medial bone graft generally consists of a composite autogenous and allogeneic graft of the first cuneiform and an allogeneic graft of the second cuneiform. The bone grafts should not extend into the intercuneiform articulations.

After adequate correction has been verified, fixation is achieved by staple insertion. Small serrated staples are very effective but often are too large. Staples may be fashioned intraoperatively using needlenose pliers. K-wires of 0.045 or 0.062 diameter are ideal dimensions for staple fabrication. The first cuneiform and the cuboid are always fixated, and a third staple is generally placed in the second cuneiform. Occasionally the third cuneiform is fixated instead of the second. Pin fixation may also be used.

Release of the abductor hallucis tendon or medial band of the plantar fascia is performed when necessary. When flatfoot correction is desired, the flatfoot procedures are performed first, followed by metatarsus adductus correction. Forefoot procedures, when necessary, are performed after midfoot correction.

I generally employ a medium ⅛-inch plastic drain with 400-mL evacuator. Topical thrombin may be used if the surgeon so desires.

The operative technique described is for a transverse plane deformity. Further wedging is performed as needed when frontal and sagittal plane deformities are also present in the midfoot region.

A three-layer closure is utilized. I prefer to use external nylon sutures for the final skin closure; however, staples or subcuticular sutures may be used instead. The drain is generally removed in 1 to 2 days. The nonweight-bearing period is approximately 8 weeks for a midfoot osteotomy that includes bone grafting. The casting period is approxi-

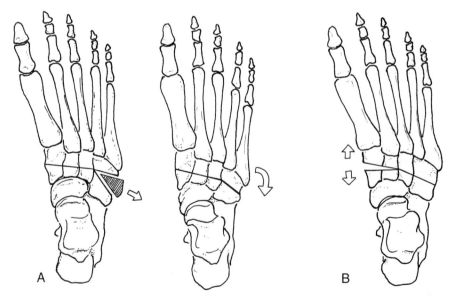

Figure 9–1. *A,* Lateral wedge resection with medial osteotomy. *B,* Medial wedge placement followed by abduction of forefoot.

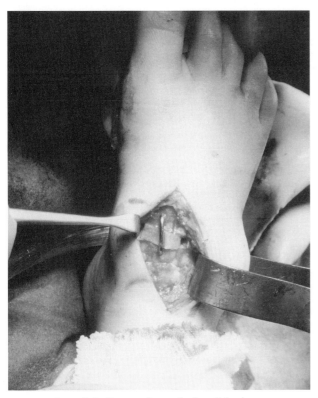

Figure 9–2. Open wedge graft of medial column.

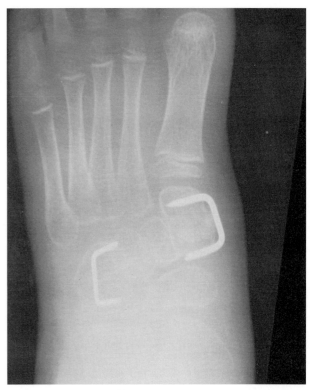

Figure 9–4. Metatarsus adductus. Postoperative anteroposterior radiograph.

mately 10 weeks. A removeable cast and early physical therapy may be employed (Figs. 9–1 to 9–4).

COMPLICATIONS

1. Osteoarthritis of intertarsal articulations may occur. For this reason, care must be taken to ensure that osseous alignment is accurate. This procedure does require detailed anatomic knowledge and advanced surgical skill. I have had one instance of osteoarthritis

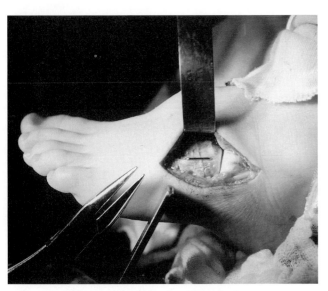

Figure 9–3. Staple fixation of lateral column.

that required articular fusion with bone grafting of the medial column.
2. Undercorrection of the metatarsus adductus deformity is very rare.
3. Nonunion of the lesser tarsal bones is also very rare.

I have used the abductory midfoot osteotomy for all metatarsus adductus corrections from 1991 to 1995. Soft tissue releases were required in approximately 10 of 40 cases. A Lepird pan metatarsal base osteotomy was performed to complete the correction in one very severe deformity.

At this time all patients past the standard recovery period are very well satisfied with the procedure and are engaging in normal and athletic activities. Two patients required reoperation other than for fixation device removal. One required joint fusion, as already mentioned, and in one child the bone graft collapsed owing to early ambulation in violation of his postoperative instructions.

SUMMARY

The abductory midfoot osteotomy has proved very effective for correction of the osseous metatarsus adductus deformity. The long lever arm of this type of correction allows correction of very severe deformities. The medial and lateral columns are treated as distinct entities, and the wedging and cardinal plane correction may differ for each. The midfoot is corrected as a unit, and submetatarsal lesions are rarely encountered postoperatively.

I suggest that the abductory midfoot osteotomy is more effective for correcting metatarsus adductus than panmetatarsal base procedures. Correction is easily achieved, and complications are few. The procedure is, however, somewhat technically demanding and requires detailed anatomic knowledge.

References

1. Mittleman G: Transverse plane abnormalities of the lower extremity. J Am Podiatr Assoc 1971; 61:1–7.
2. Yu GV, Wallace GF: Metatarsus adductus. *In* McGlamry ED (ed): Comprehensive Textbook of Foot Surgery, Vol. 2, Baltimore, Williams & Wilkins, 1987, pp. 327–351.
3. Heyman CH, Herndon CH, Strong JM: Mobilization of the tarsometatarsal and intermetatarsal joints for the correction of resistant adduction of the forefoot of the foot in congenital club foot or congenital metatarsus varus. J Bone Joint Surg 1958; 40A:299–310.
4. Thompson SA: Hallux varus and metatarsus varus. Clin Orthop 1960; 16:109.
5. Ghali NN, Abberton MJ, Silk FF: The management of metatarsus adductus et supinatus. J Bone Joint Surg 1984; 66B:376.
6. Lichtblau S: Section of the abductor hallucis tendon for correction of metatarsus varus deformity. Clin Orthop 1975; 110:227.
7. Sgarlato TF: A discussion of metatarsus adductus. Arch Podiatr Med Foot Surg 1973; 1:35.
8. Johnson JB: A preliminary report on chondrotemies. J Am Podiatr Assoc 1978; 68:808–813.
9. Saye CP: Congenital disorders. *In* Edmonsen AS, Crenshaw AH (eds): Campbell's Operative Orthopedics, 6th ed, Vol. 2. St. Louis, CV Mosby, 1980, pp. 1760–1763.
10. Bankart B: Metatarsus varus. Br Med J 1921; 2:685.
11. Ganley JV, Ganley TJ, Castellano BA: Metatarsus adductus: Neonatal management. *In* McGlamry ED (ed): Reconstructive Surgery of the Foot and Leg. Tucker, GA, Doctors Hospital Podiatry Institute Publications, 1989, pp. 219–229.
12. Peabody CW, Muro F: Congenital metatarsus varus. J Bone Joint Surg 1933; 15:171–189.
13. McCormick D, Blount WP: Metatarsus adductovarus. JAMA 1949; 141:449.
14. Fowler B, Brooks AL, Parrish TF: The cavo-varus foot. J Bone Joint Surg 1959; 41A:747–752.
15. Steytler JCS, Van der Walt ID: Correction of resistant adduction of the forefoot in congenital clubfoot and congenital metatarsus varus by metatarsal osteotomy. Br J Surg 1971; 53:558–560.
16. Berman A, Gartland JJ: Metatarsal osteotomy for the correction of adduction of the fore part of the foot in children. J Bone Joint Surg 1971; 53A:498–506.
17. Hara B, Beck CJ, Woo RA: First cuneiform closing abductory osteotomy for reduction of metatarsus primus adductus. J Foot Ankle Surg 1992; 31:434–439.
18. Benard MA: Treatment of skewfoot by multiple lesser tarsal osteotomies and calcaneal osteotomy. J Foot Ankle Surg 1990; 29:504–509.
19. Grumbine N: Cuboid osteotomy. Seminar lecture, Los Angeles, Baha Project, 1986; and personal communications, 1990 and 1994.
20. Ganley JV, Ganley TJ: Metatarsus adductus deformity. *In* McGlamry ED, Banks AS (eds): Comprehensive Textbook of Foot Surgery, 2nd ed, Vol. 1. Baltimore, Williams & Wilkins, 1992, pp. 829–852.

10

Juvenile Hallux Abducto Valgus

Richard M. Jay, D.P.M., and Elisa M. Kavanagh, D.P.M.

The etiology of juvenile hallux abducto valgus (HAV) does not have a single origin, and several elements have been suggested as predisposing to this disorder. In all of these theories there does exist one common thread—a biomechanical imbalance. The imbalance appears in all common presentations of neurologic disorders (cerebral palsy), flatfoot, metadductus, trauma, and ligament laxity. We realize that the alignment of the first metatarsophalangeal joint will be revised with any of these causes. The most important factor, however, is the understanding that no one procedure addresses the juvenile bunion alone. Biomechanic faults cause many variables along the first ray, and the appropriate procedure must be determined to avoid recurrence.

When selecting a procedure, the surgeon must determine the age of the child and the functional demands of the foot. The metatarsus adductus and the first intermetatarsal angle must be evaluated. The articular surface and the length of the first metatarsal must be determined. If one considers the hallux valgus to be either severe or mild and the first intermetatarsal angle to be less than or greater than 12 degrees, an appropriate procedure can be chosen. The four basic procedures that address correction

of the deformity are (1) first metatarsophalangeal joint soft tissue procedures, (2) first metatarsophalangeal joint soft tissue procedures with a proximal osteotomy, (3) proximal osteotomy, and (4) distal osteotomy.[1]

The child usually presents with a mild to moderate bump on the medial aspect of the first metatarsal head. This type of juvenile hallux valgus is stable. If the intermetatarsal and metadductus angle are increased, the hallux valgus angle increases, thus increasing the medial head deformity (Fig. 10–1). Chronic pain along with deformity are the indicators for surgery. Certainly cosmetic appearance plays a role, and this should be discussed openly with the parents prior to correction. Obviously, relief of pain, prevention of recurrence, and improvement in appearance are the three essential requirements for a successful outcome.

Basic surgical principles are followed in the correction of juvenile HAV. Surgery is performed at or near skeletal maturity at 11 to 15 years of age with correction of the metatarsus primus angle. The joint is preserved and should never be replaced. The sesamoid position may be in malalignment, but one should avoid sesamoidectomy. Restoration of joint alignment and reduction of the inter-

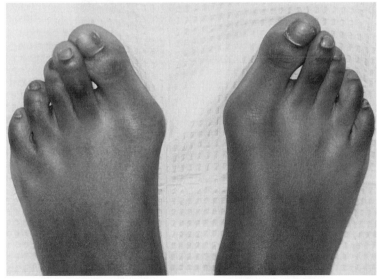

Figure 10–1. Ten-year-old child with juvenile hallux valgus. Moderate medial prominence with overriding of the second toe onto the first.

metatarsal angle prevent recurrence of the deformity. Add biomechanical control, and the likelihood of recurrence is markedly reduced.

SURGICAL PROCEDURES

Capsule Tendon Balance Procedures

These procedures have been recommended for the primary repair of juvenile HAV. However, joint alignment in the typical case of juvenile HAV is secondary to the biomechanical pull on the first toe. Simple realignment of the capsule and tendon usually is not enough to prevent recurrence. These procedures should be approached with caution in these children (Figs. 10–2 and 10–3 and Tables 10–1 to 10–3).

Epiphysiodesis

This procedure controls bone growth by arresting growth on one side of the epiphyseal plate. Compression on the lateral side allows medial bone growth and stimulates the metatarsal to grow in a lateral direction (see Chapter 11). Epiphysiodesis is indicated as an adjunctive procedure in cases of mild juvenile HAV with no significant increase in intermetatarsal angle. For females the best time for surgery is between the ages of 10 and 12, and in males the best age is from 12 to 14.

- Epiphysiodesis by bone graft. This is an irreversible technique. The amount of reduction achieved is usually inadequate for correction. Epiphysiodesis in this case is accomplished by inserting a bone graft into the lateral

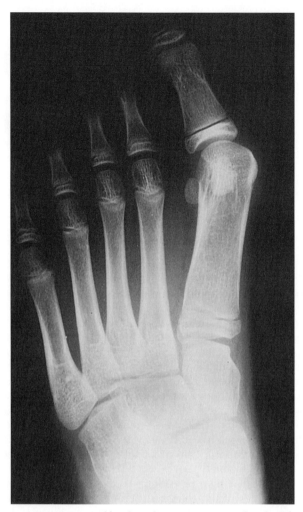

Figure 10–3. Ten-year-old with 10-degree intermetatarsal angle and 30-degree hallux abductus angle. Soft tissue corrections are indicated.

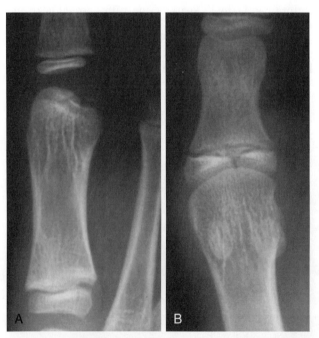

Figure 10–2. *A*, Bipartite base of proximal phalanx. *B*, Pseudoepiphysis of distal first metatarsal showing articular changes. Both conditions (in *A* and *B*) can yield an osseous deformity of the articular surface at either the base of the proximal phalanx or the head of the metatarsal.

aspect of the first metatarsal physis. Complications include a deformed first metatarsophalangeal joint that is irreversible.

- Epiphysiodesis by staple technique. This is a reversible technique. The results of this technique are not precise. Stapling is performed by placing the staple completely through the metatarsal physis from dorsal to plantar. This is important to prevent retardation of growth dorsolaterally, with potential dorsiflexion of the first ray.

Distal Osteotomies

These osteotomies are indicated for correction of mild to moderate increases in the intermetatarsal (IM) angle, an increased proximal articular set angle (PASA), and repositioning of the metatarsal over the sesamoid apparatus. These procedures are contraindicated when an open epiphysis is present at the metatarsal head (Tables 10–4 to 10–7).

Neck Osteotomies

These osteotomies are used to correct an increased PASA and also an increased IM angle.[4] The joint here is

Table 10–1. **Silver Procedure (1923)**

Radiology	Indications	Problems	Procedure	Postoperative Factors
All angles within normal limits ≤ 8	Bump pain Medial skin irritation Over first metatarsal head No sesamoid pain Neuritis	Recurrence Joint stiffness	Incision Linear capsulotomy Resect bump Closure	Surgical shoe Subcuticular nylon sutures Sneaker, 2–4 wk Early ROM exercises

Table 10–2. **McBride Procedure (1928)**

Radiology	Indications	Problems	Procedure	Postoperative Factors
IM angle of 9–10 degrees	Bump pain Pain associated with sesamoids, nerve pain, or bursitis	Hallux varus secondary to fibular sesamoid removal Recurrence Joint stiffness	Incision Dorsomedial linear capsulotomy Resect bump Adductor tendon and fibular sesamoid ligament release Excision of fibular sesamoids Adductor transfer Medial capsulorrhaphy Closure	Same as Table 10–1

Table 10–3. **Hiss Procedure (1931)**

Radiology	Indications	Problems	Procedure	Postoperative Factors
IM angle of < 12	Same as Table 10–2	Rare procedure Only procedure that uses abductor	Resect bump Dorsal transfer and advancement of abductor hallucis tendon to more dorsal, medial area	Same as Table 10–1

Table 10–4. **Reverdin Procedure (1881)**

Radiology	Indications	Complications	Procedure	Postoperative Factors
All angles within normal limits or up to 12 degrees Congruous joint Range of motion within normal limits	To reduce PASA deformity Reverdin with modified McBride	Possible sesamoid damage Avascular necrosis of metatarsal head Over/under correction Elevatus secondary to poor fixation	First cut proximal and parallel to articular cartilage Second cut made proximal to first cut Second cut perpendicular to shaft Wedge of bone removed Base of wedge medial to correct for PASA	Surgical shoe, 4 weeks Fixation remains for 4–6 wk Sneaker in 6–8 wk Early ROM exercises Physical therapy

PASA, proximal articular set angle

Table 10–5. **Reverdin/Green Procedure (1977)***

Radiology	Indications	Complications	Procedure	Postoperative Factors
PASA > 12–14 degrees IM ≤ 11 degrees	Corrects abnormal PASA Protects sesamoids and plantar articular cartilage	Elevatus Hallux varus Nonunion Sesamoiditis	Remove bump Plantar cut, medial lateral, parallel to ground starting at midportion of head Wedge cut to plantar shelf (lateral cortex intact) Medial capsulorrhaphy	Same as Table 10–4

*Distal-L and most stable of the Reverdin-type procedures. IM, intermetatarsal.

Table 10–6. **Reverdin/Laird Procedure (1977)**

Radiology	Indications	Complications	Procedure	Postoperative Factors
Corrects PASA and IM up to 12 degrees	Same as Table 10–5	Same as Table 10–5	Same as Table 10–5 Osteotomy cut through lateral cortex Capital fragment shifted laterally	Same as Table 10–4

Table 10–7. **Reverdin/Todd Procedure**

Radiology	Indications	Complications	Procedure	Postoperative Factors
Corrects increased PASA IM angle up to 12 degrees Elevatus component	Elevatus deformity Abnormal PASA	Avascular necrosis Over/under correction Sesamoid damage Disruption of plantar articular cartilage, which leads to degenerative joint disease	Wedge angled Proximal cut, proximal/plantar for correction of elevatus (plantar flexion of the head) Distal cut distal/plantar to correct dorsiflexion deformity	Same as Table 10–4

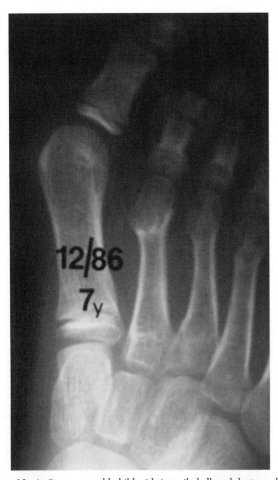

Figure 10–4. Seven-year-old child with juvenile hallux abductus valgus. The hallux abductus angle is 35 degrees. The intermetatarsal angle is less than 10 degrees. Note length pattern of metatarsals.

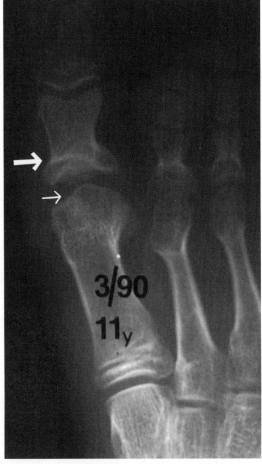

Figure 10–5. Postoperative Mitchell bunionectomy performed on child in Figure 10–4. Note that the intermetatarsal angle has decreased as well as the hallux abductus angle; however, due to the increase in pressure on the medial side, joint adaptation has occurred, yielding a deformation of the first metatarsal head.

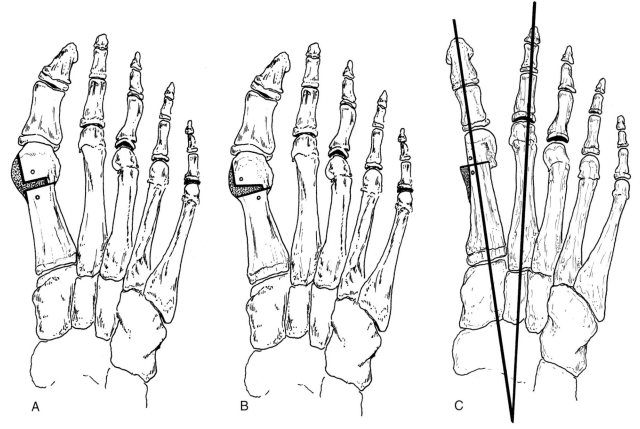

Figure 10-6. *A*, Mitchell osteotomy. Shaded area depicts the amount of bone resected. The head will shift laterally and drop approximately 2 to 3 mm, depending on the wedge removed. *B*, Mitchell osteotomy with angular cut needed to reduce proximal articular set angle. *C*, Completed position of Mitchell osteotomy with fixation and removal of medial eminence and ridge.

usually congruous or mildly deviated with a normal first metatarsophalangeal joint range of motion (Figs. 10–4 through 10–9 and Tables 10–8 to 10–13).

Base Osteotomies

Base osteotomies allow a significant degree of lateral shift and also carry the greatest risk of injury to the physis at the base of the first metatarsal. It is important to perform these procedures distal to the epiphysis. The three techniques that are commonly used are the closing base wedge osteotomy, the opening base wedge osteotomy, and the crescentic osteotomy (Figs. 10–10 and 10–11).

Opening Wedge Osteotomy of Medial Cuneiform

This procedure is indicated when a severe increase in the intermetatarsal angle is associated with an atavistic cuneiform. Radiologically, one should look for an intermetatarsal angle of greater than 18 degrees and an excessive obliquity of the metatarsocuneiform joint. The procedure consists of an initial incision between the extensor hallucis longus and the tibialis anterior tendons. This approach allows easy access to the medial cuneiform. It is important to reflect the tibialis anterior from its insertion on the medial cuneiform. The lateral cortex is left intact, and the osteotomy is wedged open medially. A bone graft is then inserted, preferably a bicortical cancellous graft that is fixated with a K-wire or staple. Common complications include lengthening of the first ray and jamming of the first metatarsophalangeal joint with hallux limitus. Osteotomies at the head may be performed in conjunction with this procedure to correct for a deviated PASA (Figs. 10–12 and 10–13 and Tables 10–14 to 10–16).

COMPLICATIONS

The main complication of juvenile bunions is that all too often they are neglected in the early stages, and it is not until the deformity becomes severe that attention is finally paid to this controllable and reducible problem. As the first metatarsal drifts medially from the retrograde force of the abducting proximal phalanx, an increase and a decrease in tension and compression take place at the metatarsal base. An increase in compression arises on the medial physis. While this medial metatarsal drift occurs, the lateral portion of the physis is pulled open, causing tension. Tension produces lateral metatarsal growth, and compression reduces medial growth. The result is a greater stimulus of growth of the first metatarsal, causing

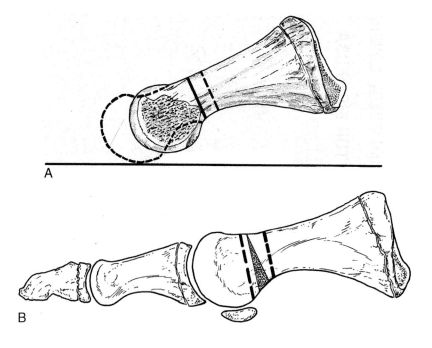

Figure 10–7. *A*, Lateral postoperative view of Mitchell osteotomy. Note elevation of metatarsal head due to the loss of 2 to 3 mm in this shift. *B*, By angulating the dorsal-plantar cut with the apex dorsally, plantarflexion of the first metatarsal can occur, eliminating the elevation of the first metatarsal head.

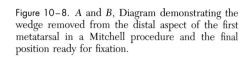

Figure 10–8. *A* and *B*, Diagram demonstrating the wedge removed from the distal aspect of the first metatarsal in a Mitchell procedure and the final position ready for fixation.

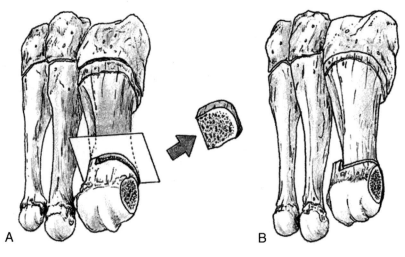

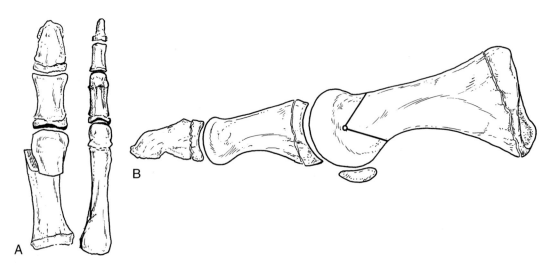

Figure 10–9. *A*, Austin chevron bunionectomy. Head of metatarsal is shifted laterally, reducing a mild intermetatarsal angle. *B*, Lateral view of first metatarsal with **V**-osteotomy of 60 degrees. Cut runs medial to lateral and head is shifted in a lateral direction. Austin chevron osteotomy.

Table 10–8. **Austin Procedure***

Radiology	Indications	Complications	Procedure	Postoperative Factors
Corrects IM angle of 12–14 degrees Normal or mildly increased PASA	IM angle of 12–14 degrees	Fracture of dorsal or plantar wing or metatarsal head Delayed union Nonunion AVN Hallux limitus Shortening Elevation of capital fragment Transfer metatarsalgia	Chevron V cut at 60 degrees with apex distal in center of imaginary circle on the medial aspect of the head Through and through cut and capital fragment shifted laterally to correct the IM angle Adductor release	Surgical shoe or slipper cast 4–6 wk, or until radiographic evidence of healing and patient comfort

*Most common and most stable. AVN, avascular necrosis

Table 10–9. **Bicorrectional Austin Procedure**

Radiology	Indications	Complications	Procedure	Postoperative Factors
IM of 12–14 degrees PASA of 12–14 degrees	Corrects moderately increased IM angle and moderately increased PASA	Same as mentioned in Table 10–8, but less stable and more difficult to perform Too much of medial wedge can cause adductus of the hallux	When making the V cut in the metatarsal head, go through 80% on top and 80% on bottom Take out wedge of bone for PASA Finish cut through and through Shift the metatarsal head over It continues to correct deformity	Same as Table 10–8

Table 10–10. **Tricorrectional Austin Procedure**

Radiology	Indications	Complications	Procedure	Postoperative Factors
IM of 12–14 degrees PASA of 12–14 degrees Need for plantar flexion	Corrects IM angle of 12–14 degrees and PASA of 12–14 degrees Corrects for plantar flexed first ray	Technically more difficult Too much of a medial wedge can cause adduction of hallux	Same as bicorrectional Austin with a tilted axis guide Apex bigger medially Plantar flex capital fragment	Same as Table 10–8

Table 10–11. **Kalish Procedure**

Radiology	Indications	Complications	Procedure	Postoperative Factors
IM of 12–15 degrees	Corrects for IM of 12–15 degrees No correction for PASA Screw fixation	Hallux varus possible due to greater degree of IM angle correction Allows for > 50% displacement Same as Table 10–10	Cut performed at 55 degrees Longer dorsal arm for fixation with 2.7-mm screws	Same as Table 10–8

Table 10–12. **Mitchell Procedure**

Radiology	Indications	Complications	Procedure	Postoperative Factors
IM of 12–16 degrees PASA of 12–16 degrees	Do this procedure only with long first metatarsal	Shortening of metatarsal (4–5 mm) Joint stiffness AVN	Rectangular wedge taken out Leave spicule laterally Capital fragment shifted laterally to correct IM angle Distal cut leaves lateral cortex Proximal cut is through and through Head shifted laterally, off stepdown shaft	Same as Table 10–8

Table 10–13. **Hohmann Procedure**

Radiology	Indications	Complications	Procedure	Postoperative Factors
IM of 12–14 degrees PASA of 12–15 degrees	Same as the Mitchell procedure	Same as the Mitchell procedure	Resect bump Trapezoidal wedge at metatarsal neck Cut through lateral cortex Capital fragment shifted laterally to correct for increased IM To correct PASA, angle transverse cut parallel to the articular cartilage	Same as Table 10–8

it to drift farther in the medial direction, increasing the intermetatarsal angle.[2] Early intervention to reduce the increased intermetatarsal angle and juvenile bunion formation reduces both the medial compressive force and the lateral tension. These forces are converted on the medial side to a tension force and on the lateral side to a compressive force. Reversing the forces on the physis decreases and eliminates the possibility of recurrence. Simple bunion procedures in children with an increasing intermetatarsal angle are contraindicated as the deforming force continues to adduct the first metatarsal. The newly distributed forces will be present after any of the intermetatarsal reducing angle procedures, and new bone growth will continue in the proper direction pending control of subtalar and midtarsal joints in their neutral position.

Shortening of the Metatarsal

Probably the most common of all complications seen with surgical correction of the juvenile bunion is shortening of the metatarsal. This can be secondary to interference in growth at the physis of the first metatarsal base. Base wedge osteotomies and epiphysiodesis are usually responsible. The shortening that results from physeal damage is unpredictable in nature and is unintentional. There are procedures that are designed to reduce the intermetatarsal angle at the cost of shortening the metatarsal. Any osteotomy, other than opening and crescentic osteotomies, has the effect of shortening the metatarsal. The Mitchell step-down osteotomy probably results in the greatest obvious shortening effect, the chevron and base wedge osteotomies to a lesser degree. When the first metatarsal is shorter than the second, the choice of a metatarsal shortening procedure is ill advised, and the surgeon should consider a length maintenance procedure, possibly the crescentic osteotomy as described in Chapter 7.

The shortening of the first metatarsal that occurs after osteotomies is not necessarily the result of direct damage to the physis. With overzealous dissection of the periosteum to expose the osteotomy site, indirect injury to the physis can occur. When performing the osteotomy it is not

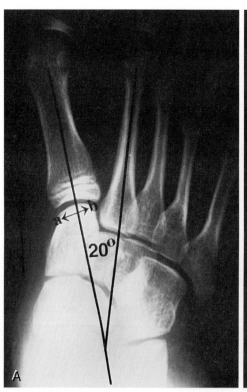
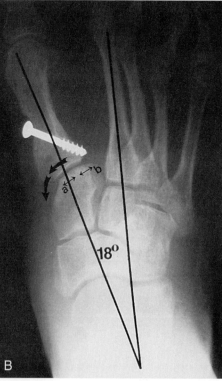

Figure 10–10. *A,* Twenty-degree intermetatarsal angle showing arced medial and distal articular surface of cuneiform. *B,* Closing base wedge osteotomy of first metatarsal. Alignment of first metatarsal is reduced; however, because the arc of the cuneiform was not addressed, the resultant decrease in the intermetatarsal angle was minimal.

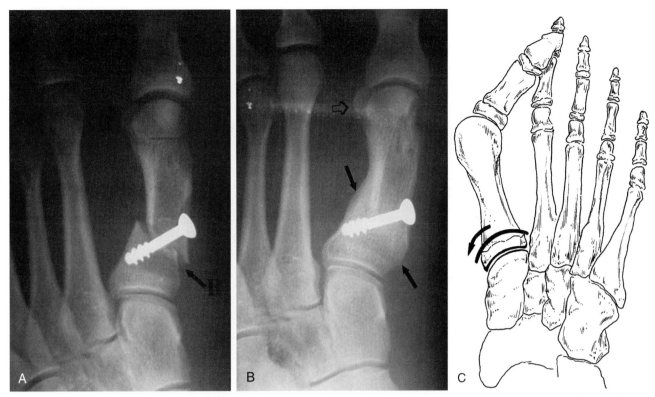

Figure 10–11. *A*, Postoperative juvenile hallux valgus deformity with shortening secondary to closing base wedge osteotomy. The medial cortex has been lost and has receded proximally. A marked shortening of the first metatarsal resulted with increased pressure on the second metatarsal. Outlined arrow depicts location of sesamoid at the articulation of the first metatarsal phalangeal joint. *B*, Immediate postoperative radiograph of fractured medial cortex along with distal osteotomy. The net result was shortening of the first metatarsal. *C*, Arced distal cuneiform articulation to metatarsal base with an increase in the medial arc. The first metatarsal can shift medially, increasing the intermetatarsal angle.

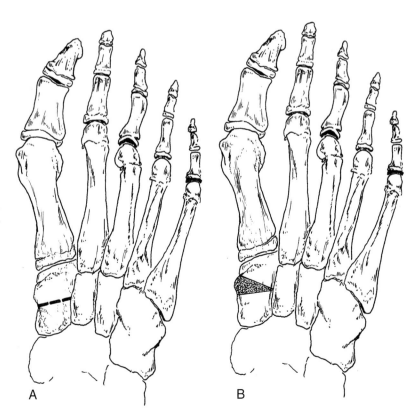

Figure 10–12. *A* and *B*, Opening wedge cuneiform osteotomy with bone implanted, reducing the distal angle of the metatarsal cuneiform joint.

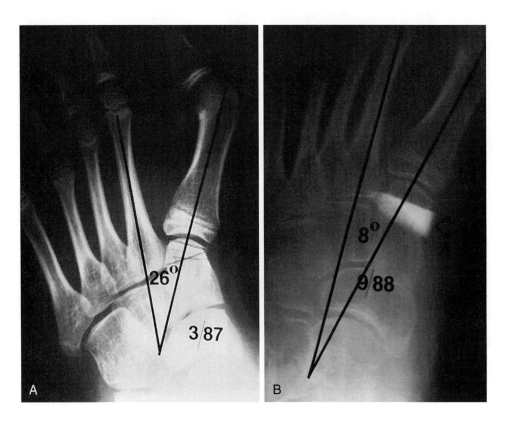

Figure 10–13. *A*, Preoperative radiograph of child with an intermetatarsal angle of 26 degrees and a hallux abductus angle of 40 degrees. The distal articular surface of the cuneiform is arced medially. A cuneiform opening wedge osteotomy was planned. *B*, Postoperative change in cuneiform that reduces the distal articular set of the cuneiform. The net result was a reduction in the metatarsal primus adductus angle.

Table 10–14. **Closing Base Wedge Osteotomy Procedure (1901)***

Radiology	Indications	Complications	Procedure	Postoperative Factors
IM of > 15 degrees No correction for PASA	Severe bunions IM of > 15 degrees	Fracture of medial cortex Elevation Nonunion Hallux limitus More shortening than oblique osteotomy but more stable	Make initial bone cut proximal Second cut distal and angled Wedge removed Keep medial cortex intact Fixate with two cross K-wires or screws	Nonweightbearing for 6 wk in below knee cast or slipper cast Partial/total weightbearing for 2 wk in cast Soft cast 1–2 wk Surgical shoe Sneaker

*Transverse cut, distal to the epiphysis.

Table 10–15. **Closing Base Wedge Osteotomy Juvara***

Radiology	Indications	Complications	Procedure	Postoperative Factors
IM angle ≥ 15 degrees No correction for PASA	Same as Table 10–14 Allows a smaller wedge to be removed	Same as Table 10–14 Less stable	Distal cut is first at 30 degrees Proximal cut at 45 degrees Cut made obliquely Screws placed perpendicular to the osteotomy site in lag fashion Base laterally Apex medial, leaving medial cortex intact First screw, compression Second screw, anchor Perpendicular to the cortex	Same as Table 10–14

*Oblique cut distal to the epiphysis.

Table 10–16. **Crescentic Procedure**

Radiology	Indications	Complications	Procedure	Postoperative Factors
IM of ≥ 18 degrees	High IM angle	Causes little shortening Difficult to fixate Elevatus Possible trauma to physis	Half moon cut peformed upon which metatarsal head swiveled Medial surface higher than lateral surface	Same as Table 10–14

advisable to locate the physis by reflecting the periosteum because this can damage the outer rim of the physis and arrest growth. The extent of shortening depends on the dissection about the physis and on the age of the child.

The periosteum in the child is much thicker and is easily reflected around the metatarsal shaft. Normally, in the adult, periosteal dissection is carried proximally until the shiny white fibers of Sharpey are noted. This is the beginning of the ligamentous attachment to the cuneiforms and is noted at the most proximal rise in the base of the first metatarsal. This is not the case in the child, in whom the ligamentous attachment from the cuneiform to the base of the first metatarsal is continuous with the thick periosteum. By the time the surgeon realizes he is at the proximal base and at the attachment of the ligament, the physis has already been passed and disturbed.[3]

It is recommended that if the surgeon is not clear about the presence or location of the physis, the surgeon should order a radiograph. In this manner the surgeon can visualize the physis and measure the distance of the physis to an established landmark. It is strongly advised that the surgeon refrain from inserting a needle to probe for the physis because this will create an insult to the outer zone of the physis and retard growth.

If the first metatarsal is shortened, the child's weight is now transfered to the lesser metatarsals. With young children this has not been a complaint; however, long-term sequelae of a short first and a longer second metatarsal can occur. The use of an orthosis to transfer weight back to the first metatarsal is mandatory, and further surgical procedures to either lengthen the first metatarsal or shorten the lesser metatarsals should not be considered until the child expresses pain or the appearance of lesions is noted.

Complications with Metatarsal Head Osteotomies

The Mitchell and chevron-type osteotomies are indicated for the reduction of a moderate intermetatarsal angle, no greater than 14 degrees, and yield excellent results with or without fixation. A major complication of concern is the possibility of partial or total avascular necrosis of the metatarsal head. Dissection is kept to a minimum, but the risk of an avascular head remains. In addition, in both procedures, the head is doomed to failure if it is not approximated on the metatarsal shaft properly and not secured. The head will either rotate off the shaft, yielding a gross malposition of the articular surface, or fail to develop proper union (nonunion, delayed union). Because the retrograde force of the proximal phalanx provides a reparative force for union, it can

also provide a postoperative deforming force. Consideration of the method of fixation is strongly recommended to minimize these complications. Absorbable pins (Johnson and Johnson, Orthopedics, Raynham, Mass.)[1] was used successfully in the fixations of chevron procedures in children. This absorbable pin is designed to prevent shear force between bones. The pins are placed obliquely to one another and are cut along the surface of the bone or cartilage pending placement. External pin fixation provides good approximation of the bone fragments but adds an additional complication in that it must be removed. In a child this can be a complicated process. Absorbable screws and stainless steel screws are also possible methods of fixation. Care must be taken to avoid disruption of the cartilage.

When performing the Mitchell or chevron osteotomy, one has the advantage not only of reducing the adduction of the first metatarsal through the osteotomy, but also of accomplishing soft tissue correction about the first metatarsophalangeal joint through the same incision. One of the major advantages of this procedure is its distance from the epiphysis at the base of the first metatarsal. The procedure does carry the complication of excessive shortening of the first metatarsal. Since the Mitchell osteotomy is a step-down procedure, certain length is lost. Through this shortening, the head is actually placed in a more dorsal position and weight is transferred to the second metatarsal, which can lead to future metatarsalgia and callus formation. The recommendation made with the Mitchell procedure is to plantar-flex the head when securing it to the shaft or to translate the head plantarly. In doing so, one can preserve the metatarsal weight-bearing parabola.

Another complication of the Mitchell procedure is that of possibly inadequate fixation of the distal fragment to the shaft (see Figs. 10–6 to 10–9). As described in the early literature, fixation is performed with suture or wire. This can result in breakage, or, since the dorsal hinge is the only area fixed, the result may be a dorsiflexed metatarsal head position. If one opts to immobilize this foot for too long a period, a stiffening of the joint does occur. For this reason, one should consider rigid fixation with either screw or pin. Screw fixation not only provides compression but also allows for earlier ambulation with a diminishing risk of joint stiffness.

The Mitchell osteotomy provides adequate results in the treatment of adolescent hallux valgus. Though the intermetatarsal angle correction is almost uniformly maintained, the incidence of recurrence of the hallux valgus deformity is high. Subjectively, metatarsalgia does not appear to be a problem in this age group, but the prevalence of second metatarsal head callosities is worrisome. The procedure may not provide adequate correction in patients with severe metatarsus primus varus and may lead to recurrence of both metatarsus primus varus and hallux valgus.[4]

CLOSING BASE METATARSAL OSTEOTOMIES

In a closing base wedge osteotomy or crescentic osteotomy of the first metatarsal, one should take care when approaching the physis. One must avoid extensive subperiosteal dissection in trying to locate the physis, since this will in fact damage the physis and create long-term sequelae. To reduce the risk of epiphyseal arrest with possible shortening of the first metatarsal, one should avoid periosteal stripping proximal to the osteotomy needed. This can be accomplished easily by taking a 27-gauge needle and gently approaching the metatarsal cuneiform joint and then moving distally to isolate the physis. Gentle handling of the periosteum can identify this epiphyseal line. The osteotomy site should be prepared distal to this physeal line. This will certainly reduce the risk of shortening because there will be no damage to the epiphysis.

CRESCENTIC OSTEOTOMY

If the metatarsus primus deformity is considered to be a transverse plane osseous deformity, the deformity must be addressed at the base of the first metatarsal. The adducted position exists in relation to the second metatarsal. When the deformity is resistant or the metatarsal is mature, surgical intervention with base wedge osteotomy is indicated. A crescentic osteotomy allows rotation at the crescentic cut, which allows the metatarsal to abduct on the transverse plane on a single axis with maximal bone contact.[2]

The advent of the crescentic blade permitted performance of an osteotomy that alleviated the problems associated with closing wedge osteotomies. The crescentic osteotomy is a procedure that is acceptable for simultaneously reducing the adducted metatarsal and maintaining the metatarsal length. The standard surgical technique for performing the crescentic osteotomy is relatively simple. Appropriate soft tissue dissection and preservation of the vital structures are much more tedious than the actual osteotomy itself. An inherent weakness of this osteotomy is the position of the cut, which is unstable in the frontal plane. Translation of the entire metatarsal can occur at the osteotomy site in the direction of dorsiflexion/plantar flexion. A similar drift of the metatarsal can cause the entire base to shift medially or laterally.[5]

Modification of the crescentic osteotomy of the base is achieved very simply to prevent drift and translation. The osteotomy is modified so that the cut is made with the crescentic blade angulated and rotated medially. The apex of the blade is positioned laterally off center to the metatarsal base. One of the most important effects of the angulated crescentic osteotomy is the intrinsic bolstering effect produced by the high medial lip on the medial side of the base. This lip of bone acts as a significant counter-force to any medially directed forces at the osteotomy site.[6] Tachdjian believes that this bolstering effect is useful when one is correcting for metatarsus adductus.[7] A shelf of bone protrudes medially into the adjacent soft tissue at the proximal cut in the shaft after the metatarsal has been manipulated into an abducted position. Manual displacement reduces the metatarsus primus adductus angle and maintains more bone-to-bone contact than does the conventional transversely placed crescentic osteotomy. Since the angulated cut is made with the medial surface higher than the lateral surface, the metatarsal is also effectively lengthened when the shaft is abducted. Because the rotation takes place in an arc, the loss of bone length secondary to the width of the osteotomy blade is prevented; length is gained because of the geometry of the cut.

Healing potential is markedly increased when this operation is performed in the proximal region of the metatarsal. If the osteotomy is performed too distally in the presence of more cortical bone and less cancellous bone, an increase in callus formation may result. In addition, a vascular insult could be initiated in the vulnerable diaphyseal blood supply, causing a possible delay in healing with the potential of nonunion.

The proximal aspect of the first metatarsal base is meticulously dissected because the epiphysis is approximately 1 cm from the metatarsocuneiform joint. The osteotomy is made another 1 to 1.5 cm proximal to the epiphysis. The epiphysis can be identified in the young child by the pale blue color that contrasts with the white bone. The periosteum is reflected carefully off all the metatarsal bases and closed after the osteotomies have been made. This minimizes large bone callus and possible intermetatarsal bone fusions. All osteotomies are made in the proximal segment to maximize reduction and increase the healing potential of the metatarsal.

Pin fixation of the proximal osteotomy is performed with a single smooth K-wire inserted through the first metatarsal to the middle cuneiform. Proper alignment and reduction of the metatarsal base is most important. The buttress effect helps in stabilization. For this reason, good visualization of the osteotomy site is mandatory. Once the pin is in place and the incision has been closed, a well-molded cast is applied. The foot is immobilized for at least 6 weeks.

References

1. Kenzora JE: Orthopedics 1988; 11:777–789.
2. Luba R, Rosman M: Bunions in children. J Pediatr Orthop 1984; 4:44–47.
3. Holden D, Siff S, Butler J. Cain T: Shortening of the first metatarsal as a complication of metatarsal osteotomies. J Bone Joint Surg 1984; 66A:582–587.
4. Canale PB, Aronsson DD, Lamont RL, Manoli A: The Mitchell procedure for treatment of adolescent hallux valgus. J Bone Joint Surg 1993; 75A:1610–1618.
5. Berman A, Gartland JJ.: Metatarsal osteotomy for the correction of adduction of the forepart of the foot in children. J Bone Joint Surg 1971; 53A:498.
6. Jay RM, Schoenhaus HD, Donohue CM: A modified crescentic osteotomy in children. J Foot Surg, 1990; 29:417–420.
7. Tachdjian MO: Pediatric Orthopedics. Philadelphia, W. B. Saunders, 1972, p. 1340.

11

Epiphysiodesis for Juvenile Hallux Abducto Valgus

Michael Seiberg, D.P.M., Richard M. Green, D.P.M., and Donald R. Green, D.P.M.

Juvenile hallux abducto valgus can be a painful deformity and a cosmetic concern in the developing child. Genetic and pathomechanical factors play an important role in its progression because often we see similar deformities in both the parents and siblings. Conservative treatment such as shoe gear changes, anti-inflammatory drugs, padding, and orthotics, although initially attempted, may provide only temporary relief of symptoms and fail to correct the deformity. As practitioners we know that structural deformities, if left untreated, tend to become more severe during development. It would seem logical to use the body's own growth potential during the developing years to aid in correcting a juvenile bunion deformity.

Many approaches to the treatment of juvenile hallux abducto valgus have been described. Unfortunately, modified McBride bunionectomies, if used alone, have been reported to have less than favorable long-term results for the treatment of this condition.[1, 2] Some authorities advise waiting until skeletal maturity and closure of the first metatarsal growth plate have occurred before addressing the deformity surgically.[1, 2] This is especially true in feet with high intermetatarsal angles, which traditionally may require a proximal first metatarsal osteotomy. Others argue that earlier treatment is more effective and advocate osteotomies distal to the first metatarsal growth plate. Epiphysiodesis of the first metatarsal growth plate can provide earlier correction and adaptation of developing osseous and soft tissue structures. In feet with larger intermetatarsal angles, epiphysiodesis can allow the body to "correct itself" with time, thus preventing the need for true first metatarsal base osteotomies, which often require a lengthy and inconvenient nonweight-bearing status.

INDICATIONS AND TIMING

Epiphyseal arrest of the lateral first metatarsal growth plate may be accomplished by a variety of methods including the use of monofilament wire, trephine bone autograft, and staples.[3–6] Staples seem to be the most logical because they are simple to insert and can be removed should overcorrection occur. Possible complications of using staples include bending of the staple, breaking, and irritation.

Epiphysiodesis of the first metatarsal base using staples is reserved for juvenile hallux abducto valgus deformity with a metatarsus primus adductus. Proper timing of the procedure is critical. The goal of the procedure is to limit bone growth on the lateral aspect of the first metatarsal base while allowing growth to continue medially, thus reducing the intermetatarsal angle during skeletal development. Epiphysiodesis performed too early can lead to overcorrection of the intermetatarsal angle, whereas performing it too late can result in undercorrection. In general, this procedure can be performed in children aged 9 to 14. Epiphyseal stapling can usually be performed earlier in the age range in females than in males owing to the earlier skeletal maturity of females.

Although epiphyseal stapling generally can be performed in children aged 9 to 14, it is more important to evaluate the patient's skeletal age than his or her chronologic age. A pedal radiographic atlas is required for this evaluation. One such atlas is Hoerr, Pyle, and Francis' *Radiographic Atlas of Skeletal Development of the Foot and Ankle.*[7] By comparing the patient's radiographs to selected maturity indicators in the atlas, the physician can determine the skeletal age. Estimation of skeletal age by radiographic comparison has been shown to be both reliable and reproducible.[8]

Once the child's skeletal age has been determined, the remaining linear growth potential of the first metatarsal must be estimated. This is accomplished by referencing a growth prediction chart. Several of these charts are available, but the most useful of them is the one devised by Nelson. Nelson's growth chart allows the physician specifically to determine the remaining first metatarsal linear growth. If the skeletal age of the patient is known, one can estimate the percentage of remaining growth by referencing Nelson's chart.[9]

PREOPERATIVE PLANNING

Certain considerations are essential in the preoperative planning for an epiphysiodesis procedure:

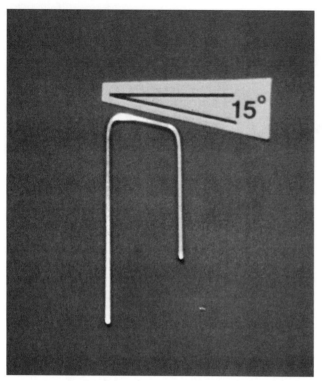

Figure 11–1. Staple fabricated with 15-degree incline to approximate declination of first metatarsal.

1. The physician must determine how much correction of the intermetatarsal angle is required to reduce the deformity. One good technique is the use of preoperative cutout templates as described by Gerbert.[10] The metatarsal is outlined on tracing paper. The metatarsal distal to the growth plate is cut along the outline. The area of the physis (growth plate) is cut from medial to lateral, leaving only the lateral proximal hinge intact. The distal metatarsal is shifted to the desired position, thus reducing the intermetatarsal angle. One then measures the medial gap created just distal to the physis. This gap is the ideal amount of growth that must occur medially, without growth laterally, to correct the metatarsus primus adductus deformity.

2. The physician must then determine the skeletal age of the patient by referring to a pedal radiographic atlas as previously mentioned.

3. The skeletal age is used to estimate the remaining growth potential of the developing first metatarsal. Nelson's growth potential chart of the first metatarsal can be used for this purpose. Nelson's chart provides a percentage of remaining growth of the first metatarsal. By measuring the length of the patient's first metatarsal and multiplying this number by the percentage shown on Nelson's chart, the amount of potential growth in millimeters is determined. This amount of future potential growth is compared with the amount of medial physeal growth needed (which was found by using Gerbert's template technique) for final correction of the intermetatarsal angle.

4. Next, the length of the patient's first metatarsal is measured, and this value is multiplied by the percentage of growth remaining that was determined in step 3. This is the amount of potential linear growth, in millimeters, that is available during skeletal development by adding length to the first metatarsal.

5. The amount of medial growth needed for correction (step 1) is compared with the potential linear growth of the first metatarsal (step 4).

Ideally, the amount of growth needed should be the same as the amount of growth remaining. Epiphysiodesis performed too early can lead to overcorrection of the intermetatarsal angle, whereas performing it too late can result in undercorrection. However, as a practical matter, epiphysiodesis should be performed a little earlier rather than later; we have not experienced any overcorrection in our series. Usually some small amount of undercorrection occurs based on what was actually estimated.

Other factors can alter bone growth and may influence the final outcome of the procedure. The stature of both parents should be considered. Uncontrolled ongoing biomechanical forces can influence the developing bones.

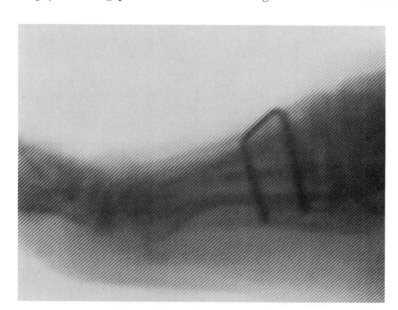

Figure 11–2. Staple should not protrude too far plantarly to avoid irritation.

Although we have not seen any overcorrection in our series, overgrowth of metatarsals has occurred in patients with von Recklinghausen's neurofibromatosis, arteriovenous aneurysms, fractures, and congenital hypertrophy disorders. Diminished bone growth has been shown to occur with pseudohypoparathyroidism and pseudopseudohypoparathyroidism, physeal plate trauma, infection, and Ollier's disease.[9] A detailed preoperative history and physical examination are therefore important.

Rarely is epiphysiodesis performed as an isolated procedure. Younger patients with a more mild deformity may simply require lateral release of the first metatarsophalangeal joint in addition to the stapling procedure. Patients with a more severe deformity may require other procedures such as a modified McBride bunionectomy. As with any foot surgery, all deforming forces need to be addressed and will vary from patient to patient. Functional foot orthoses should be used at least until adulthood.

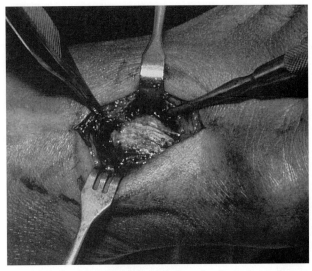

Figure 11–3. Epiphysis identified distal to the first metatarsal-cuneiform joint.

TECHNIQUE

The staples used for the epiphysiodesis procedure can be fabricated preoperatively by bending a 0.062-inch Kirschner wire into the proper shape, usually 10 to 12 mm in width. A smooth wire allows easy removal, although this is seldom necessary. Allowing a 15-degree angle in the staple from proximal to distal will help keep the staple flush on the dorsum of the first metatarsal and help minimize dorsal irritation (Fig. 11–1). The staple is placed on the lateral aspect of the first metatarsal base crossing the growth plate. The vertical arms of the staple are excessively long initially and are cut to the proper length intraoperatively.

The epiphyseal stapling procedure is performed through a 3- to 4-cm dorsolinear incision made over the lateral base of the first metatarsal between the extensor hallucis longus and extensor hallucis brevis tendons. The incision is deepened down to the level of the periosteum, which is incised linearly and reflected, thus exposing the physis (growth plate). It is important to properly identify the physis at this time because the staple must not penetrate into the first metatarsocuneiform joint nor enter the physeal plate.

Once the physis has been appreciated, a 0.062-inch K-wire is inserted proximally in a dorsal to plantar direction in the center of the lateral aspect of the epiphysis parallel to the first metatarsocuneiform articulation. A second 0.062-inch K-wire is then inserted distally from dorsal to plantar parallel to the first K-wire and at a precalculated distance that is equal to the width of the desired staple in the lateral metaphysis. These wires should be placed at the lateral 25% of the epiphysis and metaphysis. It is important for the two K-wires to be parallel to the first metatarsocuneiform joint and to each other. Proper position and length of the two K-wires can be determined with anteroposterior (AP) and lateral intraoperative radiographs or with fluoroscopy. The K-wires should just penetrate the plantar cortex of the first metatarsal. The K-wires are marked, and their lengths are measured. These measurements are compared with preoperative measurements of the lateral aspect of the first metatarsal base area. The long arms of the staple are cut to the appropriate length as measured by the K-wires. The K-wires are then removed and the 0.062 inch staple is inserted. The periosteum is then closed over the staple, and the soft tissues are closed in anatomic layers.

When performing the epiphyseal stapling procedure, one must be concerned that the staples cross both the dorsal and plantar cortices. Failure to cross the plantar cortex could result in plantar bone growth at the physis and could lead to a metatarsus primus elevatus deformity. The staple must be placed subperiosteally to help prevent dorsal dislocation. The long arms of the staple must cross the physeal plate, parallel to the physis and to each other. The staples must not penetrate the plate, joint, or lateral cortex. Finally, the staple arms should not be too long or plantar irritation may occur (Figs. 11–2 to 11–5).

Immediate weight bearing with a surgical shoe is allowed along with rest, ice, compression, and elevation following the epiphysiodesis procedure. Activity, however, should be limited for 4 to 5 weeks. Sutures are generally

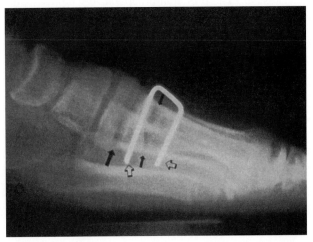

Figure 11–4. Staple position on 2-week postoperative radiograph.

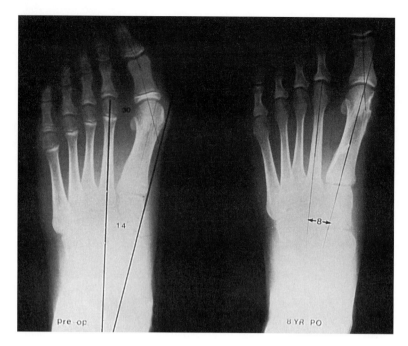

Figure 11–5. Eight-year postoperative view. There is a 6-degree decrease in the first intermetatarsal angle.

removed in 8 to 12 days. Orthotic control is mandatory shortly after the surgery to control deforming forces on the first ray that are almost always present. Hallux splinting with an interdigital foam spacer is usually continued for 3 to 4 months after surgery. Hallux night splints are used until the child reaches skeletal maturity. Regular follow-up is needed until physeal closure is obtained; the length of time will depend on the skeletal age of the patient at the time of surgery.

The staples do not need to be removed unless they become dislodged or cause irritation, or overcorrection of the intermetatarsal angle occurs. Other possible complications include improper placement or prominence of the staples, bending or breaking of the staples, inadequate bone growth available to reduce the intermetatarsal angle, overcorrection of the intermetatarsal angle, metatarsus primus elevatus, infection, and neurapraxia. Careful perioperative planning and accurate skeletal age estimates will help to minimize these complications.

Our study of nine children (15 feet) demonstrated good results.[6] The prevalent preoperative symptoms were significantly reduced postoperatively. The intermetatarsal angle decreased an average of 6.6 degrees (initial decrease was 2.7 degrees with an additional 3.9 degrees occurring over time). The hallux abducto valgus angle decreased an average of 19.6 degrees (initial decrease 10.7 degrees with an additional 8.9 degrees occurring over time). The continued improvement in the correction of the deformities is due to the dynamic nature of the procedure. These procedures were performed in conjunction with orthotic control in an attempt to neutralize the ongoing biomechanical forces. Our results are especially encouraging when one realizes that juvenile hallux abducto valgus deformities are often associated with very significant pronatory forces.

SUMMARY

Epiphyseal stapling, therefore, should be considered for juvenile hallux abducto valgus with a concomitant metatarsus primus adductus. Its greatest advantage is that the physician can use the patient's own growth potential to help correct a structural deformity. Appropriate timing of the procedure is critical, and attention should be focused on skeletal age rather than the patient's chronologic age. Preoperative templates are helpful in determining the amount of correction needed. Ancillary bunion procedures with appropriate release of tight lateral structures usually are also required.

References

1. Gebuhr P, Soelberg M, Larsen T, Niclasen B, Laursen N: McBride's operation for hallux valgus can be used in patients older than 30 years. J Foot Surg 1992; 31:241–243.
2. Helal B: Surgery for adolescent hallux valgus. Clin Orthop Rel Res 1981; 157:50–63.
3. Ellis V: A method of correcting metatarsus primus varus. J Bone Joint Surg 1951; 33B:415–417.
4. Fox IM, Smith SD: Juvenile bunion correction by epiphysiodesis of the first metatarsal. J Am Podiatr Assoc 1983; 73:448–455.
5. Marcinko D, Field N, Bryan G: Epiphysiodesis: An adjunctive surgical technique. J Am Podiatr Med Assoc 1985; 75:11.
6. Seiberg M, Green R, Green D: Epiphysiodesis in juvenile hallux abducto valgus—a preliminary retrospective study. J Am Podiatr Med Assoc 1994; 84:225–236.
7. Hoerr NL, Pyle SI, Francis CC: Radiographic Atlas of Skeletal Development of the Foot and Ankle. Springfield, IL, Charles C Thomas, 1962.
8. Graham CB: Assessment of bone maturation—methods and pitfalls. Radiol Clin North Am 1972; 10:185–202.
9. Nelson JP: Mechanical arrest of bone growth for the correction of pedal deformities. J Foot Surg 1981; 20:14–16.
10. Gerbert J: The indications and techniques for utilizing preoperative templates in podiatric surgery. J Am Podiatr Assoc 1979; 9:139–145.

12

Polydactyly

Richard M. Jay, D.P.M.

Polydactyly is a developmental anomaly in which supernumerary digits are present in the hands and/or feet. Characteristically, there is tremendous individual variation in each case. The location, anatomic configuration, and association with other anomalies and deformities are variable components.

Investigators classify polydactyly as a relatively common developmental abnormality. Ivy[1] found polydactyly to be the most common congential anomaly in nonwhites, occurring in a ratio of 1 to 258 live births, compared to 1 in 3985 in whites. Sesgin and Stark reviewed the records of all viable newborn infants in a 10-year period in a New York hospital and found that polydactyly was the seventh most common deformity.[2] It occurred in 1 in 713 births and was twice as frequent in nonwhites.[3] In his discussion of polydactyly of the foot, Venn-Watson,[4] reported an equal incidence in males and females and a 50% bilateral presentation. Interestingly, 33% of the cases cited involved polydactyly of the hand, and there was an overall incidence of 10% syndactyly. Wood,[5] discussing the treatment of central polydactyly of the hand, found a 36% incidence of associated anomalies of the feet. These consisted, for the most part, of syndactyly and polydactyly.

While no absolute statement can be made concerning the etiology of polydactyly, certainly there is strong evidence supporting hereditary transmission.[6-8] Much has been written on the hereditary aspect of polydactyly. Gillman and colleagues reported in 1948 and again in 1951 on the effects of tryphan blue in producing various congential anomalies in rats.[9] The researchers concluded that while there may be a simple dominant gene, polydactylism is often controlled by a recessive gene with incomplete entrance. Hedgekati[10] described a closely intermarried family in India consisting of 46 members, of which 23 had deformed hands.

Certainly the association of polydactyly with syndromes due to rare chromosomal aberrations lends credence to the theory of genetic transmission. Titles such as "Postaxial polydactyly, hallux duplication, absence of corpus callosum, macroencephaly and severe mental retardation: A new syndrome?" are representative of this theory.[11-13] The chromosomal aberrations and congenital abnormalities with which polydactyly is associated most frequently include Down's syndrome, congenital scoliosis plus clubfoot, congenital dislocated hip, trisomy 21, and trisomy 13 and 18. Classification of polydactyly may be discussed in terms of anatomic and etiologic criteria. Anatomic guidelines provide a simpler and more coherent system of classification than is possible with etiologic criteria.

Turek[14] classified polydactyly into three main anatomic types: *Type I* is a redundant soft tissue mass that is nonadherent to skeletal structures and is frequently devoid of bones, joints, tendons, or cartilage. *Type II* represents duplication of a digit or part of a digit that has normal components but articulates with a hypertrophic or bifid metacarpal or phalanx. *Type III* is considered rare and consists of a complete digit with its own metacarpal and all the necessary soft tissue.[15]

Temtamy and McKusick categorize polydactyly as an isolated anomaly or part of a syndrome.[16] Within this major group, polydactyly was classified as either preaxial or postaxial. Preaxial refers to the radial or tibial side of a line bisecting the long axis of the third finger or the second toe. Postaxial indicates that the deformity is present on the fibular or ulnar side of these lines.[17] There are rare cases of crossed polydactyly involving postaxial polydactyly of the hands with preaxial polydactyly of the feet (type I, crossed) or preaxial hand polydactyly and postaxial feet duplication (type II, crossed).

DISCUSSION AND SUMMARY

Surgery of polydactyly of the hand recognizes the complex nature and function of this highly specialized mobile appendage. Relatively little attention, however, has been devoted to surgical management and planning in cases of polydactyly of the foot. While similarities in the surgical approach toward polydactyly of the hands and feet do exist, essential structural and dynamic differences cannot be ignored.

The considerable weight-bearing function of the foot and the resultant transmission and distribution of force are of utmost importance. The ability to wear conventional shoes, the prevention of future deformity, and cosmetic appearance are also important criteria. Polydactyly and polymetatarsia are typically diagnosed and treated in early childhood. The unusual appearance of the affected part elicits immediate parental attention and physician diagnosis.

Correction of the polydactyly or polymetatarsia must take into account the structure, function, and cosmetic appearance. An extra toe or metatarsal joint may be easily removed, but a new function will now be present in the foot. Not only the width of the foot will be altered but also the weight-bearing shifts on the metatarsal heads. Mechanical alterations of the tendinous insertion also occur. Proper assessment of the tendon involved and metatarsal weight distribution is paramount (Figs. 12–1 to 12–7).

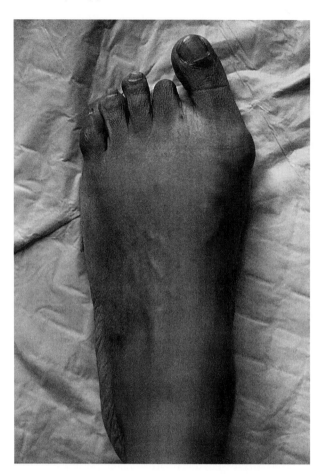

Figure 12–1. A 17-year-old patient with hallux valgus secondary to poly-metatarsia.

Figure 12–2. Preoperative radiograph of a 17-year-old child with polymeta-tarsia and secondary hallux valgus.

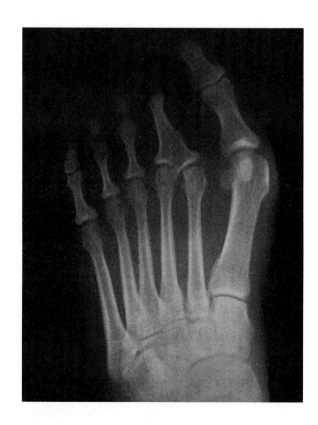

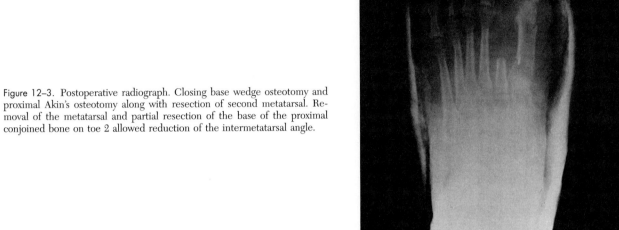

Figure 12–3. Postoperative radiograph. Closing base wedge osteotomy and proximal Akin's osteotomy along with resection of second metatarsal. Removal of the metatarsal and partial resection of the base of the proximal conjoined bone on toe 2 allowed reduction of the intermetatarsal angle.

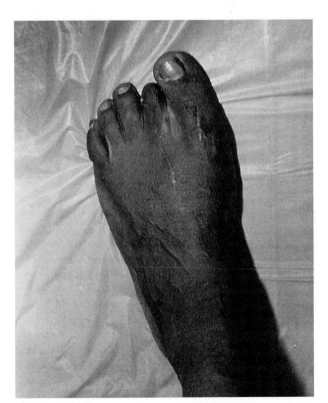

Figure 12–4. Postoperative clinical polymetatarsia with reduction of hallux valgus.

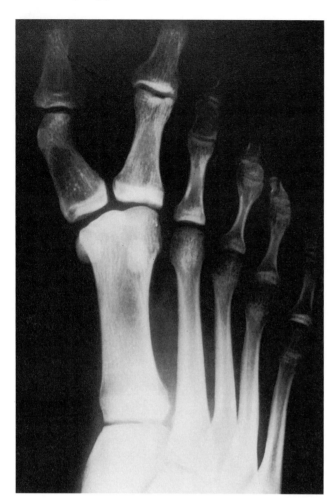

Figure 12–5. Polydactyly of great toe including the proximal and distal phalanx with Y appearance of metatarsal head 1.

Figure 12–6. Polydactyly of fifth digit and metatarsal with proposed surgical resection markers.

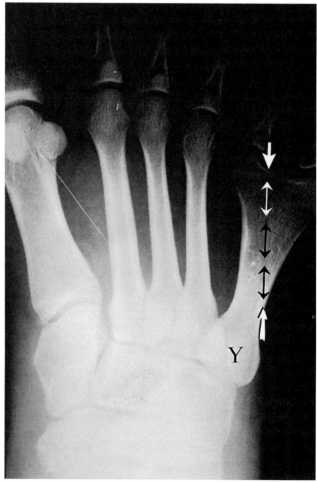

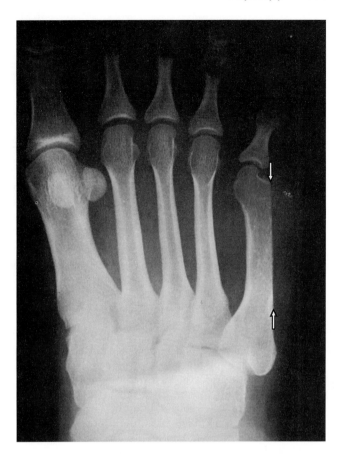

Figure 12–7. Postoperative resection of polydactyly on metatarsal 5.

References

1. Ivy RH: Congenital anomalies. Plast Reconstr Surg 1957; 20:400.
2. Sesgin MZ, Stark RB: The incidence of congenital defects. Plast Reconstr Surg 1961; 27:261.
3. Bunnell S: Surgery of the Hand, 4th ed. Revised by JH Boyes. Philadelphia, J. B. Lippincott, 1964.
4. Venn-Watson EA: Problems in polydactyly of the foot. Orthop Clin North Am 1976; 7:909–927.
5. Wood VE: Treatment of central polydactyly. Clin Orthop 1971; 74:196–205.
6. Odiorne JM: Polydactylism in related New England families. J Hered 1943; 34:35.
7. Sharma NL: Polydactylo-syndactylism with unusual skeletal anomalies in a mother and her children. Ind J Pediatr 1965; 32:233.
8. Specht E: Major congenital deformities and anomalies of the foot. *In* Inman VT (ed): Surgery of the Foot, 3rd ed. St. Louis, C. V. Mosby, 1973, pp. 58–87.
9. Gillman J, Gilbert C, Gillman T, Spence I: A further report on congential anomalies in the rat produced by tryphan blue. S Afr J Med Sci 1951; 16:125.
10. Hedgekati M: Malformed hands and feet. J Hered 1972; 30:192–193.
11. Schinzel A: Postaxial polydactyly, hallux duplication, absence of corpus callosum, macroencephaly and severe mental retardation: A new syndrome? Helv Paediat Acta 1979; 34:141–146.
12. Franciosi RV, Barney J, Kramer MF: The surgical management of polydactyly. J Foot Surg 1975; 14:103–107.
13. Dorland's Medical Dictionary, 25th ed. Philadelphia, W. B. Saunders, 1974.
14. Turek SL: Orthopaedic Principles and Their Application. Philadelphia, J. B. Lippincott, 1967.
15. Wassel HD: The results of surgery for polydactyly of the thumb. Clin Orthop 1969; 64:175–193.
16. Temtamy S, McKusick VA: Synopsis of hand malformations with particular emphasis on genetic factors. Birth Defects Orig Art Ser 1969; 5:125–184.
17. Nathan PA, Keniston BC: Crossed polydactyly. J Bone J Surg 1975; 57A:847–849.

13

Congenital Cleft Foot Deformity (Split Foot or Lobster-Claw)

William H. Mason, D.P.M.

Cleft foot deformity is a rare congenital abnormality that has a definite tendency toward hereditary transmission. In its typical form the deformity is bilateral and is characterized by the absence of two or more central rays of the foot. Historically referred to as lobster-claw or split foot, the anomaly is an inherited autosomal dominant trait that has an incidence of 1 in 90,000 live births.[1] Males are affected more often than females.

Conservative treatment for cleft foot generally consists of shoe adaptation for older patients who did not receive surgical correction and are unable to wear normal shoes. Surgical correction of the deformity should ideally be attempted at a very early age to offset the deforming forces that cause greater pathologic adaptation.[2] Surgical intervention in cleft foot is indicated to facilitate fitting of shoes and to improve the objectionable appearance.[3]

PATHOPHYSIOLOGY

The original case of lobster-claw foot, as reported in 1829,[4] was typical of cleft foot deformity in that it demonstrated congenital absence of the second, third, and fourth metatarsals bilaterally along with medial deviation of the fifth toe and hallux abductus. In general, the cone-shaped cleft in the forefoot tapers proximally to a rearfoot that is generally normal. The first metatarsal may be of normal size, or it may be broad and connected with the intermediate cuneiform at its base, representing fusion of the first and second metatarsals. The lateral digital ray may consist of only the fifth metatarsal or the fifth and fourth metatarsals.

Bilateral cleft foot occurs occasionally as an isolated deformity, but a more typical presentation may include cleft hand, cleft lip and palate, reduction in the size of the phalanges, syndactyly, triphalangeal thumb, and deafness.[5] Bilateral asymmetry, mental retardation, microcephaly, dwarfism, and spastic quadriparesis have been reported but are very rare.[1] Congenital heart disease may also be associated rarely with cleft foot and cleft hand.[6]

Unilateral deformity with no evidence of familial inheritance or other coexisting pathology is considered the less common atypical form. Congenital absence of the fibula with a cleft leg deformity consisting of a well-developed hallux and a rudimentary second toe at midcalf can occur as a bizarre variant.[7]

The embryologic genesis of cleft foot is thought to exist in a mutant gene.[8] In the second month of human gestation limb constriction appears in the limb buds at positions corresponding to future major joints. A mutant gene may cause excessive activity of the terminal portion of the limb buds, leading to duplication of rays to the hand and foot. Genes responsible for normal growth of the limb buds are not able to reverse completely the damage done by the defective mutant gene, thus leading to cleft foot and hand, triphalangeal thumb, and other digital defects such as polydactyly.[8]

CLINICAL EVALUATION

In the clinical evaluation of cleft foot the patient's age, mental and physical status, and severity of deformity are primary considerations. The family history is vital, as is a complete physical examination to determine the extent of coexisting pathology. The younger the patient the more effective surgical correction will be because the deforming forces of age and weight bearing will lead to pathologic adaptation. An older child or adult who has a medical, mental, or emotional disability may be a candidate only for conservative shoe adaptation, the historical treatment of choice for congenital cleft foot deformity.

Radiographic analysis offers the most important data the clinician can consider following the physical examination. In each case an exact understanding of the osseous pathology is paramount in the surgical consideration because small differences often exist even in the most typical deformities. Conservative as well as surgical treatment plans are often formulated based on the x-ray findings. Weight-bearing dorsoplantar, lateral, and oblique views of

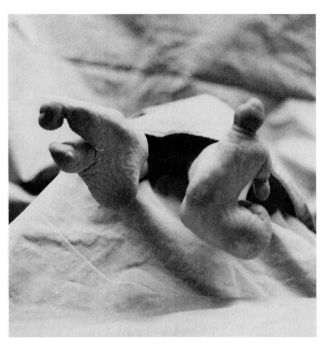

Figure 13-1. Cleft foot deformity demonstrating congenital absence of the second, third, and fourth metatarsals.

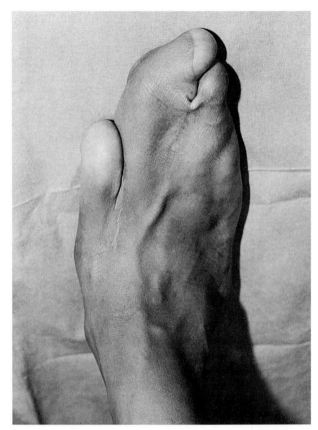

Figure 13-3. Variant of cleft foot–skin fusion with anomalous atavistic medial ray.

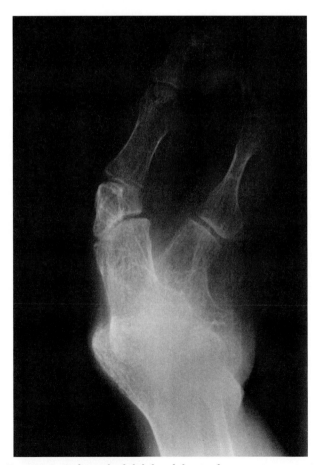

Figure 13-2. Radiograph of cleft foot deformity demonstrating congenital absence of the second, third, and fourth metatarsals bilaterally along with medial deviation of the fifth toe and hallux abductus.

the cleft foot are mandatory. The angulation of the bony deformity, radiodensity between the metatarsals and phalanges indicating possible synostoses, and the existence of digital syndactyly must be recognized[2] (Figs. 13–1 to 13–4).

SURGICAL MANAGEMENT

The ability to wear normal shoe gear, ambulation without discomfort, and prevention of psychologic problems that accompany the appearance of the deformity are the goals in surgical correction. Important surgical considerations include intervention at a very early age, the surgeon's expertise in pediatric reconstructive surgery, and a staged surgical approach. Most authors agree that surgery performed between 8 and 18 months of age leads to the best results. The family of the cleft foot patient must be told during consultation that a staged surgical approach is the management of choice.[2] Reconstruction often requires more than one operation, and it is important that the family understands that with a cleft foot deformity a cosmetically normal foot cannot be obtained. The first stage focuses on reducing the width of the foot by means of metatarsal osteotomies, excision of bony remnants, and creation of suitable skin flaps.[9] The second stage corrects digital abnormalities using desyndactylizations, toenail modifications, bunionectomies, arthroplasties, and exos-

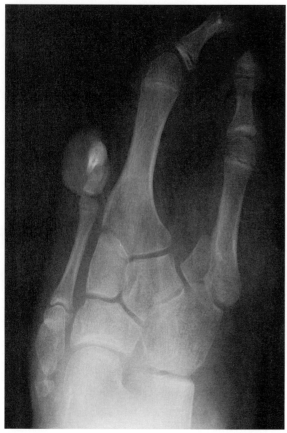

Figure 13–4. Variant of cleft foot–skin fusion with anomalous atavistic medial ray.

tectomies.[2] These procedures should be performed not less than 6 weeks later. The clinician should emphasize to the patient's family the advisability of staged surgery while also considering such factors as tourniquet time, blood loss, and tissue trauma. It is best to allow stage one procedures to heal completely before attempting digital cosmetic corrections.[2] The surgically corrected cleft foot may not resemble a normal foot in appearance, although cosmesis is an important goal.

Procedures such as the creation of toes by raising a double-pedicled flap from the cleft or by using existing redundant skin and control of splaying by holding the metatarsals together with fascia lata have been tried.[10] Most foot surgeons would agree, however, that restoration of function is the primary goal.

Five different procedures are used in cleft foot:

1. *Barsky.* This procedure was originally described for cleft hand. The incision provides a skin flap for reconstruction of the web space.
2. *Tachdijian.* This author recommends excision of the cleft, osteotomy of the adjacent metatarsals, and syndactylization of the digits adjacent to the cleft to prevent recurrent splaying of the forefoot.
3. *Giorgini.* In 1985 this author described a two-stage procedure. He used a crossed Kelikian-type incision that intersected at the center of the cleft, creating foreskin flaps.
4. *Weissman and Plaschkes.* These surgeons described a repair that is also useful in older patients with an unrepaired cleft foot. They used a transverse incision at the metatarsophalangeal joint level and then turned one of the two claw-like digits from which all nail tissue had been excised into a cleft. This procedure has not been recommended for the younger child.
5. *Sumiya and Onizuka.*[10] These authors used a two-stage technique. They considered cosmesis to be of extreme importance, and therefore this procedure has a somewhat greater morbidity.

It must be emphasized that because the cleft foot deformity occurs with wide variations in structural pathology the clinician's job is to consider different strategies of treatment to fit the various conditions.

References

1. Mason WH: Congenital cleft foot deformity (split foot or lobster claw). J Am Podiatr Med Assoc 1991; 81:575.
2. Coleman WB, Aronovitz DC: Surgical management of cleft foot deformity. J Foot Surg 1988; 27:497.
3. Tachdijian MO: The foot and leg. *In* Pediatric Orthopedics, Vol. 2. Philadelphia, W. B. Saunders, 1972.
4. Cruveilhier J: Anatomie Pathologique du Corps Humaine, Vol. 2, Part 38. Paris, Balliere, 1829.
5. Lewis T, Embleton D: Split-hand and split-foot deformities, their types, origin and transmission. Biometrika 1908; 6:26.
6. Bhat BV, Ashok BA, Puri RK: Lobster-claw hand and foot deformity in a family. Ind Pediatr 1987; 24:675.
7. Corea JR, Sankaran-Kutty M: Lobster-claw leg. J Bone Joint Surg 1989; 71B:861.
8. Phillips RS: Congenital split foot (lobster-claw) and triphalangeal thumb. J Bone Joint Surg 1971; 53B:247.
9. Du Vries HL: Major congenital deformities and anomalies of the foot. *In* Inman VT (ed): Surgery of the Foot. St. Louis, C.V. Mosby, 1973.
10. Sumiya N, Onizuka T: Seven-year survey of our new cleft foot repair. Plast Reconstr Surg 1980; 65:447.

14

Brachymetatarsia

Steven Glickman, D.P.M., Robert Cornfield, D.P.M.,
Jason Hanft, D.P.M., Richard M. Jay, D.P.M., Gary Feldman, D.P.M.,
Greg Rock, D.P.M., and John Beaupied, D.P.M.

Hypoplasia of the metatarsal is commonly seen in the fourth metatarsal bilaterally (Fig. 14–1). However, any metatarsal can be affected, and the condition can be present unilaterally (Fig. 14–2). A shortened fourth metatarsal does not cause any functional disturbance in the child. It is, however, a concern with regard to cosmesis. Most parents are more concerned about the appearance than about future functional problems. Cosmetic correction is an acceptable reason for surgery; however, the surgeon should be aware that if the condition is left untreated an increase in pressure occurs on the adjacent metatarsals. This sequela is not usually observed until the child loses the supple fat pad plantarly. Callosities de-

velop, the toes begin to override and start to contract, and it is at this point that surgery is indicated for this functional deformity.

ETIOLOGY

Brachymetatarsia is defined as premature closure of the epiphyseal plate, resulting in an abnormally short metatarsal. The most commonly affected metatarsal is the fourth, but any or multiple metatarsals can be affected. When more than one metatarsal is involved, the condition is referred to as brachymetapodia. The female-to-male

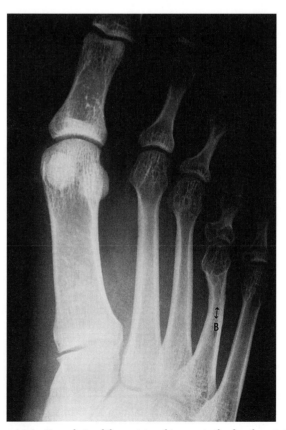

Figure 14–1. Hypoplasia of the metatarsal is seen in the fourth metatarsal. Because of the structural shortening, increased peak pressures are exerted on the adjacent metatarsal heads, creating callosities.

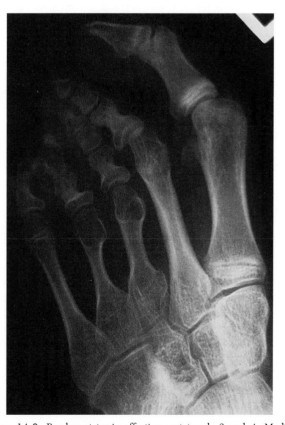

Figure 14–2. Brachymetatarsia affecting metatarsals 3 and 4. Medial drift of the hallux as well as overlapping of the adjacent digits are not uncommon.

ratio is known to be 98:4 and bilateral shortening is found in approximately 72% of all cases.[1]

The underlying cause of brachymetatarsia may be heredity, infection, trauma, infarction, neoplasm, radiation, or idiopathic factors.[2] It has been reported in the literature that brachymetatarsia may be associated with the following systemic disease processes.[3]

- Pseudohypoparathyroidism
- Pseudopseudohypoparathyroidism
- Malignancy
- Down's syndrome
- Albright's hereditary osteodystrophy
- Diastrophic dwarfism
- Multiple epiphyseal dysplasia
- Myositis ossificans
- Turner's syndrome
- Sickle cell anemia
- Basal cell nevus syndrome (Gorlin's syndrome)
- Enchondromatosis
- Marchesani's syndrome
- Epiphyseal dysostosis
- Neonatal hyperthyroidism
- Acrodysostosis

CLINICAL PRESENTATION

Congenital brachymetatarsia is usually not seen at birth, but becomes evident clinically when the patient is between 4 and 15 years old. The signs and symptoms of this condition are based on the degree of the deformity, the age of the patient, and the sex of the patient. The chief complaint of the young patient is most often one of cosmesis. Premature fusion of the epiphyseal plate may cause more of a psychologic problem than a physiologic one.[4] In many circumstances, the shortened metatarsal results in a corresponding shortened and contracted digit. This abnormal toe position results in a cosmetic disfigurement that is frequently embarrassing to the patient.[5] A short floating toe over the shortened fourth ray is present, and a sulcus or indentation can be seen beneath the involved metatarsal.[6] As the patient grows older, abnormal weight bearing produces discomfort due to the altered metatarsal length. The excessive load on the adjacent metatarsals results in painful plantar hyperkeratotic lesion formation. The weight of the patient and his or her activity level play a significant role in the degree of symptomatology. Clinically, brachymetatarsia can also present as an overlapping of the associated digit of the short metatarsal on an adjacent digit. The overlapping of the digit is a secondary response to contracture of the surrounding soft tissue. Dermatologic irritation, capsulitis, and tendinitis are among a few of the symptoms that may precipitate an inability to wear regular shoe gear. The diagnosis of brachymetatarsia is apparent both clinically and radiographically; however, the confirmatory diagnosis must be made radiographically.

NONSURGICAL TREATMENT

The approach to treatment of brachymetatarsia is dependent on the degree of metatarsal shortening, symptoms, age, and activity level of the patient. Essentially, treatment options can be divided into conservative care and surgical correction. Conservative care consists of palliative care as well as the use of orthotic or accommodative devices in the shoe to redistribute the excessive stress placed on the adjacent metatarsal heads. Conservative treatment, however, will not solve the psychologic, cosmetic, and underlying anatomic and structural problems associated with this deformity.[7, 8] Because of this fact, and because of the high percentage of patient dissatisfaction with the results of conservative care, most of the attention in treating brachymetatarsia has been directed toward surgical reconstruction.

SURGICAL TREATMENT

In selecting a surgical procedure the physician's goal is to obtain proper function first and then cosmesis. The ideal procedure should achieve adequate length of the metatarsal and preserve joint motion. Surgical correction of brachymetatarsia involves a combination of both soft tissue and osseous correction techniques.

Soft Tissue Correction

Soft tissue correction in the surgical treatment of a shortened metatarsal is imperative. The skin and underlying soft tissue, including the tendons and capsular structures, are generally contracted and often require lengthening. Various soft tissue techniques, including the V-Y skin plasty, are used to correct soft tissue contractures. The short extensor is often sectioned, while the long extensor is typically lengthened through a slide Z-plasty. A metatarsophalangeal joint capsulotomy must be performed on the dorsally displaced digit, and care must be taken to release the dorsal as well as the medial and lateral aspects of the joint capsule. The deep transverse intermetatarsal ligament must be sectioned to allow lengthening of the metatarsal. Atraumatic technique with careful anatomic dissection is especially important because the neurovascular structures are subject to compromise secondary to the lengthening process alone.[7, 8]

Surgical soft tissue procedures involving disarticulation of the fourth toe from its metatarsal, and syndactylization to the third digit have been reported to have some success; however, the fourth metatarsal remains nonfunctional because this procedure does not attempt to correct the metatarsal length.[5, 9] This surgical technique is not commonly performed today for brachymetatarsia because it reportedly is detrimental to function, often requiring later desyndactylization, and offers little cosmetic relief.[2]

Osseous Correction

The goal of the osseous component of treatment is to obtain or restore a normal metatarsal parabola. Historically, osseous correction of brachymetatarsia has been accomplished either by lengthening or plantar-flexing the involved metatarsal or by shortening or dorsiflexing the adjacent metatarsals. These procedures often require bone grafting.

Bone Grafting

Several important factors must be considered when selecting a bone graft. Autogenous bone remains the most favorable material for transplantation. It is immunologically compatible, aids in osteogenesis, and provides structural support throughout the healing process. Autogenous bone grafts result in more rapid healing because they contain viable tissues and cells that are compatible with those in the receptor site.[12] Harvesting the autograft, however, requires additional operative time and involves an increased risk of complications and a weakened donor site.

The ideal bone structure to choose when selecting a graft is one in which both cortical and cancellous bone is present. Cancellous grafts contain a high cellular component. The matrix favors neovascularization with advancement of capillary loops and microvessels across the graft. This process is termed creeping substitution and generally lasts from 5 to 20 days after the transplantation. Osteoblastic activity accelerates, replacing the transplanted trabeculae with new bone. Osteoclastic resorption of the transplanted bone occurs, and new bone infiltrates the graft site, providing strength to the graft. Autogenous cancellous bone transplantation involves the transfer of viable cells that facilitate osteogenesis, a lace-like matrix that favors neovascularization and the bathing of graft cells with nutrients and morphogenetic protein that stimulates mesenchymal cells to become osteoprogenitor cells.

Cortical bone grafts contain a dense, compact structure with few vascular channels. The cortical bone graft functions as a mechanical strut between the host tissues due to its intrinsic strength. Cortical grafts heal primarily through osteoclastic activity as the recipient tissue burrows channels through the graft to provide access for advancing vessels. Eventually, osteoblasts lay new bone around the lattice of trabeculation in the graft.[12, 13] The ideal choice of graft is one that incorporates the structural rigidity of a cortical graft, which adequately maintains graft length during healing, with the highly cellular nature of a cancellous graft, which encourages rapid osteogenesis.

The corticocancellous graft, which is most commonly obtained from the iliac crest, tibia, fibula, or calcaneus, meets these requirements. Kashuk and colleagues[10] report that the calcaneus, navicular, medial eminence of the first metatarsal, lesser metatarsals, proximal phalanx of the hallux, and the head of a lesser proximal phalanx are favorable alternative donor sites from the foot.

The bone graft should be immobilized and rigidly fixated to avoid graft displacement. Excessive compression on the graft should be avoided because it leads to excessive necrosis of the bone at the interface, resulting in gapping.[11] The potential complications of bone grafting, including graft displacement, pseudoarthrosis, malunion, and nonunion, may lead to conditions more severe than the original problem.

Bone grafts from adjacent metatarsals are placed in the distal cut shafts of the shortened metatarsal.[30, 31] The cylindrical graft is held by a longitudinally placed K-wire. I personally use a miniexternal fixator to maintain bone length and graft compression. Two screws are placed distally and proximally to the graft site. With a compressor adjusted in place, the set screw is turned gently using enough compression to hold the graft without slipping. One full turn is applied in a counterclockwise direction; this equals approximately 8 to 12 pounds of torque.

An alternative to the cylindrical bone graft is autogenous banked bone. Cancellous and cortical bone is placed in the osteotomy site, creating the desired separation without shortening of the adjacent metatarsal. Keep in mind that a dermal Z-plasty and a Z-lengthening procedure of the tendon may be necessary.

OSSEOUS SURGICAL PROCEDURES

Lengthening procedures for the treatment of brachymetatarsia have been classified by Martin and Kalish[6] into four major categories as follows:

1. Single metatarsal osteotomy with bone graft.
2. Combined lengthening and shortening metatarsal osteotomies.
3. Metatarsal osteotomy with insertion of synthetic implant.
4. Slide-lengthening metatarsal osteotomies.

Single Metatarsal Osteotomy with Bone Graft

McGlamry and Cooper[7] in 1969 were the first to describe a surgical procedure for the correction of brachymetatarsia using an autogenous cylindrical bone graft from the calcaneus as a midshaft metatarsal graft in a young female patient; they reported excellent functional and cosmetic results. Since this initial report, many cases have appeared in the literature describing use of an autogenous inlaid bone graft, with satisfactory results overall.[8, 10, 13, 14, 15, 20] Pasternack[14] reported using the hypertrophic portion of the navicular bone as an autogenous graft to lengthen the fourth metatarsal. Jinnaka[17] interposed a spindle-shaped bone graft into the metatarsophalangeal joint to lengthen the metatarsal. Urano and Kobayashi[1] used a modification of Jinnaka's procedure in a series of 82 cases. They used spindle-shaped autogenous iliac crest and tibial bone grafts to fuse the metatarsophalangeal joint without any type of fixation. The function of the joint itself, however, is lost because this procedure causes arthrodesis of the joint. Allogeneic bone grafts have also been used in the treatment of brachymetatarsia with reports of comparable success.[1, 16] Rock and associates[4] harvested bone from the proximal phalangeal heads of digits 2 and 3 and interposed the bone graft into the distal third of the hypoplastic fourth metatarsal with Kirschner wire fixation. This procedure should be reserved for feet with elongation of digits 2 and 3 in which the width of the proximal phalanx is comparable to that of the hypoplastic metatarsal.

Combined Lengthening and Shortening Metatarsal Osteotomies

Handelman and colleagues[16] described a technique in which the shortened fourth metatarsal is lengthened with an allogeneic bone graft while shortening osteotomies are performed on the adjacent third and fifth metatarsals; they reported satisfactory restoration of a normal metatarsal parabola. Autogenous bone grafts harvested from adjacent metatarsals have also been reported frequently in the literature. Kaplan and Kaplan[11] in 1978 reported correction of a shortened fourth metatarsal through an autogenous bone graft taken from the base of the second metatarsal. Chairman and colleagues[5] described surgical correction of a shortened fourth metatarsal through transplantation of a portion of the fifth metatarsal shaft and head to the shortened fourth metatarsal, reporting extreme patient satisfaction. A hemimetatarsal transposition involving transposing the distal 3.0-cm segment of bone of the fourth metatarsal with the distal 2.0-cm segment of bone of the shortened second metatarsal was performed by Beaupied and associates.[18] The gain of length in the second metatarsal was designed to establish a normal metatarsal parabola.

Metatarsal Osteotomy with Insertion of Synthetic Implant

These implants, in most cases, serve as spacers in lengthening the shortened digit and not as a functional correction to a structural deformity such as brachymetatarsia. Mah and colleagues[19] reported use of the Calnan-Nicolle implant in the metatarsophalangeal joint, again simply as a spacer. Good cosmetic as well as functional results were reported; however, some associated disadvantages include implant rejection and aseptic necrosis. This procedure is not recommended for young patients because the implant would have to be changed several times during the life of the patient.

Slide-Lengthening Metatarsal Osteotomies

Slide lengthening procedures are most commonly performed with bone grafting. Slide lengthening without bone grafts should be reserved for patients with a mild to moderate deformity that does not require excessive lengthening.[7, 8] Tabak and colleagues[20] described a case of brachymetatarsia affecting the second metatarsal that was surgically corrected using a metatarsal slide lengthening procedure. The technique used was a modification of the Giannestras step-down procedure in which no bone graft was used. Marcinko and associates[22] also described a case of post-traumatic brachymetatarsia in which a modification of the Giannestras step-down procedure was performed. The osteotomy was performed and reduced with two parallel K-wires without the use of bone grafts. Martin and Kalish[6] described a two-stage surgical technique for correction of brachymetatarsia. In the first stage the periarticular soft tissues are mobilized, including the neurovascular structures. The second stage addresses the osseous component of the deformity through a diaphyseal sliding osteotomy with rigid internal compression fixation. This technique is described as follows:

First Stage. The purpose of the first stage is to mobilize the periarticular soft tissues, including the neurovascular structures, in order to allow for osseous lengthening of the involved metatarsal. Soft tissue releases are performed through a dorsal incision extended from the proximal metatarsal shaft to the base of the proximal phalanx. Transection of the extensor digitorum brevis tendon is performed as well as a complete dorsal, medial, and lateral capsulotomy. The extensor digitorum longus tendon is generally not lengthened at this time because the stress of the gradual lengthening process would probably have detrimental effects on tendon healing. Exposure of the proximal phalanx and metatarsal is obtained. The periosteum is carefully dissected off the proximal diaphyseal portion of both bones in preparation for insertion of the external fixator. A 2.7-mm self-tapping pin is then inserted into each segment, and the external frame of the fixator device is slipped into place and locked over the two pins. Several millimeters of distraction are applied before closure. Approximately 1.5 mm of distraction is applied every other day for approximately 2 weeks to ensure adequate soft tissue lengthening without neurovascular compromise. The patient is under strict instruction to use crutches and remain nonweight bearing on the affected foot.

Second Stage. The purpose of the second stage is to effectively lengthen the shortened metatarsal to the desired length once adequate soft tissue lengthening has been obtained. This stage is generally performed approximately 3 weeks following the initial procedure. The original skin incision is used, and the external fixation device and pins are removed. The long extensor tendon is identified, and lengthening is performed in an open or sliding-7 fashion. The deep transverse intermetatarsal ligament is transected on each side of the metatarsal head. The increase in soft tissue length and mobility achieved in the first stage becomes readily apparent at this time. At this time a decision is reached about which type of osteotomy will be most appropriate. Generally, a slide-lengthening procedure of the metatarsal with internal fixation using 2.0-mm cortical screws will provide adequate fixation and lengthening; however, in more severe cases, the thickness of the shaft of the metatarsal is significantly reduced as the metatarsal is advanced distally. This makes for a highly unstable osteotomy that is prone to fracture. Therefore, in severe cases the more traditional technique of using an inlaid bone graft may be better to ensure adequate lengthening of the metatarsal.

Martin and Kalish[6] described a modified Z-type osteotomy that allows greater bone-to-bone contact and is fixated with a 2.0-mm screw. Corticocancellous inlay bone graft is used to fill the proximal metatarsal defect. This graft is fixated with an additional 2.0-mm screw. Postoperatively, the patient is placed in a below-the-knee cast and again restricted to crutches and absolute nonweight bearing for a period of 6 to 10 weeks until there is radiographic evidence of osseous union. A gradual return to weight bearing will prevent failure or disruption of the bone graft. The patient may return to full weight bearing on evidence of radiographic bone healing at approximately the fourteenth or sixteenth postoperative week. Steedman and Peterson[21] reported use of this two-stage technique in four pediatric patients with short first metatarsals. The mini-Hoffman and Orthofix external fixators were used along with subsequent fibular bone grafting to lengthen six first metatarsals with excellent results.

CALLUS DISTRACTION

An additional osseous surgical technique for the treatment of brachymetatarsia has been more recently described and is not included in Martin and Kalish's classification.[6] This technique is known as callotasis or callus distraction. It was originally described by Ilizarov and colleagues[23] and is a method of lengthening a bone without the use of bone grafting. This technique involves performing an osteotomy initially on the diaphysis of the metatarsal and then gradually elongating the callus formation with the aid of an external fixator. A minibone fixator is placed over the osteotomy site, and the screws are placed on both sides of the osteotomy. In performing the osteotomy the periosteum is carefully preserved by reflecting it around the shaft of the bone. A transverse cut is made through the entire shaft, and the periosteum is closed. Gradual distraction of the metatarsal is then performed by the patient, generally twice a day on an outpatient basis at a rate of approximately 0.25 mm per day. As with any lengthening procedure, care must be taken to prevent neurovascular compromise by avoiding overaggressive distraction. Periodic cleansing of the pin sites is important to minimize the risk of infection.[29, 32–34]

Wakisaka and colleagues[24] described a case using this technique in which the final length increase on the left fourth metatarsal was 14 mm and that on the right fourth metatarsal was 12 mm. Patients are allowed partial weight bearing, and distraction is performed as an outpatient procedure. Ferrandez and associates[25] reported that the procedure is easy to implement and leads to excellent results, both immediate cosmetic results and later on good functional results, despite its possible complications. An average of 23.7 mm of length was obtained in a study of three patients treated by callus distraction for brachymetatarsia of the fourth metatarsal. This study reported initiation of distraction 1 week after surgery; the optimal distraction rate was 0.35 mm every 12 hours, with removal of the fixator device at an average of 112.5 days after surgery. Complications included subluxation caused by tendons resisting elongation in two patients and a postoperative fracture in one patient.[26]

History

The history of limb lengthening can be traced to the late nineteenth century when several primitive techniques were attempted. However, most recent applications stem from the initial work of A. Codivilla. In 1904 he described a procedure for lengthening bone in patients with coxa vara. He called this procedure continuous extension. Codivilla's work, while instrumental, really only introduced the importance of distraction for lengthening of bone. Later research, in the early twentieth century, paved the way for today's procedures. Vitterio Putti developed an apparatus in 1918 for this procedure and described a controlled lengthening of bone. The principles of his work are the same as those that govern this process today.

As a result of the postwar work of Gavril Abramovic Ilizarov,[23] the principles of bone distraction were further modified and improved. His modular ring fixator, developed in 1952, allowed controlled lengthening through a refined technique, which also produced a more predictable response. Subsequently, in the 1970s, De Bastiani[27] modified Ilizarov's technique by stressing the need to observe radiographic evidence of callus prior to distraction. He called this procedure "callotasis" and demonstrated its success in the lengthening of upper and lower extremities.

The benefits of callus distraction in foot surgery have only recently been appreciated. In 1988, Wakisaka and colleagues[24] described a technique of lengthening a short metatarsal by callus distraction. Although other procedures for the treatment of brachymetatarsia had proved effective, this new technique proved to be the most gradual and least traumatic to the soft tissue when attempting to gain length. Since that original application in the foot, others have described this procedure in the treatment of brachymetatarsia. Callotasis has also been proposed as an alternative to bone grafting in an Evans osteotomy and in medial column lengthening as indicated for metatarsus adductus. Nevertheless, its main indication in the foot today is for the treatment of congenitally short metatarsals.

Principles and Techniques of Callus Distraction

Callotasis techniques have been utilized to treat congenitally shortened limbs and digits. Other indications include nonunion, clubfoot repair, and shortening secondary to trauma or infections. The procedure is performed through a linear incision made dorsal to the intended metatarsal. Following blunt dissection through the superficial tissues, the deep fascial layer is noted. The extensor tendon is then identified and lengthened, if desired. Martin and Kalish[6] noted that lengthening of the soft tissues with this procedure is unnecessary. The deep fascia is then incised, and all soft tissue is retracted from the periosteum. The periosteum is then incised in a linear fashion on the dorsal aspect of the metatarsal. This layer is then gently reflected, both medially and laterally, exposing cortical bone. Kojimoto and Yasui[30] showed in their study on rabbit limbs that lengthening failed if the periosteum surrounding the distraction site was removed. Therefore, careful periosteal dissection and preservation is critical.

Prior to osteotomy, four pins are placed perpendicular to the weight-bearing surface. Two pins are placed proximal and two distal to the proposed osteotomy site. After the pins have been placed the osteotomy can be performed using either power instrumentation, making sure to cool the cut bone immediately, or an osteotome.

Corticotomy may also be performed as an alternative to osteotomy. This technique allows preservation of the endosteum, which many authors believe is primarily responsible for the success of the procedure. However, recent studies have shown that the endosteal blood supply regenerates quickly, and its preservation in surgery may be unnecessary.

After osteotomy or corticotomy has been completed, the wound can be irrigated and closed. Special attention should be given to the periosteal layer, the edges of which must be well approximated. The remaining tissues are then repaired in order. Following closure, the distraction frame can be mounted onto the pins and tightened until the osteotomy site is well opposed.

Postoperatively, the patient should be kept nonweight-bearing. Lengthening should begin ideally after 21 days, thus allowing for the recovery of the endosteal circulation. After this period, distraction may begin at a rate of 0.35 to 0.50 mm per day. This procedure is usually performed every 12 hours (0.175 to 0.25 mm per 12 hours).

During the distraction period, the patient should be kept nonweight bearing. Routine radiographs will reveal little callus formation with a gap between segments. Lengthening should continue until the desired length is achieved. Following completion, most authors advocate leaving the frame intact until osseous consolidation is viewed radiographically.[6] Once this is apparent, the patient can begin bearing weight with or without the frame and pins.

Complications

As described earlier, bone grafting techniques have proved to be an excellent tool in the correction of brachymetatarsia. There are several potential complications with the use of any of the bone grafting procedures. Delayed or nonunion of the graft is one of the most common complications. This painful condition will be compounded if multiple osteotomies have been created for transplantation of the grafts. Ultimately, resorption and collapse of the graft site can lead to devastating results.

The use of implants in the correction of brachymetatarsia has been controversial, especially in the pediatric population. A synthetic implant is not designed to withstand the weight-bearing load of a shortened metatarsal. Over time, implant failure is an inevitable complication.

Another potential complication seen in brachymetatarsia surgery is that of neurovascular compromise. As the metatarsal is distracted distally for extended periods of time, constriction of the vessels follow, and irreversible gangrene is the horrific end result. Some of the more recent multiple staged techniques[6] have attempted to prevent vascular compromise by mobilizing the periarticular soft tissue structures so that the vessels can safely tolerate much greater degrees of osseous lengthening. With children, not only the general complications of any surgical procedure but also specific considerations in the pediatric population must be addressed. Special attention must be paid to the integrity of the osseous growth centers. Postoperative pain management is invariably different in the younger patient. The degree of deformity, current symptomatology, and psychologic ramifications of the deformity are some of the major considerations that must be addressed when surgical intervention is being introduced. The decision of whether to wait until skeletal maturity before performing surgery is a very important issue in the final selection of the treatment course.

References

1. Urano Y, Kobayashi A: Bone-lengthening for shortness of the fourth toe. J Bone Joint Surg 1978; 60A:91–93.
2. Nuzzo JJ, Mueller RA: Diaphyseal lengthening for brachymetatarsia. J Foot Surg 1987; 26:332–335.
3. Oreenfield OB: Radiology of Bone Diseases, 3rd ed. Philadelphia, J.B. Lippincott, 1980, p. 344.
4. Rock GD, Gaspari C, Mancuso JE: Brachymetatarsia with the use of digital arthroplastic bone. J Foot Surg 1993; 32:499–504.
5. Chairman EL, Dallalio E, Mandracchia VJ: Brachymetatarsia IV: A different surgical approach. J Foot Surg 1985; 24:361–363.
6. Martin DE, Kalish SR: Brachymetatarsia: A new surgical approach. J Am Podiatr Med Assoc 1991; 81:10–17.
7. McGlamry ED, Cooper CT: Brachymetatarsia: A surgical treatment. J Am Podiatr Assoc 1969; 59:259–264.
8. McGlamry ED, Kitting RW, Butlin WE: Prominent lesser metatarsal heads: some surgical considerations. J Am Podiatr Assoc 1969; 59:303–307.
9. Kelikian H, Clayton L, Loseff H: Surgical syndactylia of the toes. Clin Orthop 1961; 19:208–211.
10. Kaskuk KB, Hanft JR, Schabler JA, Kopelman J: Alternative autogenous bone graft donor sites in brachymetatarsia reconstruction: A review of the literature with clinical presentations. J Foot Surg 1991; 30:246–252.
11. Kaplan EG, Kaplan GS: Metatarsal lengthening by use of autogenous bone graft and internal wire compression fixation: A preliminary report. J Foot Surg 1978; 17:60–66.
12. McCarthy DJ, Hutchinson BT: Autologous bone grafting in podiatric surgery. J Am Podiatr Med Assoc 1988; 78:217–226.
13. Bartolomei FJ: Surgical correction of brachymetatarsia. J Am Podiatr Med Assoc 1990; 80:76–82.
14. Pasternack WA: Brachymetatarsia. A unique surgical approach. J Am Podiatr Med Assoc 1988; 78:415–418.
15. Jimenez AL: Brachymetatarsia: a study in surgical planning. J Am Podiatr Assoc 1979; 69:245–251.
16. Handelman RB, Perlman MD, Coleman WB: Brachymetatarsia: A review of the literature and case report. J Am Podiatr Med Assoc 1986; 76:413–416.
17. Jinnaka S: Jinnaka's Orthopaedics (Seikei gekagaku) 20th ed. revised and edited by Amako. Tokyo, Nanzando, 1972, pp. 1278–1279.
18. Beaupied JP, Carrozza LP, Brynes MF, Morreale PF: Hemimetatarsal transposition: The use of autogenous bone grafting to treat brachymetatarsia—a unique approach. J Foot Surg 1991; 30:547–552.
19. Mah KS, Beagle TR, Falkner DW: A correction for short fourth metatarsal. J Am Podiatr Assoc 1983; 73:196–200.
20. Tabak B, Lefkowitz H, Steiner I: Metatarsal-slide lengthening without bone grafting. J Foot Surg 1986; 25:50–53.
21. Steedman JT, Peterson HA: Brachymetatarsia of the first metatarsal treated by surgical lengthening. J Pediatr Orthop 1992; 12:780–785.
22. Marcinko DE, Rappaport MJ, Gordon S: Post-traumatic brachymetatarsia. J Foot Surg 1984; 23:451–453.
23. Ilizarov GA, Deviatov AA, Trokhova VG: Surgical lengthening of shortened lower extremities. Vestn Khir 1972; 107:100–103.
24. Wakisaka T, Yasul N, Kojimoto H, Takasu M, Yutaka S: A case of short metatarsal bones lengthened by callus distraction. Acta Orthop Scand 1988; 59, 194–196.

25. Ferrandez L, Yubero J, Usablaga J, Ramos L: Congenital brachymetatarsia: Three cases. Foot Ankle 1993; 14:529–533.

26. Kawashima T, Yamada A, Ueda K, Harii K: Treatment of brachymetatarsia by callus distraction (callotasis). Ann Plast Surg 1994; 32:191–199.

27. De Bastiani G, Aldegheri R, Renzi-Brivio L, Trivella G: Limb lengthening by distraction of the epiphyseal plate: A comparison of two techniques in the rabbit. J Bone Joint Surg 1986; 68B:545–549.

28. Marcinko DE, Rappaport MJ: Posttraumatic brachymetatarsia. J Foot Surg 1984; 23:451–453.

29. Kaplan EG, Kaplan G: Metatarsal lengthening by use of autogenous bone graft and internal wire compression fixation: A preliminary report. J Foot Surg 1978; 17:60–66.

30. Kojimoto H, Yasui N: Bone lengthening in rabbits by callus distraction. J Bone Joint Surg 1988; 70B:543–549.

31. Aldegheri R: The callotasis method of limb lengthening., Clin Orthop 1989; 241:137–145.

32. De Bastiani G, Aldegheri R, Renzi-Brivio L, Trivella G: Limb lengthening by callus distraction (callotasis). J Pediatr Orthop 1987; 7:129–134.

33. Biggs EW, Brahm TB, Efran EL: Surgical correction of congenital hypoplastic metatarsals. J Am Podiatr Assoc 1979; 69:241–244.

15

Macrodactyly

Richard M. Jay, D.P.M.

Macrodactyly (hyperplasia) can be seen with many conditions (e.g., neurofibromatosis, Albright's dysplasia, lymphedema, and hemangiomas). There are, however, two presentations of macrodactyly—the static and the progressive. In the static form, which is the more common, the digit is enlarged at birth and continues to increase in size fairly rapidly in the early years.[1] In the progressive form the digit continues to grow throughout childhood, not just in infancy.

This congenital condition, although rare, presents the surgeon with the complex choice of whether to operate or not. It is reported that lesions of the hand are more common but that digital growth in the foot is more progressive. Once it has been determined that the lesion is an isolated condition rather than a neurofibromatous lesion or a tumor, the difficult question of approach to treatment must be solved. In a young infant with a rather large digit, the parents are rightfully concerned about its presence, and often their choice is to remove the digit. Ablation of the digit ends the cosmetic problem but creates not only a new psychologic problem of a missing toe but also a biomechanic problem. The adjacent digits have a tendency to drift into the vacant space. If the second digit is involved, the hallux is usually the digit that drifts, creating an iatrogenically induced hallux valgus deformity. An alternative choice is to arrest the growth of the digit by epiphysiodesis of the bases of the digits. The result can be successful but is inconsistent in determining the final length of the digit. Subsequent surgical procedures are often required to adjust the length pattern. One can also recommend that the digit be left untreated until the child's bone growth reaches maturity. This brings up another problem, the psychologic impact of the deformity on the child during this sensitive developmental stage.

Ablation, epiphysiodesis, and wait and watch are accepted treatment plans.[2] The clinical sequelae of all these choices must be discussed at length with the parents because this is an ethical and psychologic decision that will directly affect the child.

DEBULKING

In the debulking procedure, sections of skin and deep tissue are removed from the surrounding enlarged digit. To avoid great neurovascular damage, this procedure can be performed at 3- to 6-month intervals. By removing a section first on the medial, then on the lateral, and finally on the distal aspects, one can reduce the size of the digit successfully without disrupting the neurovascular supply. It is recommended, however, that this procedure be delayed until the child is as close to bone maturity as possible. If the procedure is done earlier, successful debulking will result; however, the probability of continued growth is still present. The digit may continue to increase in size, leaving the surgeon with the other options for treatment or further debulking. Certainly one drawback of this particular procedure is the number of times the child is exposed to surgery, which leaves the digit with a number of scarred areas. Since the digits are small to begin with, the scarring can leave a thickened area, thus creating a stiff digit.

Debulking procedures certainly are acceptable on a large thick toe; however, in a toe that presents with large osseous structures, debulking will not be successful, and additional procedures will be required (Figs. 15–1 and 15–2).

EPIPHYSIODESIS

After creating an incision on the dorsal aspect of the toe and gaining exposure to the distal, middle, and proximal phalanx, one can isolate the growth plate by inserting a small pin. Fluoroscopy can help in identification of the site; however, the area is usually soft enough that a small pin can enter between the osseous and cartilaginous structures. When this epiphysial plate is identified, the growth plate is curetted. A small curet or a narrow side-cutting bur can be used to remove the growth plate. Care must be taken not to damage the cartilage proximally. Following the contour of this growth plate, one can arrest the growth of the digit. This procedure is performed on the proximal, middle, and distal phalanges. At this point, to better ensure arrest of the growth plate, finely crushed cancellous bone is placed in the site of curettage. Cancellous bone can be retrieved from either the iliac crest or the calcaneus, or prepared freeze-dried bone can be used. The digit at this point can be stabilized with a K-wire and held for approximately 3 to 6 weeks.

This procedure may arrest the growth of this particular hyperplastic digit, but it does not address the size of the toe. Debulking procedures may still have to be performed, or, if the digit is much too large, an additional procedure may be needed to reduce the size of the osseous and soft tissues.

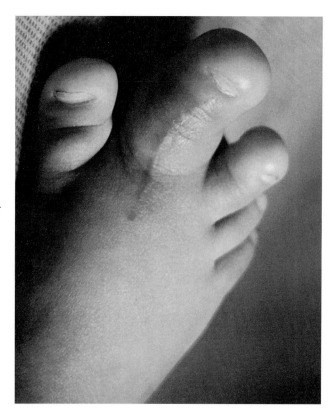

Figure 15–1. Postoperative debulking of second digit macrodactyly. Scar tissue recurred, creating a stiff large toe.

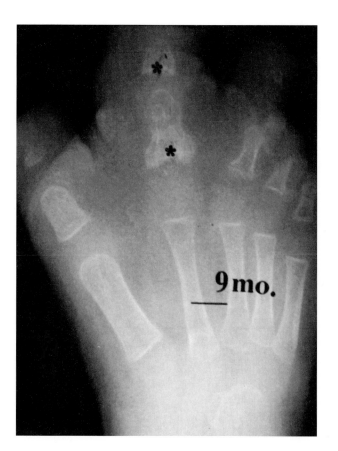

Figure 15–2. Radiograph of 9-month-old infant with second toe macrodactyly preoperatively.

DIGITAL SHORTENING

As stated earlier, macrodactyly is a perplexing problem for the child, parent, and physician. The unsightly position and size of the toe warrant attention; however, the surgeon must not fall into a false sense of security in thinking that a simple epiphysial arrest or debulking procedure will create the cosmetic appearance desired by the family. An additional procedure is that of shortening the actual digit, but part of the digit will be fused and lost with this procedure. I have found that this procedure is somewhat successful but should be reserved for the child with mature bone growth. A simple distal amputation can be performed; however, rather than amputating the distal aspect, removing both the nail and the distal tuft, a different procedure as modified by Tsuge[3] can be performed that will maintain the nail and distal aspect of the toe. The procedure is performed when the child is as close to bone maturity as possible. The inferior surface of the distal phalanx and the superior surface of the proximal phalanx are resected. The distal phalanx is then reapproximated on top of the remaining proximal phalangeal plantar shelf. The redundant skin is then excised both plantarly and dorsally.

References

1. Barsky A: Macrodactyly. J Bone Joint Surg 1967; 49A:1255–1266.
2. Kalen V, Burwell DS, Omer GE: Macrodactyly of the hands and feet. Pediatr Orthop 1988; 8:311–315.
3. Tsuge K: Treatment of macrodactyly. J Hand Surg 1985; 10A:968–969.

16

Syndactyly and Desyndactylization

David C. Puleo, D.P.M.

Syndactyly was first described by Cruveilhier in 1826 and may be defined as a coherence between one or more digits of the hands or feet with a union that may be soft tissue or bony with bridging of the adjacent phalanges. The deformity is most commonly congenital in nature, although it may be acquired by trauma following extensive burn injury. The incidence of syndactylism has been reported to be between 1 in 1000 and 1 in 3000 live births, and it has a threefold preponderance in males.[1-3]

ETIOLOGY

Congenital syndactyly is thought to be transmitted as an autosomal dominant trait. It is thought to occur at some point between the sixth and eighth weeks of fetal development owing to a failure of mesenchymal development and differentiation of the limb buds with subsequent lack of separation of the digits.[4] In the foot, this arrest of development and differentiation most frequently involves the second and third toes. More recently, it has been postulated that syndactyly may result from disruption of the digital vascular formation.[5, 6]

CLASSIFICATION

The most widely used classification system for syndactyly has been that devised by Davis and German (Table 16–1).[7]

Table 16–1. **Classification of Syndactylism**

Incomplete	Webbing of the digits does not extend to the distalmost aspect of the involved digits
Complete	Webbing extends to the distalmost aspect of the involved digits
Simple	No phalangeal (osseous) involvement
Complicated	Involvement of the phalangeal bones with abnormality or synostosis
Combination	Incomplete–simple, incomplete–complicated, complete–simple, complete–complicated

DISCUSSION

Most of the literature discussing syndactyly has been concerned with the findings and correction of digital coherence of the fingers. This is largely due to the functional and cosmetic influences of syndactyly on the hand. Syndactyly of the toes generally does not result in any significant functional alteration, although associated gait abnormalities[8] and painful digital contraction[9] have been reported. More often, the concerns of syndactyly of the toes and consideration of repair are cosmetic in nature. Physical differences among children can have significant psychologic implications, and therefore the importance of cosmetic concerns should not be disregarded.

Any consideration of a surgical repair of a syndactyly must also take into account the presence of other associated disorders. Syndactyly has been associated with an ever enlarging variety of disease states (Table 16–2).

PREOPERATIVE CONSIDERATIONS

When a surgical procedure is being considered for the correction of syndactyly, preoperative preparation and planning are perhaps just as important as the actual performance of the procedure. Several important factors must be considered to ensure the optimal functional and cosmetic result postoperatively.

The first point to be considered is the optimal age of the patient. Most authors agree that the correction should be performed before the second year of life because such timing produces the least likelihood of joint contractures.[10, 11] This age has been determined by studies on the hand and is based on the age at which independent function of the fingers occurs—normally in the first 6 months to 2 years of life.[12] An important factor in the timing of the surgery is the presence or absence of bony abnormality with bridging of adjacent phalanges. If bony involvement is present, the procedure should be carried out early in life to prevent any subsequent osseous abnormalities associated with disruption of the physis.

Additional important considerations are the pathologic anatomy of syndactyly, which may affect nearly all structural elements of the digit. In nearly all cases of syndac-

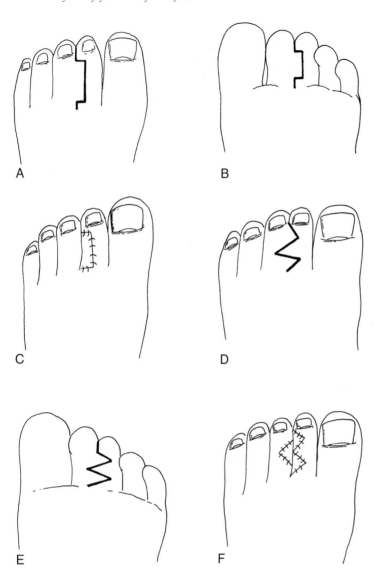

Figure 16–1. Didot modification for desyndactylization. *A*, Placement of the dorsal incisions and resultant flap extending from the point of syndactyly to the midpoint of the second toe. *B*, Placement of the plantar incisions and resultant flap extending to the midpoint of the third toe. *C*, The dorsal flap is then raised and transposed to the plantar aspect of the third toe. The plantar flap is raised and transposed to the dorsal aspect of the second toe, completing the desyndactylization. *D–F*, Cronin modification for desyndactylization. *D*, Placement of the dorsal incisions in a zigzag fashion, with two V-shaped flaps on the midline of the second toe and one flap on the third toe. *E*, Placement of the plantar incisions in a zigzag fashion, with two V-shaped flaps on the midline of the third toe and one flap on the second toe. *F*, The dorsal and plantar flaps are then raised and transposed, completing the desyndactylization.

tyly, the skin present about the circumference of the digits and the web space is less than that required to cover the exposed surfaces following separation, and this discrepancy may be as high as 57%.[13] Tissue expanders have been inserted in the hand and are recommended to be left in place for a 2-month period to provide additional skin for coverage and closure without skin grafting.[14, 15] To date, there is no report of the use of such devices in reconstruction of syndactyly in the toes.

Table 16–2. **Diseases Associated with Syndactylism**

Oculodental dysplasia	Noonan's syndrome
Trisomy 13	Polydactyly
Metatarsus varus	Apert's syndrome
Down's syndrome	Fraser's syndrome
Pfeiffer's syndrome	Trisomy 21
Orofaciodigital syndrome	Aplasia cutis congenita
Trisomy 18	Poland's syndrome
Craniofacial syndromes	Intracranial arteriovenous
Klippel-Trénaunay	malformation
syndrome	
Cleft palate	
Talipes equinovarus	

There can be an abnormality of the neurovascular bundle, most commonly resulting in distal migration of the bifurcation of the common digital vessels and nerves into the aberrant web space.[13, 14, 16] There may also be an abnormality in the anatomy of the extrinsic and intrinsic tendons and their insertions.[17] The osseous deformity has been well documented and may be primary, with congenital bridging of the adjacent phalanges, or secondary, with changes resulting from the deforming forces of the syndactyly.

When planning a surgical procedure, it is important to consider whether the design of the chosen skin flaps will provide adequate coverage or not. If the chosen flaps fail to come together, it must be decided whether to allow secondary wound healing or to use a split-thickness skin graft. Also, great care must be taken to avoid creating sharp corners within the flap, which may be more susceptible to necrosis and dehiscence.

SURGICAL PROCEDURES

Historically, a multitude of surgical procedures has been devised dating back to ancient times. Initially, sim-

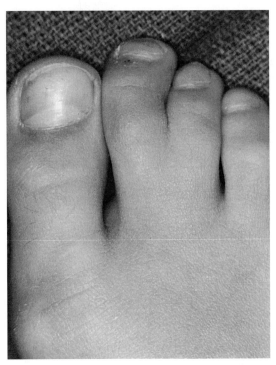

Figure 16–2. Syndactyly of the second and third toes.

The disadvantage is that the orientation of the flaps may not provide complete soft tissue coverage, and there is a higher risk of joint contracture postoperatively due to straight line incisional scarring. The Cronin procedure (Fig. 16–1 D–F) utilizes a Z-shaped incision dorsally and plantarly, which provides V-Y capabilities with mobilization of the skin and subsequent superior soft tissue coverage with less likelihood of joint contracture. The procedure described by Weinstock has the advantage of ease of dissection without the use of skin flaps but requires the use of a full-thickness graft taken from the region of the lateral opening of the sinus tarsi to cover the entire desyndactylized site.

Park[21] recently described a modification of the Radulesco skin flap method used in hand surgery. A dorsolateral skin flap is used to close the medial side of the lateral toe. Then a long linear incision is made in the the middle of the syndactylized toes (Figs. 16–2 and 16–3) extending plantarly to the proximal toe crease where a rhomboid-shaped plantar skin flap is used to close the lateral side of the medial toe. The two flaps are transposed to create a new web space.

ple procedures involving splitting of the webbed digits were performed; these undoubtedly resulted in a high rate of recurrence. Refinement of surgical techniques has resulted in the development of a variety of flaps that have the goal of maximal soft tissue coverage and development of a normal interdigital web space. Current surgical procedures used to desyndactylize toes are modifications of procedures described by Didot,[18] Cronin,[19] and Weinstock.[20] In any instance, consideration must be given to the fact that the skin available is not usually sufficient to provide complete coverage and skin grafting may be necessary. The procedure devised by Didot involves the elevation of rectangular flaps along the dorsal and plantar aspect of the digits (Fig. 16–1 A–C). The advantage of this procedure is the ease of development of the flaps.

Operative Technique

The choice of anesthetic is at the discretion of the surgeon, and the surgery may be performed under general or intravenous sedation with local anesthesia. A pneumatic tourniquet at the level of the thigh or ankle is recommended for better visualization of the neurovascular bundles.

Preoperatively, the planned incisions and flaps should be drawn out prior to proceeding. Once incised, the flaps are raised full thickness, and sutures are placed through the flaps, which allows for gentle retraction and exposure. The flaps should be handled with care, and the surgeon should avoid the use of pickups or other instruments, which may cause vascular embarrassment to the flaps. The soft tissue dissection must be precise, and the neurovascular bundles to each digit should be located prior to complete separation of the toes. The dissection should be

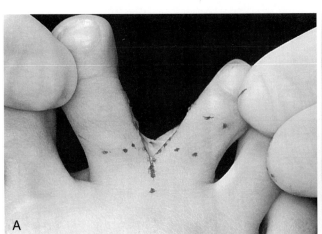

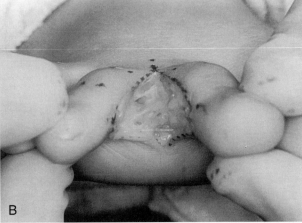

Figure 16–3. Alternative linear incision. A, Anteroposterior view; B, frontal view. Incision is deepened to the depth of the neurovascular structures. Incisional closure assumes the 3:1 ratio of a semi-elliptical closure to approximate skin edges.

carried to the level of the bifurcation of the common digital vessels and nerves.

Closure of the desyndactylization can present a challenge to the surgeon because the skin provided often is not sufficient to close the exposed soft tissue entirely. Dissection and excision of the fatty tissue about the toes, taking care not to disrupt the neurovascular bundles, can aid in better skin coverage of the defects. The tourniquet should be deflated prior to closure, and hemostasis must be achieved to prevent hematoma formation under the flaps, which will lead to failure. The site may be closed using simple and apical sutures of either absorbable or nonabsorbable 6–0 sutures. The viability of the flaps must be assessed, and any tight sutures must be loosened to allow the flaps to become pink and healthy.

If there are small deficits that are not covered, these may be allowed to close secondarily. Larger deficits require full-thickness skin grafts, which can be obtained from the region of the lateral opening of the sinus tarsi, the dorsum of the forefoot, or the medial aspect of the medial column in the midfoot; once harvested, the sites can be closed primarily. Full-thickness skin grafts are generally preferred to split-thickness grafts because they are associated with less likelihood of joint contraction, although split-thickness grafts have been used successfully.[9]

Postoperatively, the site is covered with a mildly compressive nonadherent dressing, and the toes are bandaged separated. The toes are immobilized with a posterior splint, and, if possible, the patient is kept nonweight-bearing for a 3-week period to maximize flap and skin graft viability. Postoperative complications of the procedure include infection, necrosis of the flaps with dehiscence, and sloughing of the skin leading to resyndactylization, hypertrophic scarring with joint contracture, web creep (distal migration of the corrected web space), and graft failure. The most common complication is sloughing of the flaps, which can result in an open wound. Wet to dry saline dressings with bandaging to separate the digits are indicated to allow secondary wound healing to occur. Once healthy granulation tissue forms, a split-thickness skin graft can be applied to complete the closure.

References

1. Mondolfi L: Syndactyly of the toes. J Plast Surg 1983;71:212.
2. McGlamery ED: Comprehensive Textbook of Foot Surgery. Baltimore, Williams & Wilkins, 1987.
3. Ruby L, Goldberg M: Syndactyly and polydactyly. Symposium on birth defects and the orthopedic surgeon. Orthop Clin North Am 1976;7:363.
4. Entin MA: Syndactyly of the upper limb: Morphogenesis, classification, and management. Clin Plast Surg 1976;3:129–140.
5. Hoyne HE, Jones KL, VanAllen MI: Vascular pathogenesis of transverse limb reduction defects. J Pediatr 1982;101:839–843.
6. VanAllen MI: Fetal vascular disruption mechanisms and some resulting birth defects. Pediatr Ann 1981;10:219–233.
7. Davis JS, German WJ: Syndactylism (coherence of the fingers or toes). Arch Surg 1930;21:32.
8. Cisco RW, Pitts TE, Cicchinelli LD, Caldarella DJ: Bilateral syndactyly. J Am Podiatr Med Assoc 1993;11:645–650.
9. Dowdy NL, Puleo DC: Desyndactylization: A unique case report. J Foot Surg 1991;4:340–343.
10. Bauer TB, Tondra JM: Technical modification in repair of syndactylism. J Plast Reconstr Surg 1956;17:835.
11. Morreale PF, Carnozza LP, Byrnes MF: A complicated incomplete syndactylism. J Foot Surg 1988;5:428–432.
12. Dobyns JH, Doyle JR, Von Gillern TL: Congenital anomalies of the upper extremity. Hand Clin 1989;3:321.
13. Eaton CJ, Lister GD: Syndactyly. Hand Clin 1990;4:555–575.
14. Gudushauri OH, Tvaliashvili LA: Local epidermoplasty for syndactyly. Int Orthop 1991;1:39–43.
15. Ogawa Y, Kasai K, Doi H: The preoperative use of extra tissue expander for syndactyly. Ann Plast Surg 1989;6:552–559.
16. Mantero R, Rosello MI, Grandis C: Digital subtraction angiography in preoperative examination of congenital hand malformations. J Hand Surg 1985;10A:754.
17. Flatt AE: Practical Factors in the Treatment of Syndactylism. Symposium on Reconstructive Hand Surgery, Vol. 9. St. Louis, C.V. Mosby, 1970.
18. Didot A: Note sur la separation des doigts palmes, er sur un nouveau procede anaplastique destine a prevenir la reproduction de la difformite. Bull Acad R Belge 1849;9:351–366.
19. Cronin JD: Syndactylism: Experience in its correction. Tristate Med J 1943;15:2869–2884.
20. Weinstock RE, Bass SJ, Farmer MA: Desyndactylization: A new modification. J Am Podiatr Assoc 1984;74:458–461.
21. Park S, Tomoaki E, Tokioka K, Minegishi M: Reconstruction of incomplete syndactyly of the toes using both dorsal and plantar flaps. Plast Reconstr Surg 1996;98:534–537.

17

Digital Deformities

Edwin Harris, D.P.M.

The management strategies used for digital deformities in young children differ from treatment plans used for the same problems in adults. Although the deformities are as evident objectively in children as they are in adults, most children are remarkably free of subjective symptoms when the parents first become aware that a problem exists. In fact, these children rarely experience pain and discomfort from their toe deformities until the end of the first decade of life. Because these abnormalities are not subjectively problematic and because treatment advantages are afforded by the immature skeleton, the most appropriate reparative procedures for these children are designed to reconstruct the soft tissue components of the condition in anticipation of more normal growth after the deforming forces have been altered. For this age group, techniques that spare the bones and joints are usually selected.

The bioplastic properties of the child's skeleton are unique. Bones grow in the direction determined by the forces placed on them. Persistent static changes develop as a result of long-standing positional abnormalities and muscular forces placed on the developing bone and cartilage. The presence of growth plates allows the immature skeleton to change shape.

Because of the capabilities for altering shape, the approach to the treatment of pediatric digital deformities uses these remodeling potentials to the surgeon's advantage. More attention is placed on manipulating soft tissue and less on surgically modifying bones and joints directly. This is particularly advantageous if one considers the technical difficulties associated with bone-cutting procedures performed on structures that measure only millimeters in size. Joint preservation is critical for continued bone growth.

Soft tissue abnormalities are more likely to be the primary cause of digital deviations in the child. Reestablishment of normal soft tissue anatomy can prevent additional deformity and restore anatomy to an acceptable state. Complete surgical correction is usually the goal. In some situations, surgical intervention may be indicated for the sole purpose of preventing progression of a minimal deformity that does not need radical correction at that time. In other situations, the goal may be to halt progression of a severe deformity that cannot be fully corrected at the time of intervention.

THE HALLUX

Congenital Hallux Varus

Transverse deviation of the hallux at the metatarsophalangeal joint from birth is called congenital hallux varus. Even though it is present in early infancy, the deformity is usually identified only when the infant begins to walk. Congenital hallux varus may occur in isolation or in association with other conditions. These include preaxial polydactyly, longitudinal epiphyseal bracket, talipes equinovarus, and metatarsus adductus.

Hallux Varus Associated with Polydactyly

This form of hallux varus is associated with some variation of preaxial polydactyly. This may take the form of a fully developed vestigial toe. Hallux varus may also be associated with a fibrous remnant tethering the medial aspect of the first proximal phalanx to the medial tarsus. This is regarded as an incompletely expressed preaxial polydactyly. There is no recognizable additional ray in this second variant.

Hallux Varus Associated with Longitudinal Epiphyseal Bracket of the First Metatarsal

Hallux varus may be associated with longitudinal epiphyseal bracket. This is an anomaly of growth plate formation that occurs in bones having single epiphyses located at the proximal ends. In the foot this anomaly occurs only in the first metatarsal and the toe phalanges. When it is associated with hallux varus, the aberrant epiphysis brackets the medial side of the first metatarsal diaphysis. It also extends as a continuous unit distally and proximally to encompass the articular ends of the involved bone. This configuration causes abnormal growth of the first metatarsal that results in both shortening and varus angulation. The distal metatarsal articular surface deviates medially to produce a negative proximal articular set angle.

Hallux Varus Associated with Abnormality of the Abductor Hallucis

Most frequently, there are two divisions in the insertion of the abductor hallucis. The inferolateral fibers insert into the medial sesamoid along with the medial tendon of the flexor hallucis brevis. These two tendons continue together distally to insert onto the plantar and medial tubercle at the base of the proximal phalanx. The superior and medial fibers insert into the medial portion of the extensor hood. The tendon does not usually insert independently into the medial aspect of the proximal phalanx of the hallux as described incorrectly in some anatomy texts.[19] Basmajian and Kerr (quoted in Thompson) identified five variations of insertion.[22] In the first form the tendon continues medially to insert independently into the medial side of the first proximal phalangeal base. With this type of insertion, the muscle acts as a pure adductor of the hallux. In the second form the tendon of the abductor hallucis and the medial head of the flexor hallucis brevis may conjoin to insert into the tibial sesamoid in such a way that the abductor hallucis acts as a plantar flexor. In the third form the tendon of the abductor hallucis may pass medial and plantar to the tibial sesamoid without inserting into it. In the fourth form a tendinous slip leaves the lateral side of the abductor hallucis and goes to the tibial sesamoid. This slip comes off just before the abductor inserts onto the proximal phalanx. In the fifth form there is a common insertion of the abductor hallucis and the medial head of the flexor hallucis brevis into the tibial sesamoid. Basmajian and Kerr's fourth variant most closely matches the configuration depicted by Sarrafian when he describes the superomedial fibers attaching to the extensor expansion and the inferolateral fibers attaching to the medial sesamoid.[19]

The three abnormalities of the abductor hallucis that can result in medial deviation of the hallux on the transverse plane are abnormal insertion, contracture of the muscle, and abnormal tone in the muscle.

Abnormal Insertion. The superior and medial portion of the tendon of insertion can be the dominant segment. The tendon courses much higher on the medial side of the metatarsophalangeal joint and can actually run superior to the joint axis. Its major insertion also occurs farther distally on the dorsomedial side of the proximal phalanx. The inferolateral insertion may be absent. The muscle's action becomes pure adduction in the transverse plane.

The course of the tendon can be palpated by placing proximal traction on the muscle through the skin. Alternatively, the muscle can be tested by transcutaneous electrical stimulation over the muscle belly. Either technique allows preoperative mapping of both the course of the tendon and its point of insertion. There is a high correlation between the results of preoperative assessment and the course of the tendon actually visualized during surgical exploration.

Contracture of the Abductor Hallucis. The abductor hallucis may lack sufficient length. This condition is almost always associated with other forefoot adduction deformities. For example, forefoot adduction is common to both metatarsus adductus and talipes equinovarus. When the forefoot malposition is corrected, the distance between the origin and the insertion of the abductor hallucis becomes greater. Contracture results if the abductor hallucis does not elongate on its own. The effect is adduction and plantar flexion of the hallux (Fig. 17–1).

Altered Tone in the Abductor Hallucis. Inappropriate activity of the abductor hallucis can cause medial deviation of the great toe. Some of the movement disorders associated with cerebral palsy and other forms of encephalopathy can produce altered tone, hyperreflexia, and improper activity patterns. Over a period of time, the abductor hallucis may develop myostatic contracture resulting in anatomic shortening.

Consequences of Hallux Varus

The first metatarsal head in very young children with hallux varus is round and is not deformed. The base of the proximal phalanx is abnormally positioned on the medial side of the head. It is possible to reposition the hallux on the first metatarsal because the head shape has not yet become permanently altered. If the abnormal adducted position is maintained long enough, the articular surface of the head will remodel to form a negative proximal articular set angle (Fig. 17–2). If this occurs, the adduction deformity becomes permanent. This can lead to shoe-fitting problems and joint pathology.

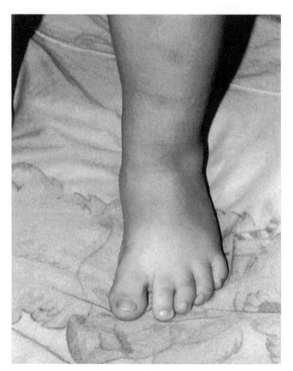

Figure 17–1. A 2-year-old girl had successful closed reduction of metatarsus adductus by serial casting. Although the metatarsal deformity was corrected, the hallux remained adducted at the metatarsophalangeal joint. On surgical exploration, the tendon of the abductor hallucis was located much more medial than normal and inserted predominantly into the base of the proximal phalanx.

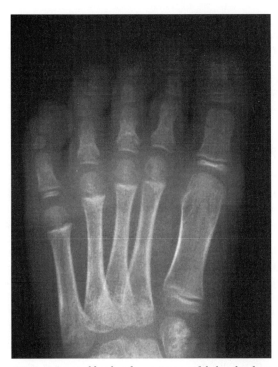

Figure 17–2. A 5-year-old girl underwent successful closed reduction for metatarsus adductus during infancy. At age 4, her parents noted adduction of the hallux. This was dynamic, and was most obvious when the child was walking. An AP radiograph of the foot shows medial rotation of the usable cartilage of the first metatarsal head.

Hallux varus may play a role in the cause of the primary metatarsal or forefoot deformity. Since forefoot conditions such as metatarsus adductus and talipes equinovarus are associated with hallux varus, it has been theorized that persistent hallux varus could cause recurrence of the forefoot deformity after it has been corrected by other means.

Although there are no data to support this contention, it has been argued that some cases of juvenile hallux valgus may be the result of hallux varus. Medial pressure from shoes against the hallux could cause attenuation of the medial capsule of the first metatarsophalangeal joint and the tendon of the abductor hallucis. The adductor hallucis then would become mechanically advantageous and contract to rotate the hallux into valgus. Movement of the abductor hallucis and the sesamoid apparatus in a lateral direction would follow, destabilizing the first metatarsophalangeal joint.[8]

Treatment for Hallux Varus

There is no nonoperative treatment for hallux varus. The decision to intervene surgically is based on the severity of the deformity, subjective complaints, the potential for worsening, additional associated deformities, and family preferences.

Preaxial Polydactyly

Whenever possible, reconstruction of a biphalangeal first toe should be attempted. This may not be possible in all cases. First ray function, cosmetically acceptable medial foot contour, and shoe wear then become the concerns. Farmer described a technique for repair of preaxial polydactyly and hallux varus that combines excision of any preaxial components with creation of a flap to reposition the hallux transversely. The first web space can be reconstructed if possible, or the first and second toes can be syndactylized.[5]

Occasionally, a vestigial preaxial ray may be represented only by a fibrocartilage band running from the medial side of the first toe to some point in the tarsus. The medial side of the first ray should be explored, and any fibrous band encountered should be excised. The insertion of the abductor hallucis should then be reconstructed.

Longitudinal Epiphyseal Bracket

Longitudinal epiphyseal bracket is a progressive problem resulting in both varus angulation of the metatarsal head and metatarsal shaft shortening by interference with longitudinal growth.[10, 14] Magnetic resonance imaging (MRI) of the first metatarsal demonstrates the extent of the bracket. It is possible to excise the physeal bridge. The void is filled with fat to prevent the bridge from reforming. At an appropriate time, lengthening of the first metatarsal can be achieved by Z-lengthening, intercalary grafting, or distraction corticotomy. Osteotomy of the first metatarsal to correct the reversed proximal articular angle may also be indicated.

Insertion Abnormalities and Contracture

Four types of procedures are designed for this deformity: excision of the abductor hallucis, distal tenotomy, midbelly and proximal release, and distal tendon transfer. Thompson first recommended excision of the entire abductor hallucis for metatarsus adductus.[22] He believed that the abductor hallucis and the adductor hallucis were unimportant muscles. Other surgeons have adopted his procedure as a treatment for hallux varus. There are a number of problems with this operation. First, complications can result from intraoperative and postoperative injury to the medial and lateral plantar neurovascular bundles. Second, the alteration of the medial contour of the foot is cosmetically unacceptable. Third, transverse medial control of the first metatarsophalangeal joint is lost. The result is severe acquired hallux abducto valgus unless the adductor hallucis insertion is detached. Thompson also noted keloid formation in the incision line as a complication.

Jones and McCrea recommended closed tenotomy of the abductor hallucis muscle and its fascia through a dorsal incision 1.5 cm proximal to the metatarsophalangeal joint as a treatment for hallux varus.[7] While I do not recommend this procedure in isolation, I do have experience performing combined midbelly tenotomy and myotomy as a component of other procedures. When performing capsulotomy of the tarsometatarsal joints for unresolved metatarsus adductus, I section the fascia and incise the abductor hallucis muscle just distal to the first metatarsal base. Great care must be taken to avoid injuring the neurovascular structures.

During medial release for clubfoot, I detach the origin of the abductor hallucis and free it distally to the first metatarsal base. This facilitates medial dissection and releases this tight structure. I do not repair the abductor hallucis proximally. Despite this wide release, hallux varus persists in some children following otherwise successful clubfoot repair.

Tenotomy of Abductor Hallucis

Tenotomy of the abductor hallucis can be performed through a small plantar and medial incision.[11] This releases the distal portion of the muscle. However, this procedure neither releases the aponeurosis of insertion from the medial plantar skin nor normalizes an anomalous insertion of the abductor hallucis, thus allowing the possibility of recurrence.

Transfer of Abductor Hallucis

It is easy to explore the insertion of the abductor hallucis with the intent of reconstructing any abnormal insertion. This is done through a conventional bunion incision made longitudinally over the first metatarsophalangeal joint medial to the extensor hallucis longus tendon (Fig. 17–3A). The dissection is carried out in a plantar direction on the medial side of the first metatarsophalangeal joint. Care is taken to preserve the dorsomedial nerves. The muscle belly of the abductor hallucis is identified. If it cannot be found, it was probably carried in a plantar direction during the skin dissection because its distal fascia is intimately adherent to the plantar skin. The aponeurosis of insertion is followed distally. It can be determined visually if the insertion is abnormal or if the tendon is contracted. If the tendon inserts normally, it can be lengthened in Z-fashion. If it inserts abnormally, it is followed distally into the toe to gain as much length as possible. The inferolateral portion is separated from the medial head of the flexor hallucis brevis. The abductor fascia is separated from the skin (see Fig. 17–3B), and the tendon is detached distally. Excess tendon length is trimmed, and the tendon is sutured to the medial sesamoid and the medial head of the flexor hallucis brevis (see Fig. 17–3C). The medial capsule and the site of the former abductor hallucis bed are carefully incised subtotally in a vertical plane. Care is taken to not completely incise the capsule; the joint should not be entered. The choice of closure is the surgeon's preference. The child is placed in a walking cast for 2 weeks to allow the tendon to adhere to its transferred position and to protect the wound from the young child. This technique is preferred because it restores normal insertion.

THE SECOND DIGIT

The two most common deformities of the second toe are flexion deformity in the sagittal plane and deviation in the transverse plane. Flexion deformity may occur at the proximal interphalangeal articulation, the distal interphalangeal articulation, or both sites. The more common of the two is flexion deformity at the distal interphalangeal joint. Transverse deviation may be adductory or abductory. This deformity usually occurs at the level of the middle phalanx.

Sagittal Plane Deformity

It is unusual for sagittal plane deformity of the second toe to be congenital. Most cases begin at about age 6 or 7 years. Once started, the condition progresses rapidly. Axial rotational deformity is not likely to be associated with sagittal deformity. The abnormality is usually flexible in the beginning, and the interphalangeal joint can be passively repositioned in full extension. Flexor digitorum longus pulls the distal segment of the toe into sharp plantarflexion. With time, the distal interphalangeal joint capsule undergoes contracture. Fixed contracture causes subjective complaints and objective findings, of which keratosis at the distal aspect of the toe is the most common. Traumatic nail deformity follows. Pain from pressure of the distal aspect of the toe against the weight-bearing surface results from the fixed flexion deformity.

Transverse Plane Deformity

Transverse plane deformity may consist of medial or lateral deviation; lateral deviation is the most frequent. The apex of the deformity is at the middle phalanx. X-ray studies often show an absence of the physis at the base of the middle phalanx. Although not as frequent as lateral deviation, medial displacement does occur.

Subjective complaints resulting from transverse plane deformities are very rare in early childhood. The deformity is not likely to progress, although increased lineal length of the toe with growth may make the deformity appear worse. Discomfort may be caused by abutment of the second and third toes. Interdigital lesions may form owing to the close proximity of the two toes.

The parents become concerned about the physical appearance of the toe. It should be pointed out that some degree of lateral deviation of the second toe is commonly associated with flexion and varus deformity of the third toe. On occasion, the parents single out the second toe when the deformity is actually due to the third toe underlapping the second toe. The parents may interpret this configuration as crossing over of the second and third toes.

Treatment for Second Toe Deformities

Taping and splinting second toe deformities in infancy and childhood is not effective in modifying the natural history of the deformity. Any morbidity associated with this technique is conjectural, but the technique is difficult to perform in infants and very young children. It is possible that contact dermatitis may develop from prolonged

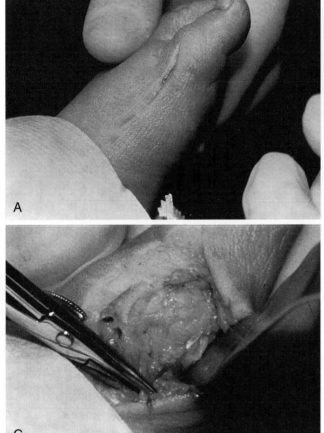

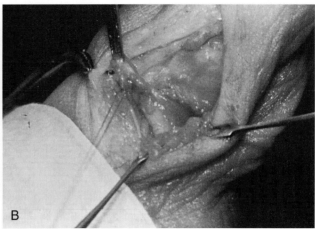

Figure 17–3. *A,* Transfer of the abductor hallucis tendon. The abductor hallucis is approached through a standard dorsomedial bunion incision. *B,* The abductor tendon is detached from its insertion into the base of the proximal phalanx. It is freed from the skin and from the first metatarsal. The tendon and the muscle belly are freely mobilized. *C,* The abductor tendon is sutured into the medial sesamoid and the medial head of flexor hallucis brevis *(arrow).*

application of tape. Anecdotal stories suggest that strangulation of the toe is a possibility, although I have never encountered such a case.

Flexor tenotomy and flexor tendon transfers are the main surgical procedures performed for sagittal plane deformity. A number of reports advocate both surgical approaches. The long and short flexor tendons can be identified and retrieved from an appropriately placed plantar incision. Tenotomy of both tendons is performed transversely. The tendons are not repaired or lengthened. Care should be taken not to place the incision in such a way that contracture of the skin of the plantar crease results.

Simple flexor tenotomy has a number of advantages. It is easy to perform. Postoperative management is simple, and very minimal morbidity is associated with the procedure. The biggest disadvantage is largely theoretical: Since there may be abnormal insertion of the long flexor tendon, the problem may recur because the tendon may reconstitute itself.

Transfer of the long flexor tendon to the extensor tendon is also advocated for this deformity. The details of this procedure are discussed in the next section on congenital third and fourth curly toe deformity. This procedure demands greater surgical skill than simple tenotomy. Since it is performed through an open dorsal exposure, interphalangeal capsulotomy and other soft tissue proce-

dures can easily be performed at the same time (Fig. 17–4).

Currently, I recommend flexor digitorum longus tendon transfer for flexion deformity of the second toe for children who are neurologically intact. In other cases, simple tenotomy does have some clear indications. For example, children with cerebral palsy may require a palliative procedure to deal with painful second toe contractures. This technique is especially suitable for nonambulatory children. Simple tenotomy for this group is the procedure of choice. It should be noted that the deformity can recur following simple tenotomy.

Most transverse plane deformities do not require any surgical intervention. When necessary, surgical treatment is limited to osteotomy of the middle phalanx followed by Kirschner wire fixation. For obvious technical reasons, the middle phalanx must be of substantial size to perform an osteotomy. This procedure is reserved for older children and adolescents (Fig. 17–5).

VARUS DEFORMITY OF THE THIRD AND FOURTH TOES

This deformity goes under the names congenital hammertoe, varus toe, and congenital curly toe. The deformity is present at birth in most cases (Fig. 17–6). It may be

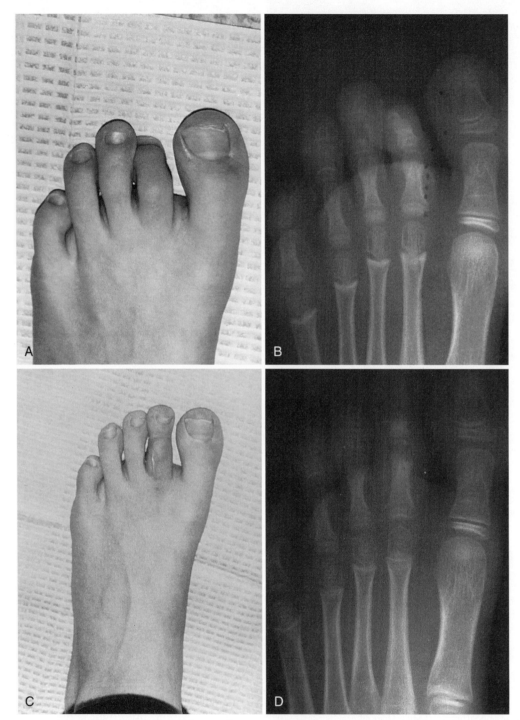

Figure 17–4. *A,* A 10-year-old boy had a 15-month history of progressive flexion deformity of the second toe. *B,* Preoperative radiograph of the left foot of the boy shown in Figure 17–4*A.* Note that the second toe has three separate phalanges and that there is a flexion deformity at the distal interphalangeal joint. *C,* Postoperative appearance of the boy shown in *A* after flexor-to-extensor tendon transfer. *D,* Postoperative radiograph following flexor-to-extensor tendon transfer in the second toe.

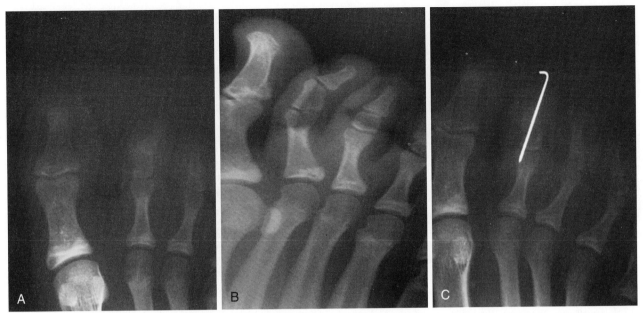

Figure 17–5. *A* and *B*, A 14-year-old skeletally mature boy had lateral deviation of the right second toe for many years. He developed keratosis on the lateral side of the second toe. AP and oblique radiographs show obliquity of the middle phalanx of the second toe. *C*, The deformity was treated by osteotomy and Kirschner wire fixation of the middle phalanx.

missed early in life only to become worse at age 2 or 3 years. In other cases, the deformity develops at around 2 to 3 years of age.

There is mild hyperextension at the metatarsophalangeal joint, flexion at the proximal and distal interphalangeal joints, and varus rotation of the involved toe. The affected toe underlaps the next medial toe (Fig. 17–7).

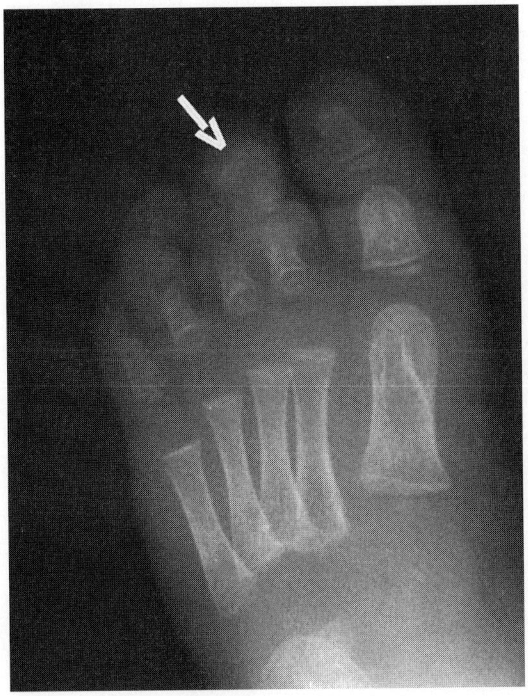

The involved toe is usually longer than anticipated, as can be seen when the toe is passively extended and derotated. It almost always appears longer than the next medial toe. The parents should be advised before surgery that this will result (Fig. 17–8).

Subjective symptoms in infancy and early childhood are uncommon. As the child becomes older, discomfort is experienced on the distolateral end of the toe as it rubs on the shoe. In longstanding cases, the nail changes shape because of the abnormal pressure.[17] The child may develop pain in the next medial toe because the varus toe underlaps it.

As is the case with second toe deformity, there is no benefit in taping and strapping the affected toes.[20] Simple tenotomy has been described for the repair of curly digits, but I prefer to treat the problem with flexor digitorum

Figure 17–6. A male infant had had curly digit deformity of the third toe since birth. The distal phalanx of the third toe completely underlaps the second toe so that the third toenail is completely covered by the second toe (*arrow*).

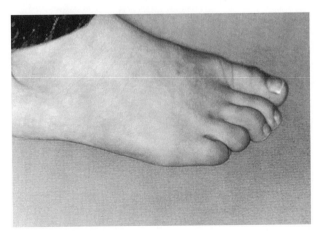

Figure 17–7. A 7-year-old boy with an underlapping right fourth toe (congenital curly toe deformity). There is marked varus rotation of the distal segment. The tip of the fourth toe is completely rotated under the third toe.

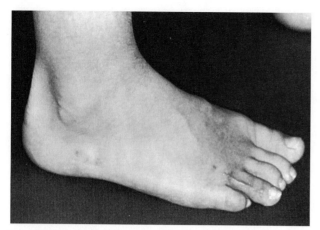

Figure 17–8. Same child shown in Figure 17–7. The position of the toe has been corrected by a flexor-to-extensor tendon transfer. Usually the distal phalanx regains its normal sagittal flexion curve when the short flexor tendon resumes function.

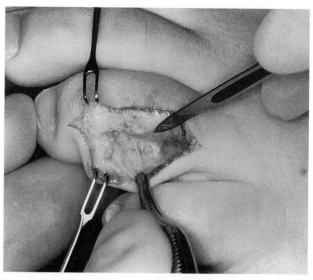

Figure 17–10. The dissection is carried on in a plantar direction along the lateral sides of the phalanges. The neurovascular bundle is easily seen and protected. It is carried down with the skin.

longus tendon transfer to the extensor hood. The exact pathologic anatomy of the deformity may vary from child to child, but the flexor digitorum longus becomes the deforming force when flexor digitorum brevis imbalance produces axial rotation. The goal is to neutralize the effect of the long flexor tendon on the distal phalanx while at the same time preserving flexion of the metatarsophalangeal joint. This is accomplished by transferring the long flexor tendon from the plantar side of the base of the distal phalanx to the lateral side of the extensor hood.

Surgical Technique

A longitudinal incision is made on the dorsolateral surface of the affected toe. It begins at a point just proximal to the eponychium. It is carried proximally to the level of the web space (Fig. 17–9). The incision is deepened along the lateral side of the phalanges. Careful dissection preserves the neurovascular bundles and allows them to be taken laterally with the skin (Fig. 17–10). The

lateral side of the flexor tendon sheath is identified plantar to the head of the proximal phalanx. It is incised at the level of the distal third of the proximal phalanx. A hook is placed in the sheath, and the long flexor tendon is delivered into the wound (Fig. 17–11). The tendon is followed distally and is detached from the base of the distal phalanx. It is best to tag it with a suture in the event that it retracts into the wound during the remainder of the dissection. The tendon is sutured into the lateral aspect of the extensor expansion just proximal to the head of the proximal phalanx. If the tendon has sufficient length, it can be used for a tenodesis of the proximal interphalangeal joint by carrying it dorsally over the capsule (Fig. 17–12). If the distal interphalangeal joint is

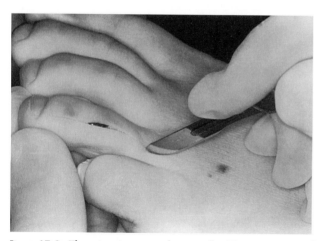

Figure 17–9. Flexor-to-extensor tendon transfer. Exposure is gained through a dorsolateral longitudinal incision extending from the web space to a point just distal to the distal interphalangeal joint. The nail matrix should not be violated.

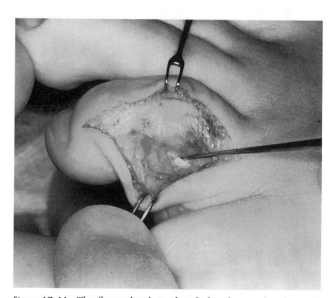

Figure 17–11. The flexor sheath is identified and opened in line with the long axes of the phalanges. Flexor digitorum longus is identified in the sheath and withdrawn into the wound. It is tagged with a suture and detached as far distally as possible to maximize its length for transfer.

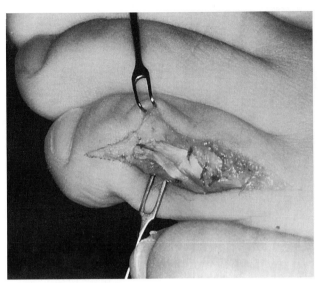

Figure 17–12. The flexor digitorum longus is sutured into the lateral aspect of the extensor hood. If there is enough residual length, the remaining flexor tendon can be used for tenodesis of the proximal interphalangeal joint. If necessary, the incision can be extended distally to allow capsulorrhaphy of the distal interphalangeal joint to maintain extension.

contracted, an ellipse of capsule can be excised from the dorsum. Repair of the capsular excision holds the distal interphalangeal joint in extension.

Children under the age of 3 usually do not need any fixation. In children over age 3, the toe is fixated in extension with a smooth Kirschner wire. This is followed by placement of a short leg walking cast. The cast and the Kirschner wire remain in place for 2 weeks; no additional splinting is necessary. In young children, remodeling of slight residual varus is to be expected (Fig. 17–13). On very rare occasions, the middle phalanx fails to remodel. In these cases, an osteotomy of the middle phalanx can

be used to correct this residual deformity. This salvage procedure can be done only when the middle phalanx is large enough for osteotomy (Fig. 17–14).

FIFTH TOE DEFORMITIES

Simple Varus Rotation

Some degree of varus rotation of the fifth toe is so common that it is considered normal. Of course, there are extremes of varus that are clearly pathologic. These extremes are so infrequently seen in children that the deformity is not an important pediatric issue. Parents notice this physiologic position and occasionally seek an opinion about treatment. In the vast majority of cases, management consists of parental reassurance.

Pathologic Varus Rotation

Treatable varus deformity occasionally develops following open reduction of talipes equinovarus. It is most likely to occur if there has been a radical plantar release of the first and second layer of plantar muscles. In the single case referred to me for surgical intervention, a flexor digitorum longus transfer to the extensor hood restored alignment.

Digiti Quinti Varus

Overriding of the fifth toe on the fourth toe is a frequently encountered pediatric deformity. Overriding fifth toe, cock-up toe, congenital elevation of the fifth toe, digitus minimus varus, and digiti quinti varus are the terms most frequently used to describe this condition. In

Figure 17–13. *A*, Preoperative radiograph of a 4-year-old boy with varus deformity of the left fourth toe. The interphalangeal flexion approached 90 degrees. *B*, Postoperative radiograph of the child shown in *A*. He underwent flexor-to-extensor tendon transfer without Kirschner wire fixation. There is no physis for the middle phalanx. Despite this, the residual varus was completely remodeled within a year.

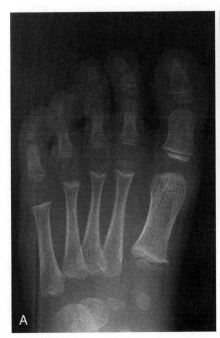
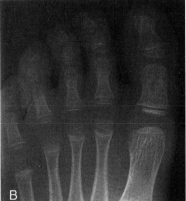

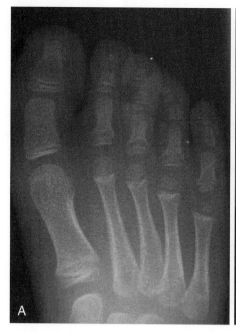

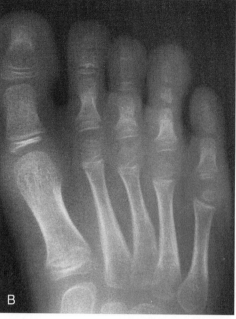

Figure 17–14. *A,* A 5-year-old boy underwent a flexor-to-extensor tendon transfer at age 30 months. The varus deformity never fully remodeled. He had discomfort in the fourth toe. *B,* The child shown in *A* underwent a simple abducting displacement osteotomy of the middle phalanx. The osteotomy was fixated with a Kirschner wire for 5 weeks. Alignment improved greatly, and the discomfort resolved.

this deformity, the fifth toe is extended at the interphalangeal joints. On occasion, symphalangism involving the middle and distal phalanges may be seen. The metatarsophalangeal joint is hyperextended. The fifth toe is deviated medially, rotates into varus, and overrides the fourth toe. The skin of the web space is shortened in response to this abnormal configuration, and the skin on the dorsum of the foot is also contracted (Fig. 17–15).

This abnormality has a wide range of clinical expression extending from simple hyperextension at the metatarsophalangeal joint without significant overlap to extreme adduction with 90 degrees or more of varus rotation. Several authors have proposed that digiti quinti varus deformity is hereditary.[1, 2, 9] The deformity may exist in isolation or as a component of a broader clinical picture. I have noted an association of digiti quinti varus deformity with Charcot-Marie-Tooth syndrome. Another common association is with postaxial polydactyly.

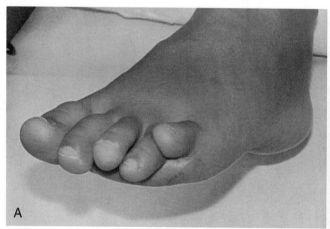

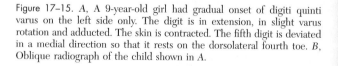

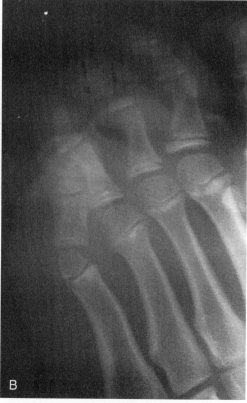

Figure 17–15. *A,* A 9-year-old girl had gradual onset of digiti quinti varus on the left side only. The digit is in extension, in slight varus rotation and adducted. The skin is contracted. The fifth digit is deviated in a medial direction so that it rests on the dorsolateral fourth toe. *B,* Oblique radiograph of the child shown in *A.*

Exploration of the deeper anatomy shows a number of consistent abnormalities. The extensor digitorum longus tendon for the fifth toe is contracted. This abnormality involves the tendon, its sheath, and the proximal portion of the extensor hood. The capsule is dorsally contracted. The tendons of the flexor digiti minimi and the abductor digiti minimi ride high along the lateral side of the fifth metatarsophalangeal joint; in some cases, their course is superior to the fifth metatarsophalangeal joint axis. When this happens, these muscles become dorsiflexors of the metatarsophalangeal joint. As a result of longstanding malposition, the head of the metatarsal adapts in response to the abnormally located base of the proximal phalanx. This creates a congruous joint in an undesirable position but should not be confused with a subluxed joint. The proximal phalanx naturally seeks this position until the metatarsal head remodels.

Surgical Repair

The large number of surgical procedures available to correct this deformity can be grouped into two classes. In the first group are those procedures designed for primary repair. These include Z-plasty of the skin with deep soft tissue release, Wilson's V-Y skin plasty, and the Butler procedure. The second group comprises procedures designed for salvage.

Current thought in the pediatric surgical literature is that surgical treatment in children should be directed toward soft tissue release and sparing of bone.[16] More aggressive procedures involving bone excision should be reserved for patients in whom soft tissue release alone is likely to fail. This group includes patients in whom previous soft tissue procedure have failed, those with digital developmental anomalies (polydactyly, complex polysyndactyly), and adults undergoing repair later in life.

Primary Soft Tissue Repair

Soft tissue repair planning must take into account the dorsal skin contraction as well as the abnormal tendon, ligaments, and capsular anatomy. Any procedure that does not address the skin tightness will almost certainly fail to achieve and maintain correction.

In 1964, Hulman described a procedure in which the abnormal skin crease on the lateral side of the fourth web space and the medial side of the fifth toe is excised.[6, 12] Through that incision, a capsulotomy and extensor tenotomy are performed. I have no experience with this procedure. Illustrations suggest that it should be selected for children with short fifth toes and shallow web spaces.

Z-Plasty of the Skin and Deep Release

Appropriately configured multiple Z-plasty or Z-Y incisions may be used in cases of mild contraction of the skin. They should be used only if the web space is not contracted. If planned correctly, the capsulotomy and tenotomy can be performed through one of the more lateral limbs of the incision.[3]

V-Y Plasty of the Skin and Deep Release

In 1953, Wilson described a V-Y incision technique that addressed the skin contracture and allowed access to the fifth metatarsophalangeal joint.[23] The medial limb of the incision can be carried well into the web space to release the skin contracture. The carefully raised flap allows deep access. There are two potential problems with this incision. First, because the flap is not physiologically based on an adequate blood supply, vascularity of the flap is dependent on distal blood vessels. Careful handling minimizes the potential for flap necrosis.[13] Second, the amount of distal advancement is limited. Currently, I use the Wilson procedure only for very mild deformities. Paton reported recurrence of the deformity and 60% poor results with this technique[15] (Fig. 17–16).

Rotational Transposition

In 1968, Cockin credited Butler posthumously with the description of a useful technique for repair of digiti quinti varus.[2] This procedure is best thought of as a vascularized repositioning toe flap. The skin, nail, bone, and cartilage are transferred as a vascularized unit based on the digit's own neurovascular bundles. Ellipses are made on both the medial and lateral sides of the fifth toe. The initial incisions on the plantar surface are designed in such a way that the apex can be advanced proximally by extending the incision laterally toward the rearfoot.

After the initial incisions are made, the dorsal and distal flap is raised in full-thickness fashion. The sheath and tendon of the extensor digitorum longus for the fifth toe are encountered. Although it is possible to lengthen this tendon in Z-fashion, the current recommendation is to perform an en bloc excision of 1 cm of the tendon and its sheath just proximal to the metatarsophalangeal joint.

The capsule of the metatarsophalangeal joint is identified and incised medially, dorsally, and laterally. Both the medial and the lateral collateral ligaments are sectioned. It is important also to incise the tendon insertions of the abductor digiti minimi and the flexor digiti minimi because they course superior to the axis of the metatarsophalangeal joint. The plantar plate of the metatarsophalangeal joint is usually left intact. In some cases, release of the plantar plate is needed to fully mobilize the toe.

In preparation for rotation, the incision lines are deepened along their full extent by blunt dissection. All four neurovascular bundles are preserved. The plantar incision is extended proximally to allow advancement of the plantar flap to derotate the toe in the sagittal plane. It is very often necessary to excise a triangular area of skin from both sides of the proximal extension to allow the distal flap to fit properly.

The toe is manually placed in the corrected position, and the web space is repaired with simple interrupted absorbable sutures. The toe is then fixated from its distal end across the metatarsophalangeal joint with an appro-

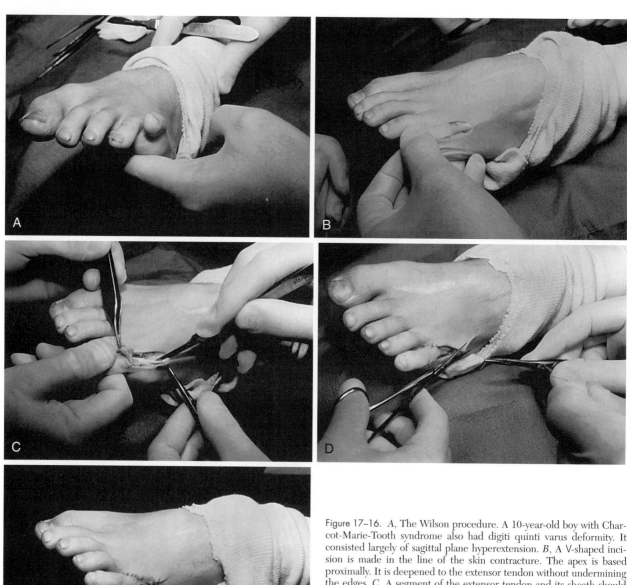

Figure 17–16. *A,* The Wilson procedure. A 10-year-old boy with Charcot-Marie-Tooth syndrome also had digiti quinti varus deformity. It consisted largely of sagittal plane hyperextension. *B,* A V-shaped incision is made in the line of the skin contracture. The apex is based proximally. It is deepened to the extensor tendon without undermining the edges. *C,* A segment of the extensor tendon and its sheath should be excised completely. I no longer recommend Z-plasty of the extensor tendon because of the higher incidence of recurrence of the deformity. *D,* The proximal limb of the incision is closed to form the long arm of a Y. The distal limbs are closed to form the short arms. *E,* The final closure converts the V-shaped incision into a Y-shaped incision.

priately sized smooth Kirschner wire. The plantar incisions are closed with the plantar flap advanced proximally in a Y-to-V technique. The dorsal incision is closed by changing its original V shape to a Y configuration (Fig. 17–17). A short leg cast is then placed. The cast and the Kirschner wire remain in place for 4 weeks (Fig. 17–18).

Salvage Procedures

McFarland is credited with describing excision of the base of the proximal phalanx of the fifth toe with surgical syndactyly of the fifth toe to the fourth toe for the management of digiti quinti varus.[4] This technique was popularized by Kelikian and is attributed by some to him. I have never found a situation in which this technique was indicated as the primary procedure in a pediatric patient.

In 1954 Ruiz-Mora described a technique for the management of digiti quinti varus.[18] An elliptical incision is made on the plantar surface of the fifth toe extending back proximally toward the metatarsal head area. The proximal portion of the incision is carried medially to help approximate the fourth and fifth toes after closure. Through this incision, the entire proximal phalanx is excised. The elliptical incision is closed from end to end and then from side to side to shorten the plantar surface of the fifth toe.

Earlier, in 1942, Lapidus had described a procedure

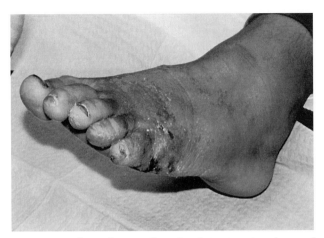

Figure 17–17. The Butler procedure. Initial postoperative photograph of the child shown in Figure 17–15. The incision totally isolates the toe. The original dorsal incision is shown. It is closed in V-Y fashion to move the distal flap even more distally. The plantar incision is initially Y-shaped. It is closed in Y-V fashion to advance the distal flap in a proximal direction.

for the correction of digiti quinti varus.[9] The incision is made on the dorsal surface of the fifth toe in serpentine fashion from the distal interphalangeal joint medially toward the web space. It is continued laterally across the fifth metatarsophalangeal joint and along the distal and lateral fifth metatarsal shaft. A separate proximal incision is made over the middle of the fifth metatarsal to allow tenotomy of the extensor digitorum longus tendon of the fifth toe. The distal tendon is brought out of the distal wound and is freed to its insertion. A subcutaneous tunnel is made by blunt dissection, starting dorsomedially distally under the phalanges and ending on the lateral side of the metatarsophalangeal joint. The tendon is passed through this tunnel and sutured under tension into the flexor digiti quinti and abductor digiti quinti tendons. This plantar-flexes and derotates the toe at the same time.

Amputation of the fifth toe is not a good alternative treatment for digiti quinti varus. Alteration in forefoot load bearing and pressure against the fifth metatarsal

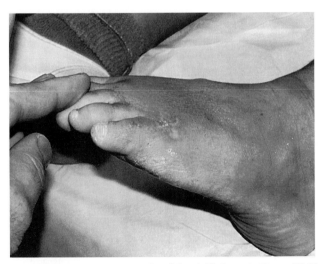

Figure 17–18. Postoperative results of the child shown in Figure 17–15 after the Butler procedure.

head cause subjective and objective problems that are worse than the original difficulty. Every attempt should be made to preserve the fifth toe.

SOME PERSONAL OBSERVATIONS

Hallux Varus

About half of the cases of hallux varus occur in the absence of any other pathology. In most patients the anatomy of the insertion of the abductor hallucis tendon is abnormal. In most of these, the dorsal and medial portion of the tendon is dominant, so that it acts as a one-plane adductor of the hallux. Some children simply have a tight muscle. I have found it useful to explore the insertion and transfer the tendon proximally into the area of the tibial sesamoid in both of these situations.

Deformities of the Lesser Toes

Transverse plane deformities of the second toe are usually so mild that they do not justify surgical intervention. For those symptomatic cases, osteotomy of the middle phalanx works well. These bones are usually so small that an off-set osteotomy is the only practical technique.

Tenotomy or Transfer

There are two very vocal schools of thought on tenotomy of the flexor tendons as opposed to transfer of these tendons. Those favoring tenotomy cite the simplicity of the procedure and the resultant supple toes as the advantages of this procedure. Those favoring tendon transfer cite a more physiologically sound procedure and resultant supple toes as advantages. In my personal experience, there is no stiffness or rigidity following flexor digitorum longus tendon transfer into the extensor hood.

Perhaps a review of the literature may give some insight into this problem of stiffness and rigidity. Taylor popularized the flexor-to-extensor transfer.[21] However, he transferred both the long and the short tendons into the extensor expansion. Most surgeons performing this procedure today transfer only the long flexor tendon. This allows the flexor digitorum longus to continue to function as a plantar flexor of the metatarsophalangeal joint. At the same time, the flexor digitorum brevis continues to act as a plantar flexor on the middle and distal phalanges. This may explain the lack of stiffness following flexor tendon transfer as performed today.

Flexor transfer works well both for sagittal plane deformity of the second toe and for varus rotation of the third and fourth toes. I routinely reroute the flexor along the lateral side of the toe. The single exception in my experience was transfer to the medial extensor expansion for correction of a severe varus deformity of a fifth toe.

Digiti Quinti Varus

In general, I have not been enthusiastic about the long-term results of Wilson's procedure for digiti quinti varus because the problem tends to recur. This is most likely due to the limitation of skin advancement resulting from the incision technique. For this reason, this procedure should be used only for milder deformities.

Butler's technique is preferable because of its greater potential for correction. The dorsal incision should be modified from that in the original description. Rather than a racquet-handle shape, it should begin dorsally with a V-shaped incision. This closes better and does not require any additional plastic repair. The greatest disadvantage of this procedure is the possibility of vascular catastrophe and potential loss of the toe. With delicate tissue handling, this should not be a problem.

SUMMARY

Most digital deformities are caused by abnormality of the soft tissues. If there is growth potential remaining, correction of the soft tissue abnormality will naturally lead to remodeling. Of course, each case must be judged on its own merits. Remodeling potential is finite and is a function of the child's developmental age.

Bone- and joint-sparing procedures are indicated for this age group, and mutilative procedures should be avoided. Particularly, every attempt possible should be made to avoid amputation of a toe.

Last, some problems seen in early childhood are mild. However, they have a known natural history of progression that leads to more serious disease later in life. It is perfectly acceptable to perform surgery designed to prevent progression of a mild deformity. In many cases, it is not necessary or advisable to fully correct a deformity with a very low potential for morbidity. The cure might be worse than the disease.

References

1. Black G, Grogan D, Bobechko W: Arthroplasty of the adducted fifth toe. J Pediatr Orthop 1985;5:439–441.
2. Cockin J: Butler's operation for an over-riding fifth toe. J Bone Joint Surg 1968;50B:78–81.
3. Crawford ME, Dockery GL: Use of Z-skin plasty in scar revisions and skin contractures of the lower extremity. J Am Podiatr Med Assoc 1995;85:28–35.
4. Crenshaw AH (ed): Campbell's Operative Orthopaedics, 4th ed. St. Louis, C. V. Mosby, 1963, pp. 1656–1657.
5. Farmer AW: Congenital hallux varus. Am J Surg 1958;95:274–278.
6. Hulman S: Simple operation for the overlapping fifth toe. Br Med J 1964;11:1506–1507.
7. Jones RA, McCrea J: Tenotomy of the abductor hallucis for correction of resistant metatarsus adductus. J Am Podiatr Assoc 1980;70:40–43.
8. Koop SE: Adolescent hallux valgus. *In* Drennan JC (ed): The Child's Foot and Ankle. New York, Raven Press, 1992, pp. 418–419.
9. Lapidus PW: Transplantation of the extensor tendon for correction of the overlapping fifth toe. J Bone Joint Surg 1942;24:555–559.
10. Light TR, Ogden JA: The longitudinal epiphyseal bracket: Implications for surgical correction. J Pediatr Orthop 1981;1:229–305.
11. McCrea JD: Pediatric Orthopedics of the Lower Extremity: An Instructional Handbook. Mount Kisco, NY, Future Publishing Co, 1985, pp. 313–314.
12. Morris E, Scullion J, Mann T: Varus fifth toe. J Bone Joint Surg 1984;64B:99–100.
13. Nilson RZ, Dockery GL: V-Y plasty and its variants. J Am Podiatr Med Assoc 1995;85:22–27.
14. Ogden JA, Light TR, Conlogue GJ: Correlative roentgenography and morphology for the longitudinal epiphyseal bracket. Skel Radiol 1981;6:109–117.
15. Paton R: V-Y plasty for correction of varus fifth toe. J Pediatr Orthop 1990;10:248–249.
16. Rang M: Other feet. *In* Wenger DR, Rang M (eds): The Art and Practice of Children's Orthopaedics. New York, Raven Press, 1993, p. 186.
17. Ross ERS, Menelaus MB: Open flexor tenotomy for hammer toes and curly toes in childhood. J Bone Joint Surg 1984;66B:770–771.
18. Ruiz-Mora J: Plastic correction of overriding fifth toe. Orthop Letters Club, 1954.
19. Sarrafian SK: Anatomy of the Foot and Ankle. Philadelphia, J.B. Lippincott, 1983, p. 227.
20. Sharrard WJW: Paediatric Orthopaedics and Fractures. Oxford, Blackwell Scientific Publications, 1971, pp. 295–299.
21. Taylor RG: The treatment of claw toes by multiple transfers of flexor into extensor tendons. J Bone Joint Surg 1951;33B:539–542.
22. Thompson SA: Hallux varus and metatarsus varus. A five year study (1954–1958). Clin Orthop 1960;16:108–118.
23. Wilson JN: V-Y correction for varus deformity of the fifth toe. Br J Surg 1953;41:133–135.

18

Nail Procedures

Richard M. Jay, D.P.M., and Michael Chung, D.P.M.

All too often the treatment of ingrown nails in children takes the path of least resistance. An ingrown nail in the child causes no less discomfort or deformity than in the adult. For this reason, the approach to treatment should be identical. The rate of recurrence of ingrown nails is as high as 80% after a simple avulsion.[1] These procedures have been repeated in children as often as three or four times. This rate of recurrence could be reduced if the nail problem were treated originally with a cauterization procedure of phenol and alcohol or by excising the matrix.

It is a matter of concern to the treating physician and the parent that injections can be a traumatic experience for a child. The use of a 27-gauge needle on a 1.8-mL dental syringe produces minimal pain due to the decrease in barrel pressure on the small needle size. However, the risk of repeated anxiety in a child with a recurring nail problem can be reduced by confronting the situation properly the first time. Of course, each situation is different, and for this reason each patient must be approached individually.

PREOPERATIVE CONSIDERATIONS

A thorough evaluation and identification of the cause of a pediatric ingrown toenail should be performed before any definitive action is taken. Evaluation may include radiographs isolating the digit to rule out any underlying bony pathology such as subungual exostosis, osteochondroma, enchondroma, or even the possibility of malignancy. Also, proper vascular assessment is warranted preoperatively, especially if a digital tourniquet is to be used. Any underlying systemic disease should also be considered in regard to healing potential and risk of complications. The surgical area should be scrubbed and painted with Betadine, and aseptic technique should be maintained.

PARTIAL NAIL REMOVAL

When only one nail border is affected and conservative slant-back techniques have failed, a surgical partial nail avulsion is indicated. After proper anesthetic block and preparation of the surgical area, the digit is exsanguinated, and a Penrose drain and hemostat tourniquet are applied. The nail plate is then split using an English nail splitter approximately a quarter inch from the lateral nail border.

Utilizing a straight nail clipper or a No. 62 Beaver blade, the nail is then split proximally to the proximal border of the nail plate at the margin of the extensor ridge of the distal phalanx. The split fragment is then stabilized with a straight hemostat and freed up by pulling it distally while slightly turning the fragment inward away from the affected nail border. Curettage of the lateral nail groove can then be performed to remove any remaining debris.

PARTIAL MATRICECTOMY

Phenol and Alcohol

At this point, a permanent partial matricectomy can be performed by various techniques. The choice of chemical or surgical matricectomy depends on the surgeon's preference. The most popular type of chemical matricectomy involves the use of an 89% liquefied phenol solution with alcohol washes. A sterile cotton swab dipped in the phenol solution is applied to the lateral nail groove under the proximal nail fold to destroy the germinal nail matrix. This is followed by a swab of alcohol solution to flush the area and neutralize the phenol, preventing it from burning the surrounding tissues. This procedure is repeated twice for a total of three phenol (30-second) and alcohol applications. It is quite effective in permanently preventing the ingrown nail. However, it is important to ensure that adequate hemostasis is present and no active infection exists. These factors can neutralize the phenol before it accomplishes its purposes. The surgical area can be dressed with antibiotic ointment and sterile gauze. Daily saltwater soaks and dressing changes with antibiotic ointment are recommended.

Winograd Procedure

Surgical partial matricectomies are an effective solution to the problem of onychocryptosis as well. One of the earliest procedures, described by Winograd[2] in 1929, involves making a semi-elliptical incision as well as a straight incision through the nail bed to excise the lateral nail fold and the lateral portion of the matrix (Fig. 18–1). This procedure is effective, especially when a paronychia involves proud flesh along the lateral nail border. The skin is undermined and is closed with several simple sutures.

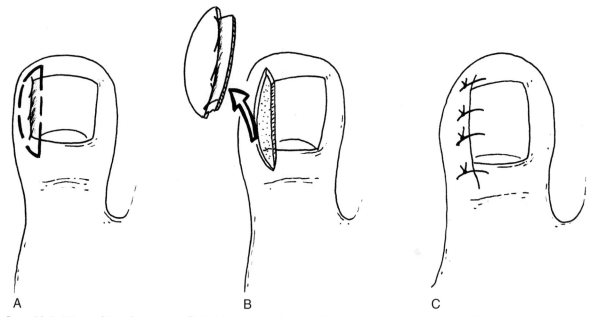

Figure 18–1. Winograd Procedure. *A*, An elliptical type incision is made through the nail and the hypertrophic nail fold. *B*, The entire wedge of skin and nail is removed. A Freer elevator is used to lift the nail bed and matrix. *C*, The skin is closed with nylon suture, coapting the skin and nail borders.

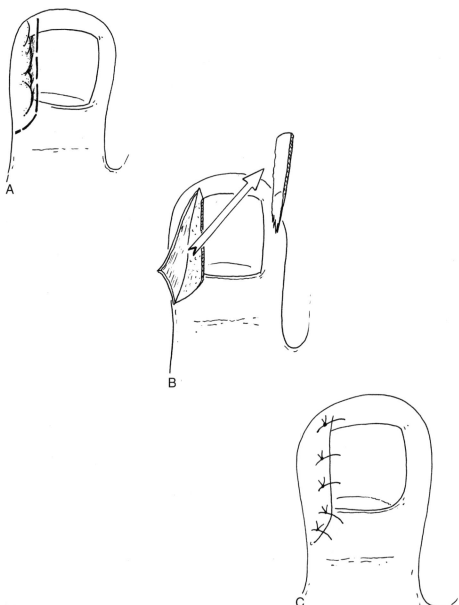

Figure 18–2. Frost Procedure. *A*, An L-type incision is made in the nail and proximally through the skin and matrix. *B*, A Freer elevator lifts the nail, nail bed, and matrix. The skin fold is left intact. *C*, The skin is closed by suturing the skin fold to the nail plate.

Frost Procedure

Frost[3] described a similar procedure involving a single incision in line with the partial nail avulsion and then bending the proximal arm of the incision laterally into a hockey stick configuration (Fig. 18–2). This allows better access for the surgical matricectomy. Several different techniques for suture closure have been described including drilling holes through the remaining nail plate through which to pass the suture. However, because the nail plate is relatively dirty even after proper antiseptic preparation, this step can lead to an increase in infection rates.

Postoperative care begins with the application of a povidone-iodine (Betadine)-soaked gauze or Adaptic dressing reinforced by sterile gauze and wrapped with Kling or Coban. It is also imperative to check the return of baseline capillary refill following release of the tourniquet. The patient is instructed to elevate the limb and keep the dressing clean, dry, and intact. The first dressing change can be performed within a week, and daily dressing changes with antibiotic ointment are recommended thereafter. Postoperative concerns include continued drainage, erythema, edema, and pain, all of which are normal and expected following a partial matricectomy. Postoperative complications can include infection, recurrence of the problem, dehiscence, and inclusion cyst formation.

BULBOUS DISTAL SKINPLASTY

Sometimes a child develops an ingrown nail deformity at the distal nail plate. This may be secondary to a traumatic event or even the use of shoes that are too small. The condition is very common in newborns, and treatment should be conservative. In the newborn usually just placing an elevator under the distal nail is enough to encourage the nail to override the bulbous tip. If the nail plate begins to grow into the bulbous formation of skin at the distal nail fold, a distal skinplasty is performed to bring down the excess tissue (Fig. 18–3). Two semi-elliptical skin incisions are made at the distal pulp of the

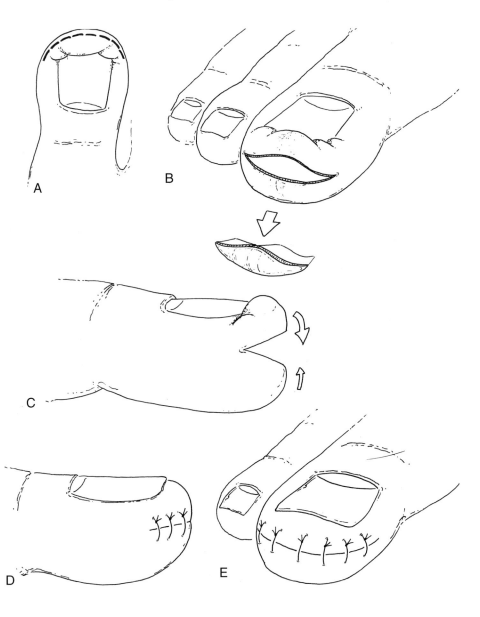

Figure 18–3. Bulbous Distal Skinplasty. A, The first incision is made from the medial to lateral border of the nail distally. B, An elliptical incision plantar to the first incision allows a wedge to be removed. C, The dorsal and distal aspect of the toe is debulked and lowered to meet the plantar fold of skin. D and E, Nylon or absorbable sutures are used for skin closure of the ellipse.

toe. The incisions are deepened through the subcutaneous fat, and the wedge of tissue is removed. The dorsal tissue is undermined and then sutured to the plantar flap, thus pulling the bulbous tissue plantar to the nail plate.

TOTAL NAIL AVULSION AND MATRICECTOMY

When both nail borders are affected by onychocryptosis, it is often secondary to an underlying exostosis or osteochondroma that results in formation of a pincer nail. To remove the offending ingrown nails and gain access to the underlying osseous pathology, a total nail procedure is indicated. After proper anesthetic block and tourniquet application, a Freer elevator can be used to push the soft tissue away from the borders of the nail plate. Then a hemostat is used to stabilize and remove the nail plate by pulling it distally while gently teasing the nail from medial to lateral.

The bottle cap method is an alternative procedure for total nail avulsion using only a Freer elevator (Fig. 18–4). After bluntly loosening the tissue around the nail plate, the eponychium is pushed back proximally away from the nail. Then the Freer elevator is slid under the proximal nail border with the concave side up. While a retrograde force is applied to the distal nail border, the nail plate is pulled off in a proximal to distal direction. Curettage of

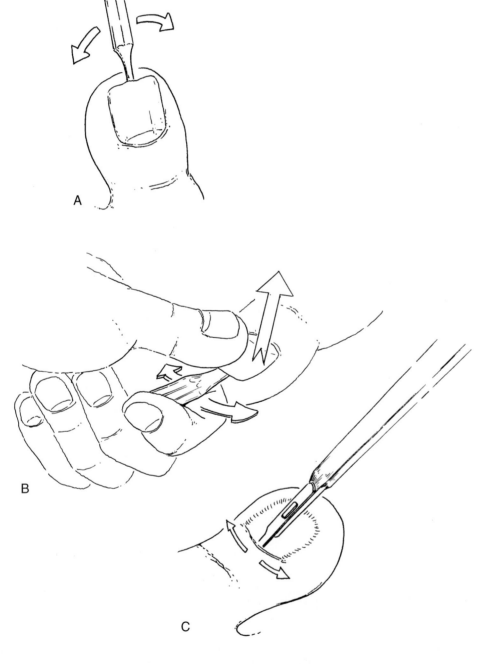

Figure 18–4. Total Nail Avulsion. *A*, A Freer elevator is used under the nail plate. The tissue around the nail plate and the eponychium is loosened bluntly. *B*, The Freer elevator is slid under the proximal nail border with the concave side up. By applying a retrograde force to the distal nail border, the nail plate can be pulled off from proximal to distal. *C*, The nail groove and nail bed can then be removed by curettage or cutting.

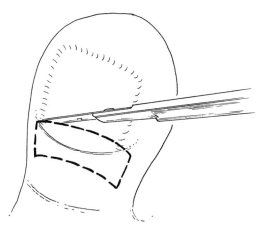

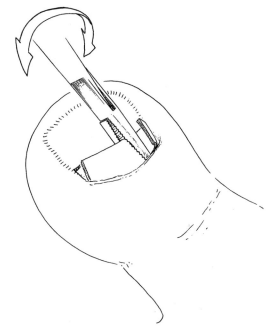

Figure 18–5. Acisional Matricectomy. The matrix is cut transversely medially while curving the blade along the contour of the bone. Then the blade is placed back in the center ridge directed laterally, and the matrix is cut again. Next, another transverse semi-elliptical incision is made just distal to the lunula and into the corners of the nail grooves.

the nail groove and nail bed is then performed to remove any remaining debris.

Figure 18–7. Acisional Matricectomy. The matrix is clamped with a hemostat and a "sardine-type" twisting method is used to remove the matrix.

ACISIONAL MATRICECTOMY

When no underlying osseous pathology is present, an acisional technique is indicated for removal of the matrix. A No. 15 blade is slid sideways beneath the proximal nail fold back to the extensor ridge of the distal phalanx. This is the proximal margin of the nail matrix. With the blade placed firmly against the bone, the matrix is cut transversely medially while the blade is curved along the contour of the bone. Then the blade is placed back in the center ridge directed laterally, and the matrix is cut again. Next, another transverse semi-elliptical incision is made just distal to the lunula and into the corners of the nail grooves. Finally, a Freer elevator is used to loosen the wedge of matrix from the underlying periosteum. The matrix is clamped with a hemostat, and a "sardine type" method of twisting can be used to remove the matrix. Curettage of any remaining matrix is performed, and the open surgical area (Figs. 18–5 to 18–8) is packed with Gelfoam or sutured closed.

ZADIK PROCEDURE

When a subungual exostosis or osteochondroma is present, the surgical procedure most often used is the H-shaped incision described by Zadik.[4] Two longitudinal linear incisions are made on each side of the nail, and a transverse incision is then made just distal to the matrix to connect the two previous incisions (Fig. 18–9). As a result, a proximal and distal flap are created to allow excellent exposure of the nail matrix for adequate resection. The matrix is sharply dissected free, and a hemostat is then used to twist the matrix out of the corners. If necessary, the linear incisions can be extended distally to provide exposure for removal of any osseous pathology. Furthermore, the nail bed is saved to allow primary closure over the distal phalanx. Great care should be taken to keep all surgical incisions distal to the interphalangeal joint.

Postoperative care begins with application of a nonadherent dressing followed by Betadine-soaked gauze, dry

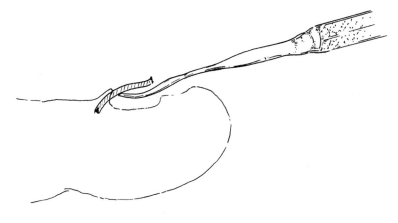

Figure 18–6. Acisional Matricectomy. A Freer elevator is used to loosen the wedge of matrix from the underlying periosteum.

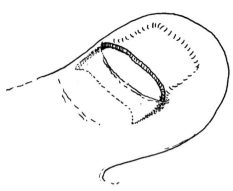

Figure 18–8. Acisional Matricectomy. The remaining matrix is removed by curettage, and the open surgical area is packed with Gelfoam.

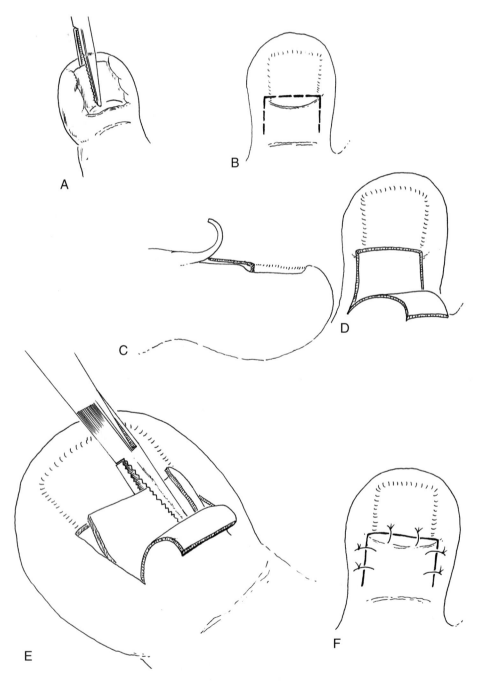

Figure 18–9. Zadik Procedure. *A*, Nail is avulsed in standard fashion (see Fig. 18–4). *B*, Two longitudinal linear incisions are made on each side of the nail, and then a transverse incision is made just distal to the matrix to connect the two previous incisions. *C* and *D*, A proximal flap is created to expose the nail matrix to allow adequate resection. *E*, The matrix is sharply dissected free, and a hemostat is utilized to twist the matrix out of the corners. *F*, The flap is closed with either nylon or absorbable suture.

gauze, and Kling or elastic wrap. The digit should be evaluated for return of baseline capillary refill time. The patient is instructed to elevate the limb and keep the dressing clean and dry until the first follow-up visit in 1 week. The patient can then begin daily dressing changes using antibiotic ointment. Sutures can be removed after 10 to 14 days depending on clinical evaluation. Postoperative complications can include recurrence, inadequate resection, infection, dehiscence, and osteomyelitis.

References

1. Murray WR, Bedi BS: The surgical management of ingrowing toenail. Br J Surg 1975;62:409–412.
2. Winograd AM: A modification in the technic of operation for ingrown toenail. JAMA 1929;91:229–230.
3. Frost LA: A surgical correction for incurvated nails. Chirop Rec 1952;35:17–23.
4. Zadik FR: Obliteration of the nail bed of the great toe without shortening of the terminal phalanx. J Bone Joint Surg 1950;32B:66.

Three

Rearfoot

19

Introduction to the Flatfoot

Richard M. Jay, D.P.M.

ETIOLOGY

The cause of a flatfoot, which is due to excessive subtalar joint pronation, may be muscular, osseous, ligamentous, neurologic, or a combination of these. Flatfoot has been referred to as a weak foot, strained and flaccid foot, valgus foot, and extremely relaxed foot. More common terms used today are convex pes valgus, collapsing-type pes valgoplanus, and calcaneovalgus.[1, 2] There is a good consensus on two types of flatfoot when considering the correction: pathologic and physiologic. The pathologic forms often require treatment, usually an operative approach. Pathologic forms include congenital forms such as calcaneovalgus, vertical talus, tarsal coalition, the Z-foot of compensated metatarsus adductus, and the short Achilles tendon hypermobile flatfoot as well as acquired forms of flatfoot such as those resulting from trauma and neuromuscular disorders.

The common physiologic form requires no intervention. Physiologic flatfoot is probably the single entity and deformity of the foot that receives the greatest amount of discussion about both conservative and surgical approaches. This pronated foot type has been discussed and argued about by many physicians, and the discussions all center around whether or not treatment is justified. The problem with the physiologic flatfoot is that the parent usually brings the child to the physician for an opinion about a treatment plan. Recommendations usually are presented in the following way: (1) Do nothing and watch the child grow as the deformity diminishes on its own. (2) Control the child's foot conservatively in a functional orthosis. Maintaining the foot in proper alignment will cause it to grow in the correct position. (3) Intervene surgically to realign the osseous structures mechanically to obtain better foot function.

There is no absolute answer. The old adage First do no harm is appropriate, but doing no harm does not mean ignoring or dismissing a parent's concerns about a child's deformity. The question should rather be, Should a conservative approach be undertaken and maintained with no surgical intervention, or should surgical intervention follow the conservative approaches if these methods fail? The answer is obvious. All flatfoot deformities, not excluding physiologic flatfoot, should be conservatively con-

trolled and maintained in a corrected position to allow normal bone growth. If symptoms continue and there is difficulty with ambulation that includes fatigue, pain, awkward gait, or unusual shoe wear, then surgical intervention is warranted.[3–5]

Many factors are involved in the flexible flatfoot. These can be divided into factors that have a direct influence on the foot (referred to as intrinsic factors) and those attributed to suprastructural influences (extrinsic factors). Among the suprastructural factors are such conditions as scoliosis, lumbar lordosis, coxa vara and coxa valga, genu varum and genu valgum, and congenital dislocated hip (CDH). Torsional and rotational deformities of the femur and tibia, muscle imbalance, or neurologically induced dysfunction leading to subtalar joint instability and deformation are extrinsic suprastructural influences that also induce a flatfoot.[6] Any factors that normally contribute to the stability of the foot also have an effect. These include the various ligamentous laxity disorders such as Ehlers-Danlos syndrome and Marfan's syndrome, osseous deformity, equinus deformity, midtarsal syndrome,[7] calcaneovalgus, and subtalar valgus and varus. Other etiologic conditions include gastrocnemius contracture, ankle dorsiflexor activity, and abnormalities of the peroneal tendons. Kidner identified the position of the tibialis posterior as a major contributing factor.[8] Other causes implicated in the formation of calcaneovalgus include lack of ontogenic development of talar neck torsion, tibial torsion, and conditions such as forefoot varus, forefoot valgus, equinus, and muscle imbalances (weak supinators). Other factors contributing to flatfoot may be imposed by trauma and neuropathologies such as spastic paralysis of muscles. Flatfoot deformity may be caused by any one or a combination of these factors.

The flatfoot of the untreated calcaneovalgus foot is exacerbated by the child during weight bearing. This is the time in which true deformity can occur because the pressure on the foot that normally helps in concluding ontogenic rotation and formation of cartilage in weight-bearing articulations serves to deform the foot further. As the talus assumes a more vertical and medial position, the calcaneus is forced to rotate posterolaterally from its position under the talus. The sustentaculum tali loses its supporting position beneath the neck of the talus as the calcaneus subluxates laterally.

The contracted heel cord or a laterally inserted heel cord can create a tendency toward hyperpronation and pes planus. The equinus problem must be dealt with if it is part of the deformity. Because the hind part of the foot cannot be dorsiflexed, dorsiflexion occurs at the midfoot. A breech of the midpart of the foot or a rocker-bottom foot may result, putting the hind part of the foot in a valgus angulation and the fore part in abduction.

EVALUATION

A complete clinical and roentgenographic examination should be performed when the child is 3 years of age. Clinical signs of flatfoot include an excessively everted calcaneal stance (heel valgus), severe depression of the longitudinal arch, midtarsal subluxation, or medial talar head bulge. Hypermobility symptoms can include foot and heel pain, plantar fasciitis, excessive foot fatigue, and other similar complaints. Evaluation of the flatfoot deformity is accomplished by: (1) evaluation of the positions of the ankle and subtalar and midtarsal joints; (2) evaluation of the motion of the ankle and subtalar and midtarsal joints; and (3) roentgenographic studies of the foot in the standing and, weight-bearing positions.

Radiography

The common radiographic models used are the lateral and anteroposterior (AP) views. These involve measurement of the articulation percentages between the navicular and the talar head, which are abnormal in the calcaneovalgus foot owing to the lateral drift of both the calcaneus and the forefoot. The dorsoplantar (AP) view generally shows an increase in Kite's angle (talocalcaneal deviation) with a 50% or less articulation between the talar head and the navicular. The lateral view generally shows a plantargrade or decreased calcaneal inclination angle, an anterior break in the cyma line, and a naviculo-cuneiform break of varying degree.

Neutral Position

For visualization of the foot in neutral position on a lateral weight-bearing roentgenogram, the posterior articular margin of the talus and the middle of the nose of the talus are marked with dots. A line drawn from the dot at the back of the talus through the dot in the middle of the anterior nose of the talus and continued distally should bisect the middle of the navicular bone and then continue through the cuneiforms and the middle of the shaft of the first metatarsal bone. This is known as the talometatarsal angle. If this line drops below the middle of the first metatarsal bone, the foot is labeled planus. If it is above the middle of the first metatarsal bone, the foot is labeled cavus. In either case, a dot is placed distally at the middle of the first metatarsal head, and a second dot is placed at the midpoint of the visualized base of the first metatarsal bone. A line is then drawn between these dots and extended proximally until it intersects the talar

line. The angle between these lines is then measured and recorded as a positive angle for cavus and a negative angle for planus. In my experience, an angle of +4 degrees to −4 degrees indicates a neutral foot. On the anteroposterior view, a dot is placed at each margin of the articular nose of the talus, and the midpoint of this articular surface is marked. Dots are then placed at each margin of the receiving articular surface of the navicular bone, and its midpoint is marked. The distance between these midpoints is measured and recorded in millimeters. In the neutral nonweight-bearing foot the distance between these two points is about 0, and the talus is directed in a more or less straight line with the first metatarsal bone. In the neutral weight-bearing foot the nose of the talus deviates medially and articulates in congruity with the navicular. In the flatfoot, the forefoot has a supinated position in relation to the rearfoot, the heel goes into eversion, and the foot is considered hyperpronated.[9] During radiography, the child should be in the standing position with the feet relaxed in the normal angle of gait.[10] Talar declination, calcaneal inclination, and a talocalcaneal angle on the lateral view and Kite's talocalcaneal angle on the AP view are considered prerequisite values for the decision to undertake surgical correction.

Mechanical Aspects of Flatfoot

Probably the greatest contributor to the integrity of the arch of the foot is the development of a satisfactory sustentaculum tali. The second strongest factor in support of the arch is probably the integrity of the posterior tibial tendon. The deltoid ligament of the ankle, especially the deep portion, also helps to support the arch. A well-placed inferior calcaneonavicular ligament is supportive. The plantar aponeurosis, with its anchorage to the toes and the os calcis, creates a very strong fibrous windlass effect. A standing lateral talometatarsal angle is used to evaluate the deformity roentgenographically. With the foot in hyperpronation, the Harris-Beath views show a 0-degree or negative angle of the sustentaculum tali in its relationship to the long axis of the os calcis. Inman has also shown that the sustentaculum tali should show a positive angle of 5 to 15 degrees in the neutral foot.[9] A Harris-Beath view yields valuable information about the posterior and middle subtalar facets and is usually performed when surgical correction has been decided on. Normally, the subtalar joint, which is mildly supinated during swing phase, pronates 4 to 6 degrees following heel contact. Elftman explained the mechanism, describing the transverse tarsal joint as composed of the talonavicular and calcaneocuboid joints.[11] When the hindfoot and midfoot are in supination, the axes of these joints are angled away from each other, and this part of the foot is "locked." After heel strike and eversion of the heel, the subtalar and midtarsal joints "unlock" to the limit of the range of the restricting ligaments.

Pronation provides proper shock absorption for the stresses of standing, walking, jogging, and splinting. When pronation is restricted (as in the cavus foot), the forces of weight bearing, failing dissipation within the foot, are transmitted upward through the ankle joint, knee joint, hip joint, pelvis, and spine until they are dissipated. As shown by Inman, in the person with flatfoot the weight-bearing force to each leg increases from body weight with an additional 20% for a slow walk to as much as three to four times that with sprinting.[9] Disabling secondary deformities can result. Problems such as hallux abducto valgus, plantar keratosis, metatarsalgia, hammer digit syndrome, neuromas, plantar fasciitis, heel spur syndrome, postural pains of the foot and leg, and arthrosis deformans of the midtarsal and subtalar joints may be directly related to the pronated foot.[12] Hyperpronation inevitably develops, particularly in patients who have static deformities in the knees or hips (e.g., genu valgus). Also, tenosynovitis of the posterior tibial tendon frequently occurs and may ultimately result in rupture or stretching of the tendon and subsequent, rather fixed hyperpronation and pes planus.

In closed kinetic chain pronation, the calcaneus everts, and the talus adducts and plantar-flexes. The reactive force of gravity may then cause subluxation of the talonavicular or naviculocuneiform joint (or both), resulting in the midtarsal fault syndrome.[7] Parallelism of the longitudinal axes of the talonavicular and calcaneocuboid joints allows unlocking of the midtarsal joint with subsequent dorsiflexion of the forefoot on the rearfoot and hypermobility of the metatarsals during the propulsive phase of gait when they should be stable.[13] The end result of this chain of events is a stressed pronated foot with multiple deformities and symptomatology in the rearfoot and forefoot. These problems include hallux abducto valgus, hammertoes, tailor's bunions, neuromas, and plantar keratosis. The clinical pattern is predictable and consistent with either forefoot varus or subtalar valgus foot types. Compression forces retard longitudinal bone growth of the affected bones according to the Heuter-Volkmann law.[14, 15] Compression forces are dorsal and lateral and result in a decrease in longitudinal endochondral growth in these regions as well as a relative increase in plantar and medial growth. If not treated, this imbalance leads to a structurally based and fixed pronated foot, probably a permanently pronated foot.

TREATMENT

Treatment includes both conservative and surgical methods. Conservative methods include reduction of the dislocated navicular from the talus and moving the calcaneus back under the talus with adduction of the forefoot. This correction is performed in a serial manner and only with resistance. The correction is held in place with serial casting and advanced at weekly intervals. Correction is halted when the foot is just slightly past neutral and held with night splinting. The casting technique is most effective when the child is under the age of 18 months, after which the force of correction will not reduce the deformity but instead will cause motion at the midfoot and further advancement of the flatfoot. In the ambulating child, an orthotic is necessary to control the foot and limit operation at end-stage pronation. Some authors advocate no treatment unless the patient is symptomatic.

The child who has undergone corrective casting should also have an orthotic device to control growth in the foot.

Once skeletal maturity has been attained (13 years of age in girls and 15 years in boys),[16] no treatment is recommended unless the hypermobile flatfoot deformity is painful and limits the child's activities. In this situation, attempts to relieve the difficulty should include inserts or the use of prescription orthotic devices. Surgery is considered only if these devices do not alleviate the difficulty and the patient is incapacitated. Surgical procedures are designed to correct the structural abnormalities without fusing the joints in an attempt to restore the normal position and motion of the components of the foot (see Chapter 21).

When conservative orthotic control fails in children who have a severely pronated, painful, or deformed foot, surgical correction is the only means of correcting the condition. When the deformity is corrected, the calcaneus must be realigned beneath the talus and maintained in a neutral relationship. The talar declination must be reduced and the forefoot placed in correct alignment with the talus in both the transverse and frontal planes (Figs. 19–1 and 19–2). Ideally, the deformity should be corrected in young children before it becomes fixed and adaptive osseous changes have occurred. These are the goals of flatfoot treatment.

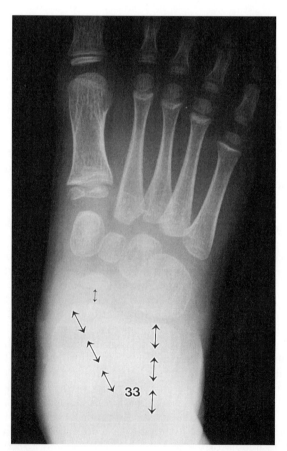

Figure 19–1. Subtalar joint unlocking with bisection of the calcaneus and talus. Kite's angle is 33 degrees. With increased separation at the talocalcaneal joint, a transverse plane deformity is noted by the drift of the navicular laterally on the talar head.

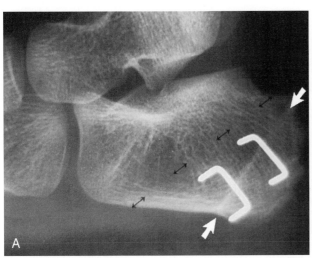
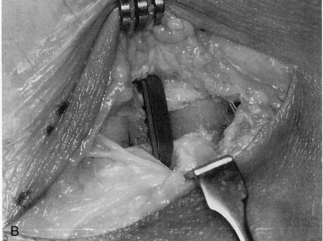

Figure 19–2. *A*, Closing wedge Dwyer osteotomy of the calcaneus with staple fixation. Ideally, the cut should be parallel to the peroneal tendons to attain the maximum degree of frontal plane correction. *B*, Opening wedge osteotomy of the calcaneus with graft inserted and staple fixation.

KIDNER FOOT

The Kidner foot is divided into three types. Type I (Fig. 19–3) has small sesamoids sitting within the tendon of the tibialis posterior; the sesamoid is separated from the navicular. Type II (Fig. 19–4) has an accessory navicular connected to the navicular with a fibrous or fibrocartilaginous bond. Type III has an elongated medial horn of navicular appearing cornuate (Fig. 19–5). The presenting symptoms are usually pain on the medial tuberosity of the navicular. Pain is usually reduced by conservative approaches. Any orthotic that will supinate the foot will reduce the symptoms. However, if there is a concomitant equinus, the medial arch will collapse further, and the pain will become more acute. If the foot can be controlled with an orthosis paired with a rearfoot varus post but pain continues, surgical options can be considered. The standard procedures used to reduce the medial prominence with or without tibialis posterior transfer usually have little effect on the elevation of the arch. The physician should plan on adjunctive procedures if reduction of the flatfoot deformity is needed (Figs. 19–6 to 19–12).

Figure 19–3. Type I Kidner foot. Two sesamoids rest within the body of the posterior tibial tendon at the insertion of the tibial tuberosity of the navicular.

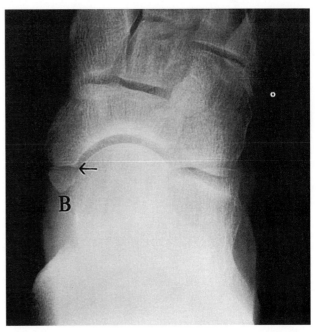

Figure 19–4. Type II Kidner foot. A large secondary ossification center is noted just medial and plantar to the curvature of the tuberosity of the navicular.

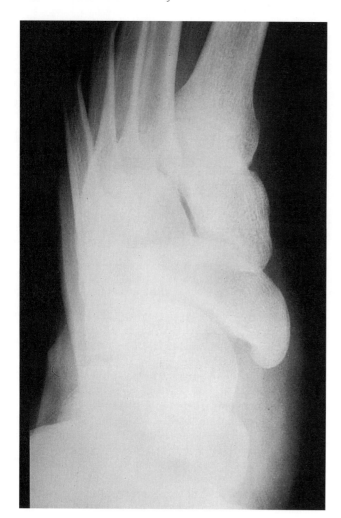

Figure 19–5. Cornuate navicular in type III Kidner foot deformity.

Figure 19–6. The attachments of the posterior tibial tendon into the navicular and cuneiform are primary with extensions into all of the lesser tarsal bones as seen in this figure.

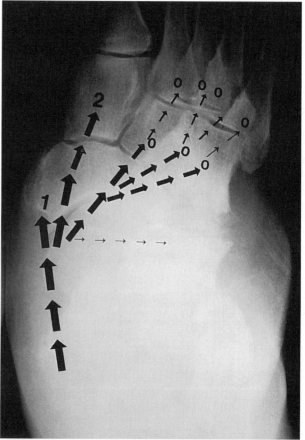

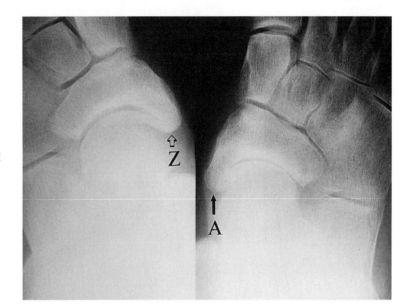

Figure 19–7. Two variations (Z and A) of Kidner type III navicular deformities.

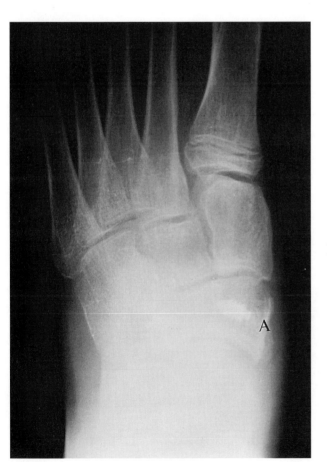

Figure 19–8. Insertion of bone anchor (A) to provide tenodesis of posterior tibial tendon. Anchor is inserted into the resected medial tuberosity of the navicular to achieve reduction of a Kidner foot.

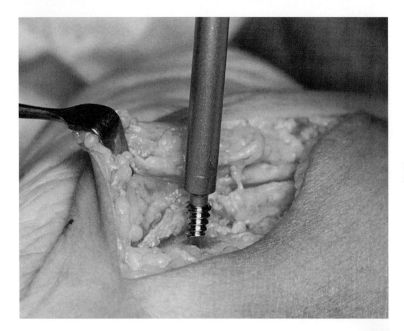

Figure 19–9. Bone anchor being driven into plantar medial aspect of the resected surface of the navicular.

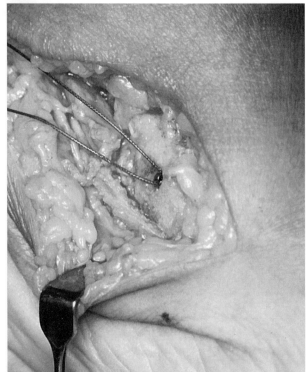

Figure 19–10. Insertion of bone anchor into medial aspect of the tuberosity of resected navicular. The suture ends will be tied to the tibialis posterior.

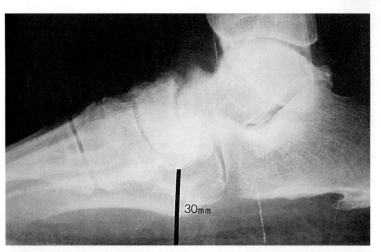

Figure 19–11. Preoperative Kidner foot. Note 30-mm arch height.

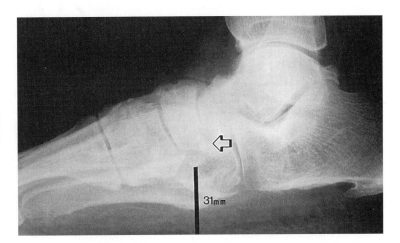

Figure 19–12. Postoperative Kidner foot procedure with insertion of bone anchor *(arrow)* to stabilize posterior tibial tendon. The height of the medial arch is unchanged at 31 mm.

References

1. Ganley JV: Calcaneovalgus in children. J Am Podiatr Med Assoc 1975;65:405–421.
2. Ferciot CF: The etiology of the developmental flatfoot. Clin Orthop 1972;85:7.
3. Crego CH, Ford LT: An end result study of various operative procedures for correcting flat foot in children. J Bone Joint Surg 1952;34A:183.
4. Jones BS: Flatfoot—Preliminary report of an operation for severe cases. J Bone Joint Surg 1975;57B:279.
5. Ozonoff MB: Pediatric Orthopedic Radiology. Philadelphia, W.B. Saunders, 1979, p. 300.
6. Elftman H: Torsion of lower extremity. Am J Physiol Anthropol 1945;3:255–265.
7. Gamble FC, Yale I: Clinical Foot Roentgenology, 2nd ed. Huntington, NY, Robert Kreiger Publishing, 1975, pp. 209–212.
8. Kidner FC: The prehallux in relation to flat foot. J Bone Joint Surg 1929;11:831.
9. Inman VT: Joints of the Ankle. Baltimore, Williams & Wilkins, 1977.
10. Bordelon RL: Correction of hypermobile flatfoot in children by molded insert. Foot Ankle 1980;1:143.
11. Elftman H: The transverse tarsal joint and its control. Clin Orthop 1960;16:41–46.
12. Root ML, Orien WP, Weed JH, et al: Biomechanical examination of the foot. Los Angeles, Clinical Biomechanical Corporation, 1971, p. 34.
13. Steindler A: Kinesiology of the Human Body. Springfield, IL, Charles C Thomas, 1955, p. 413.
14. Heuter C: Anatomische Studien an den Extremitatengelenken Neugeborener und Erwachsener. Virchows Arch 1862;25:572.
15. Volkmann R: Chirurgische Erfahrungan über Knochenverbiegurgen. Arch Path Anat 1862;24:512.
16. Hoerr NL: Radiographic Analysis of Skeletal Development of the Foot and Ankle. Springfield, IL, Charles C Thomas, 1962.

20

Symptomatic Juvenile Flatfoot Condition

Gary L. Dockery, D.P.M.

Being flatfooted does not necessarily mean that symptoms will be associated with this condition. In fact, many people with low or flat arches never experience any form of discomfort or pain and are functionally stable when performing most activities. However, juvenile patients with symptomatic flatfoot condition do exist, and in this chapter that foot type is described by the terms symptomatic flexible juvenile pes planovalgus. This pathologic condition is also referred to as congenital hypermobile flatfoot and is described radiographically as lateral peritalar subluxation or peritalar dislocation. Several factors must be considered in the symptomatic juvenile flatfoot condition. These include a family history of a similar problem, an associated calcaneal eversion at midstance, a complete collapse of the midfoot, a widened or adducted gait, an associated tightness of the gastrocnemius tendon or the entire Achilles tendon, and, most important, whether the condition is flexible or rigid. A rigid flatfoot condition needs a completely different conservative and surgical treatment approach than the flexible hypermobile flatfoot.

There are many types of congenital and acquired flatfoot conditions that may begin with or progress to symptoms during standing and walking. Most of these symptomatic feet are best treated by a variety of conservative methods. It should be stated that, in these cases, all forms of conservative care, including organized and properly executed stretching of the posterior lower leg muscle group (triceps surae), strengthening regimens for the anterior tibial and posterior tibial tendons, functional orthotic devices to help stabilize the foot and verticalize the heel, decreasing participation in all physical activities that increase the symptoms, and use of corrective or protective shoe gear should be tried. Only when these have failed to alleviate the patient's symptoms should surgical treatment be considered. A small percentage of patients with symptomatic flatfeet continue to experience increasing symptoms after an extended trial of aggressive conservative care. It is these patients that are considered candidates for surgical intervention.

CLINICAL CRITERIA[7–9, 15, 17, 32]

Contrary to popular belief, there is no single clinical finding that defines the symptomatic juvenile flatfoot con-

dition. The following combination of affirmative findings on physical examination and diagnostic procedures are commonly found in the 3- to 18-year-old patients who present with specific positive clinical and radiologic findings:

1. A relatively normal appearing foot and arch in the nonweight-bearing position, which then collapses on weight bearing with complete loss of the medial longitudinal arch (Fig. 20–1).
2. Midstance (weight-bearing) calcaneovalgus or heel eversion, which returns to vertical or inverts significantly when the patient stands on tiptoes (Fig. 20–2).
3. A positive toe extension test of Jack (also generally known as the Hubscher maneuver) (Fig. 20–3).
4. Midtarsal abduction.
5. Mild to moderate metatarsal abduction (or in some cases compensatory metatarsal adduction as the foot tries to stabilize the excessive pronation) (Fig. 20–4).
6. Forefoot varus greater than 8 degrees (or fixed forefoot supinatus).

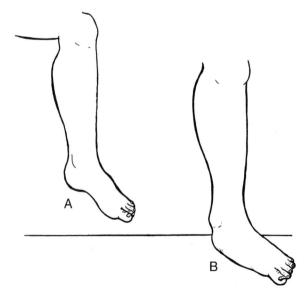

Figure 20–1. *A*, The foot has a normal contour and medial longitudinal arch appearance in the nonweight-bearing position. *B*, The medial arch is flattened on full weight bearing.

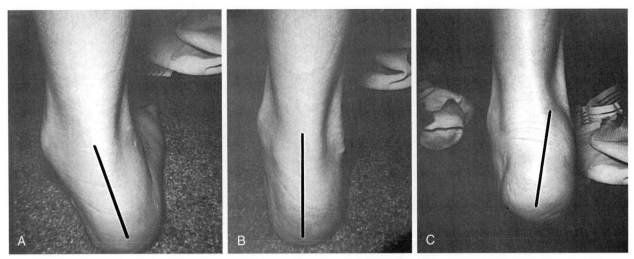

Figure 20–2. *A*, Flexible midstance calcaneal valgus (heel eversion). *B*, The heel returns to vertical with external rotation of the tibia. *C*, The heel inverts significantly when the patient stands on tiptoes.

7. Limited ankle joint dorsiflexion caused by tightness of the gastrocnemius tendon (Fig. 20–5) or the entire Achilles tendon (Fig. 20–6).

8. Weight-bearing radiographs taken in the angle and base of gait position that show peritalar subluxation. This is manifested radiographically as an increased talocalcaneal angle on the dorsoplantar x-ray view with uncovering of the talar articular surface (positive medial deviation). The lateral radiograph shows a plantar deviation of the talus (an increased talar declination angle) as well as a naviculocuneiform sag or "fault" (Fig. 20–7). In the older

child, the lateral radiograph shows an increased talar declination angle with "faulting" or a breach of the talonavicular joint, the naviculocuneiform joint, or both the talonavicular and naviculocuneiform joints (Fig. 20–8). Additionally, a calcaneal axial view should be performed to evaluate the subtalar facets and the alignment of the calcaneus (Fig. 20–9).[33–35, 37, 44, 45]

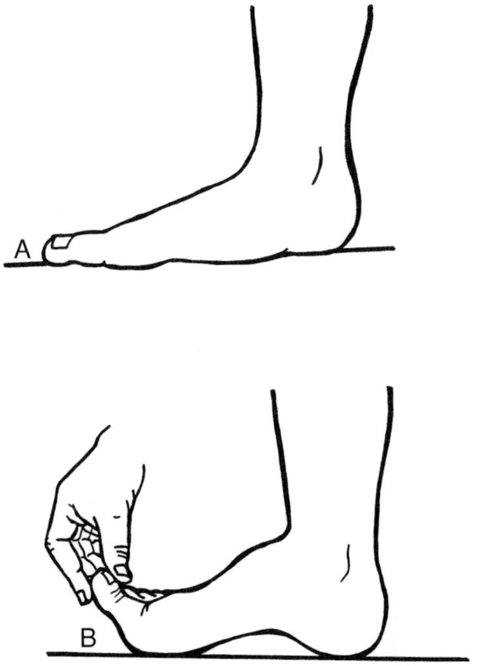

SURGICAL PROCEDURES

In this section, a preferred group of surgical procedures is evaluated for the treatment of the symptomatic juvenile flexible flatfoot condition. Not all of these procedures are performed on the same foot, but the operations are selected by planal dominance of deformity and can be combined to give the best long-term results. The procedures discussed include the following:

Figure 20–3. Jack's test or great toe extension test. *A*, Full weight bearing with collapse of medial longitudinal arch, talar prominence, and calcaneal valgus. *B*, Passive dorsiflexion (extension) of the hallux causes rise of the medial arch, supination of the foot, and external rotation of the tibia with inversion of the heel. When this occurs, it indicates a flexible flatfoot condition.

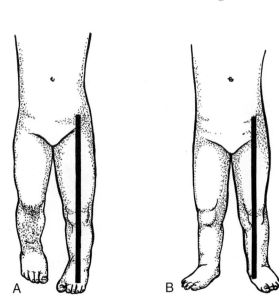

Figure 20–4. *A*, Mild to moderate metatarsal abduction (sometimes referred to as a duck walk by parents). *B*, Mild compensatory metatarsal adduction as the foot tries to stabilize the excessive pronation.

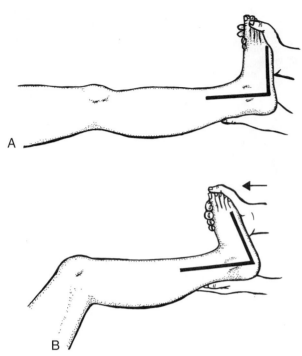

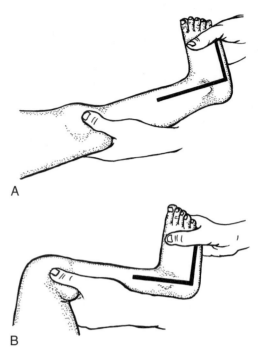

Figure 20–5. The Silfverskiold test for gastrocnemius equinus. A, With the knee in full extension, the range of dorsiflexion of the foot while the calcaneus is held vertical or in slight varus and the forefoot is held in a supinated position, is limited (less than 50). B, With the knee flexed, the range of dorsiflexion of the foot is increased (greater than 100).

Figure 20–6. The Silfverskiold test for triceps equinus. A, With the knee in full extension, the range of dorsiflexion of the foot is limited (less than 50). B, With the knee flexed, the range of dorsiflexion is still limited (less than 50).

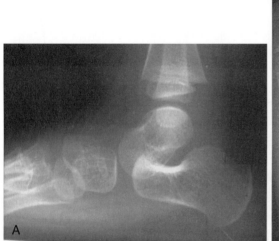

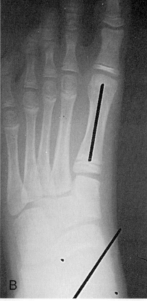

Figure 20–7. A, Lateral weight-bearing radiograph of a young child in the base and angle of gait position, which shows an increased plantar deviation of the talus (an increased talar declination angle) as well as a decreased calcaneal inclination angle secondary to compensation for equinus. B, Dorsoplantar view of an older child depicting an increased talocalcaneal angle (Kite's angle) with uncovering of the talonavicular articular surface (positive medial talar deviation).

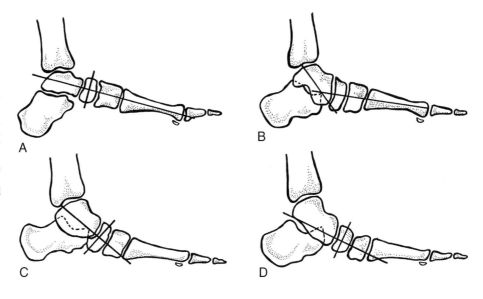

Figure 20–8. Lateral standing views in the base and angle of gait position. *A*, Normal angle of talonaviculocuneiform articulation. *B*, Decreased talus and calcaneus angle with a talonavicular breach. *C*, Decreased talus and calcaneus angle with naviculocuneiform faulting. *D*, Decreased talus and calcaneus angle with both a talonavicular and naviculocuneiform joint breach.

I. Lateral subtalar joint arthroereisis
  A. Silastic custom plug
  B. Smith STA-Peg implant
  C. Maxwell-Brancheau arthroereisis (MBA) implant
II. Calcaneal osteotomy
  A. Complete calcaneal relocational osteotomy (modified Koutsogiannis's procedure)
  B. Varus opening wedge osteotomy with bone graft (modified Silver's procedure)
  C. Lateral column lengthening calcaneal osteotomy with bone graft (modified Evans procedure)
III. Medial column reconstruction (osseous procedures)
  A. Arthrodesis of the naviculocuneiform joints (modified Hoke's procedure)
  B. Arthrodesis of the naviculocuneiform joints and the first metatarsocuneiform joint (modified Miller's procedure)
  C. Midbody navicular plantarflexory closing wedge osteotomy (modified Barouk's procedure)
  D. Midbody medial cuneiform dorsal opening wedge osteotomy with bone graft (modified Cotton's procedure)
IV. Medial column reconstruction (soft tissue procedures)

A. Osteoperiosteal flap transposition under the anterior tibial tendon and suture plication and tightening of the medial aspect of the plantar calcaneonavicular ligament (modified Giannestras procedure)
B. Rerouting of the anterior tibial tendon through a slot in the navicular with advancement of the posterior tibial tendon beneath the navicular bone (modified Young's procedure)
C. Excision of accessory navicular (os tibiale externum) and any hypertrophy of the navicular with transposition of the posterior tibial tendon insertion under the navicular bone (modified Kidner's procedure)
D. Tendon balancing or transfer procedure with distal advancement of the posterior tibial tendon, split portion of the anterior tibial tendon transferred to the posterior tibial tendon, and, in many cases, transfer of the flexor digitorum longus to supplement the posterior tibial tendon
V. Posterior equinus release
  A. Gastrocnemius recession
  B. Tendo Achillis lengthening procedure
VI. Procedures for symptomatic Z-foot correction
  A. Medial cuneiform opening wedge osteotomy with bone graft (modified Fowler's procedure)
  B. Closing wedge cuboid osteotomy (modified Tachdjian's procedure)
  C. Abductor hallucis tenotomy (modified Lichtblau's procedure)
  D. Sectioning of abductor hallucis (modified McCauley's procedure)

Indications

1. The most important indication for consideration of surgical treatment is complete failure of all conservative treatments to reduce the patient's symptoms or prevent progression of the deformity.

2. Another major consideration is persistent pain. This may be described as dull, aching, throbbing, cramping, or

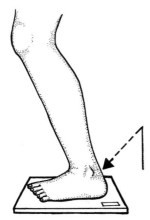

Figure 20–9. Position of foot needed to obtain a calcaneal axial radiograph to assess the shape of the heel and the subtalar joint facets.

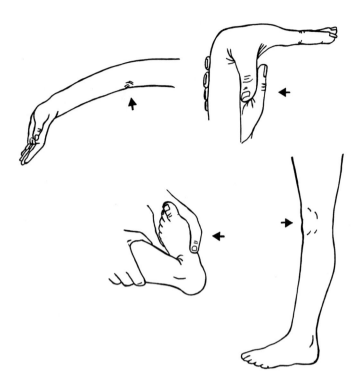
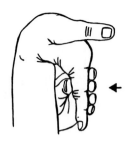

Figure 20–10. Wynne-Davies test for ligamentous laxity. Hyperextension of the elbow; hypermobility of the thumb, allowing it to touch or go beyond the arm; total hyperextension of the metacarpophalangeal joints; excessive motion of the foot in dorsiflexion; and genu recurvatum of the knee.

generalized fatigue. Pain commonly involves the medial longitudinal arch, lateral sinus tarsi region, medial or plantar heel, and posterior calf. This is one of the most common combinations of symptoms and is often referred to by pediatricians as "growing pains."

3. Callus formation or ulceration under the head of the plantar-flexed talus (more common in patients with cerebral palsy).

4. Difficulty in walking or running secondary to the excessive valgus attitude of the foot and the usually present equinus condition.

5. General inactivity of the patient with poor participation in physical activities that require running or jumping (including decreased regular play compared with organized sports activities). Parents frequently describe this as an inability to "keep up" with other children of the same age group during activities.

6. Excessive distortion and wear of shoe gear with breakdown of the medial heel counter and medial plantar forepart of the sole. This condition is frequently present but is the least important reason for surgery.

Goals

1. To decrease symptoms (pain, aching, throbbing, cramping, or generalized fatigue) of the feet and legs.

2. To improve overall function: standing, walking, and running more efficiently.

3. To improve the position of the foot and its general appearance.

4. To prevent long-term degenerative changes in the abnormally positioned joints of the foot and ankle.

Contraindications

Besides the standard contraindications to any surgery, such as an unhealthy or medically compromised patient, inadequate family support network, and concurrent infections, specific contraindications to this combination surgical treatment of the flexible flatfoot include:

1. Rigid plantar-flexed (or vertical) talus.

2. Osseous ankle equinus, confirmed by diagnostic radiographs.

3. Excessive ligamentous laxity (Fig. 20–10).

4. Tarsal coalition anomalies (Fig. 20–11).

5. Severe tarsal arthritis.

6. Excessive obesity.

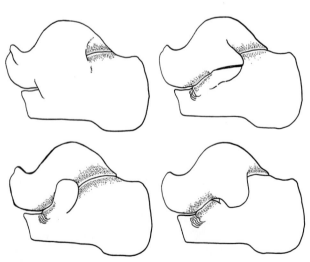

Figure 20–11. Tarsal coalition (subtalar or calcaneonavicular) is a contraindication to flexible flatfoot surgery.

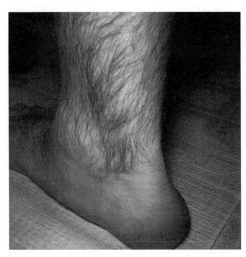

Figure 20–12. Rigid flatfoot condition that is not flexible with the external tibial rotation test or the extension toe raise test of Jack.

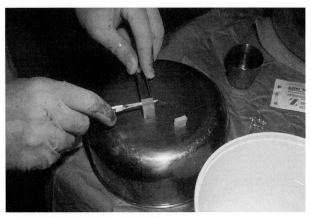

Figure 20–13. Silastic plug arthroereisis. The implant is fashioned during the surgical procedure from medical grade Silastic.

7. Rigid flatfoot uncorrected by Hubscher's maneuver (Jack's test) (Fig. 20–12).

8. Osseous procedures are generally not recommended for children under the age of 6 years.

Many other appropriate surgical procedures are available to treat the conditions and patients listed above.

Techniques[1, 6, 21, 24–26, 42, 43, 49]

Lateral Subtalar Joint Arthroereisis

Silastic Custom Plug. A 2- to 4-cm incision is made following the natural skin lines over the lateral sinus tarsi area. Care must be taken to protect the peroneal tendons and the intermediate dorsal cutaneous nerve during the skin incision. The incision is deepened into the subcutaneous layer, and several vessels traversing the area may be retracted or cut and ligated. If the superficial branch of the peroneal nerve cannot be adequately protected, it is usually sacrificed by sharp dissection. Once the fat layer is retracted there should be good exposure of the deep fascial layer and the inferior extensor retinaculum. A linear incision is made, or a U-shaped flap is created with the base attached superiorly. The flap is elevated, and the cervical ligament (external talocalcaneal ligament) is identified and transected from the floor of the sinus tarsi. The deep fat plug (Hoke's tonsil)[*18] is then removed from within the sinus tarsi, and the capsule of the posterior facet of the subtalar joint is opened. Next, the deep interosseous talocalcaneal ligament is identified and transected completely. During this portion of the procedure, the soft bone and cartilage should be protected from damage by the scalpel or other sharp instruments. Once the deep interosseous ligament has been transected, there is usually a noticeable increase in the range of motion of the calcaneus in inversion. Failure to cut this ligament

completely may cause extrusion of the custom Silastic plug from the sinus tarsi during weight bearing. This occurs when the deep ligament acts like the string of a bow and the custom plug becomes the arrow during functional weight bearing. This is sometimes referred to as the "bow and arrow" style of implant extrusion.

The appropriate-sized plug is then fashioned from a block of sterile medical-grade Silastic material (Fig. 20–13). This coffin-shaped plug should fit into the lateral sinus tarsi well enough to block the anterior leading edge of the talus as it descends from the posterior calcaneal facet, thus preventing talar subluxation. The plug is secured in the sinus tarsi by using two straight needles with 2–0 nonabsorbable sutures (Fig. 20–14). The threaded needles are run through the plug and passed through the sinus tarsi from lateral to medial and out through the medial aspect of the foot, where they are tied over the medial deltoid ligament (Fig. 20–15). Care should be taken to avoid the medial neurovascular structures (posterior tibial vein, artery, and nerve). After the custom Silastic plug has been positioned correctly within the sinus tarsi, the foot is moved through supination and pronation, and the amount of correction is assessed (Fig. 20–16). If the size of the implant is adequate, the talar declination

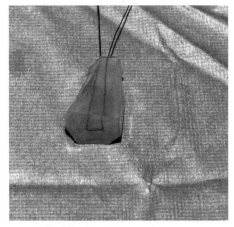

Figure 20–14. Silastic plug arthroereisis. The coffin-shaped implant is prepared for implantation by passing a 2–0 nonabsorbable suture through it using straight Keith needles.

---

[*]Hoke's tonsil is the term given to the tissue removed from within the lateral sinus tarsi.

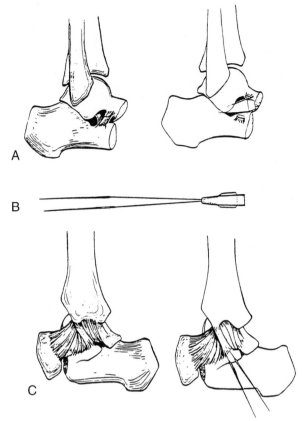

Figure 20–15. Silastic plug arthroereisis. *A*, The lateral ligaments are severed, and an appropriate-sized implant is fitted into the sinus tarsi joint. *B*, Sutures are passed through the implant using two Keith needles. *C*, The needles are passed through the subtalar joint from lateral to medial and sutured to the deltoid ligament on the medial aspect of the foot.

is improved and the calcaneus is more vertical in alignment. At this point, the linear or U-shaped capsular incision is closed with simple interrupted 3–0 absorbable sutures. This is followed by closure of the subcutaneous layer with 4–0 absorbable suture and final closure of the skin with 5–0 absorbable intradermal suture. The securing layer suture technique and the sequence of tissue layer closure also help to prevent lateral extrusion of the custom plug during early weight bearing.

The Smith STA-Peg Procedure.[38–40] The surgical approach for the angled STA-Peg implant is very similar to

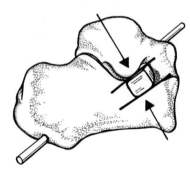

Figure 20–16. Silastic plug in place in lateral sinus tarsi. The foot is moved through supination and pronation, and the amount of correction of the talus is noted.

that described for the custom plug. However, there is no need to sever the deep interosseous talocalcaneal ligament in this procedure because the implant stem secures the STA-Peg in place (Fig. 20–17A). It is very important to place the implant in the floor of the sinus tarsi in the correct position to ensure optimal function and correction. The posterior edge of the implant body should be flush with the anterior leading edge of the posterior subtalar joint facet of the calcaneus. The stem of the implant should be vertical within the drill hole in the calcaneus, and the implant should be set firmly in place without rocking. The hole for the implant stem is made by using the drill and drill guide provided by Wright Medical Technology. Polymethylmethacrylate bone cement is not used unless the STA-Peg implant is loose or unstable.

The Maxwell-Brancheau Arthroereisis (MBA) Implant. This new implant offers the latest technology and design for correction of pediatric pes valgus as well as adult posterior tibial dysfunction deformity. The location and surgical approach for the MBA implant are similar to those described for the STA-Peg implant except that the incision is much smaller in length, usually 2 cm or smaller. The procedure does not require resection of any cartilage or bone and is relatively noninvasive. The implant is constructed of premium grade titanium alloy and has excellent biocompatibility characteristics. The implant is a soft-threaded device designed to be inserted between the anterior and middle facets of the subtalar joint (Fig. 20–17B). It acts as a block to anterior and inferior displacement of the talus, thus allowing normal subtalar joint motion while blocking excessive pronation. The implant's cannulated design allows precise alignment and proper placement during surgery. It is radiopaque and has a unique slotted design to absorb peak shock and impact stress while allowing fibrous ingrowth to buttress the subtalar joint (Fig. 20–17C). This implant is supplied in four sizes and comes with a teaching tape supplied by the company.

Calcaneal Osteotomy[2, 20, 27, 31, 36]

Relocational Calcaneal Osteotomy. The Koutsogiannis displacement osteotomy[23] of the calcaneus is performed through a lateral incisional approach. The osteotomy is made in a slightly curved oblique fashion beginning at the superior border of the calcaneus, just posterior to the talus, and extending to the inferior border of the calcaneus (Fig. 20–18). The posterior fragment is relocated medially until it lies beneath the sustentaculum tali and is displaced inferiorly to increase the height of the arch. Once the posterior fragment is in the corrected position, it is fixated with K-wires or screws placed through a percutaneous posterior approach.

Varus Opening Wedge Calcaneal Osteotomy. The Silver calcaneal osteotomy is performed through a slightly curved skin incision on the lateral heel just posterior to the peroneal tendons. The incision is deepened to the calcaneus with reflection of the peroneal tendons superi-

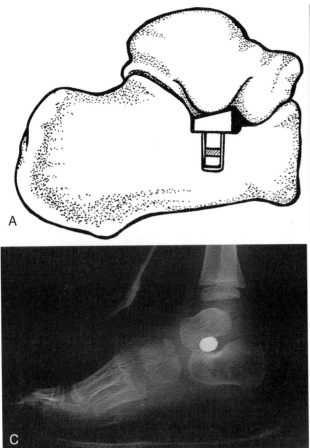

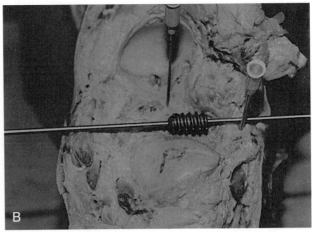

Figure 20–17. *A*, The Smith STA-Peg implant in place in the floor of the sinus tarsi of the calcaneus. *B*, The cannulated MBA implant placed between the anterior facet (central needle) and posterior facets of the subtalar joint. The lateral needle is at the calcaneal edge. *C*, Lateral radiograph demonstrating radiopaque MBA plug.

orly. The lateral sural nerve should be protected throughout the procedure. The soft tissues and the calcaneal periosteum are incised laterally and reflected to provide adequate exposure for the osteotomy. The more anterior the osteotomy is performed, the greater is the correction obtained. The osteotomy is performed with either a straight osteotome or bone saw, leaving the medial cortex of the calcaneus intact. The osteotomy site is opened, and an allogeneic iliac crest bone graft, ranging from 4 mm to 1 cm in width, is placed in the lateral opening (Fig.

20–19). The medial cortical hinge will provide adequate compressive forces to prevent graft displacement. If the graft does not appear to be locked in place it may be stabilized with a lateral bone staple or K-wire fixation.

Lateral Column Lengthening Osteotomy with Bone Graft. The modified Evans calcaneal osteotomy is designed to lengthen the lateral column in patients with pes valgus by inserting a transverse bone graft into the distal portion of the calcaneus (Fig. 20–20).[12] The procedure is

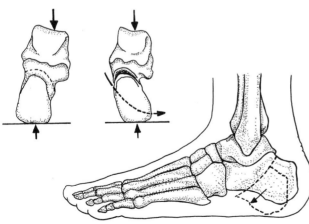

Figure 20–18. Koutsogiannis' displacement calcaneal osteotomy. The posterior fragment is relocated medially below the sustentaculum tali and then displaced inferiorly to increase the calcaneal angle.

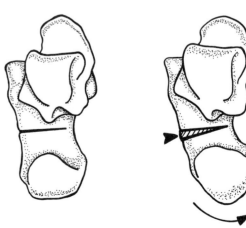

Figure 20–19. Posterior view of the rearfoot complex demonstrating the Silver varus producing calcaneal osteotomy with bone graft wedge placed laterally.

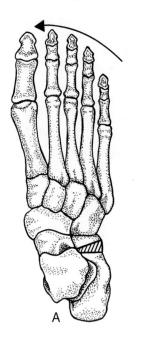
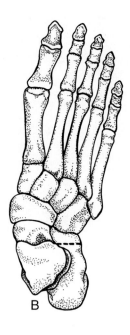

Figure 20–20. Modified Evans osteotomy. *A*, Proper tarsometatarsal alignment for the osteotomy. Distal calcaneal bone cut is placed approximately 1.5 cm proximal to the calcaneocuboid joint. *B*, Lateral lengthening is accomplished by placing a bone graft in the osteotomy site, which produces realignment of the midtarsal joint.

Figure 20–21. A long curved incision is placed over the medial aspect of the foot centered over the naviculocuneiform joint from the base of the first metatarsal to the base of the talus.

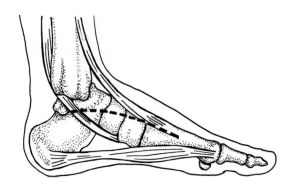

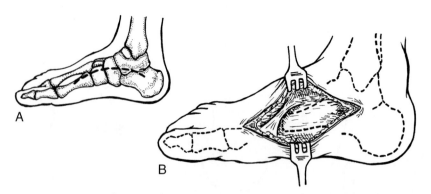
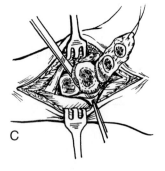

Figure 20–22. *A* and *B*, Once the incision is made, a U-shaped flap is sharply created with its base proximal, extending as far under the insertion of the anterior tibial tendon as possible. *C*, Using a straight osteotome, the periosteal-osteal flap is then raised from the proximal medial aspect of the first metatarsal, the medial cuneiform, and the navicular bone, exposing the underlying talonavicular, naviculocuneiform, and the first metatarsocuneiform joints.

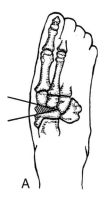

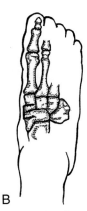

Figure 20–23. *A,* The articular cartilage from the opposing surfaces of the navicular and the medial and intermediate cuneiforms is excised; slightly more subchondral bone is removed from the medial and plantar aspects. *B,* The naviculocuneiform joint is closed and fixed with one or two bone staples.

Medial Column Reconstruction (Osseous Procedures)[2, 4–6, 19, 28–30, 37]

Naviculocuneiform Arthrodesis. This modification of the Hoke procedure involves the surgical fusion of the medial and intermediate naviculocuneiform joints with correction of the transverse and sagittal plane deformities by adduction and plantar flexion of the forefoot. The procedure begins with a long curved incision (convex dorsally) placed over the medial aspect of the foot and centered over the naviculocuneiform joint from the base of the first metatarsal to the talonavicular joint (Fig. 20–21). The incision is then carried directly to the deep fascia, where multiple perforating veins from the dorsal venous arch are encountered. The crossing veins are cut and ligated. The inferior extensor retinaculum is identified and incised and suture-tagged for later closure. The tendon sheath of the anterior tibial tendon is identified and freed of adjacent attachments down to its point of insertion. A long U-shaped incision is then made with its base proximal and extending as far under the insertion of the anterior tibial tendon as possible. The plantar portion of the flap should include portions of the plantar calcaneonavicular ligament and posterior tibial tendon. Using a straight osteotome, a periosteal-osteal flap is raised from the proximal medial aspect of the first metatarsal, the medial cuneiform, and the navicular, thus exposing the underlying talonavicular, naviculocuneiform, and the first metatarsocuneiform joints (Fig. 20–22). Caution must be exercised to avoid damage to the epiphysis of the first metatarsal base and the head of the talus by the osteotome during the creation of this flap.

The articular cartilage from the opposing surfaces of the navicular and the medial and intermediate cuneiform bones is resected, slightly more subchondral bone being removed from the plantar aspect. The naviculocuneiform joint is held open during this part of the process by using a self-retaining retractor such as the small lamina spreader. The foot and the distal end of the first metatarsal are placed in equinus while the hallux is dorsiflexed. This maneuver closes the osteotomy site. The osteotomy site is then fixated with one or two bone staples across the naviculocuneiform joints (Fig. 20–23). The periosteal-osteal flap is pulled distally and relocated under the anterior tibial tendon while the foot is held supinated. It is then sutured under slight tension to the first metatarsal base and medial cuneiform soft tissues, thus advancing the insertion of both the flap and the tendon-ligament complex. Final periosteal-osteal closure is performed with nonabsorbable sutures (Fig. 20–24). The subcutaneous

performed through an oblique skin incision placed over the lateral calcaneocuboid joint. The extensor digitorum brevis is freed from its insertion at the sinus tarsi, and the peroneal tendons are freed and retracted inferiorly. The vertical osteotomy is made in the distal calcaneus 1.5 cm proximal to the calcaneocuboid joint. The osteotomy may be complete or may leave the medial hinge intact. Autogenous or allogeneic bone is used and is cut into a wedge-shaped graft and fitted into the osteotomy site. In most cases, fixation is not required unless the bone graft or the distal segment of the calcaneus is unstable. Fixation is with crossing K-wires, a staple, or a screw.

Figure 20–24. *A,* The periosteal-osteal flap is advanced under the freed anterior tibial tendon while the foot is held in a corrected position. *B,* Final suture closure of the advanced periosteal-osteal flap using nonabsorbable suture material.

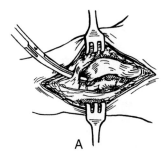

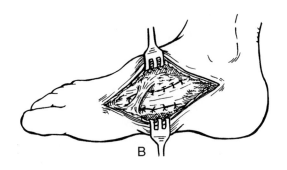

layer and the skin are then closed individually with absorbable sutures. The end-result of this procedure is to stabilize the fault at the naviculocuneiform joint, bring the first ray down to the ground, and create a visible arch structure to the foot (Fig. 20–25).

Naviculocuneiform and Cuneiform–First Metatarsal Arthrodesis. This medial column stabilization operation is a modification of the Miller procedure and involves the surgical fusion of the naviculocuneiform joint as well as the medial cuneiform–first metatarsal joint (Fig. 20–26). The incisional approach and the medial periosteal-osteal flap are performed just as in the modified Hoke procedure. The modified Miller procedure is performed instead of the modified Hoke procedure only when ligamentous laxity at the first metatarsocuneiform joint or metatarsus primus elevatus is present.

Closing Wedge Plantar Flexion Navicular Osteotomy. The modified Barouk navicular osteotomy is used when the medial column joints are not severely collapsed but significant visual flattening of the arch is still present. It is also used in older patients when arthrodesis of the medial column joints may be unsuitable. The procedure is performed through a skin and soft tissue approach using the medial periosteal-osteal flap as in the modified Hoke procedure. The navicular bone is identified, and the adjacent ligaments are left intact. Any prominence of the medial navicular bone may be removed to leave a flat

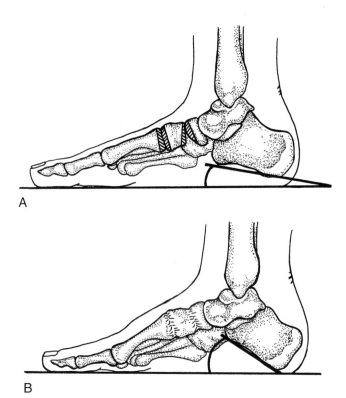

Figure 20–26. Modified Miller's procedure. *A,* The naviculocuneiform and first cuneiform–first metatarsal joints are resected with the base made wider plantarly. *B,* The osteotomies are closed and fixed with K-wires, staples, or screws.

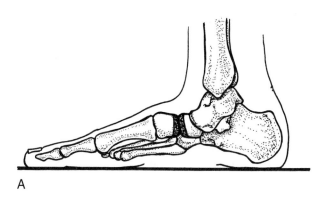

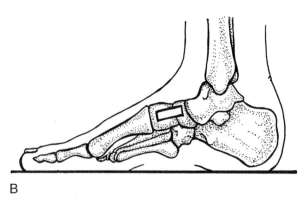

Figure 20–25. Modified Hoke's procedure. *A,* Dark areas represent bone and joint to be removed. *B,* The naviculocuneiform arthrodesis stabilizes the faulting that occurs and brings the first ray to the ground, thereby providing a visual increase in the arch. This procedure is never performed in isolation and is always used in combination with other procedures.

bone surface. A midbody closing and plantarflexory wedge osteotomy is performed using a combination of bone saws and osteotomes (Fig. 20–27). The resected midportion of the navicular may be removed after careful planning and execution of the cuts. This procedure brings the forefoot medially and plantar-flexes and stabilizes the first and second rays. This repositioning dramatically improves the function and visual appearance of the foot. I use this procedure for patients with pes planovalgus and in older patients with pes cavovalgus. The osteotomy is fixated with K-wires or bone staples.

Opening Wedge Plantar Flexion Osteotomy of the Medial Cuneiform. The modified Cotton dorsal opening wedge osteotomy of the medial cuneiform with bone graft is designed to produce plantar flexion of the medial column. This procedure is generally limited to deformities in which additional plantar flexion of the medial column is required after medial arch suspension, subtalar arthroereisis, and posterior equinus release have already been performed. The procedure is performed in a fashion similar to that used for the modified Barouk technique. The medial cuneiform is identified, and the adjacent ligaments are left intact. The midbody dorsal osteotomy of the cuneiform is performed with osteotomes and power bone saws. The osteotomy is carried plantarly with preservation of the plantar cortex. The osteotomy is opened with a smooth lamina spreader, and a wedge-shaped bone graft is placed in the dorsal opening (Fig. 20–28). Either autogenous or allogeneic bone may be used as the graft material for this procedure. Fixation is usually not neces-

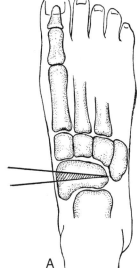

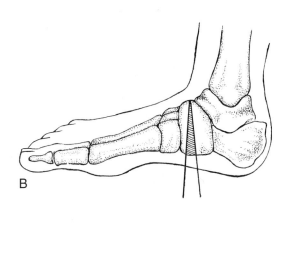

Figure 20–27. Modified Barouk's procedure. The navicular plantar flexion closing wedge osteotomy produces a result similar to that obtained with the modified Hoke procedure without sacrificing the tarsal joints.

sary, but if the graft appears unstable it may be fixated with K-wires, screws, or staples.

Medial Column Reconstruction (Soft Tissue Procedures)

Flap Transfer. A medial arch soft tissue reconstruction procedure with a periosteal-osteal flap (as described in the modified Hoke procedure) but without the joint fusion is performed, transposing the flap under the anterior tibial tendon. This is combined with suture plication and tightening of the medial aspect of the plantar calcaneonavicular ligament. This procedure is used with the subtalar arthroereisis procedure or the calcaneal osteotomy procedure when most of the deformity is in the rearfoot and mild collapse of the arch is present.

Rerouting Anterior Tibial Tendon. The modified Young tenosuspension procedure involves rerouting the intact anterior tibial tendon through a slot created in the medial navicular (Fig. 20–29).[48] Once this is accomplished, the posterior tibial tendon is advanced distally and reattached plantarly beneath the navicular bone with nonabsorbable suture. This procedure is generally recommended for children 10 years of age or older and is indicated to stabilize the medial column in patients with

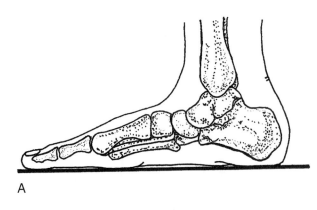

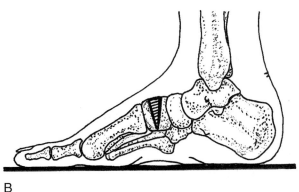

Figure 20–28. Modified Cotton's procedure. The cuneiform opening wedge osteotomy with bone graft is used with soft tissue medial column procedures to assist in plantar flexion of the medial column.

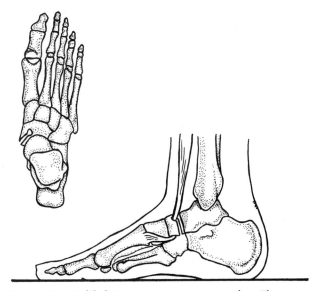

Figure 20–29. Modified Young's tenosuspension procedure. The anterior tibial tendon is freed to its insertion and rerouted through a slot in the medial navicular bone, effectively elevating the medial arch.

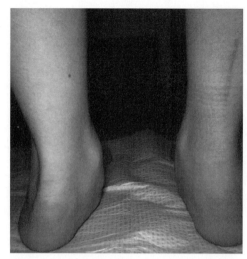

Figure 20–30. Gastrocnemius tendon recession and modified Kidner's procedure on the right greatly improved this patient's symptoms but had virtually no effect on the clinical appearance of the foot.

flexible sagittal plane deformity. Plantar flexion of the first ray usually occurs, which helps to reduce residual frontal plane varus or supinatus.

Excision of Accessory Navicular Bone. This operation is usually performed in patients with a symptomatic accessory navicular (os tibiale externum) with a very mild pes planovalgus foot condition. The modified Kidner procedure involves excision of the accessory navicular and resection of any hypertrophy of the navicular tuberosity with transposition of the posterior tibial tendon insertion to the inferior aspect of the navicular. This procedure is not advocated as a definitive procedure for the treatment of the symptomatic flatfoot because it is unable to sustain correction of the transverse plane component of pes valgus. Most patients undergoing a modified Kidner procedure show a decrease in the presenting symptoms but no visible improvement in the radiographic or clinical appearance of the foot (Fig. 20–30).

Tendon Balancing Procedures. The posterior tibial tendon insertion point on the medial and plantar arch area may be advanced distally and sutured into the soft tissues or bone.[22] In many cases, the anterior tibial tendon is split at its insertion site, and the inferior proximal arm of the tendon is brought down to the plantar medial calcaneonavicular ligament and posterior tibial tendon region and sutured in place to reinforce the arch. Additional tightening or shortening of these tendon and ligament structures may also be performed by plication during final closure. The flexor digitorum longus tendon may also be transected deeply in the arch and the distal end rerouted to the posterior tibial tendon insertion site; it is sutured in place with nonabsorbable suture.

Posterior Equinus Release[3, 10, 11, 13, 14]

Gastrocnemius Tendon Recession. When only gastrocnemius equinus is present (limitation of dorsiflexion of the foot at the ankle with the knee extended but not with the knee flexed), the gastrocnemius portion of the Achilles tendon is lengthened. With the patient in the prone position, a 5- to 7-cm linear incision (depending on the size of the child) is made on the inferior portion of the posterior calf slightly medial to the midline to avoid the neurovascular structures. This incision is placed approximately 5 to 7 cm proximal to the superior border of the posterior calcaneus. Blunt and sharp dissection is carried down through the deep fascia to the underlying Achilles paratenon. A linear incision is made through the sheath layers, which are gently retracted and tagged with suture for later closure. The plantaris tendon is identified on the medial aspect and lengthened or severed. The gastrocnemius aponeurosis is separated from the underlying soleus muscle and tendon, and a tongue-in-groove recession is performed (Fig. 20–31). The superior medial and lateral third of the aponeurosis are severed while the foot is held in a dorsiflexed position. The foot is then plantar-flexed, and the distal central third is then severed either transversely or with a V-shaped cut. With the knee extended, the foot is held in a corrected position and dorsiflexed to the desired amount. Ankle joint dorsiflexion should not exceed 100 with the knee extended. Once the lengthening has been performed the loose ends of the tendon may be secured with suture, and the deep fascia and paratenon layers are closed and sutured with absorbable materials. Final closure of the subcutaneous superficial fascia and skin is then completed with absorbable suture material.

Tendo Achillis Lengthening (TAL). In patients who have a significant combined equinus (triceps surae) with a negative amount of dorsiflexion of the foot at the ankle in both knee flexed and knee extended positions, a lengthening procedure of the Achilles tendon is performed.[46]

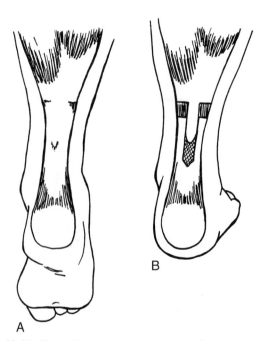

Figure 20–31. Tongue-in-groove gastrocnemius tendon recession procedure. *A,* The incisions are placed through the aponeurosis. *B,* The foot is dorsiflexed allowing the tendon to lengthen by a slide technique.

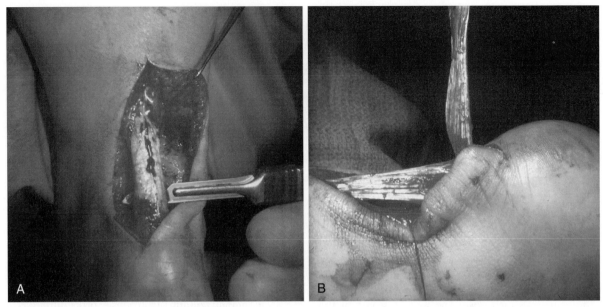

Figure 20–32. Open frontal plane Achilles tendon lengthening procedure. *A*, Posterior view. The distal portion of the tendon is divided into two equal halves. *B*, Lateral view. The most superficial half is transected proximally and the deep half is transected distally. The foot is dorsiflexed to the desired level of correction, and the tendon is sutured.

This may be accomplished with a percutaneous tenotomy, an open sagittal or frontal plane Z-lengthening procedure, or, preferably, a low tongue-in-groove procedure similar to the gastrocnemius recession described earlier. The percutaneous tenotomy may be performed in a number of different ways, but I prefer the modified White tenotomy procedure. This is a simple and relatively consistent procedure that involves sectioning the anterior two thirds of the distal end of the tendon and the medial two thirds of the tendon 3 to 5 cm proximal to this point, depending on the size of the child.

The open Z-lengthening procedure is performed in either the sagittal plane or the frontal plane (Fig. 20–32). The procedure is performed through a 5- to 7-cm linear skin incision placed either medial or lateral to the tendon on the posterior lower leg from just above the heel proximally. The incision is carried down to the deep fascia and paratenon, which are then opened in a linear fashion. The plantaris tendon is identified and lengthened or cut. The Achilles tendon is lengthened in the sagittal or frontal plane. The foot is then dorsiflexed and the separated ends of the tendon are repositioned and sutured into the corrected position. Layer closure is then performed.

The final open procedure is the tongue-in-groove lengthening of the Achilles tendon (Fig. 20–33). This procedure is performed in the same fashion as the gastrocnemius recession except that the cuts are made more distally and are carried completely through the conjoined Achilles tendon. Of these Achilles lengthening procedures, the low tongue-in-groove procedure for triceps surae equinus has been found to give more consistent results with less complications and fewer cases of recurrence. If a limitation of ankle joint dorsiflexion persists after Achilles tendon lengthening, release of the posterior ankle and subtalar joint capsules may be necessary (Fig. 20–34).

Adjunctive Procedures[41]

In children with a serpentine or Z-foot condition, additional procedures may be necessary to achieve the best long-term results. In most cases, the procedures are designed to eliminate forefoot adduction, hallux varus or adductus, or metatarsus adductus. These procedures include a medial cuneiform opening wedge with bone graft, an opening bone graft in the naviculocuneiform arthrodesis site, a lateral closing wedge osteotomy of the cuboid bone, and a medial release of the abductor hallucis tendon.

Medial Opening Wedge Bone Graft. The medial procedures are designed to decrease the forefoot adduction seen in cases of Z-foot. They may be performed independently, as in the modified Fowler procedure, or in conjunction with the modified Hoke medial naviculocu-

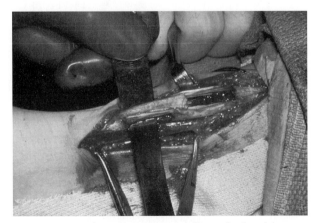

Figure 20–33. Distal tongue-in-groove Achilles tendon lengthening procedure. Heel is to the left.

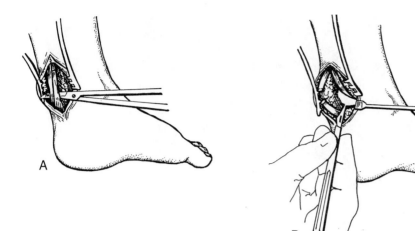

Figure 20–34. Lengthening of the Achilles tendon and posterior ankle and subtalar joint release. *A*, Through a posterior inferior incision, the Achilles tendon is lengthened with a **Z** incision. *B*, The deep compartment is entered with retraction of the flexor hallucis longus tendon, and the posterior ankle joint capsule is incised. The foot is then dorsiflexed to gain additional correction. Sectioning of the posterior subtalar joint capsule may also be done at this time if necessary.

neiform arthrodesis procedure. The medial cuneiform opening wedge osteotomy with bone graft is performed through an incision made over the medial aspect of the foot, extending from the base of the first metatarsal to just inferior and posterior to the navicular bone. The medial cuneiform is identified and exposed subperiosteally, taking care to preserve the anterior tibial tendon insertion. If the tendon cannot be preserved and retracted, a portion may be detached to aid in exposure. The osteotomy is performed centrally with either a bone saw or an osteotome, and the osteotomy is opened with a smooth lamina spreader. A wedge-shaped autogenous or allogeneic bone graft is then placed in the opening (Fig. 20–35). Because the cuneiform osteotomy is intrinsically stable and under compression, fixation is often not necessary. However, if the bone graft or adjacent cuneiform portions appear to be unstable, the osteotomy and

bone graft may be stabilized by K-wires or threaded pins for 6 weeks to prevent collapse of the osteotomy site.

If a medial column arthrodesis procedure has been planned in the patient with a Z-foot, the bone graft may be placed in the resected naviculocuneiform joints (Fig. 20–36). The incisional and deep surgical exposure are performed as described under the modified Hoke procedure. In most cases, the graft is simply incorporated into the fusion site, and fixation is accomplished with staples. The shape and placement of the graft can help to increase the overall correction obtained by accentuating the plantar flexion of the medial forefoot and decreasing the metatarsus adductus component.

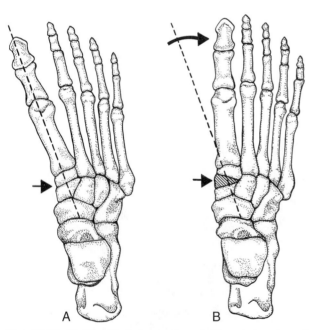

Figure 20–35. Modified Fowler's procedure. *A*, The osteotomy is made through the central portion of the medial first cuneiform bone. *B*, A wedge-shaped bone graft is then inserted into the osteotomy site with abduction of the forefoot.

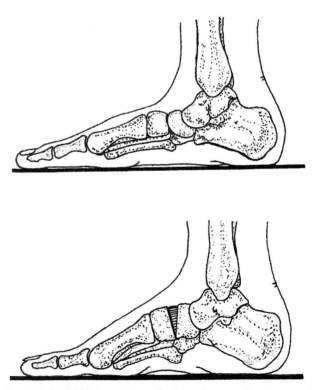

Figure 20–36. Medial opening and plantar-flexor wedge bone graft added to the naviculocuneiform arthrodesis site assist in creating an arch and prevent excessive adduction of the forefoot in a patient with a Z-foot.

Closing Wedge Cuboid Osteotomy. In the older child with skewfoot, the lateral column of the foot may have to be shortened as part of the flatfoot surgical correction. In these cases, a modified Tachdjian cuboid osteotomy is performed through a curvilinear lateral skin incision placed over the cuboid bone. The osteotomy is performed with a bone saw or osteotome, and the wedge resection is performed in the midline of the cuboid with removal of the central third of the bone (Fig. 20–37). Care should be taken not to remove too large a wedge of bone because otherwise the osteotomy site may be difficult to close. Once the laterally based wedge has been removed from the cuboid, the foot is manipulated, bringing the forefoot into marked abduction. When the osteotomy site is firmly closed it may be secured by a small staple or K-wire fixation. The bone removed from the cuboid may be used to graft the medial cuneiform osteotomy or the naviculocuneiform arthrodesis site described earlier.

Abductor Hallucis Release. In many cases of Z-foot the abductor hallucis muscle appears to be involved, at least in part, in the metatarsus adductus or the hallux adductus deformity. The abductor hallucis may be examined by holding the heel vertically and correcting the metatarsus adductus component of the forefoot. At the same time, the tendon of the abductor hallucis may be palpated (Fig. 20–38). This is frequently referred to as the Lichtblau test. Release of the abductor hallucis is performed with either a pure tenotomy (modified Lichtblau's procedure) or a resection of a portion of the tendon and muscle (modified McCauley's procedure). The tenot-

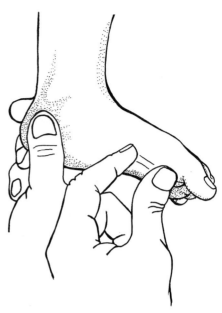

Figure 20–38. Lichtblau's test. Examination of the abductor hallucis tendon is performed with the heel held vertical and any forefoot adductus corrected.

omy procedure is made through a short linear incision on the medial aspect of the foot just proximal to the first metatarsal head. Careful dissection toward the metatarsal exposes the tendon of the abductor hallucis muscle (Fig. 20–39). The tendon is identified and sharply tenotomized. Subcutaneous and skin layers are closed with appropriate suture technique. The modified McCauley procedure is performed through an incision placed slightly more proximal than that used for the tenotomy procedure. Using a technique similar to that used in the tenotomy procedure, the tendon and muscle (myotendinous junction) of the abductor hallucis is exposed with deep dissection. A tenomyotomy is then performed, resecting a section of muscle and tendon of approximately 1 cm. Closure is performed in layer fashion. In this procedure, a compression dressing over the incision site is recommended because there tends to be more bleeding when the muscle is cut. As mentioned earlier, these procedures are designed to be used as adjunctive measures with other corrective flatfoot procedures in patients with the serpentine or Z-foot condition.

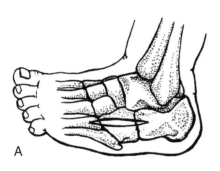

A

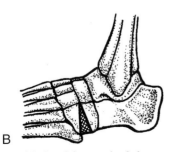

B

Figure 20–37. Modified Tachdjian's cuboid closing wedge osteotomy. *A*, Incisional area. *B*, The shaded area represents the bone to be removed. The osteotomy site may be fixated with K-wires or staples.

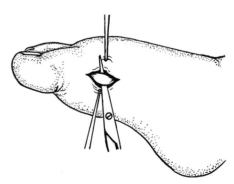

Figure 20–39. Modified Lichtblau's procedure. Tenotomy of the tight abductor hallucis tendon is performed through a small incision on the medial aspect of the foot.

JUSTIFICATION OF PROCEDURES

In theory, three major foot joint axes are considered in the evaluation of flatfoot: the subtalar joint axis, the midtarsal joint oblique axis (lateral column of the foot), and the midtarsal joint longitudinal axis (medial column of the foot). When subtalar joint compensation is due primarily to excessive transverse plane deformity with a high subtalar joint axis, the forefoot is abducted on the rearfoot while the rearfoot adducts. When this associated rearfoot adduction-eversion is present, an opening wedge anterior calcaneal osteotomy is the preferred procedure to lengthen the lateral column of the foot. In the older child, however, this procedure usually does not completely correct the forefoot varus or fixed supination, nor does it correct the naviculocuneiform sag (which is secondary to the deforming forces of the equinus and the forefoot varus or supinatus) owing to the adaptive changes that have already taken place. The Evans procedure corrects a significant amount of the frontal plane eversion and greatly improves the calcaneal inclination angle. Flatfoot conditions in which the calcaneus is located lateral to the weight-bearing line of the ankle (heel valgus) are corrected by an opening calcaneal osteotomy with bone graft. If the calcaneus is also plantar-flexed, the modification of the Koutsogiannis calcaneal relocation osteotomy may be a better choice. When the deforming force of the subtalar joint is in the frontal plane, it may be more appropriate to use a subtalar joint (STJ) arthroereisis plug or a Smith STA-Peg implant procedure.

The lateral STJ arthroereisis plug procedure was developed as an alternative to the extra-articular arthrodesis of the subtalar joint, and it has had good long-term success. This procedure involves the use of a custom carved plug from extra-firm, medical-grade Silastic material, the use of the stems cut from great toe Silastic implants, or a spherical ball of Silastic to block abnormal subtalar joint motion.

The STA-Peg implant procedure uses a stemmed implant made of a high-molecular-weight polyethylene. The implant was originally designed to be secured with the aid of polymethylmethacrylate bone cement into the floor of the lateral sinus tarsi of the calcaneus. The current model has an angled surface that makes contact with the anterior leading edge of the talus as it moves down the posterior facet of the subtalar joint. This allows for easier application and better fit than the original flat-surfaced implant.

This STA-Peg subtalar implant procedure effectively positions the calcaneus vertically and relocates the talus on top of the calcaneus in a corrected attitude. If the forefoot varus or supinatus is reducible, this stabilization of the subtalar joint results in a more effective sling for the peroneus longus to function on the longitudinal axis. This process plantar-flexes and helps stabilize the first ray. During the 6 to 8 months following surgery the flexible forefoot supination usually is reduced significantly. Once again, if articular and muscular adaptive changes have occurred, the forefoot imbalance may not be reduced. The results of this procedure, when performed alone, are characterized by an improved calcaneal stance position with a clinically low arch. In other words, the heel may appear vertical, but there may be no visible improvement of the pes planus condition. When the medial column instability remains uncorrected, a combination of osseous stabilization with fusion of the naviculocuneiform joints and/or soft tissue reconstruction of the medial arch is necessary. It is important to point out that arthrodesis of the naviculocuneiform joints is *never* performed independent of other procedures and is used as an adjunctive procedure for the total surgical correction of this particular type of flatfoot condition. When performed alone, the medial arch fusion may yield poor results over the long term.

The choice between a custom-made arthroereisis implant plug carved from extra-firm, medical-grade Silastic or a prefabricated Smith STA-Peg implant is a difficult one. I believe that correction of talar declination is more consistent with the STA-Peg implant and that the risk of lateral extrusion is much reduced with the implant compared with the custom-made plug. Methylmethacrylate bone cement is not used with most STA-Peg implants unless there is obvious movement of the implant or it appears very unstable when the leading edge of the lateral process of the talus contacts the superior aspect of the implant during pronation. In such cases, a small amount (0.25 to 1.0 mL) of bone cement is used to help secure the implant stem in place within the drill hole of the calcaneus. There is a relatively higher incidence of silicone detritus synovitis with the custom plug compared with the polyethylene STA-Peg.

The custom plug appears to have a much softer impact when the talus contacts it during weight bearing. The custom plug is also easier to put in and does not require remodeling of the posterior facet of the subtalar joint or the drill hole in the floor of the sinus tarsi of the calcaneus. It also has the advantage of being sized more accurately, since any shape or size can be custom-fitted to the patient.

The decision of whether or not to perform specific osseous procedures, such as opening or closing wedge osteotomies with or without bone grafting, depends on the deformity present in each individual bone or joint complex. For example, calcaneal osteotomy procedures are designed to accomplish different end results. The Evans anterior calcaneal osteotomy is useful for treatment of the foot with a vertical subtalar joint axis (transverse plane dominant pes valgus). This type of flatfoot compensates for the biomechanical deforming forces that are present predominantly in the transverse plane. When the anterior osteotomy and bone graft are performed, the lateral column is lengthened, and the midtarsal joint is realigned. Heel valgus is also reduced secondary to the change in the midtarsal joint and the retrograde effect on the subtalar joint. Forefoot varus and supinatus are usually not reduced, and some other type of medial column repair is necessary to address these conditions. This procedure is not recommended in patients with compensated metatarsus adductus because it will worsen this condition. Varus-producing or relocational posterior calcaneal osteotomies such as the modified Silver opening wedge calcaneal osteotomy and the modified Koutsogiannis displacement osteotomy are designed to treat the frontal plane dominant flatfoot. Additional medial column procedures are generally performed along with the calcaneal osteotomies.

Opening and closing wedge osteotomies of the cuboid, navicular, and cuneiform bones are performed to assist in the final correction of foot deformity by increasing adduction, abduction, plantar flexion, and so on. These procedures are almost never performed alone but are very important in helping to stabilize the foot.

The modified Young tenosuspension and the Kidner soft tissue procedures have their specific place in the treatment of symptomatic juvenile flatfoot conditions. For example, in a foot with a symptomatic accessory navicular bone, the modified Kidner procedure may be performed independently or may be combined with a posterior equinus release procedure. Or the modified Young tenosuspension procedure might be performed in a patient who has a STA-Peg implant but a supinatus or forefoot varus continues to be present. However, I use these procedures only rarely and mostly in cases in which there is minimal faulting of the naviculocuneiform joints. When the modified Kidner or Young procedures are performed, they are adjunctive to other corrective procedures such as equinus release, calcaneal osteotomy, lateral arthroereisis, or other osseous procedures.

The correction of the posterior equinus condition is based simply on whether the problem is due to inadequate length of the gastrocnemius tendon alone (gastrocnemius equinus) or to inadequate length of the entire posterior group (triceps surae equinus). When solitary gastrocnemius tendon tightness is identified, a modification of the tongue-in-groove procedure is performed approximately 5 to 7 cm above the calcaneal insertion point. When a combined triceps surae equinus is present, a percutaneous tenotomy, open Z-plasty, or low tongue-in-groove tendo Achillis lengthening is performed approximately 2 to 5 cm above the calcaneal insertion point.

SUMMARY

Children with symptomatic flatfeet may present with varying symptoms and complaints of disability, such as an inability to keep up with their friends in walking or running, recurrent aching of the feet or calves, generalized lower extremity fatigue, and excessive shoe or heel wear. When symptoms do not respond to conservative care, surgical treatment should be considered. In younger patients there may be no actual complaints, but the parents can usually highlight the amount of disability present. The parents have often been told repeatedly by their family physician or pediatrician not to worry and that the child will outgrow the condition. Older children have a greater tendency to report pain and disability and are much more specific about their complaints than younger children.

I prefer the combination of procedures described for treatment of the specific symptomatic flexible flatfoot condition with posterior equinus, calcaneal valgus, forefoot varus or supinatus, and naviculocuneiform sag. It is recognized that other procedures are available for the treatment of this problem and for other types of flatfoot conditions. Long-term experience with this combined surgical procedural approach suggests that, in properly selected patients, the results are fairly predictable and provide good to excellent relief of symptoms as well as improvement of function and appearance.

References

1. Addante JB, Chin MW, Loomis JC, et al: Subtalar joint arthroereisis with Silastic silicone sphere: A retrospective study. J Foot Surg 1992; 31:47–51.
2. Anderson AF, Fowler SB: Anterior calcaneal osteotomy for symptomatic juvenile pes planus. Foot Ankle 1984; 4:274–283.
3. Baker LD: A rational approach to the surgical needs of the cerebral palsy patient. J Bone Joint Surg 1954; 38A:313–317.
4. Barouk LS: Navicular Osteotomy for Correction of Flatfoot. Presented at the World Congress for Foot and Ankle Surgery, Philadelphia, October 22, 1995.
5. Cohen-Sobel E, Giorgini R, Velez Z: Combined technique for surgical correction of pediatric severe flexible flatfoot. J Foot Ankle Surg 1995; 34:183–194.
6. Cotton FJ: Foot statistics and surgery. N Engl J Med 1936; 214:353–362.
7. Dockery GL: Perioperative management of the infant and child. Clin Podiatr Med Surg 1984; 3:645–665.
8. Dockery GL: Surgical treatment of the symptomatic juvenile flexible flatfoot condition. Clin Podiatr Med Surg 1987; 1:99–117.
9. Dockery GL: Symptomatic juvenile flatfoot condition: Surgical treatment. J Foot Ankle Surg 1995; 34:135–145.
10. Downey MS, Banks AS: Gastrocnemius recession in the treatment of nonspastic ankle equinus. J Am Podiatr Med Assoc 1989; 79:159–174.
11. Downey MS: Ankle equinus. In McGlamry ED, Banks AS, Downey MS (eds): Comprehensive Textbook of Foot Surgery, 2nd ed. Baltimore, Williams & Wilkins, 1992, pp. 687–730.
12. Evans D: Calcaneo-valgus deformity. J Bone Joint Surg 1975; 57B:270–278.
13. Fowler SB, Brooks AL, Parrish TF: The cavo varus foot. J Bone Joint Surg 1959; 41A:757.
14. Fulp MJ, McGlamry ED: Gastrocnemius tendon recession. J Am Podiatr Assoc 1974; 64:163–171.
15. Giannestras NJ: Foot Disorders: Medical and Surgical Management, 2nd ed. Philadelphia, Lea & Febiger, 1973, pp. 108–133.
16. Grice DS: An extra-articular arthrodesis of the subastragalar joint for correction of paralytic flat feet in children. J Bone Joint Surg 1952; 34A:927–935.
17. Hawksley JC: The nature of growing pains and their relation to rheumatism in children and adolescents. Br Med J 1939; 155–157.
18. Hoke M: An operation for the correction of extremely relaxed flat feet. J Bone Joint Surg 1931; 13:773–783.
19. Jack EA: Naviculocuneiform fusion in treatment of flat foot. J Bone Joint Surg 1955; 35B:75–81.
20. Jacobs AM, Oloff LM, Visser HJ: Calcaneal osteotomy in the management of flexible and nonflexible flatfoot deformity: A preliminary report. J Foot Surg 1981; 20:57–66.
21. Jacobs AM, Oloff LM: Surgical management of forefoot supinatus in flexible flatfoot deformity. J Foot Surg 1984; 23:410–419.
22. Kissel CG, Blacklidge DK: Tibialis anterior transfer "into talus" for control of the severe planus pediatric foot: A preliminary report. J Foot Ankle Surg 1995; 34:195–199.
23. Koutsogiannis E: Treatment of mobile flatfoot by displacement osteotomy of the calcaneus. J Bone Joint Surg 1971; 53B:96–100.
24. Lanham RH: Indications and complications of arthroereisis in hypermobile flatfoot. J Am Podiatr Assoc 1979; 69:178–185.
25. LeLievre J: The valgus foot: Current concepts and correction. Clin Orthop 1970; 70:43–55.
26. Lundeen RO: The Smith STA-Peg operation for hypermobile pes planovalgus in children. J Am Podiatr Med Assoc 1985; 75:177–183.
27. Marcinko DE, Lazerson A, Elleby DH: Silver calcaneal osteotomy for flexible flatfoot: A retrospective preliminary report. J Foot Surg 1984; 23:191–198.

28. Miller OL: A plastic flat foot operation. J Bone Joint Surg 1927; 9:84–89.
29. Miller GR: The operative treatment of hypermobile flatfeet in the young child. Clin Orthop 1977; 122:95–101.
30. Miller SJ: Collapsing pes valgoplanus (flexible flatfoot). *In* Levy LA, Hetherington VJ (eds): Principles and Practice of Podiatric Medicine. New York, Churchill Livingstone, 1990, pp. 893–929.
31. Mosca VS: Calcaneal lengthening for valgus deformity of the hindfoot. J Bone Joint Surg 1995; 77A:500–512.
32. Oloff-Solomon J: Radiographic evaluation in the pediatric patient. Clin Podiatr Med Surg 1987; 4:21–36.
33. Page JC: Symptomatic flatfoot: Etiology and diagnosis. J Am Podiatr Assoc 1983; 73:393–399.
34. Pascarella EM, Estrada RJ: Pes cavo-valgus foot. J Foot Surg 1991; 30:553–557.
35. Powell HDW, Cantab MB: Pes planovalgus in children. Clin Orthop 1983; 177:133–139.
36. Sangeorzan BJ, Mosca V, Hansen ST Jr: Effects of calcaneal lengthening on relationships among the hindfoot, midfoot, and forefoot. Foot Ankle 1993; 14:136–142.
37. Seymour N: The late results of naviculocuneiform fusion. J Bone Joint Surg 1967; 46B:558–562.
38. Smith SD: The STA Operation: A New Surgical Approach to the Pronated Foot in Childhood. Chicago, Fifth Annual Northlake Surgical Seminar, 1975.
39. Smith SD, Millar EA: Arthroereisis by means of a subtalar polyethylene peg implant for correction of hindfoot pronation in children. Clin Orthop 1983; 181:15–23.
40. Smith SD, Wagreich CR: Review of postoperative results of the subtalar arthroereisis operation: A preliminary study. J Foot Surg 1984; 23:253–260.
41. Spinner S, Caseate F, Long DH: Criteria for combined procedure selection in the surgical correction of the acquired flatfoot. Clin Podiatr Med Surg 1989; 6:561–575.
42. Subotnick SI: The subtalar joint lateral extra-articular arthroereisis: A preliminary report. J Am Podiatr Assoc 1974; 64:701–711.
43. Subotnick SI: The subtalar joint lateral extra-articular arthroereisis: A follow-up report. J Am Podiatr Assoc 1977; 67:157–171.
44. Tachdjian MO: Pronated feet. *In* Pediatric Orthopedics. Philadelphia, W.B. Saunders, 1972, p. 1397.
45. Tax HR: Flexible flatfoot in children. J Am Podiatr Assoc 1977; 67:616–619.
46. White JW: Torsion of the Achilles tendon: Its surgical significance. Arch Surg 1943; 46:784–787.
47. Wynne-Davies R: Family studies and the cause of congenital clubfoot—talipes equinovarus, talipes calcaneovalgus and metatarsus varus. J Bone Joint Surg 1964; 46B:445–451.
48. Young C, Charles S: Operative treatment of pes planus. Surg Gynecol Obstet 1939; 68:1099–1102.
49. Yu GV, Boberg J: Subtalar arthroereisis. *In* McGlamry ED, Banks AS, Downey MS (eds): Comprehensive Textbook of Foot Surgery, 2nd ed. Baltimore, Williams & Wilkins, 1992, pp. 818–828.

21

Calcaneovalgus

Richard M. Jay, D.P.M.

Calcaneovalgus is the most common congenital foot deformity. Wynne-Davies calculated that it occurs in about 1 in 1000 live births.[1] Unfortunately, it is perhaps the least recognized and least treated foot abnormality. The calcaneovalgus foot type is identifiable at birth, but it continues to go untreated due to perpetuation of the myth that no treatment is necessary. Parents are commonly reassured that "They will grow out of it" or "All babies are born with flat feet." Consequently, conservative methods of correction are not attempted during the first year of life, the time when these methods are most effective.

Congenital deformities do not usually occur before the twentieth week of the gestational period. They occur in the last 10 weeks of pregnancy because of the relationship between the size of the fetus and the amount of amniotic fluid present. Extrinsic constraining factors, not inherent in the fetus, that influence deformities are intrauterine compression (as seen in a multiple fetus pregnancy) and the presence of uterine fibroids. Extrauterine compression affecting fetal development may arise from tight abdominal muscles, which are present during the first pregnancy, or from any bony structure (e.g., the lumbar spine). Extrauterine compression may also be due to the small size of the mother's pelvis. Uterine compression contributes to congenital deformation when the fetus increases in size and the amniotic fluid pressure increases.[2]

The vertex position of the fetus during the last period of gestation uses uterine space efficiently and allows normal development and functional rotation of the limbs. Any rotational change in the position of the fetus increases the compressive forces against the body from the head to the toes.

A child that is examined immediately after delivery rests in its position of comfort. The baby assumes this abnormal position easily and resists any attempt to reduce the position of comfort. Early examination may reveal certain congenital deformities and provides better insight into the treatment of these deformities. Early detection of these congenital problems allows reduction of deformities with simple conservative measures.[3]

When the forces of growth and development can be directed, one can properly address and redefine the direction of growth into an accepted normal position. It is also understood that if an abnormal force is applied to any growing child, a deformity will result.[4] Wolff's law describes this reaction of bone to forces acting upon it:

"Every change in the form and function of bones or their function alone is followed by certain definite changes in their normal internal structure and equally definite changes in their external configuration in accordance with mathematical laws."[5] Forces of weight bearing and the action of muscles reshape and remodel the bone, gradually correcting the deformity. Bone can thus change its architecture in response to altered mechanical loads.

Immediate recognition and correction of the calcaneovalgus foot type is necessary during the first year of life while the bones and soft tissue structures are still amenable to change and before abnormal joint relationships have formed. Correction is easily obtained through serial manipulative casting. If left untreated, the flexible flatfoot may lead to disabling secondary deformities and symptoms that may emerge in adolescence and early adulthood. The majority of these problems, including metatarsalgia, hammertoe syndrome, neuromas, plantar fasciitis, heel spur syndrome, postural pains of the foot and leg, and arthrosis deformans of the midtarsal and subtalar joints, may be directly related to the pronated foot.[6] The untreated calcaneovalgus foot becomes a pronated foot. Therefore, one must act early and definitively to prevent the known consequences of pronated feet in adult life.[7]

ETIOLOGY

Intrinsic and extrinsic environmental factors that affect the position of the calcaneovalgus foot may cause or maintain varying degrees of deformity. A genetic factor may also exist to some degree. Giannestras' study of 82 patients showed a hereditary predisposition in 68%.[7] The majority of valgus foot deformities probably result from fetal malposition in which the placental wall acts as an extrinsic force in maintaining a calcaneovalgus attitude. This is readily demonstrable in the neonate. The fetal "position of comfort" unfortunately becomes the habitual sleeping position in the first year of life. Children with a concomitant neuromuscular deformity have a greater predilection to extrinsic factors.[8] In this attitude of deformity, the ossification which takes place produces an unstable platform (valgus foot) upon which the child's first steps are taken.[9]

There are many extrinsic environmental factors that may induce a calcaneovalgus foot before birth. These include a small uterus, a large fetus, tight amniotic membranes, and an intrauterine breech or transverse lie pre-

Table 21–1. **Extrinsic Factors**

Small uterus
Tight amniotic membranes
Intrauterine breech or transverse lie
Sitting and sleeping positions that force the foot outward—sleeping in
   prone position with feet outward; reverse tailor-sitting position with
   feet forced outward
Large fetal size
Early walking and crawling
Shoes (may maintain abnormal position)

Table 21–2. **Intrinsic Factors**

Muscular imbalances (hyperinnervation, hypoinnervation)
Weak ligaments (Ehlers-Danlos syndrome, Marfan's syndrome)

sentation at birth. The fact that this disorder often occurs in successive births may be explained by the fact that certain environmental factors are the same (e.g., small uterus). After birth, sitting and sleeping positions that force the foot outward will maintain the deformity. Examples include sleeping in a prone position with the feet spread outward or the reverse tailor-sitting position with the feet forced outward. Shoes may also maintain the abnormal position.

One intrinsic environmental factor is muscular imbalance. Muscle is a dynamic tissue that affects both motion and position at the joint level. Muscular imbalance between opposing muscle groups can deform the body architecture. This imbalance may be due to hyperinnervation or paralysis. In calcaneovalgus, certain muscles overpower the weaker muscles and drive the foot into an outward position. In cerebral palsy, in which a tendoachilles muscle spasticity is present, compensation occurs at the midtarsal joint because the muscles maintaining an arch are weaker than the tendoachilles and a mechanical advantage is given to the comparatively stronger muscles (peroneus brevis and tibialis anterior).

The chief supinator of the forefoot is the anterior tibial muscle. Its antagonist is the chief pronator of the forefoot, the peroneus longus muscle. The chief evertor of the heel is the peroneus brevis muscle, and the chief supinator of the rearfoot is the tibialis posterior. In the calcaneovalgus foot type, the anterior tibial tendon becomes shorter

because its origin and insertion are brought closer together. This maintains dorsiflexion and pulls the flexible forefoot into a supinated position. The peroneus longus muscle is greatly overstretched and is essentially functionless except when the foot is in extreme dorsiflexion. The heel cord and tibialis posterior muscles are also elongated. The peroneus brevis muscle becomes active at about 4 to 6 weeks of age and pulls the heel into marked eversion and abduction secondary to the position of the calcaneovalgus foot.

A second intrinsic environmental factor is "weak ligaments." Bones follow the course of least resistance. If an abnormal force is applied to a loose joint, the bone deforms in the direction of the applied force. In the presence of a lax joint (e.g., in Ehlers-Danlos syndrome, Marfan's syndrome, hypertonia, or trisomy 21) the joint responds to extrinsic pronatory forces. In time, the muscles acting around the joints further change the bones' positions, and the bones themselves change their shapes. All these factors, both instrinsic and extrinsic, result in a condition of dislocation of the talonavicular joint. The navicular articulates with the dorsal aspect of the talus, locking it into a vertical to plantar-flexed position (Tables 21–1 and 21–2).[6]

CLINICAL SIGNS

The calcaneovalgus foot type is most often described as an "up and out" position of the foot relative to the leg (Fig. 21–1). In fact, the dorsum of the foot lies in close proximity to the anterolateral aspect of the leg. This dorsiflexed and abducted position leaves the foot in a calcaneus position. The foot and heel are in complete

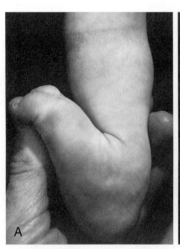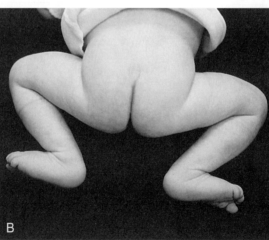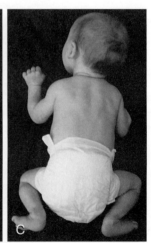

Figure 21–1. The dorsum of the foot lies in close proximity to the anterolateral aspect of the leg. This dorsiflexed and abducted position leaves the foot in a calcaneus position. The foot and heel are in complete valgus. *B*, Four-month-old child in typical calcaneovalgus position. The hip is externally positioned, and external tibial torsion is present. The feet are in an up-and-out position. In the creeping reflex, the foot dorsiflexes further to maintain the calcaneovalgus position. *C*, Three-month-old child demonstrating the up-and-out position and frog leg attitude as seen in calcaneovalgus.

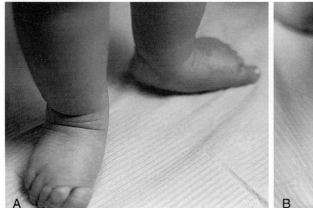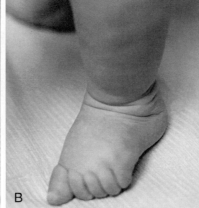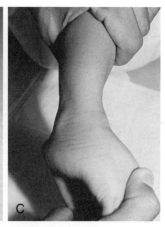

Figure 21–2. *A*, The calcaneovalgus foot is extremely abducted with marked flattening of the medial column. A talar bulge is present along with excessive and redundant skin folds on the lateral side of the foot over the sinus tarsi. *B*, Six-month-old child with calcaneovalgus. Note marked increase in skin folds and transverse plane position. When the child is held in a weight-bearing attitude, the foot increases its abduction and dorsiflexion components in the subtalar and midtarsal joints. *C*, A calcaneovalgus foot held in forced plantar flexion. Note the increased darkening of the lateral skin folds over the ankle and sinus tarsi region. Also noted is the limitation of plantar flexion of the foot on the leg. The foot should be a complete extension of the leg, and there should be no limitation of plantar flexion in the young infant.

valgus. If the leg is held and the foot is rapidly shaken and then released, the foot immediately returns to a dorsiflexed everted position relative to the leg. (The normal foot rests at a neutral to plantar-flexed attitude in relation to the leg.) Redundant skin folds are commonly seen along the lateral border of the foot in the area of the sinus tarsi. The skin about the medial aspect of the ankle appears stretched. The skin lines in the lateral ankle area blanch when the foot is plantar-flexed and inverted. This tightness suggests that the anterior and lateral soft tissue structures are already adapting to the position of deformity. The calcaneovalgus foot is described as banana-shaped due to the lateral deviation present. The Achilles tendon is stretched and excessively long, the talar head is prominent medially, and the longitudinal arch is flattened (Fig. 21–2).

Clinically, one may also detect an abnormal range of motion consisting of excessive dorsiflexion and eversion and limited plantar flexion and inversion. These limitations of motion depend on the degree of the deformity. The foot often can only plantar-flex to reach a right angle. Calcaneovalgus is a *flexible* deformity. Neutral position can be reached, restoring the normal architecture of the foot and its joint relationships (Fig. 21–3).

The congenital calcaneovalgus foot is often confused with the convex pes valgus (vertical talus). Vertical talus involves complete dislocation of the talonavicular joint, the navicular articulating with the talar neck dorsally. The two have similar clinical characteristics (dorsiflexed and everted foot) but can be distinguished by the fact that the convex pes valgus foot type is rigid (Fig. 21–4). The normal architecture cannot be restored by forced plantar flexion as is possible in the calcaneovalgus foot. Another distinguishing feature is that the Achilles tendon is tight in convex pes valgus. The convex pes valgus foot often breaks down in the midfoot and develops a rocker-bottom flatfoot.

PATHOMECHANICAL FACTORS

With a knowledge of the clinical signs and etiology, the osseous malposition of calcaneovalgus is better understood. The ankle joint is a strong mortis joint that primarily allows the talus to move in a sagittal direction (dorsiflexion and plantar flexion). If one were to crank the foot in a transverse abductory direction at the metatarsals, little twist would take place in the ankle joint. The net result is that the calcaneus moves outward or rather abducts and pivots under the talus. Since the calcaneocuboid joint is a strong locked joint, the cuboid follows the calcaneus outwardly, and the entire lateral column abducts. In the meantime, the talus remains locked within the ankle joint mortis. One must remember that the spring ligament (the plantar calcaneonavicular ligament)

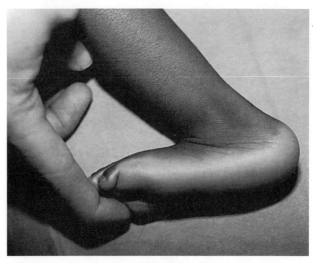

Figure 21–3. The foot is easily dorsiflexed with a minimal degree of plantar flexion available.

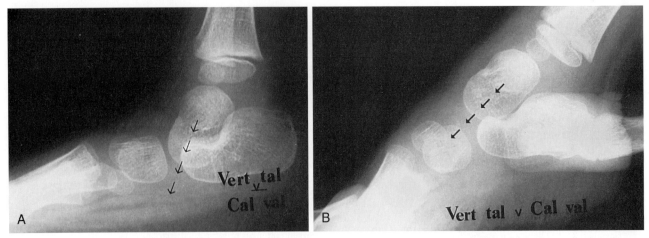

Figure 21–4. *A* and *B*, Calcaneovalgus and vertical talus can be radiographically distinguished by actively plantar-flexing the foot. In both conditions the talus appears to be plantar-flexed in the neutral position, and with plantar flexion the talus remains plantar-flexed in relation to the calcaneus. In calcaneovalgus the forefoot realigns with the talus when the foot is plantar-flexed.

spans the calcaneus and the navicular. With the abductory drift of the calcaneus and cuboid, the navicular abducts off the talar head. The spring ligament also supports the talus. When the navicular moves laterally, bringing the spring ligament with it, the talus plantar-flexes because it is no longer supported by the ligament. Now the foot is in an abducted position due to a transverse force. The transverse plane motion forces the entire lateral column to abduct, which forces the calcaneus to abduct; the spring ligament pulls on the navicular, which also moves laterally, bringing with it the first ray. This allows the talus to plantar-flex (Figs. 21–5 to 21–7).

The cervical ligament of the sinus tarsi occupies the space from the anterior calcaneus laterally and travels superiorly to the inferior surface of the medial talus in the sulcus of the sinus tarsi. This ligament is responsible for limiting inversion of the subtalar joint. The interosseous ligament, also known as the axial ligament, is a very thick, fibrous, and strong ligament. It prevents abduction and dorsiflexion of the calcaneus from under the talus.[10, 11] In calcaneovalgus with its strong transverse abductory

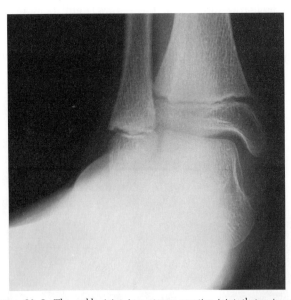

Figure 21–5. The ankle joint is a strong mortise joint that primarily allows the talus to move in a sagittal direction. With a transverse rotational drive through the foot, abduction occurs in the foot excluding the talus. Torque is exerted through the ankle joint, but no actual motion occurs in the direction of abduction. The talus remains locked in the ankle joint mortise.

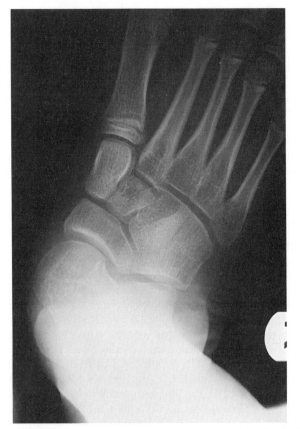

Figure 21–6. With abductory drift of the calcaneus and cuboid, the navicular abducts off the talar head. The spring ligament also supports the talus. When the navicular moves laterally, bringing the spring ligament with it, the talus plantar-flexes because it is no longer supported by the ligament. Now the foot is in an abducted position due to a transverse force.

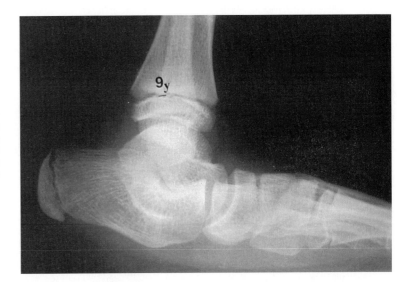

Figure 21–7. The transverse plane motion forces the entire lateral column to abduct, which in turn forces the calcaneus to abduct; the spring ligament pulls on the navicular, which also moves laterally, bringing with it the first ray. The plantar medial support of the talar head is lost by the lateral drift, and the talus further plantar-flexes.

forces, the axial ligament is stretched and weakened; if the foot is not realigned early, the ligament always remains lax and allows the subtalar joint to continue to pronate as the child ages.

RADIOLOGIC EVALUATION

One must be aware that calcaneovalgus is determined by clinical evaluation at an early age, not by radiographic evaluation. However, if the condition is severe enough to warrant therapy with casting or surgery, a radiograph can be taken to determine the degree of the deformity. With a young child it is obvious that the bones are not fully matured; therefore, interpreting the navicular position on the head of the talus is impossible since the navicular's primary ossification center does not appear until at least 2 to 3 years of age. However, on a lateral radiograph, one can determine the degree of talar declination by bisecting the talus through the cuboid.[12] In a lateral projection of a calcaneovalgus foot, the talus appears plantar-flexed, and the line bisecting the talus extends far below the plantar surface of the cuboid. One should also notice the overlapping of the head of the talus on the anterior-superior surface of the calcaneus. The talus, which gives the appearance of a shortened talar neck, appears to be smaller owing to the plantar medial position of the head on the calcaneus. The bone itself is not shortened; this is only a radiographic finding. Since the navicular is locked toward the calcaneus by the spring ligament, the navicular now lies lateral to the talar head. This is evident in the increased talocalcaneal angle on the anteroposterior radiographic view of the foot (Figs. 21–8 and 21–9).

Owing to the continual abductory force on the foot, the osseous structures eventually adapt to the new positions. The navicular resting lateral to the bisection of the talar head becomes deformed by the pull of the spring ligament; it appears as a wedge as it twists laterally. Because the navicular now has less and less contact with the rounded head, the nonarticulating surface of cartilage starts to thin out, and the head takes on a conical appearance. The end result is a talar head that appears squared

off and leads to a rigid deformity. The degree of drift determines the severity of rigidity and its age of onset (Figs. 21–10 and 21–11).

CONSERVATIVE REDUCTION

A conservative approach to the reduction of calcaneovalgus is usually all that is needed as long as it is attempted early. In an infant younger than 12 months the deformity can be greatly reduced with this conservative approach.

Prior to cast immobilization, the infant's foot is gently manipulated into the corrected position. The small heel is held gently, and teased into an inverted position. At the same time, the foot is plantar-flexed at the ankle. The parents are instructed in this simple maneuver to reduce cast time. It is recommended that gentle and gradual manipulation be continued for 1 week prior to cast appli-

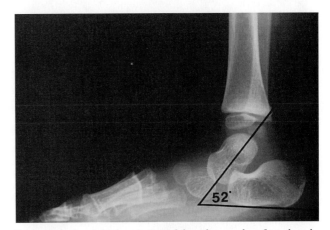

Figure 21–8. In a lateral projection of the calcaneovalgus foot, the talus appears to be plantar-flexed and the line bisecting the talus extends far below the plantar surface of the cuboid. Also notice the overlapping of the head of the talus on the anterior-superior surface of the calcaneus. Note that the talus, which has the appearance of a shortened talar neck, appears to be smaller because of the plantar medial position of the head on the calcaneus. The bone itself is not shortened; it merely appears shortened on the radiograph.

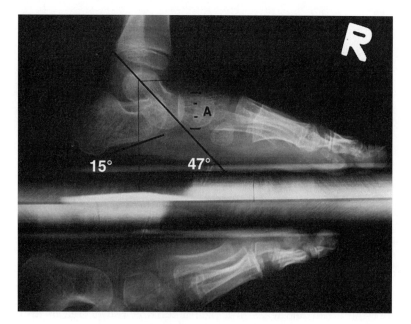

Figure 21–9. The cartilaginous structure of the talar head is not complete in the young child. Using the relationship of the bisection to the cuboid helps in determining the degree of deformity. The cuboid is divided into thirds. If the bisection lies in the lower third, pronatory changes are maximal. If the bisection rests in the upper third, pronatory changes are minimal.

cation. Exact reduction and final manipulation are accomplished using the following cast techniques.

If concomitant external tibial torsion is present, the cast is applied from the toes to the proximal segment of the thigh. If an isolated calcaneovalgus is present, then only a below-the-knee cast is necessary. Stockinette is applied to the forefoot and proximally on the leg to a point just below the knee. Two-inch Webril (Johnson and Johnson, Raynham, MA) is then wrapped smoothly and snugly over the foot up to the proximal segment. Obviously, the purpose of the cast is to maintain the position of the foot, but if the Webril is too thick or too loose, the cast will not completely control the foot in the desired position, and the foot will wobble within the cast; usually

two layers of Webril are sufficient. A little extra Webril is placed at the heel because the infant kicks on the supporting surface while in a supine position.

The assistant holds the child's toes with one hand while stabilizing the thigh with the other. Plaster roll, 2 or 3 inches wide, depending on the child's size, is applied from

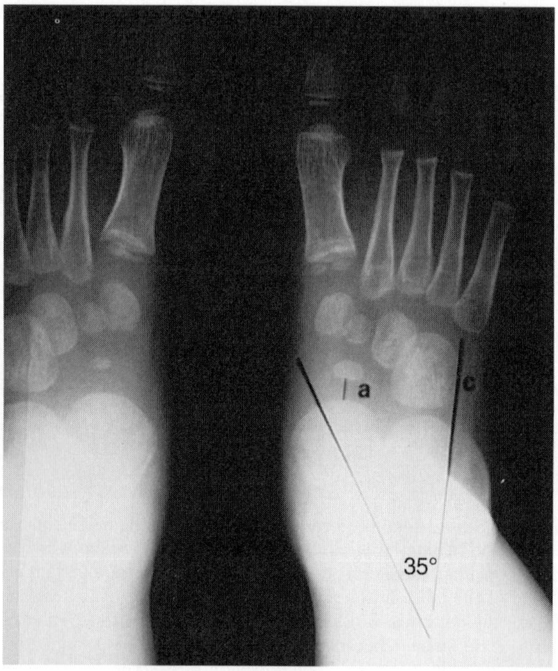

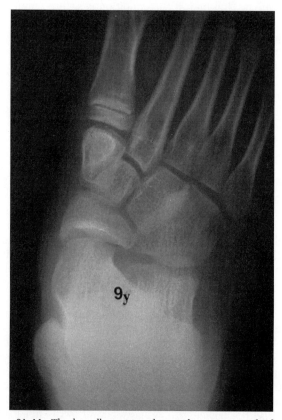

Figure 21–11. The laterally positioned navicular appears wedged with loss of the round talar head. With loss of medial cartilage of the talar head, the talus becomes conical. The motion of the navicular on the talar head is limited owing to the squared-off angles of the talar head.

Figure 21–10. The navicular is lateral to the bisection of the talus.

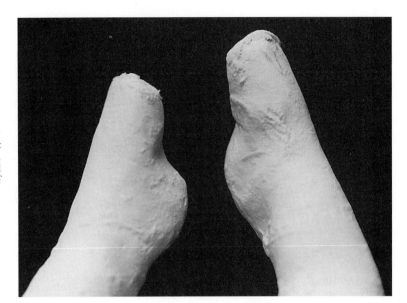

Figure 21-12. Plaster cast material applied to the calcaneovalgus foot. The finished product should show the foot plantar-flexed at the ankle, plantar-flexed at the first ray, heel inverted, and forefoot adducted. The cast should extend past the toes but allow visualization of the tips of the digits.

the toes to the proximal aspect of the leg or thigh. Flexible Scotchrap (3M Healthcare Products, St. Paul, MN) cast material can also be used; in fact, Scotchrap is easier to apply and remove than the plaster. Soaking or cast cutters are not necessary with the flexible material.

Casting should completely reverse the direction of the existing deformity. One can simply reduce the position of the foot and the tendons and ligaments that maintain the deformity by stretching out those tightened components. With the foot up and out, the peroneus brevis and lateral ankle ligaments are tight. In addition, the dorsiflexed position is maintained by the tightened anterior tibial tendon and the anterior ankle ligaments. One begins by stretching out the anterior ankle by plantar-flexing the foot at the ankle. The tight peroneus brevis is further lengthened by inverting the calcaneus and adducting the forefoot. The tibialis anterior is stretched by plantar flexion of the ankle, but by additionally plantar-flexing the first ray, the tibialis anterior tendon is isolated, and an even greater increase in length is attained. The cast is molded to maintain these positions. The soft tissue and osseous structures adapt to the new position over a 4- to 12-week period of casting.

The cast should be changed weekly until the foot is brought into the desired position. It is recommended that the cast be held in position an extra week to achieve slight overcorrection because the foot has a tendency to draw back in the direction of its original position. After the foot has gained its correct position, a cast is applied to the foot alone in a gently dorsiflexed attitude on the leg. Giannestras believes that prolonged casting in a plantar-flexed position induces an equinus. If the foot is maintained in this position of correction, the heel cord is stretched out and the pronatory effects of equinus are prevented.[7] If the foot does not present with equinus after the cast has been applied, additional casting of the foot alone in dorsiflexion is not indicated.

To remove the cast, the parents should soak the plaster by allowing the infant to sit in warm water for about 30 minutes. One ounce of vinegar added to the water aids

in softening the plaster. The parents then unravel the plaster without using any sharp instruments to avoid injury to the infant. If Scotchrap is used, the unravelling can be performed during office hours. Cast removal and application should be performed weekly (Figs. 21-12 and 21-13).

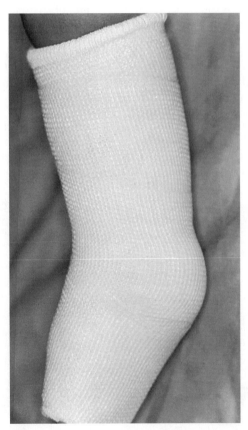

Figure 21-13. Scotchrap flexible cast material in place on a calcaneovalgus foot. Because this material is not as rigid or as moldable as plaster, it should be used in infants who do not have a severe deformity.

AFTER CAST MAINTENANCE

Ganley Splint

Now that the deformity is reduced, the entire foot-leg relationship must be maintained in a corrected position. The Ganley splint (J. Ganley, Norristown, PA) is used to reduce tibial torsion, talipes equinovarus, metadductus, and calcaneovalgus. In the correction of calcaneovalgus the Ganley splint is the device that achieves the desired position most accurately. Although the splint can be easily affixed to the shoe by the practitioner, I have found that either a shoemaker or orthotist can do an excellent job of securing the splint to the shoe by using cinching nails. The splint is a maintenance device that is applied directly to the child's leather soled Oxford shoe; it consists of a transverse torsion bar connected to plates placed on the bottom of the shoe. The forefoot plate is attached to the rearfoot plate by a shank bar that allows rotation on the frontal plane, thereby creating a rearfoot varus or valgus and also allows transverse plane maintenance through the longitudinal axis of the foot. The torsion bar allows transverse plane maintenance as well but also influences the entire foot-leg relationship. Adjustments are made by rotating and applying torque to the shanks and bars.

The plate of the shoe as well as the medial and lateral vamps are cut along the transverse plane of the shoe to allow motion of the forefoot against the rearfoot. The torsion bar is set to a length equal to that of the anterior superior iliac spine, which in a young child is usually between 6 and 8 inches. For correction of calcaneovalgus the torsion bar is bent to create an internal or medial rotation of the foot to the long axis of the body. External tibial torsion usually occurs secondary to calcaneovalgus because the foot is cranked on the transverse plane in an up-and-out direction. It should be understood that an external rotatory force is being exerted on the foot. If the force is significant, it can be translated through the ankle and into the leg. The result is an extremely torqued tibia.

When the torsional bar is set internally, an internal alignment is maintained rather than an external rotatory force through the foot. With the use of bending irons the shank bar is also bent inward, adducting the forefoot on the rearfoot. At the same time, the rear heel plate is inverted to maintain the subtalar joint in a neutral position. Because of the inverted or varus position of the rearfoot to the forefoot, a plantar flexion of the first ray on the rearfoot has been created.

In the initial application of the splint, it is a good idea to gradually exert torque on the bars and shanks rather than applying maximum correction. The foot should not be cranked any farther than the point of first resistance; the shoe will become uncomfortable, and the child will not want to wear the device. The device is intended to be used during sleep only and is not intended for wear during walking or sitting during the day (Fig. 21–14).

Unibar

The Unibar (Spectra Industries Corp., Yeadon, PA), a universal joint placed on the shoe-mounting plate, allows internal and external rotation as well as inversion and eversion of the rearfoot. When used for correction of a calcaneovalgus deformity, the Unibar maintains position in the transverse plane by internally positioning the universal joint. The rearfoot is set at 10 degrees of inversion, and the plate is internally rotated 10 degrees. In correction of metatarsus adductus, the foot is abducted approximately 25 degrees, and the rearfoot is maintained in inversion approximately 10 degrees. One should be aware that the Unibar does not address the foot deformity of calcaneovalgus or metatarsus adductus; its purpose is to maintain the internal or external attitudes that are secondarily present with those two diagnoses. The Unibar maintains the correction obtained by casts. An inflared or standard shoe can be used with this device to maintain the foot position. The bar prevents the infant from rotating the foot outward during sleep and nap time. Discouraging the outward migration of the foot enhances the possibility of full reduction of the deformity.

Fillauer Bar and Denis Browne Bar

The Fillauer Bar (Durr-Flower Medical Inc., Orthopedic Division, Chattanooga, TN) and the Denis Browne

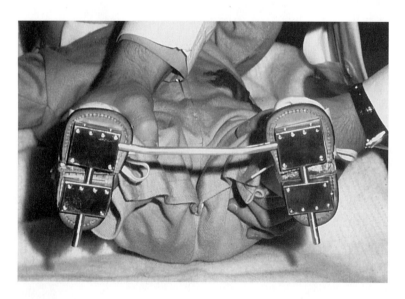

Figure 21–14. The Ganley splint set for the reduction of a calcaneovalgus foot. The transverse leg bar is positioned mildly internal (10 degrees), and the longitudinal foot plate bar is adducted to the required amount of correction. The rearfoot plate is inverted (10 degrees), and the shoe is split in the center of the sole.

Bar (Durr-Flower Medical) also maintain the transverse plane position of the foot in relation to the axial segment. They do not address the foot deformities of metatarsus adductus or calcaneovalgus directly but maintain an external attitude in dealing with tibial torsion. Care must be taken with the use of any of these splints and devices; if the child has an internal hip deformity, it will only become worse with the use of these splints and bars. Children sitting in a reverse tailor position experience an internal rotation at the hip while the leg is maintained externally. Therefore, these splints should be used only at night or whenever the child is sleeping. They are not intended to correct any of these deformities but only to maintain the present position or prevent increasing the present malposition.

Counter Rotational System

The Counter Rotational System (CRS) (Langer Laboratories, Deer Park, NY) is a dynamic orthosis that can replace the use of the rigid Fillauer or Denis Browne Bar. This system is a flexible parallelogram that allows rotation on the transverse plane and motion and freedom in the leg, hip, and knee. At the same time, it maintains the foot in an internal or external position depending on the diagnosis. In patients with calcaneovalgus, the foot plate should be set at approximately 10 degrees internal; with metatarsus adductus, it should be placed at approximately 25 to 35 degrees external. The CRS has a diagonally split sole plate that allows forefoot frontal plane motion. By splitting the sole of the shoe along the same axis, the first ray can be plantar-flexed. The CRS thus acts in the same way as the Ganley splint with regard to frontal plane motion, but it has no effect on transverse plane motion. This device allows more dynamic motion and stimulates normal muscle development by allowing movement during both night and day; the child can wear the splint for a greater amount of time compared to the conventional rigid devices. Although this device allows more mobility, it is recommended that the child wear a shoe without the system at first, and then when the child is asleep, the system can be placed on the shoe. Thus, the child can get used to the positional changes gradually.

Bebax

The innovative Bebax device (Inter Axial France, Sallanches, France) provides triplaner control in the foot. A double universal joint, one on the rearfoot segment and the other on the forefoot, controls the position of the foot. The two segments are held together by a longitudinal bar. Calcaneovalgus can be obtained by inverting the rearfoot and adducting and everting the forefoot. Translation of the forefoot on the rearfoot can be attained by lowering the distal plate at both universal joints. Bebax provides excellent control after immobilization for this type of deformity. The shoe is available in various infant sizes.

THE AMBULATING CHILD

Orthotics

A Roberts plate, calcaneal brace, or rigid molded acrylic orthosis that stabilizes the rearfoot is mandatory for treatment of the child with calcaneovalgus with or without prior casting. The orthosis should be used as early as possible; control can be gained with an orthotic device as early as 24 months. The orthosis is placed directly into a running sneaker and is replaced when the child's foot grows approximately two shoe sizes.

Ideally, an orthotic device such as the Roberts plate stabilizes the rearfoot by placing it in varus; inverting the rearfoot locks the midtarsal joint and the subtalar joint. One side extends laterally but stops at the cuboid and fifth metatarsal base to secure the lateral side of the foot and at the same time stabilize the rearfoot in its slightly inverted 5-degree position. This position is maintained by a 5-degree inverted post (versus a 5-degree inverted heel seat). The lateral flange limits calcaneal abduction on the transverse plane. A medial flange extends up to the first metatarsal neck and prevents midtarsal and subtalar joint breakdown. The stabilizing effect depends on the severity of the deformity and the amount of equinus present.

Actually, a standard orthotic device offers a negligible amount of stability because the heel seat is too low to control a child's fat-covered calcaneus. It is necessary to use a deep-seated heel cup with the addition of a Plastizote (BXL Plastics Ltd., Croydon, UK) or PPT (Langer Laboratories, Deer Park, NY) flange to extend the depth of the heel seat and protect it from irritation on the medial talar bulge. By approximately 7 or 8 years of age, the child cannot tolerate this very deep flanged orthosis and requires an orthosis without the lateral flange. The younger child can tolerate the flange extending as far distally as the fifth metatarsal head because of the extra fat present in the early years. With the older child it is necessary to decrease the depth of the heel seat, but one should maintain enough depth to control the calcaneus in an inverted position. This device, discussed next, dynamically stabilizes the rearfoot and the forefoot.

DSIS

The design concept of the DSIS (Dynamic Stabilizing Innersole System; Langer Laboratories, Deer Park, NY) incorporates a deep offset heel seat that cups the calcaneus and maintains it in the correct alignment (approximately 5 degrees of varus) relative to the ground. It is well recognized that the position of the heel has an extended controlling capacity on the midfoot-midtarsal joint region and the longitudinal arch. The calcaneus and the midfoot are also controlled through two flanges that continue along the sides of the foot to the level of the first and fifth metatarsal necks. Normal pronation and resupination occur with restriction on excessive transverse and sagittal plane motion.

The lateral and medial flanges of the device extend to the neck of metatarsals 1 and 5, and their function is based on the mechanics of the foot—the calcaneus and

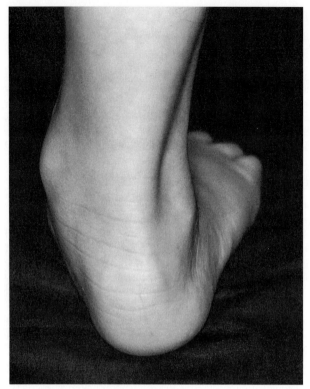

Figure 21–15. Marked transverse plane motion as noted by the abduction of the lateral column with depression of the medial longitudinal arch and an appearance of heel valgus.

cuboid and the entire forefoot abduct with pronation and the talus adducts. The medial and lateral flanges are split to allow the medial and lateral columns of the foot to function independently in the transverse plane. A stiff lateral counter extending to the neck of the fifth metatarsal prevents lateral shifting, while adduction of the talus is maintained by the medial flange and the off-set varus heel. This provides complete stabilization in the transverse plane, which cannot be accomplished with standard orthotic devices.

Flattening of the arch in all three planes is also addressed by the DSIS. (Fig. 21–15). The sagittal and frontal planes are controlled by the inverted position of the heel as well as a rise on the medial side of the device corresponding to the arch and extending to the first metatarsal neck. The deep heel seat, which is offset to maintain the calcaneus in an inverted position, allows normal pronation to occur. All other orthotic devices, in an attempt to invert the heel, approach the foot from the plantar aspect of the insert itself or from the shoe. The DSIS

design concept of offsetting the calcaneus within the interior of the cup, on the other hand, provides direct contact control. It is essential to control all aspects of foot contact with the ground. During walking, the heel is placed in an inverted position at heel strike so that the foot is controlled from the point of contact. As the walking cycle continues and the foot contacts the ground, weight is transferred from the heel to the midfoot and finally to the forefoot, resulting in propulsion. The DSIS thus addresses the position of the calcaneus, the talus, the midfoot, and the arch.[13–22]

References

1. Wynne-Davies R: Clubfoot deformities in children. J Bone Joint Surg 1964;46B:445.
2. Clarren SK, Smith DW: Congenital deformities. Pediat Clin North Am 1977;24:665–677.
3. Browne D: Congenital deformities of mechanical origin. Proc R Soc Med 1936;29:1409–1431.
4. Jay RM: Don't worry, your child will outgrow it (editorial). J Foot Surg 1990;29:412.
5. Wolff J: Das Gesetz der Transformation der Knochen. Berlin, Hirschwald, 1892.
6. McGlamry ED: Comprehensive Textbook of Foot Surgery. Baltimore, Williams & Wilkins, 1987, p. 381.
7. Giannestras NI: Foot Disorders, Philadelphia, Lea & Febiger, 1973, pp. 108–120.
8. Jay RM: Orthoses for cerebral palsy patients. J Curr Podiatr Med 1989;38:26–27.
9. Ganley J: The treatment of calcaneovalgus. J Am Podiatr Med Assoc 1975;65:405–421.
10. Viladot A, Lorenzo JC: The subtalar joint: Embryology and morphology. Foot Ankle 1984;5:54–66.
11. Schmidt HM: Shape and fixation of band systems in the human sinus and canalis tarsi. Acta Anat 1978;102:184.
12. Subotnick SI: The subtalar lateral extra-articular arthroeresis. J Am Podiatr Assoc 1974;64:701–711.
13. Otman S: Energy cost of walking with flatfeet. Prosthet Orthot Int 1988;73–76.
14. Wickstrom J: Shoe corrections and orthopedic foot supports. Clin Orthop 1970;70:30.
15. Cowell H: Shoes and shoe corrections. Pediatr Clin North Am 1977;24:791.
16. Gould N: The development of the toddler arch. Foot Ankle 1989;9:241.
17. Gould N: Shoes versus sneakers in toddlers. Foot Ankle 1985;6:105.
18. Menkveld SR: Analysis of gait patterns in normal school-aged children. J Pediatr Orthop 1988;8:263–267.
19. Doxey GE: Clinical use and fabrication of molded thermoplastic foot orthotic devices. Phys Ther 1985;1679–1682.
20. Smith LS: The effects of soft and semi-rigid orthoses upon rearfoot movement in running. J Am Podiatr Med Assoc 1986;76:227–233.
21. Minns RJ: A study of foot shape, underfoot pressure patterns, lower limb rotations and gait of children. Chiropodist 1986;89–99.
22. Johnson GR: The effectiveness of shock-absorbing insoles during normal walking. Prosthet Orthot Int 1988;12:91–95.

22

Subtalar Extra-articular Arthrodesis

Richard M. Jay, D.P.M.

The original extra-articular arthrodesis procedure was used to fuse the subtalar joint in the area of the sinus tarsi to create a stable position for the foot.[1] By performing the fusion extra-articularly in the canal, growth of the foot is allowed to continue. Basically, the procedure avoids delay in treatment and thus avoids the need for a triple arthrodesis in which large segments of bone are resected to realign the progressively deformed foot. Arthritic changes will develop in the adjacent joints with a triple arthrodesis; however, with the Grice procedure the calcaneocuboid and the talonavicular joints are not fused. If degenerative joint changes progress to adjacent joints, a fusion can always be performed when the child is older. Extra-articular arthrodesis is indicated for the child with the valgus foot type, which includes paralytic calcaneovalgus, nonparalytic calcaneovalgus, congenital vertical talus, coalitions, and severe flatfoot as seen in children with cerebral palsy.

PROCEDURE

Complete evacuation of the sinus tarsi is performed, using an approach similar to that used for the extra-articular arthroereisis procedure. The inferior surface of the talus and the superior surface of the calcaneus are identified. With a side-cutting bur or a narrow blade on a sagittal saw, a trough is created on both the superior and inferior aspects of the canal. This trough will house the graft. The trough should not be too deep or the graft will impact too far and correction will be lost. Attention is then paid to the graft used for insertion. This graft should be modeled to fit snugly between the talus and the calcaneus within the trough. The foot is inverted at the rearfoot, thus opening the floors of the subtalar joint. The graft is inserted so that the joint maintains and resembles a neutral rearfoot position. A staple or two K-wires (6.2) inserted on both sides of the struts through the talus and calcaneus secure the fragment (Fig. 22–1). The child is placed in nonweight-bearing casts for at least 6 to 8 weeks. Dynamic Stabilizing Innersole System (DSIS) (Langer Laboratories, Deer Park, NY) or UCBL are dispensed with compressible posts to absorb shock.

COMPLICATIONS

Overcorrection

The most common complication of the procedure is inadvertent overcorrection of the valgus rearfoot, creating a supinated rearfoot in a varus position.[2, 3] The graft struts are placed in the sinus tarsi and wedged between the talus and calcaneus. The struts are cut to a length equal to the height of the canal when the foot is held in a neutral position, not supinated. When an oversized graft is used, an increase in talar height occurs, reducing the

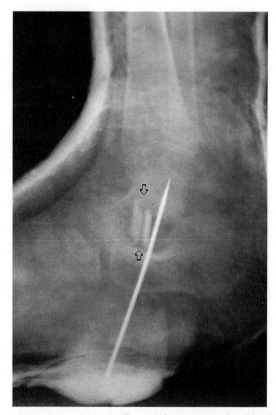

Figure 22–1. Two corticocancellous grafts (arrows) placed within a trough in the sinus tarsi. Two K-wires stabilize the grafts and keep them from twisting out of the trough.

179

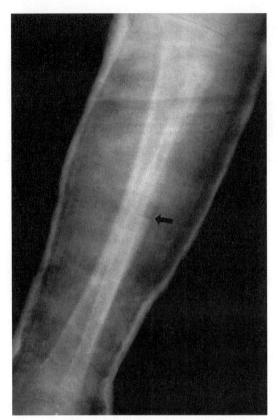

Figure 22–2. Graft from proximal tibia *(arrow),* showing potential weakening of the shaft that may lead to fracture.

talocalcaneal angle too much and creating a supinated subtalar joint. The result is a varus rearfoot. The operation has eliminated the subtalar motion but has increased lateral ankle instability. The creation of chronic ankle instability with its continual sprains tends to lead to further osseous changes in the ankle joint and the adjacent joints.

Canal Complications

Additional complications include failure of the arthrodesis with loss of position and resorption of the graft. Sometimes the strut placed in the sinus tarsi partially fuses with either the superior surface of the calcaneous or the inferior surface of the talus. This type of partial fusion creates an arthritic condition because the nonunited border forms a pseudarthrosis.

When the graft is resorbed, the original collapsed talar position will recur. The graft should fuse the superior calcaneal sulcus to the inferior talar sulcus in a neutral position. Anything less than this position produces an unacceptable result. The fused foot should assume this neutral attitude if motion is to be sacrificed.

Grafts

The donor graft site is also subject to possible complications. Care must be taken when selecting the donor site. The distal fibular graft has a high rate of graft failure.[4] Lancaster and Pohl, however, state that the fibula

provides good healing potential and that the tibia is too weak.[5] The lateral support column is disrupted by resection of the distal fibular graft, creating the conditions for the possible complication of ankle valgus. Considering that with these severely pronated valgus and paralytic feet an ankle valgus is usually present anyway, use of the fibular graft will only increase this deformity.

The proximal tibia provides good cortical and cancellous bone and can be harvested fairly easily. Drill holes used as safety points in the four corners of the graft site reduce the possibility of stress fractures. The recommendation for using an osteotome to make the cuts in the tibia is good; however, a slow power saw with flush using plenty of water provides a clean straight cut with no bone border necrosis (Figs. 22–2 and 22–3).

GRAFTS

Allografts may be used, and the difference between them and autogenous grafts may not be discernible in their healing properties. The graft must have the ability to support the opened talocalcaneal joint. The cortical bone part of the graft supplies the strength, and the cancellous portion allows vascular ingrowth with good osteogenesis. The graft must be placed perpendicular to the axis of Henle within the sinus tarsi. Proper placement of the graft locks the subtalar joint, and the graft becomes well seated in the canal and does not slip out. If the double-strutted corticocancellous graft is placed in an angular fashion the graft will collapse with loss of fusion, or fusion will occur with a return to the original valgus position. It is a good idea to use a Kirschner wire running

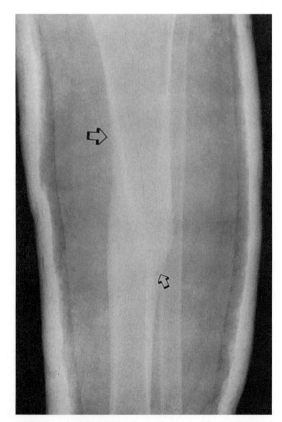

Figure 22–3. Fractured tibial graft site *(arrow)* with resultant malunion.

anterior to the graft to further protect against slipping and turning of the graft.[6–8] When placing the graft, it is preferable, no matter what type of graft is used, to be able to visualize the entire canal of the sinus tarsi.[9] It is important here to avoid entering the articular surfaces of the subtalar joints to reduce the risk of intra-articular arthritis and shortened bone growth. It must also be emphasized that a double strut of corticocancellous bone of substantial thickness be placed in the sinus tarsi; it should encompass a good percentage of the space. By this means, the shear force that is present will not splinter the bone as the grafted site matures, whereas if too thin a strut or graft is used, failure is imminent.

The best bone to use as a graft is the bone that (1) allows proper osseous alignment and (2) guarantees perfect osteogenesis with no risk of failure in union. Unfortunately, this type of bone does not come easily packaged. A great deal of thought must be given to selection of the proper graft material. Cancellous bone provides a greater amount of osteogenesis and cortical bone provides strength, but where do we get the bone? Autogenous bone is best, but where should it be harvested (hip, tibia, fibula, calcaneus, or bone from an adjacent surgical site)? The choice can also be allograft, freeze-dried banked bone. The alternatives for grafting all have intrinsic risks, and the selection truly depends on the choice of the family and the surgeon.

Both autogenous bone and allografts can provide the necessary elements of a good graft, which should maintain structural stability at the graft site and act as a bridge through which bone develops by creeping substitution, eventually completely replacing the bones. There is little or no difference in the host response to either of these bone grafts.

ARTHRODESIS-ARTHROEREISIS COMBINATION

Arthrodesis-arthroereisis in the child over 6 years old, also called the Grice arthroereisis, has been a mainstay in the child with flatfoot secondary to cerebral palsy. However, the Grice procedure should not be considered in patients under 6 years old. The results are unpredictable. A combination arthrodesis and arthroereisis—that is, a raising of the subtalar joint to allow upper function of the joint—can be recommended in the child under 6 years of age. This procedure is performed in children who have a severe valgus deformity located in the subtalar joint that can be manually reduced into a neutral position in which the talar sits high on the calcaneus. This qualification can be determined by taking a weight-bearing lateral view of the foot while supinating the foot by externally rotating the limb.

The procedure for raising the subtalar joint is performed by releasing the talus at its articulation with the calcaneus. The calcaneus is then repositioned inferiorly. This allows the talus to role up on the calcaneus and decreases the plantar deformity in the sagittal plane. The talus assumes a greater dorsiflexed position in relation to the forepart of the foot. At the same time, a tendo Achillis lengthening is necessary because there is tightness in the posterior group that causes the calcaneus to plantar-flex as well. Once the talus is in this accepted position, a staple is placed across the subtalar joint entering from the lateral aspect of the foot. This staple is placed in the inferior third of the talus and the superior third of the calcaneus. The staples should be parallel to the tibia and perpendicular to the weight-bearing surface. The child is then placed in a below-the-knee cast and maintained in this position for approximately 6 weeks. The subtalar joint should not be placed in a maximum varus attitude because too much pressure during weight bearing will be created on the lateral surface of the subtalar joint and ankle. The subtalar joint should be placed in a mild valgus attitude. In this position, more pressure is exerted medially, allowing the foot at heel strike and midstance to gently pronate out of the midtarsal joints rather than the subtalar joints. This pronation allows equal distribution of weight on the plantar aspect of the foot and diminishes the amount of shock exerted on the subtalar joint. When the Achilles tendon is lengthened, a greater amount of dorsiflexion out of the ankle joint is present, thus decreasing the demand for subtalar joint pronation and midtarsal joint pronation. The risk of developing a rocker-bottom foot is minimized.

With the subtalar joint held in this neutral position, the tendons on the medial and lateral aspect of the ankle joint can now support the foot and allow a normal gait. If there are additional spasticities in the surrounding musculature, tendon transfers and lengthenings can be performed. Because the subtalar joint is in this neutral position, normal ontogeny can occur within the talus. The entire medial column can go through its normal valgus rotation, allowing the first ray to be stabilized on the supporting surface of the ground with the aid of the stable cuboid to allow passage of the peroneus longus tendon.

The staple can be removed once normal muscle function and normal bone growth have occurred in sufficient volume to support this. If weakness secondary to cerebral palsy is present, the staple may remain.[10]

References

1. Grice D: The role of subtalar fusion in the treatment of valgus deformities of the feet. Instr Course Lect 1959;16:127–150.
2. Bacardi BE: Complications of the Grice-Green operation. J Foot Surg 1989;28:325–332.
3. Moreland JR, Westin GW: Further experience with Grice subtalar arthrodesis. Clin Orthop 1986;207:113–121.
4. McCall RE, Lllich JS, Harris JR, Johnston FA: The Grice extraarticular subtalar arthrodesis: A clinical review. J Pediatr Orthop 1985;5:442–445.
5. Lancaster SJ, Pohl RO: Green-Grice extraarticular subtalar arthrodesis: Results using a fibular graft. J Pediatr Orthop 1987;7:29–33.
6. Russotti GM, Cass JR, Johnson KA: Isolated talocalcaneal arthrodesis. A technique using moldable bone graft. J Bone Joint Surg 1988;70A:1472–1478.
7. Mallon WJ, Nunley JA: The Grice procedure: Extra-articular subtalar arthrodesis. Orthop Clin North Am 1989;20:649–654.
8. Scott SM, Janes PC, Stevens PM: Grice subtalar arthrodesis followed to skeletal maturity. J Pediatr Orthop 1988;8:176–183.
9. Hsu LCS, Jaffray D, Leong JCY: The Batchelor-Grice extra-articular subtalar arthrodesis. J Bone Joint Surg 1986;68B:503–510.
10. Crawford AH: Subtalar stabilization of the planovalgus foot by staple arthroereisis in young children who have neuromuscular problems. J Bone Joint Surg 1990;72A:840–845.

23

Arthroereisis-Subtalar

Richard M. Jay, D.P.M.

An arthroereisis procedure is defined as an operative limitation of the motion in a joint that is abnormally mobile due to paralysis.[1] The term arthroereisis has been commonly used to identify procedures that have some form of blockage or impingement in the sinus tarsi to restrict abnormal pronatory components of a flexible flatfoot.

The arthroereisis limits subtalar motion by the insertion of a Silastic or polyethylene plug. The process of fusing the subtalar joint, as in the Grice procedure, creates an arthrodesis of the joints and eliminates motion. The Grice procedure is indicated in patients with a calcaneovalgus flatfoot with a forefoot supinatus deformity. The sagittal plane deformity is reduced by elevating the talus on the calcaneus and limiting the end-range pronatory motion of the subtalar joint. By realigning the subtalar joint to neutral and increasing the range of dorsiflexion of the ankle joint, the peroneus longus can function under a stable cuboid. Plantar flexion of the first ray occurs and reduces the supinatus. Usually present with this deformity is a primary or secondary gastrocnemius equinus deformity that may be addressed when the arthroereisis of the subtalar joint is performed (see description of procedure later under Adjunct Procedures: Tendo Achilles-Gastrocnemius Lengthening).

The procedure involves the insertion of a Silastic or polyethylene plug into the lateral sinus tarsi (Fig. 23–1). Various techniques of insertion and types of plugs have

been described (e.g., STA-Peg, high-density silicone, Richard's Buck plug, MBA).[2–19]

PROCEDURES

In the pathologic flatfoot excessive pronation occurs at the subtalar joint. This abnormal motion sets off a series of multiple pathologic motions including eversion of the calcaneus beyond the perpendicular, shifting of the talonavicular and calcaneocuboid joints to a more perpendicular alignment, and unlocking and pronation of the midtarsal joint. The dominant plane of the deformity is determined by the planar alignments of the axes of the subtalar and midtarsal joints. A more vertical alignment of the axes produces more transverse plane motion, whereas a more horizontal alignment produces more frontal plane motion.[20] Arthroereisis procedures in general attempt to limit this excessive subtalar joint pronation through a variety of mechanisms. Often these procedures may only affect specifically one plane of subtalar joint motion; however, as Root and Orien note, correction of one plane of subtalar motion produces correction in all three planes.[21] Three basic categories based on their mechanism of action are classified as follows:

1. Self-locking wedges (Viladot, Valenti, Addante, Buck plug, Valgus stop procedure, MBA). These devices

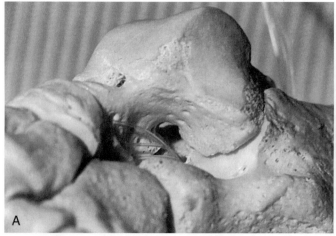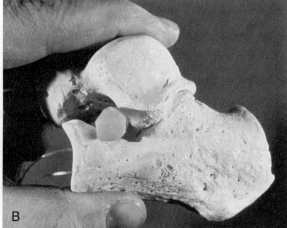

Figure 23–1. *A*, Entrance of sinus tarsi from the lateral aspect of the foot. The canal follows from anterior-lateral to posterior-medial. *B*, Example of Silastic plug in the sinus tarsi elevating the talus on the calcaneus. As the talus rises, it also adducts, reducing the talocalcaneal angle.

decrease the pronatory range of motion of the subtalar joint to neutral or varus by preventing the lateral process of the talus from contacting the sinus tarsi floor.

2. Axis-altering devices (STA-Peg). Through their insertion into the calcaneus, these devices in effect create an artificial higher middle calcaneal facet, thereby raising the axis of the subtalar joint. This in turn decreases frontal plane eversion of the talus, thus resulting in triplanar correction.

3. Direct impact of subtalar joint motion (Sgarlato, Pisani).

INDICATIONS

The subtalar arthroereisis with Silastic or polyethylene implants should be reserved for flexible flat feet. The procedure is indicated for the uncontrolled, reducible rearfoot valgus foot that has a calcaneal stance position of greater than 7 degrees everted (Table 23–1). Arthroereisis may be performed alone or in conjunction with other flatfoot procedures. There are numerous short-term retrospective studies on the arthroereisis procedure with its potential complications of inversion sprains and implant extrusion. It is incumbent on the surgeon to clearly inform the patient of the additional risks in the use of any of these implants.[22, 23]

The surgery should be reserved for flexible flat feet in which there is abduction of 35 degrees and not less than 20 degrees of adduction. This surgery should not be performed when the patient has only a few degrees of abduction motion or when there is not enough flexibility of the forefoot to allow the plantar surface to make full contact with the ground after the abnormal range of abduction has been reduced.

Arthroereisis candidates have a flexible triplane deformity in which the prominent feature is a rearfoot valgus. A rigid flatfoot deformity is also a contraindication due to the fact that there may be a coalition within the tarsus.

I do not recommend arthroereisis alone when a forefoot varus is present. Such a procedure may produce a partially compensated forefoot varus and result in a coxa vara-genu valgum deformity.

Table 23–1. **Indications for Subtalar Arthroereisis: Ages 2–4 Years to Early Adolescence**

Uncontrolled but reducible rearfoot valgus
Flexible forefoot varus
Metatarsus adductus with rearfoot valgus
Calcaneovalgus deformity
Congenital vertical talus
Tibialis posterior weakness or faulty insertion
Neuromuscular disease
Ligamentous laxity
Radiographic considerations including:
  Kite's angle greater than 30 degrees
  Subluxed talonavicular joint, less than 50% articulation on a
    dorsoplantar view
  Talar declination angle greater than 40 degrees
  Midtarsal joint collapse with talonavicular joint fault
  Low calcaneal inclination angle

The implant does not allow hyperpronation in the foot during the midstance and propulsion phases. In the hyperpronated foot during the midstance and propulsion phases, the foot pronates past the neutral position into pronation; this unlocks the forefoot from the plane of the rearfoot and thus produces an apropulsive gait.

SURGICAL TECHNIQUE

General

Exposure of the sinus tarsi is achieved through a 3- to 4-cm lateral incision following Langer's skin lines. Dissection is carried down to the extensor digitorum brevis (EDB) muscle, which is identified from its origin; if necessary to gain access to the superior surface of the calcaneus, the proximal fibers of the EDB are retracted. Care is taken during the dissection to avoid incising the sural nerve, which usually runs just below the incision site. Most authors then incise the talocalcaneal ligament. Hoch's tonsil (fat pad in the sinus tarsi) is also removed by many authors. A self-retaining retractor or large flat probe is then inserted into the sinus tarsi to separate the articular facets of the subtalar joint (STJ) in a supinatory manner. For most procedures not involving implantation of a device into the calcaneus itself, an appropriately sized homogeneous or polyethylene implant is then firmly seated into the sinus tarsi region. For procedures involving the Smith STA-Peg, MBA, and Viladot staple implants, the involved devices are implanted into the calcaneus according to the procedures described later in this chapter. Closure of the surgical site, including reattachment of the EDB muscle, then progresses in a retrograde fashion using appropriately sized sutures (usually absorbables sutures are preferred). Steri-Strips and an appropriate sterile dressing are then applied. A Jones compression dressing may also be used to minimize postoperative edema. In most patients a plaster cast is not applied unless adjunct procedures are performed. A gradual return to full weight bearing over a period of several weeks aids in the prevention of postoperative complications. With procedures involving implantation of a bone graft wedge into the calcaneus, weight bearing is based on radiologic evidence of osteogenic healing. Range of motion (ROM) exercise is implemented. Both active and passive ROM exercises are performed for the direction of adduction, not abduction.

LeLievre's Procedure

In patients aged 3 to 6 years a Blount staple is used in LeLievre's procedure. The outer talar and calcaneal articular surfaces are separated, and a Blount staple is inserted to maintain the corrected position. The staple is removed 2 years later, and the articular surfaces are reapproximated. In adults the correction is obtained by driving an unfixed bone graft into the sinus tarsi, performing a tendoachilles lengthening, and tightening the tibialis anterior and tibialis posterior tendons.

Exposure of the sinus tarsi is gained through a lateral

skin incision. The talocalcaneal ligament is resected, and the talus is aligned on the calcaneus. A pyramidal or cone-shaped bone graft of fresh homograft or allograft is driven into the medial portion of the sinus tarsi with its base facing laterally. The graft should be seated firmly; otherwise a Blount staple is used to stabilize the graft. The upper arm of the staple is driven into the lateral part of the talar neck, and the lower arm is driven into the calcaneus. The staple is removed 4 months later.

Lanham's Procedure

In patients aged 2 to 5 years the cut stem from a Swanson size 2 great toe prosthesis is used; for patients aged 6 to 11 a stem cut from a Swanson size 3 great toe implant is used. The interosseus ligament is palpated and completely severed. The cone-shaped stem is inserted with the apex pointed plantarly and medially into the sinus tarsi from a dorsolateral oblique approach. The capsule is closed, and the remaining soft tissue and skin are closed last.

Addante's Procedure

The implant is sized using a measurement of the diameter of the sinus tarsi as seen on a radiograph, usually a medial oblique view. Sphere implant sizes range from 12.5 to 17.0 mm. The sinus tarsi is exposed and burred using a drill slightly smaller than the diameter of the selected sphere. The sphere is then forcibly inserted.

STA-Peg Arthroereisis

Surgical Procedure. The anterior leading edge of the calcaneal facet is exposed and squared off. The flat surface of the drill guide is placed flush against the remodeled edge, and a drill hole is made. Plugs are color-coded for easy determination of size. The plug is then inserted with cement. Once the cement has dried, the area is irrigated. The extensor digitorum brevis is relocated and the wound is closed. No casting or immobilization is needed.

Mechanics and Philosophy. The STA-Peg procedure is used to eliminate abnormal pronation, to correct heel valgus, and to produce an increase in the medial arch. It does this by limiting the anterior motion of the talus and stopping the triplane motion of pronation, creating a stable fulcrum for the peroneus longus muscle. The operation produces a force vector that enables the peroneus longus muscle to plantar-flex the medial pillar of the foot to the weight-bearing surface, thus increasing arch height and reducing forefoot varus. It also allows secondary bony and soft tissue adaptation, which becomes permanent at maturity, creating a foot capable of normal function.

Valente's Procedure

A sizer, an instrument with a series of graduated cylinders on the shaft, is inserted into the sinus tarsi with mild-moderate pressure using a twisting motion. The sizer is passed through the foot until the desired restriction of eversion is obtained. The numbered cylinder on the sizer is noted, and the corresponding size implant is obtained. The proper implant is then locked onto the inserting tool, which screws the implant into the sinus tarsi in the interosseous ligaments. The implant should be large enough to restrict eversion to the degree desired but not so large that the capsule of the sinus tarsi and the deep fascia cannot close.

Viladot's Procedure

A lateral incision identical to that described earlier under general technique is made. A 3- to 4-cm incision 1 cm anteromedial to the medial malleolus is added to allow a medial capsulorraphy. Insertion of the cup-like orthosis occurs through the latter incision.

Subotnick's Procedure

In this procedure a wedge of bone is inserted into the floor of the sinus tarsi.

Chambers' Procedure

The tissue immediately in front of the sinus tarsi is cleared, but the fibers of the interosseous ligament are not disturbed. The foot is then placed in neutral position, and an estimate is made of the area of posterior calcaneal facet that remains uncovered by the talus. The primary bone flap is made from the area of the uncovered facet plus about ¼ to ⅜ inch of the floor of the sinus tarsi. The cut is made while the foot is held in adduction. The bone flap is raised and held in the appropriate position permanently by placing a bone graft wedge underneath the flap. The source of the bone chip or wedge can be the tibia or the calcaneus; I prefer to use bone from the calcaneus. A secondary reinforcement flap is turned under the primary flap with additional chip grafts from the calcaneus and lightly impacted with a broad nail punch. The foot is then taken through a range of motion between abduction and adduction. The bone block should not be too large or it will interfere with adduction motion. Excess abduction should be reduced, not lost entirely.

ADJUNCT PROCEDURES

Tendo Achillis-Gastrocnemius Lengthening

The pathologic flatfoot is made worse by equinus, which prevents normal dorsiflexion. As the talus assumes a more vertical and medial position, the calcaneus is forced to rotate posterolaterally from its position under the talus. The sustentaculum tali loses its supporting position beneath the neck of the talus as the calcaneus subluxates laterally. Because the hind part of the foot cannot be dorsiflexed, dorsiflexion occurs at the midfoot. A breach of the midpart of the foot (a rocker-bottom foot) may result, with the hind part of the foot in valgus angulation and the fore part in abduction.

Determination of ankle joint dorsiflexion range of motion is performed with the patient in the supine or prone position. If dorsiflexion is less than 10 degrees beyond the perpendicular, the muscles producing the equinus are identified by the Silverskiold test (knee straight versus flexed to 90 degrees; at 90 degrees the effect of the gastrocnemius is eliminated). When ankle dorsiflexion with the knee flexed is adequate, gastrocnemius lengthening alone is performed.

Young's Tenosuspension

This procedure is described as a rerouting of the tibialis anterior tendon through the navicular, which reinforces the medial tarsometatarsal and plantar naviculocuneiform ligaments. Ultimately, the goal is to increase the declination angle of the first ray.

Kidner's Procedure

The Kidner procedure involves resection of an accessory navicular bone, if present, together with a repositioning of the tibialis posterior tendon insertion plantarly. The purpose of the procedure is to increase the mechanical advantage of the tibialis posterior tendon in elevating the medial arch. The procedure is also effective in removing a prominent navicular.

Hoke's Procedure

This procedure plantar-flexes and fuses the medial column (navicular through first metatarsal), using a wedge-shaped corticocancellous graft implanted into the naviculocuneiform joint as well as a transfer of the tibialis posterior tendon distally.

Talar and Navicular Osteotomies

These procedures may be used to shorten an elongated medial column bone deformity or stabilize a hypermobile medial column. Such procedures aid in the realignment of normal articular congruity to stabilize the rearfoot and midfoot. Associated soft tissue procedures such as the Pisani desmoplasty are usually required to tighten and reposition stretched or weakened structures.

Calcaneal Osteotomies

These procedures may be indicated when the calcaneal inclination angle is significantly decreased or when sig-

nificant rearfoot valgus is present, beyond the amount that can be corrected through arthroereisis procedures alone. A tendo Achilles lengthening is often performed in conjunction with each of these procedures. Lindholm has classified these procedures and their general indications as follows:

Anterior

Evans Procedure. A bone graft wedge is inserted just posterior to the calcaneocuboid joint, creating significant forefoot abduction, which is favorable if a significant adductus component is present. This procedure helps to reposition the talus on top of the calcaneus and addresses the transverse component of pronation. In his original description, Evans[27] stated that this procedure may be indicated for a short lateral column.

Extra-articular Procedures

These procedures are rarely performed in conjunction with an arthroereisis procedure because their mechanisms of action are somewhat similar.

Chambers' Procedure. This was perhaps the first arthroereisis procedure. It involves use of a bone graft to elevate the floor of the sinus tarsi.

Baker-Hill Procedure. This procedure involves use of a bone graft inserted posterior to the posterior facet of the subtalar joint to induce a supinatory component.

Selkaovich's Procedure. This procedure is described as a wedge of bone placed posterior to the sustentaculum tali, creating an anteromedial advancement and effective elevation of the subtalar axis. Very few practitioners now use this procedure.

Posterior

Koutsogiannis Type. This procedure involves a through-and-through crescentic osteotomy of the calcaneus, posterior to the subtalar joint and peroneal tendons. The posterior aspect of the calcaneus is then shifted in a plantar-medial direction. No bone wedge is removed or added. Advantages of this procedure are an increased supinatory mechanical advantage of the Achilles tendon with a minimal loss of bone and retention of the subtalar joint range of motion.

Dwyer's Procedure. This procedure uses a closing wedge in the medial aspect of the calcaneus to introduce a varus component.

Silver's Procedure. This procedure also introduces a varus component into the calcaneus by an oblique insertion of a bone wedge laterally from just posterior to the posterior facet inferiorly to just proximal to the calcaneocuboid joint.

Gleich's Procedure. This procedure has been described as a plantar-oblique closing wedge with an ante-

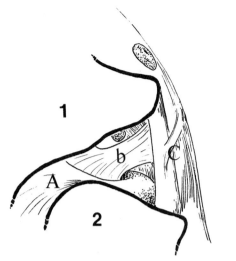

Figure 23–2. Ligaments of the sinus tarsi. (1) Talus, (2) calcaneus, (A) cervical, (B) interosseus, (C) peripheral.

rior advancement to introduce a varus attitude to the calcaneus.

Cuboid Osteotomies

These procedures generally involve the insertion of a wedge-shaped bone graft. They may be indicated for a plantar-flexed lateral column and used in conjunction with many other column extra-articular osteotomies. Results of such procedures are not always predictable.

Subtalar Arthrodesis

This type of procedure is often necessary when arthritic joint changes are present or when there is contin-

ued subluxation of the rearfoot and midfoot involving the subtalar and midtalar joints. Subtalar joint arthrodesis procedures are also used in cases of sectioning or rupture of the tibialis posterior tendon. Bony repositioning or additional joint fusions may be needed with these procedures. Repositioning procedures may include calcaneal displacement to correct elements of varus or valgus or equinus calcaneus in the deformity.

Soft Tissue Release

The cervical ligament, interosseous ligament, and calcaneocuboid ligaments may be released if excessive tightness is present.

COMPLICATIONS

Plug Extrusion

Arthroereisis is a means of limiting subtalar motion rather than eliminating motion via fusing as in the arthrodesis procedure. The indication is the hypermobile flatfoot with a forefoot supinatus deformity. This is a sagittal plane deformity that will be reduced by the elevation of the talus on the calcaneus, thus limiting the end-range pronatory motion of the subtalar joint. Usually present with this deformity is a primary or secondary gastrocnemius equinus deformity, which may have to be addressed at the time of arthroereisis of the subtalar joint. With the realignment of the subtalar joint to neutral and an increase in the range of dorsiflexion of the ankle joint, the peroneus longus can function under a stable cuboid. Plantar flexion of the first ray occurs, reducing the supinatus. The procedure is designed to allow the insertion of a Silastic or polyethylene plug into the lateral sinus tarsi. Various techniques have been described for the insertion and the type of plug used (STA-Peg, MBA, high-density silicone, and Richard's Buck plug). With all these variations of techniques and materials, the most common complication is extrusion of the plug.

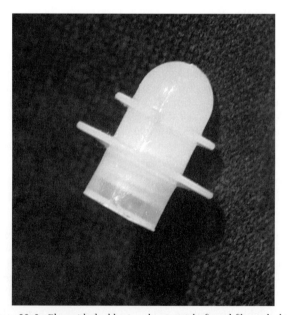

Figure 23–3. Plug with double ring showing tight fit and fibrous locking within the sinus tarsi.

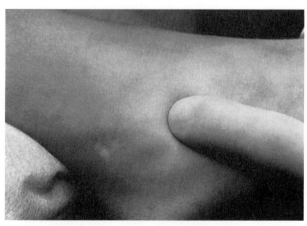

Figure 23–4. Palpation of the sinus tarsi.

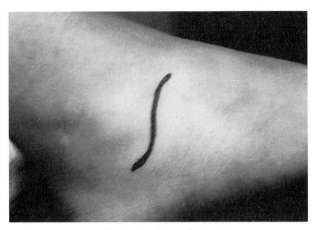

Figure 23–5. Curvilinear skin incision.

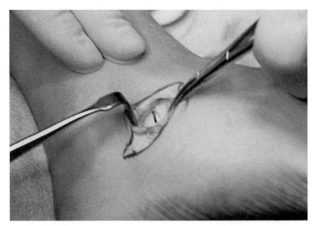

Figure 23–7. Peripheral ligaments can be separated to allow entrance of the implant and later closed to protect against extrusion.

Anatomy

The sinus tarsi anatomy must be understood to comprehend the reason for this complication. The canal is cone-shaped with the apex positioned medially; the internal ligaments guard against excessive inversion and eversion, thus stabilizing the subtalar joint. In the flexible flatfoot the interosseous ligament limits eversion and is not doing its job, allowing deforming forces to take their toll on the subtalar joint. The cervical ligament, whose purpose is to limit inversion of the subtalar joint, begins to become taut and further limits inversion[24] (Fig. 23–2). Some authors perform the procedure by severing the interosseous and cervical ligaments, but this destroys all the inherent stability we are trying to restore, and the subtalar joint is left unchecked. One can open the sinus tarsi floor with greater ease, however, by incompletely addressing the etiology of the flatfoot by allowing the talus and calcaneous to pronate on one another, since the interosseous ligament is no longer present to prevent eversion. The situation is further complicated by the cone-shaped canal. With no failsafe mechanism present to prevent excessive inversion of the subtalar joint, the plug can be forcibly squeezed out of the canal like a cherry pit between the fingers.

Buck Plug and MBA

By not cutting the ligaments and addressing the etiology of the excessive pronation, one can eliminate the possibility of plug extrusion. In addition, the risk of cutting the arterial supply to the talar neck, which is a reported complication, is also reduced. Because of concern about the continuing forces that can still force the plug out, other techniques to stabilize the plug have been suggested. The use of the Richard's Buck plug, devised by C. Mammas, limits the possibility of extrusion by the built-in design of the plug. The two rings of the plug are locked into the canal with fibrous union (Figs. 23–3 to 23–12). Another technique that limits the possibility of extrusion is to tie the implant through to the medial side as Viladot[25] has recommended. The procedure is sound in the young child but is not advised in the older mature child because irritation to the surrounding tissue can occur, creating a synovitis in the peripheral ligaments of

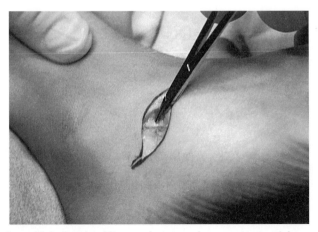

Figure 23–6. Peripheral ligament kept intact by separating it with hemostat in a longitudinal direction.

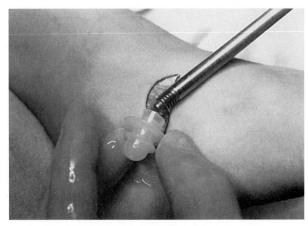

Figure 23–8. Plug being placed on impactor.

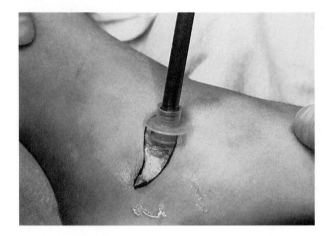

Figure 23–9. Approximation of implant through peripheral ligaments. The outer ring and total length usually need to be modified.

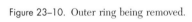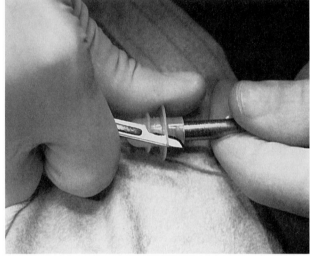

Figure 23–10. Outer ring being removed.

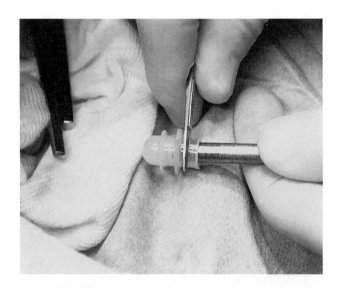

Figure 23–11. Length is reduced to avoid protrusion from sinus tarsi.

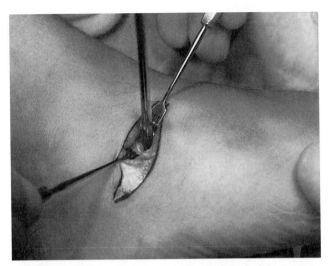

Figure 23–12. Plug enters the sinus tarsi with the aid of the impactor. Ligaments can be removed from the canal with the aid of a pituitary rongeur. This allows the implant to sit nicely in the sinus tarsi.

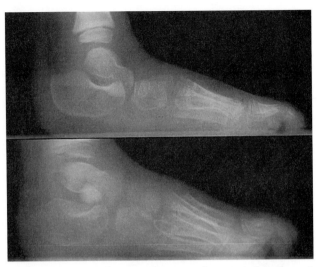

Figure 23–14. Six-month postoperative view of extra-articular arthroereisis. Note the reduction of the talar declination and of the forefoot component.

the sinus tarsi, which in turn warrants removal of the plug. The synovitis decreases immediately when the plug is removed and causes no permanent changes on the osseous surface (Figs. 23–13 to 23–16).

STA-Peg

Traumatic insults to the foot have been reported to cause complications with the STA-Peg. However, it is the shear factor from the talus on the calcaneus that is most significant. It is the translation of force from the body weight and the converted force of the internal torque during the gait cycle that makes the shear factor so significant. When an object such as a plug is placed in the sinus tarsi, it is under great compressive pressure, torque and shear. If this plug is secured in the roof of the calcaneus, as with the STA-Peg, the shear force on the

implant is high, and no motion is possible through which the implant can yield or adapt to the converted torque. The result is a weakening of the implant at the stem, leading to fracture of the stem. If the stem is not secured in the calcaneus, the implant is forced to glide out of its insertion and jams beneath the talus[26] (Fig. 23–17). To ensure the placement of the implant and to protect the foot against further pronatory changes, a functional orthosis is recommended. In young children after the sinus tarsi implant and adjunctive procedures are performed, a deep-seated orthosis is used to guarantee position. This is used for the first 3 to 6 months, and then the flanges are reduced.

Other Complications

In addition to complications associated with any surgical procedure (e.g., wound dehiscence, infection, etc.),

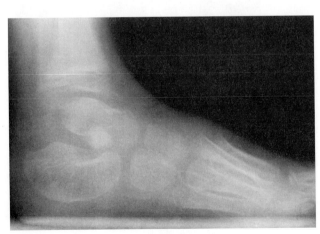

Figure 23–13. Sinus tarsi plug inserted with reduction of talar declination.

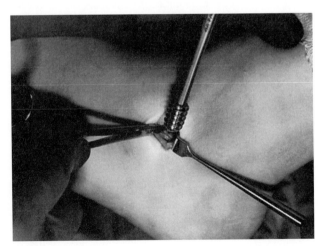

Figure 23–15. MBA plug on driver ready to be implanted into the sinus tarsi.

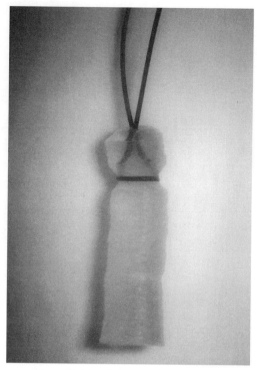

Figure 23–16. Viladot-type Silastic implant.

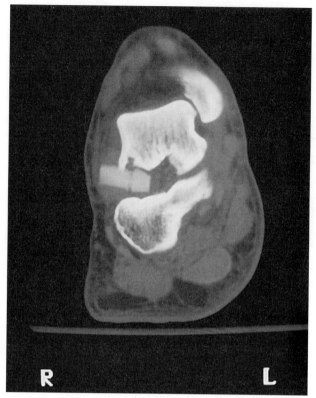

Figure 23–17. Extrusion of plug with chipping of the lateral wall of the talus after the child twisted her ankle.

the potential complications associated with correction of flatfoot may include the following:

1. Overcorrection (with introduction of a varus component)
2. Avascular necrosis (due to vascular embarrassment)
3. Possible subluxation of the implanted device (particularly with the Silastic sphere)
4. Migration of the implant (particularly with the Staple procedure)
5. Nerve damage (through poor anatomic dissection or excessive retraction)
6. Implant extrusion into soft tissue (combined technique)
7. Fragmentation (due either to implant failure from chronic degradation or acute breakage as in a fall) (Fig. 23–18)
8. Dislocation
9. Synovitis
10. Pain
11. Swelling
12. Local or systemic reactions to polymethylmethacrylate bone cement including formation of loose bodies resulting from extrusion of excess bone cement into the joint space, loosening of an implanted device owing to improper application, cement hepatitis (symptoms: hyperpyrexia, nausea, rapid rise in gamma glutamyl transpeptidase liver enzymes), pulmonary leak (pulmonary edema resulting from a hypersensitivity reaction), thermal necrosis with subsequent loosening of the implant
13. Biomaterial reaction or failure
14. Joint arthritis or stiffness
15. Peroneal contracture
16. Additional support required
17. Calf stiffness with cramping due to changes in muscular function and demands
18. Radiolucency or sclerosis of calcaneus and talus (especially with the STA-Peg device)
19. Osteomyelitis
20. Undercorrection or recurrence of problem
21. Detritic synovitis secondary to implant fragmentation and giant cell reaction to minute silicone particles
22. Flattening of the lateral talar process

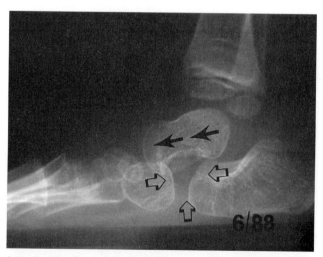

Figure 23–18. The plug placed in the sinus tarsi was too large. The talus has forced the entire foot to become dislocated. Note that the plug is resting within the calcaneocuboid articulation. This plug was eventually removed, and a smaller plug was inserted.

23. Spur formation at the point of contact of the lateral process with the polyethylene peg

References

1. Dorland's Illustrated Medical Dictionary, 28th ed. Philadelphia, W.B. Saunders, 1994.
2. Addante JB, Chin MW, Loomis JC, Burleigh W, Lucarelli JE: Subtalar joint arthroereisis with Silastic silicone sphere: A retrospective study. J Foot Surg 1992;31:47–51.
3. Addante JB, Ioli JP, Chin MW: Silastic sphere arthroereisis for surgical treatment of flexible flatfoot: A preliminary report. J Foot Surg 1982;21:91–95.
4. Peters PA, Sammarco GJ: Arthroereisis of the subtalar joint. Foot Ankle 1989;10:48–50.
5. Langford JH, Bozof H, Horowitz BD: Subtalar arthroereisis. Clin Podiatr Med Surg 1987;4:153–61.
6. Lanham RH: Indications and complications of arthroereisis in hypermobile flatfoot. J Am Podiatr Assoc 1979;69:178–185.
7. Lepow GM, Smith SD: A modified subtalar arthroereisis implant for the correction of flexible flatfoot in children: The STA-Peg procedure. Clin Podiatr Med Surg 1989;6:585–590.
8. Smith DK, Gilua LA, Totty WG: Subtalar arthroereisis: Evaluation with CT. AJR 1990;154:559–562.
9. Smith RD, Rappaport MJ: Subtalar arthroereisis: A four-year follow-up study. J Am Podiatr Assoc 1983;73:356–361.
10. Smith SD: The STA-Peg operation for the pronated foot in childhood. Clin Podiatr 1984;1:165–173.
11. Smith SD: STA-Peg subtalar arthroereisis implant (Smith design). Product manual. Wright Medical Technology, Inc. 1993, pp. 1–6.
12. Smith SD, Milar EA: Arthroereisis by means of a subtalar polyethylene peg implant for correction of hindfoot pronation in children. Clin Orthop Rel Res 1983;181:15–23.
13. Subotnick SI: The subtalar joint lateral extra-articular arthroereisis: A follow-up report. J Am Podiatr Assoc 1977;67:157–171.
14. Subotnick SI: The subtalar joint lateral extra-articular arthroereisis: A preliminary report. J Am Podiatr Assoc 1974;64:701–711.
15. Sullivan RW: Correction of the hypermobile flatfoot by the subtalar arthroereisis procedure. Mil Med 1985;150:546–548.
16. Tompkins MH, Nigro JS, Mendicino S: The Smith STA-Peg: A 7-year retrospective study. J Foot Ankle Surg 1993;32:27–33.
17. Viladot A: Surgical treatment of the child's flatfoot. Clin Orthop Rel Res 1992;283:34–38.
18. Smith RD, Wagreich CR: Review of postoperative results of the subtalar arthroereisis: A preliminary study. J Foot Surg 1984;23:253–260.
19. Lundeen RO: The Smith STA-Peg operation for hypermobile pes planovalgus in children. J Am Podiatr Med Assoc 1985;75:177–183.
20. Yu GV, Boberg J: Subtalar arthroereisis. In McGlamry ED, Downey MS, Banks AS. (eds): Comprehensive Textbook of Foot Surgery, 2nd ed. Baltimore, Williams & Wilkins, 1993.
21. Root ML, Orien WP: Normal and Abnormal Function of the Foot. Los Angeles, Clin Biomech Corp., 1977.
22. Lanham RH: Indications and complications of arthroereisis in hypermobile flatfoot. J Am Podiatr Assoc 1979;69:178–185.
23. Oloff LM, Naylor BL, Jacobs AM: Complications of subtalar arthroereisis. J Foot Surg 1987;26:136–140.
24. Schmidt HM: Shape and fixation of band systems in the human sinus and canalis tarsi. Acta Anat 1978;102:184.
25. Viladot A, Lorenzo JC: The subtalar joint: Embryology and morphology. Foot Ankle 1984;5:54–66.
26. Kuwada GT, Dockery GL: Complications following traumatic incidents with STA-Peg procedure. J Foot Surg 1988;27:236–239.
27. Evans D: Calcaneovalgus deformity. J Bone Joint Surg 1975;57A:270.

24

Evans Procedure

Richard M. Jay, D.P.M.

Evans originally described this procedure to elongate the lateral column. He believed that the flatfoot presented with a shortened lateral column that was the reverse of a clubfoot. In his clubfoot procedure a wedge was removed to shorten the elongated lateral column, thus allowing the foot to abduct. By reversing this technique in the flatfoot the lateral column would extend and adduct with the insertion of a wedge. By elongating the lateral column, he was able to preserve the articulation between the calcaneus and the cuboid.[1] The lateral column consists of the calcaneus, the cuboid, and the fourth and fifth metatarsals. If this column is shorter than the medial column, the navicular, cuneiforms, and metatarsals 1, 2, and 3 are abducted to the talus, and the foot rests in valgus. This is a transverse plane deformity, and with an osteotomy of the distal calcaneus and insertion of a wedge, the lateral column is adducted along an arc, thus reducing the abduction deformity (Fig. 24–1). The navicular now realigns with the talus. The function of the

peroneus longus is regained from its weakened attitude so that it can function under an adducted, locked, and stable cuboid. The peroneus longus now plantar-flexes the first ray, reducing the sagittal plane deformity.

COLUMNS

The indication for the Evans procedure is a flexible flatfoot with an excessive transverse plane motion as exhibited by the abducted excursion of the midtarsal joint. This is fairly visible on the anterioposterior (AP) radiograph, which demonstrates a foot with a prominently abducted lateral border and an increased talocalcaneal angle. Two variations are present on radiographic interpretation that dictate the procedure needed to reduce the abducted forefoot. (1) It is important that the lateral and medial columns be equal in length. If the lateral column is significantly shortened as seen on the AP view,

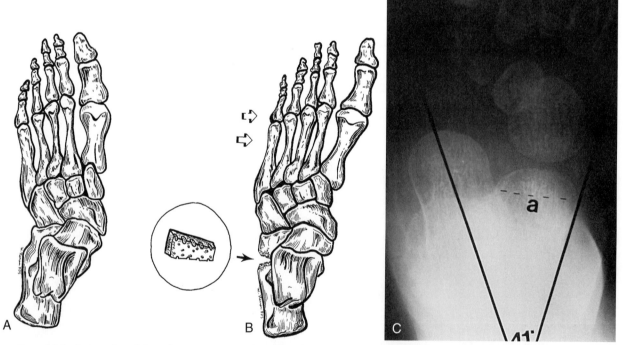

Figure 24–1. A through-and-through osteotomy is performed in the distal calcaneus to allow the insertion of a trapezoidal graft. The graft provides length in the lateral column and rotates the lateral column medially about the arc of the medial calcaneal cut. If the calcaneocuboid and the talonavicular joint align equally on the transverse plane, a wedge can be inserted instead of the trapezoidal graft. (a, osteotomy site in calcaneus.)

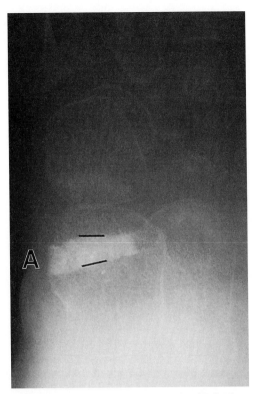

Figure 24–2. Trapezoidal allograft in place in the distal calcaneus. The C-C joint and the T-N joint are now aligned, and transverse rotation of the lateral column can occur without jamming.

the cuboid will not rotate properly in an adducted fashion and will jam into the talus. It is then necessary to lengthen and equalize the lateral column to ensure the proper adductory rotation and reduce the abducted forefoot. When evaluating the AP radiograph, the calcaneocuboid joint may be located proximally to the talonavicular joint. With this variation the calcaneocuboid joint must be advanced distally to equal the talonavicular joint position. When this is done, the distal calcaneal fragment allows rotation to occur in adduction with no jamming of the cuboid into the talus. (2) If the columns are of equal length, a simple wedge is placed in the anterior aspect of the calcaneus 1 cm proximal to the calcaneocuboid joint (Fig. 24–2).

FIXATION

Proper visualization is required to prevent the distally cut fragment from migrating too high or too low after the graft has been placed. Fixation methods include pin fixation to guard against this migration. When inserting a Kirschner wire to secure the distal calcaneal fragment and graft, it is most difficult to avoid the articular surface. Care must be taken to place the pin through the calcaneocuboid joint correctly the first time. The pin runs from the cuboid through the joint into the calcaneus. The graft can also be made to supply its own integral fixation by creating a T-shaped cut in the calcaneus and graft. The graft is then locked into place and is prevented from migrating dorsally or plantarly on the body of the calca-

neus. The graft must not rise because it will then project into the talus and either prevent motion or cause a natural wearing away of the periosteum, thus creating fusion at the anterior calcaneal surface. When dissecting the lateral surface to visualize graft placement, it is a good idea to avoid the capsule of the calcaneocuboid joint. Releasing the capsule and ligaments about this joint causes a greater loss of stability of the distal fragment.

Since the graft is wedged into the lateral surface of the calcaneus and force is needed to distend the bone fragment, fixation is rarely needed as long as no instability is noted about the graft site (Fig. 24–3). Once the osteotomy has been made the distal osseous fragment has a tendency to rise, especially when the fragment is distracted distally. This will occur if the calcaneocuboid joint is opened. When making the osteotomy in the distal calcaneus, it is advisable to free the plantar ligament because this ligament prevents the fragment from moving anteriorly.[2]

WEDGE

The grafts used should not be oversized because this will cause overcorrection of the deformity in a medial direction. A supinated foot will ensue, and with a concomitant metatarsus adductus, the in-toe position will be significantly increased; a metatarsal procedure must be considered at this time to avoid a serious complication. If the forefoot is allowed to drift too far in the adducted position by elongation of the lateral column, the peroneals will become taut and tendinitis will result. Care must be taken when inserting the graft laterally to ensure that the final position of the graft lies flush with the calcaneal surface to avoid the possibility of tendon impingement of the peroneals.

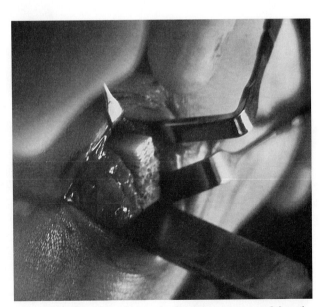

Figure 24–3. Allograft in place at the distal osteotomy site of the calcaneus. If the C-C joint is left intact, the pull of the peroneals creates a compressive effect at the graft site, obviating the need for fixation. The corticocancellous graft provides strength and allows vascular ingrowth. If necessary, the graft can be fenestrated to increase osteogenesis through a thick graft.

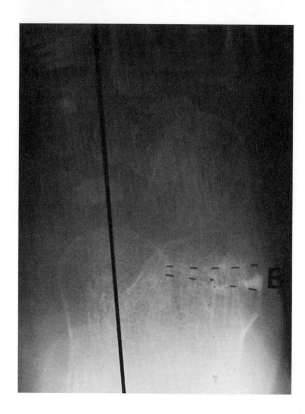

Figure 24–4. Evans procedure 1 year postoperatively. Graft is incorporating within the calcaneus. (B, site of graft incorporated in calcaneus.)

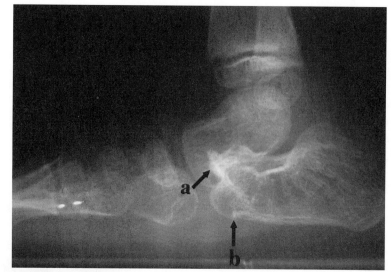

Figure 24–5. Graft placed too far distally, resulting in avascular necrosis. (a, graft slipped dorsally impinging on talus; b, remnant of distal calcaneus.)

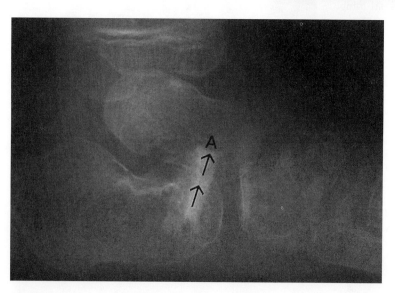

Figure 24–6. Graft placed too far proximally, resulting in slippage and impingement into the talus. (A, graft rising out of osteotomy site.)

The use of allografts is an acceptable approach; the graft consists of corticocancellous bone. The graft can be fenestrated to allow good vascular ingrowth and promote osteogenesis. With creeping substitution, the graft will be incorporated into the surgical site (Fig. 24–4). The cortical portion of the bone graft provides a strong strut that keeps the cut surfaces apart and maintains the adducted alignment.[3, 4]

PLACEMENT

The wedge is placed 1 cm proximal to the calcaneocuboid joint. If the graft is placed too far anteriorly, the distal surface of the calcaneus will develop avascular necrosis (Figs. 24–5 to 24–7). A graft placed too far proximally will invade the medial facet and guarantee arthritic changes.

The sural nerve runs along the lateral surface under the lateral malleolus and becomes the lateral dorsal cutaneous nerve. This is the nerve that one encounters with the skin incision because it lies within the superficial fascia. Cutting this nerve is an error in tissue handling; sensory loss will result, and in a child undergoing an elective procedure this result is considered unacceptable.

Strict attention should be given to cast application because the position of the foot is critical. The foot must be maintained in a neutral position; however it should not be actively dorsiflexed above its neutral position or the graft will slip. The same is true in that the foot should not be inverted and plantar-flexed or the graft will become loose and may be dislodged.

When applying the cast one starts with the foot by maintaining it in a neutral position as when applying a cast for orthotics. The leg segment follows but only to its neutral position; the leg should not be overly dorsiflexed. After 3 to 4 weeks the cast is changed to a walking cast, and the foot is kept in a neutral position for another 5 to 6 weeks. When the child is removed from the walking cast he or she is allowed to ambulate in a neutral Dynamic Stabilizing Innersole System (DSIS) or orthotic device. It is a good idea to measure the child for these devices at the third week cast change. This will allow enough time

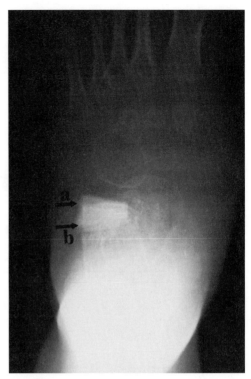

Figure 24–7. Loss of distal articular surface of calcaneus. Necrosis occurred in the distal cancellous fragment. (a, distal site of graft; b, proximal site of graft.)

for the laboratory to complete the insert and be ready for the final cast removal.

References

1. Evans D: Calcaneo-valgus deformity. J Bone Joint Surg 1975; 57B:270.
2. Gauley JV: Flatfoot: Evans procedure. *In* Jay RM: Current Therapy in Podiatric Surgery. Toronto, B.C. Decker, 1989, pp. 251–253.
3. Kite JH: Errors and complications in treating foot conditions in children. Clin Orthop 1967; 53:31–38.
4. Dollard MD, Marcinko DE, Lazerson A, Elleby DH: The Evans calcaneal osteotomy for correction of flexible flatfoot syndrome. J Foot Surg 1984; 23:291–301.

25

Medial Displacement Osteotomy of the Posterior Calcaneus for Flatfoot Deformity

Alan R. Catanzariti, D.P.M.

Flatfoot or pes planus is a term used to describe a foot characterized by a decrease in longitudinal arch height, which may be accompanied by hindfoot valgus, forefoot abduction, or both. Which cases of flexible pes planus become symptomatic and therefore demand treatment is unknown. Unfortunately, there are no clearly defined patterns for the type and degree of pes planus. Additionally, the best therapeutic approach for symptomatic pes planus is unknown. In specific situations, a combination of various procedures may be used to correct a symptomatic flatfoot. One such procedure is calcaneal osteotomy.

Calcaneal osteotomies can be classified as anterior, posterior, and extra-articular (Table 25–1).[1] The posterior calcaneal osteotomy is used to address functional abnormality of the subtalar joint. Medial displacement of the posterior calcaneus results in dynamic redirection of the force of the gastrocnemius-soleus muscle group in a pronatory to a supinatory direction (Fig. 25–1). Patients experiencing longstanding flatfoot deformity develop functional adaptation of the hindfoot. Longstanding calcaneal eversion secondary to subtalar joint pathology may result in hindfoot valgus. Unfortunately, the calcaneus maintains this everted position throughout the midstance phase of gait. Normal resupination during late midstance never takes place. The posterior muscle group, therefore, acts as a pronator rather than a supinator during the stance

phase of gait. The Achilles tendon may become contracted and maintains this position thereafter. Medial displacement of the posterior calcaneus permits the elimination of a deforming pronatory force and creates an active supinatory moment about the subtalar joint. Additionally, the osteotomy creates a structural reconfiguration of the calcaneus, essentially displacing subtalar joint motion in a supinatory direction. Also, Jacobs and colleagues observed the reduction of forefoot supinatus following posterior calcaneal osteotomy.[2] As the calcaneus is inverted and the subtalar joint supinates, the midtarsal joint becomes locked. The lateral column becomes stable to allow the peroneus longus tendon to gain a mechanical advantage. The result is plantar flexion of the first ray, creating a normal-appearing arch.

SURGICAL TECHNIQUE

The ideal position for performing this procedure is the lateral decubitus position. If the patient must be supine, a beanbag under the ipsilateral hip is recommended to allow better access to the lateral aspect of the foot. The incision is placed approximately 1 cm inferior to the tip of the lateral malleolus and 1 to 2 cm anterior to the insertion of the Achilles tendon. In this manner, both the sural nerve and the peroneal tendons should be dorsal to the incision site. The incision begins just anterior to the Achilles tendon above the calcaneus and is made obliquely downward to the plantar aspect of the foot so that its inferior edge meets the margin between the dorsal and plantar skin (Fig. 25–2). Dissection is carried through the subcutaneous tissue with care being taken to ligate any appropriate vessels. Additionally, the sural nerve may be identified in this layer; if it is identified, it should be retracted dorsally

Table 25–1. **Classification of Calcaneal Osteotomies for Flatfoot Deformity**

Extra-articular calcaneal osteotomy	Posterior calcaneal osteotomy
Baker-Hill type	Gleich type
Chambers type	Dwyer type
Selakovich type	Silver type
Anterior calcaneal osteotomy	Koustogiannis type
Evans type	

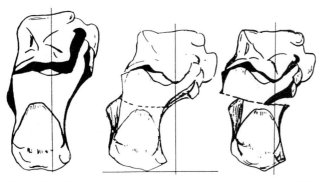

Figure 25–1. The osteotomy creates a structural reconfiguration of the calcaneus, essentially displacing subtalar joint motion in a supinatory direction.

Dissection

A moistened sponge or Metzenbaum scissors may be used to mobilize some of the subcutaneous tissues from the deep fascia and periosteum. Prior to the periosteal incision, the posterior facet of the subtalar joint should be identified dorsally, and the calcaneal tubercle should be identified plantarly. A deep fascia-periosteal incision is made beginning posterior to the posterior facet dorsally and ending anterior to the plantar tubercle. The periosteal tissue is then dissected away from the calcaneus approximately 1 cm on both sides of the proposed osteotomy site. Additionally, it is important to dissect the periosteum both dorsally and plantarly. Curved elevators seem to work well for both dorsal and plantar dissection.

The calcaneal osteotomy is then performed with a large sagittal saw. The osteotomy should be performed in line with the skin incision. The osteotomy should begin posterior to the posterior facet of the subtalar joint and should finish plantarly anterior to the plantar tuberosity of the calcaneus. It is important to actually see the saw exit both the dorsal and plantar cortices. Appropriate retraction both dorsally and plantarly is important to avoid

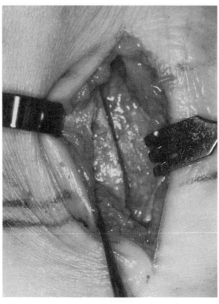

Figure 25–3. Osteotomy site is cut through to the medial cortex.

soft tissue damage from the sagittal saw. Once the medial cortex is encountered, it is important not to overextend the saw into the medial soft tissue structures because injury to the posterior tibial nerve and artery may result. After the entire medial cortex has been osteotomized, the posterior segment of the calcaneus is shifted medially into the desired position (Fig. 25–3). It is important to either divide or stretch the periosteum on the medial aspect of the calcaneus, especially in patients with severe hindfoot valgus. The periosteum may limit the surgeon's ability to translate the posterior segment in a medial direction. A sharp osteotome may be used to divide the medial periosteum, or a lamina spreader may be used to stretch the periosteum about the medial aspect of the osteotomy (Fig. 25–4).

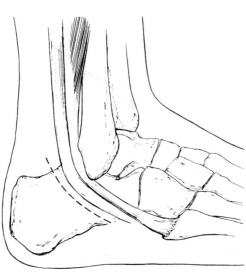

Figure 25–2. The incision is placed approximately 1 cm inferior to the tip of the lateral malleolus and 1 to 2 cm anterior to the insertion of the Achilles tendon. In this manner, both the sural nerve and the peroneal tendons should be dorsal to the incision site.

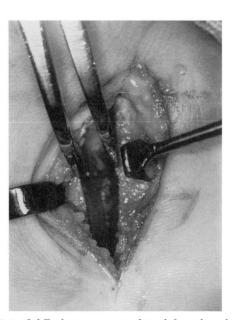

Figure 25–4. If difficulty is encountered in shifting the calcaneus, a laminar spreader is used to loosen the surrounding structures.

The posterior segment of the calcaneus is translated in a medial direction approximately half to a third the width of the entire calcaneus (Fig. 25–5). An intraoperative axial radiograph may assist in determining the appropriate amount of medial translation. Another guideline is to translate the posterior segment medially until it lines up with the sustentaculum tali. The posterior segment may also be rotated or twisted in a medial direction to further displace the insertion of the Achilles tendon in a medial position. Additionally, the posterior segment may be displaced plantar to increase the pitch of the calcaneus.

Provisional fixation is provided with a guide pin from the 6.5-mm cannulated cancellous screw system. This may be placed under fluoroscopy. The guide pin is placed just inferior to the insertion of the Achilles tendon in a percutaneous fashion. Additionally, the pin is placed perpendicular to the osteotomy site to obtain maximum compression. It is important to ensure that the guide pin does not invade the subtalar joint. The shorter 16-mm thread pattern is used. Typical length of the screw is between 55 and 66 mm. The periosteal tissue is closed with 2–0 absorbable suture. Skin is usually reapproximated with 4–0 monofilament nylon sutures.

When an Achilles tendon lengthening is being performed in conjunction with the medial displacement osteotomy, the lengthening is performed *first*. After the Achilles tendon has been incised, the posterior calcaneal osteotomy is performed. Following fixation of the posterior calcaneal osteotomy, the Achilles tendon is then placed at the desired length and sutured in that position. This ensures that the equinus deformity is not recreated after displacement of the posterior calcaneus in a plantar direction. A Hemovac is recommended for at least 24 hours because the osteotomized calcaneus tends to bleed profusely.

Postoperatively, the patient is placed in a below-knee, nonweight-bearing cast or a posterior splint for 6 weeks. However, other authors have recommended a nonweight-bearing cast for 10 days followed by a short leg walking cast for 4 weeks.[3]

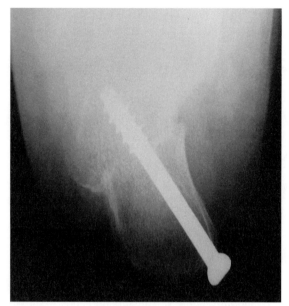

Figure 25–5. A 6.5-mm cannulated screw maintains and compresses the fragments.

SUMMARY

Medial displacement osteotomy of the posterior calcaneus may be used in surgical management of flatfoot deformity. Its primary benefit is to convert the function of the posterior muscle group from pronation to supination. This has a direct effect on the subtalar joint by reducing hindfoot valgus and indirectly affects the longitudinal axis of the midtarsal joint by reducing a flexible forefoot supinatus. These patients must be evaluated on an individual basis, and posterior muscle group lengthening may be needed to address any existing equinus.

Medial displacement osteotomy is a technically simple procedure. Additionally, it has the advantage of avoiding arthrodesis, thereby preserving hindfoot motion; it requires no bone grafting and no implantation of foreign materials and directly affects the existing pathology at the subtalar joint.

References

1. Jacobs AM, Oloff L, Visser JH: Calcaneal osteotomy in the management of flexible and nonflexible flatfoot deformity: A preliminary report. J Foot Surg 1981;20:54–66.
2. Jacobs AM, Geistler P: Posterior calcaneal osteotomy. Clin Podiatr Med Surg 1991;8:647–657.
3. Saxby T, Myerson M: Calcaneus osteotomy. *In* Myerson M (ed): Current Therapy in Foot and Ankle Surgery. St. Louis, B. C. Decker, 1993, pp. 159–162.

26

Subcapital Talar Osteotomy for Transverse Plane Structural Deformities

John H. Walter, Jr., D.P.M.
and Michael A. Bailey, R.P.H., D.P.M.

When presented with a flatfoot deformity, one must determine the predominant plane or planes in which the abnormalities exist. Multiple planal deformities are common and must be identified by performing a thorough clinical and radiographic evaluation. Any combination of frontal, sagittal, and/or transverse plane abnormalities may be present; although a single plane deformity may dominate and may be responsible for the clinical appearance of a flatfoot.[1]

Historically, transverse plane flatfeet have been identified as being problematic and generally not amenable to functional orthoses therapy.[2-4] Therefore, surgical correction of transverse plane deformities in patients with flatfeet has been the focus of attention. Surgical procedures addressing the osseous and soft tissue abnormalities have been mentioned extensively in the literature.[5-8] Kidner in 1923 was the first to identify the need for soft tissue reorientation as playing a vital role in correction of transverse plane flatfoot. Realignment of the osseous structures in the transverse plane by lengthening the lateral column was proposed by Evans.[6] Through an opening wedge osteotomy of the anterior calcaneus, he hoped to provide stability by reducing pronation in the midtarsal joint.

These procedures, although often effective when used individually and in combination, may not provide the desired amount of correction in the transverse plane. Identification and correction of the structural deformity in the head and neck of the talus is essential if reconstructive surgery is to be successful. Angular relationships between the head, neck, and body of the talus may exist due to a congenital abnormality, as in clubfoot deformity.[9, 10] Similar secondary changes occur in the structural adaptation of the functional flatfoot. In the mid 1980s, it was proposed that the subcapital region of the talus was a viable site for surgical correction of talar head and neck deviations. Early studies were performed on congenital clubfoot deformities with encouraging results.[9-11] Preliminary studies on the use of talar neck osteotomies for correction of structural flatfoot had been performed in 1978. Initially, the procedure was performed to correct sagittal plane deviations of the talar head and neck.[3] Due to the previous success in correcting transverse plane deviations in patients with congenital clubfeet, the subcapital talar osteotomy was viewed as a procedure that could potentially correct transverse plane structural flatfoot deformity.

CLINICAL APPEARANCE

The chief concern of the patient with this type of flatfoot deformity is bilateral medial arch and leg pain

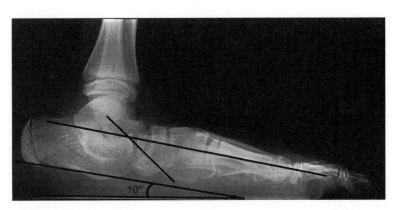

Figure 26–1. Congenital flatfeet develop alterations in the osseous architecture as form follows function. A severe congenital flatfoot deformity with a negative calcaneal inclination angle of 10 degrees is shown here.

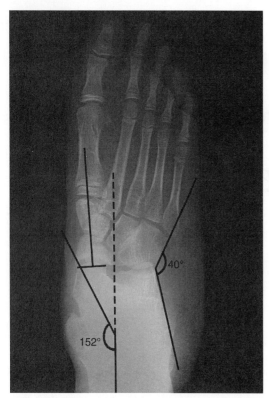

Figure 26-2. The deviation of the talar head in flatfoot deformities resembles the abductory deviation of the articular cartilage of the first metatarsal head in hallux valgus. This font demonstrates pathologic adduction of the talus with abduction of the articulating surface of the talar head.

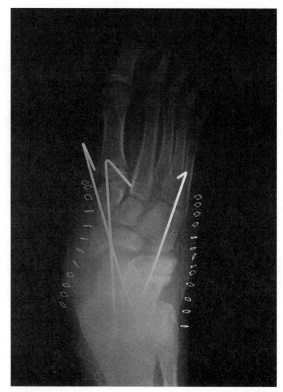

Figure 26-4. Fixation of the osteotomy for 4 to 6 weeks minimizes the risk of slippage or delayed union of the capital fragment. Congruency has been returned to the talar navicular joint, and the lateral column has been lengthened.

when walking long distances, and when pain is present in a child engaged in athletic activities, the talar osteotomy is indicated. Functional orthoses are recommended; if minimal relief of symptoms is seen surgery should be considered. On weight bearing, the abducted forefoot position increases. An apropulsive gait with early heel-off is noted during gait analysis.

Dorsoplantar radiographs of the patient's foot in angle and base of gait views reveal a talocalcaneal angle of greater than 140 degrees and a calcaneal-cuboid angle of greater than 40 degrees of abduction. The articular surface of the talar head appears to have structurally adapted to the abducted forefoot position. Lateral radiographs reveal a calcaneal inclination angle of −10 degrees and

no appreciable medial column fault (Figs. 26–1 and 26–2).

A sagittal plane open Z tendo Achillis lengthening procedure is performed to address the equinus deformity. An Evans open calcaneal osteotomy, using a hand-carved wedge of freeze-dried tricortical iliac crest, is performed to reduce forefoot abduction. A single 0.062 Kirschner wire is used to secure the allograft (Fig. 26–3).

Attention is then directed to the medial aspect of the foot, where a curvilinear incision is placed from the tip of the medial malleolus to the dorsomedial aspect of the first metatarsal base. Once the deep fascia has been incised and reflected, the tibialis posterior tendon is identified and its dorsal and distal insertions are released, while the inferior portion of the insertion is left intact. The tendon is then reflected plantarly to increase visualization

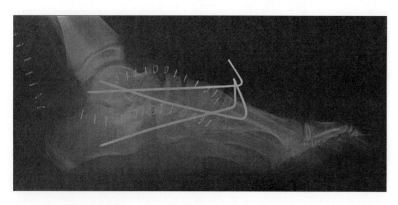

Figure 26-3. Correction of talar head deformities through a medial incision involves performing a stable adductory wedge osteotomy in the metaphyseal bone just proximal to the articular cartilage. Pin fixation maintains the adductory wedge at the talar head and the bone graft in the opening osteotomy of the calcaneus.

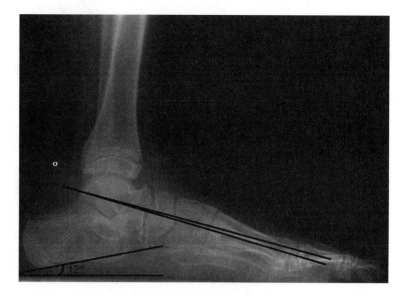

Figure 26–5. A rectus foot type has been achieved 8 months after surgery. The talar osteotomy has healed, and the calcaneal allograft is well incorporated. Calcaneal inclination is now 12 degrees, a 22-degree improvement. Medial arch reconstruction, tendo-Achilles lengthening, and calcaneal lengthening osteotomy with bone graft are other procedures commonly performed with the talar head adductory wedge osteotomy.

of the talonavicular joint and the spring ligament. An L-shaped capsulotomy of the talonavicular joint is performed, and the distal attachment of the spring ligament is transected. At this time the talar head and neck is inspected, and it is noted that the medial aspect of the talar head is devoid of any articular cartilage.

The articular cartilage of the remaining articular surface of the talar head is intact and has adapted laterally. Minimal periosteal reflection is then performed at the medial and dorsodistal subcapital regions of the talar head. A sagittal saw is then used to create an adductory wedge osteotomy with its base medial, immediately proximal to the articular surface of the talar head, and preserving the lateral cortex. Following reduction, crossed 0.062 Kirschner wires are placed across the osteotomy to maintain correction (Fig. 26–4). Following the subcapital talar wedge osteotomy, the abducted forefoot position is reduced to rectus. A modified Young's tendosuspension is then performed to enhance medial column stability, and the distal attachments of the spring ligament and tibialis posterior are advanced distally and secured, A long leg plaster cast is then applied with the knee bent at 30 degrees of flexion and the ankle at 90 degrees.

POSTOPERATIVE COURSE

After 3 weeks, the long leg nonweight-bearing cast is replaced with several short leg fiberglass casts for a total of 12 weeks. During the final 9 weeks of casting, the patient is gradually converted from nonweight bearing to full weight bearing. The calcaneal inclination angle is increased to 12 degrees from −10 degrees while the calcaneocuboid angle is reduced from 40 degrees to 13 degrees (Fig. 26–5). The talar declination angle is restored to normal from its previous adducted and plantar-flexed position. A rectus forefoot is observed, and the talar articular bisection is now parallel with the long axis of the talar neck.

SUMMARY

The goal of the subcapital talar adductory wedge osteotomy is to realign the articular surface of the talar head to restore a normal relationship with the talar neck. By adducting the capital portion of the talus, the bisection of the talar head articular surface may more closely parallel the long axis of the talar neck. However, in some cases these axes may not be parallel, but a more normal talar declination angle is produced which is a quantitative measurement. Adductory wedge osteotomies of the talar head shorten the medial column and complement lateral column lengthening achieved by the Evans procedure, producing a rectus forefoot.

References

1. Green DR, Carol A: Planal dominance. J Am Podiatr Assoc 1984;74:98–103.
2. Bleck EE: Persistent fetal medial deviation of the neck of the talus: A common cause of intoeing in children. J Bone Joint Surg 1976;58A:724.
3. Grumhine NA: Talar neck osteotomy for the treatment of severe structural flatfoot deformities. Clin Podiatr Med Surg 1987;4:119–136.
4. McGlamry ED, Mahan KT, Green DR: Pes valgo planus deformity, Part I. In McGlamry ED (ed): Comprehensive Textbook of Foot Surgery, Vol. 1. Baltimore, Williams & Wilkins, 1987, pp. 403–445.
5. Beck EL, McGlamry ED: Modified Young tendosuspension techniques for flexible flatfoot. J Am Podiatr Assoc 1973;63:582.
6. Evans D: Calcaneovalgus deformity. J Bone Joint Surg 1975;57B:270–278.
7. Kidner FC: The pre-hallux (accessory scaphoid) in its relationship to flatfoot. JAMA 1923;81:1500.
8. Tachdjian MO: The Child's Foot. Philadelphia, W.B. Saunders, 1985.
9. Hielmstedt A, Sahlstedt B: Talar deformity in congenital clubfoot. Acta Orthop Scand 1974;45:628.
10. Hielmstedt A, Sahlstedt B: Talo-calcaneal osteotomy and soft tissue procedures in the treatment of clubfeet. Acta Orthop Scand 1980;51:349–357.
11. Hielmstedt A: Correction osteotomy of the talus in congenital clubfoot. Acta Orthop Scand 45:978, 1984.

27

Tibialis Anterior Transfer "Into Talus" for Control of Severe Pes Planus

Charles G. Kissel, D.P.M.

In the normal foot the talus has no muscular attachments; however, it is responsible for the function of the entire foot. The position of the talus is controlled indirectly by its joints and the extrinsic muscles of the foot. The talus allows the foot to be both a mobile adapter and a rigid lever depending on its relationship with the calcaneus and the navicular. In the abnormally pronated foot, the talus becomes anteriorly displaced with adduction and plantar flexion. In the pediatric patient this can result in a very hypermobile foot depending on the severity of the deformity. Control of the talus by surgical intervention has been well documented in the literature.

I have used the transfer of the tibialis anterior to control the pediatric flatfoot in selected symptomatic patients with severe talar declination and subluxation (Fig. 27–1). The tibialis anterior is transferred through the talus from dorsal lateral to plantar medial for direct talar control. The remaining tendon end is sutured to the plantar medial foot to form a strong ligament, which also helps to control plantar talar subluxation (Fig. 27–2). This procedure has been used in combination with other commonly employed flatfoot procedures to restore the medial column deformity of the flexible flatfoot with severe talar declination. Other components of the pes planus deformity, such as equinus, must also be addressed with ancillary procedures (Figs. 27–3 and 27–4).

PROCEDURE

The patient is taken to the operating room and placed in the supine position; general anesthesia with endotracheal intubation is administered. The involved foot is prepared and draped in the usual aseptic manner. Following adequate elevation and exsanguination, a well-padded pneumatic thigh tourniquet is inflated.

Attention is then directed to the medial aspect of the foot where a curved incision is made beginning at the tip of the medial malleolus and extending dorsally over the

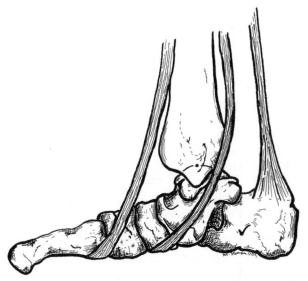

Figure 27–1. Severe pediatric flatfoot deformity with declination of the talus.

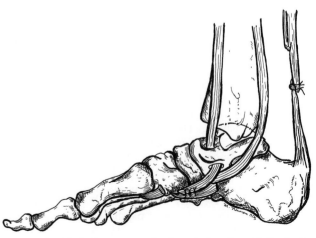

Figure 27–2. Tibialis anterior transfer through the talus with distal reinforcement of the medial column as a "ligament."

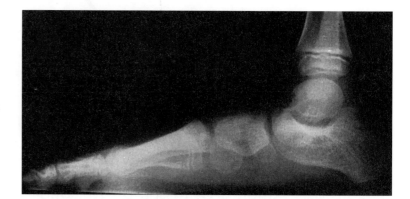

Figure 27–3. Eight-year-old male preoperatively.

navicular tuberosity and then plantarly to the base of the first metatarsal. The incision is carried deep through layers using both blunt and sharp technique. All superficial vessels are identified and cauterized or ligated as needed. All vital structures are gently retracted.

Dissection is continued until the tendons of the tibialis posterior and anterior are completely exposed. The tibialis anterior is released from its tendon sheath to the level of the ankle joint and is sectioned just proximal to its insertion. The tibialis posterior is freed from its attachments to the navicular tuberosity and retracted inferiorly. Blunt dissection is carried out to expose the talar neck dorsally and plantar medially. A 3-mm bone trephine is used to create a hole in the talar neck from plantar medial to dorsal lateral. A 2–0 suture is placed in the distal end of the tibialis anterior tendon to facilitate its transfer from dorsal to plantar through the talus. The talonavicular joint is reduced by dorsal lateral pressure on the talar head while the transferred tibialis anterior is pulled plantarly. (It is usually necessary to perform an Achilles tendon lengthening prior to this procedure to mobilize the talus.) Soft tissue release about the talus is performed as necessary to ensure complete reduction of the deformity. While plantar-flexing the medial column on the talus, the spring ligament and talonavicular joint capsule are plicated, the tibialis posterior is advanced, and the tibialis anterior is sutured distally along the plantar medial column. If possible, it is also reattached distally near its insertion. Absorbable sutures are used for this part of the procedure.

At this point stable restoration of the medial column should be noted. The surgical site is irrigated and closed in layers. Local anesthetic is then infiltrated to control postoperative pain. A dry sterile compressive dressing is applied followed by deflation of the tourniquet. A below-the-knee cast is applied while maintaining the foot in a supinated position.

Additional indicated procedures such as calcaneal osteotomy or Achilles tendon lengthening are performed prior to the medial column restoration.

POSTOPERATIVE MANAGEMENT

A below-the-knee cast is maintained on the leg. Depending on the child's size and age, the patient is kept nonweight-bearing for 3 to 6 weeks. If osteotomies are performed as part of the reconstruction, an additional 1 to 2 weeks of a weight-bearing cast may be required.

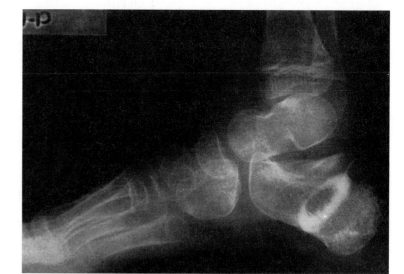

Figure 27–4. Eight-year-old male 20 weeks postoperatively.

28

Triplane Correction of the Flexible Flatfoot

Charles G. Kissel, D.P.M., and Troy J. Boffeli, D.P.M.

Surgical restoration of the flexible flatfoot requires realignment of the rearfoot with concurrent reduction of the midfoot and forefoot deformities. We advocate combining a posterior calcaneal osteotomy with allogeneic graft, anterior tibial tenosuspension, and Achilles tendon lengthening to achieve correction of all three components. The senior author has repaired over 60 feet using this combined operation between 1982 and 1992 at Hutzel Hospital. Fifteen randomly selected operations have been retrospectively evaluated, and an outline of the procedures used and our rationale for their use is presented here along with long-term subjective and radiographic results.

Surgical restoration of the recalcitrant symptomatic flexible flatfoot requires neutralization of the pathologic pronatory forces. Major components of pronation seen in the flexible flatfoot are heel valgus, medial column subluxation, and posterior equinus. These imbalances, which can be either primary or secondary, accentuate one another in a cyclic manner, producing an uncontrollable foot. Surgical intervention should therefore be directed at these specific components. Theoretically, a synergistic effect may be obtained when the pathologic cycle is interrupted at multiple points. Numerous procedures have been described to "correct" the flexible flatfoot.[1-15] We advocate combining a Silver type[8, 10] calcaneal osteotomy with a tibialis anterior tenosuspension and Achilles tendon lengthening.

BIOMECHANICS

The heel valgus component can be a primary etiologic deformity or a mechanism that compensates for an equinus. The Silver type calcaneal bone graft repositions the posterior aspect of the calcaneus medially, thus decreasing the pronatory lever arm around the subtalar joint axis. The ground reactive force and the pull of the Achilles tendon then produce less pronatory torque. Secondarily, less forefoot supinatus is required to compensate for the valgus heel.[16]

Pathologic pronation of the subtalar joint leads to subluxation and collapse of the medial column in the sagittal and transverse planes. During growth, the soft tissues and osseous structures adapt to this subluxed position and may eventually become nonreducible. Tenosuspension of the medial column in a fashion similar to that described by Young[6] repositions the midfoot by reducing the forefoot supinatus. Realignment of the articular structures may decelerate osseous adaptation. Once tenodesis occurs, the section of the tibialis anterior tendon that connects the plantar navicular to the first metatarsal base acts as a strong plantar ligament supporting the medial arch. This procedure is further enhanced by advancing the tibialis posterior tendon and by the improved effectiveness of the peroneus longus tendon.

The gastrocnemius-soleus equinus can be a primary etiologic force or a secondary contraction in the flexible flatfoot. When this abnormality occurs as a primary deformity, the foot pronates in an effort to allow the heel to reach the ground. A secondary equinus may occur in patients with longstanding pronation due to the decreased origin-to-insertion distance of the gastrocnemius-soleus complex.[16] Regardless of the cause, the Achilles tendon is lengthened to allow complete mobilization of the talocalcaneal complex and secondarily the medial arch. Optimal effectiveness of the associated procedures is obtained once these structures are mobilized. The equinus component is not always evident on clinical examination. Excessive talar declination and diminished calcaneal inclination often indicate a hidden equinus deformity.

INDICATIONS

The goal of surgical treatment of the flexible flatfoot is to decrease the pathologic pronatory forces that cannot be controlled by conservative means. Prevention of progressive arthrosis and the ultimate occurrence of a dysfunctional rigid collapsed foot are primary objectives. Surgical intervention is therefore indicated in the presence of a severe and uncontrollable deformity that will inevitably result in degenerative arthrosis. Surgical candidates represent a small percentage of patients who have flatfoot complaints. Physical activities, social interaction, endurance, and performance must be considered when evaluating symptomatology.[17]

The operation described here is ideally performed be-

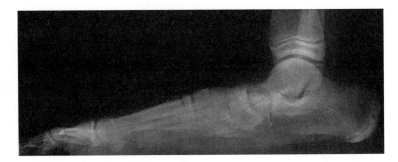

Figure 28–1. Preoperative lateral radiograph of patient No. 2, left foot. Note midfoot subluxation, No. 2, left foot. Note talonavicular subluxation and cuboid abduction.

tween the ages of 9 and 10; however, acceptable results are seen in both younger and older age groups. The tibialis anterior tenosuspension is best performed when adequate ossification of the navicular has been achieved. The operation is best performed prior to adolescence so that growth will aid in correction rather than accentuate the deformity. In older patients, the tenosuspension is intended to augment the dysfunctional and symptomatic tibialis posterior tendon rather than to reduce the medial column deformity.

PROCEDURE

The operation is begun in the prone position if the Achilles tendon is to be lengthened. The Achilles tendon is lengthened through two transverse incisions approximately 2 cm in length, one at the insertion of the tendon and the second 5 to 10 cm proximal to it depending on the amount of correction needed. The incisions are placed more medial than lateral to avoid the sural nerve. Proximally, a No. 11 blade is inserted from posterolateral to anteromedial to bisect the tendon. The blade is then rotated to transect the posteromedial two thirds of the tendon fibers. The blade is then inserted transversely through the tendon in the distal incision and rotated to transect the anterior two thirds of the tendon fibers. The tendon is then slide lengthened approximately 2 cm by dorsiflexing the foot in the supinated position with the knee maximally extended.

The calcaneal osteotomy is performed through an oblique incision made 0.5 to 1 cm posterior and parallel to the peroneal tendons. The skin incision extends from the dorsal to the plantar aspects of the calcaneus. The periosteum is incised obliquely and is minimally elevated. A 9-mm blade on an oscillating saw is used to obliquely osteotomize the calcaneus leaving a medial hinge intact.

The osteotomy is made posterior to the posterior facet and distal to the plantar tuberosity. An osteotome is then used to weaken the hinge and pry open the osteotomy. A wedge-shaped allogeneic implant formed from a lyophilized tibial segment is then prepared at the back table using auxillary power equipment. A 3- to 4-cm circular wedge with a 5- to 7-mm base is fashioned from the allogeneic bone. The size of the alloimplant varies and can be measured intraoperatively. The wedge is carefully tapped into place. Two percutaneous 0.062-inch Kirschner wires are driven across the alloimplant from posterior to anterior, avoiding the subtalar joint (Figs. 28–1 and 28–2).

The patient is then rotated into the supine position. The Young tenosuspension is performed through an incision made from the first metatarsal base to the tip of the medial malleolus curving dorsally over the navicular tuberosity. Dissection is carried to the deep fascia, retracting venous structures dorsally. The deep fascia is incised in an inverted T fashion. The plantar arm extends from the first metatarsal base to the head of the talus along the superior edge of the posterior tibial tendon. The vertical arm crosses the navicular from the tuberosity and extends dorsally. The tibialis posterior tendon is retracted plantarly, and the periosteum is elevated to expose the dorsal and plantar navicular. The tibialis anterior tendon is removed from its sheath and mobilized to the ankle level. The attachment at the base of the first metatarsal is preserved. The distal medial insertion of the posterior tibial tendon is then released. A 4-mm trephine is driven through the navicular from proximal dorsal to distal plantar. An oscillating saw is then used to complete the keyhole in a proximal medial direction. The foot is then placed in the dorsiflexed and supinated position, and the tibialis anterior tendon is drawn into the keyhole and held in place while the capsule and periosteum are repaired. Nonabsorbable 2–0 suture is then used to anteriorly ad-

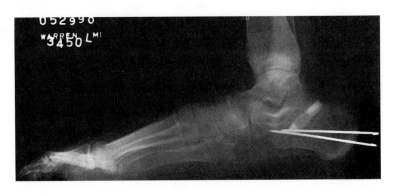

Figure 28–2. Lateral radiograph of patient No. 2, left foot, 6 weeks postoperatively. Note percutaneous Kirschner wire fixation and allogenic bone graft with plantar incorporation.

vance the tibialis posterior tendon on the plantar portion of the tibialis anterior tendon.

POSTOPERATIVE CARE

A below-the-knee cast is applied in the operating room with the rearfoot supinated and dorsiflexed and the medial column plantar-flexed. Nonweight bearing is continued until radiographic consolidation of the calcaneal bone graft is noted plantarly, which usually occurs in 6 to 8 weeks. The percutaneous Kirschner wires are removed at this time. Progressive weight bearing in an athletic shoe is then allowed.

MATERIALS AND METHODS

Patients were selected for follow-up based on availability, elapsed time since the operation, and combination of procedures. Questionnaires were used to determine subjective complaints and any activity limitations present before and after surgery. Long-term satisfaction was also measured.

Radiographic measurements were obtained from anteroposterior and lateral radiographs taken in the standard angle and base of gait views. Preoperative and postoperative angular relationships were compared to evaluate subtalar joint pronation. The talar declination angle, calcaneal inclination angle, and talo-first metatarsal angles were evaluated on lateral radiographs. The talocalcaneal angle and talonavicular joint congruity were evaluated on anteroposterior radiographs.[18] Patients included in this study were those for whom both subjective questionnaire and radiographic results were available.

Fifteen feet in 10 patients were evaluated. Five patients underwent bilateral operations staged an average of 8 months apart with a range of 4 to 12 months. The average age at the time of surgery was 13 years with a range of 8 to 20 years. Seven of the 10 patients were female. The average follow-up period was 36 months with a range of 15 to 66 months. All patients underwent the aforementioned combination of procedures with the exception of four patients who did not require Achilles tendon lengthening.

RESULTS

Preoperative complaints ranged from discomfort with heavy activity to severe pain after minimal activities that significantly limited the patient's lifestyle. The most common preoperative complaint was marked frequent pain that caused avoidance of common activities. Postoperative complaints ranged from no pain to mild discomfort with heavy activity that did not limit participation in such activities. The most common postoperative complaint was an occasional slight ache that occurred only after heavy activity.

Patients rated their satisfaction with postoperative pain relief and activity level as very satisfactory in 4 feet and satisfactory in 11. Foot appearance was rated very satisfactory in 2 feet, satisfactory in 11 feet, and unsatisfactory in 2 feet (one patient). Nine of ten patients stated that they would have this operation again. Subjective rating of overall improvement ranged from 75% to 100% with an average of 88%.

Results of radiographic evaluations and normal values are listed in Table 28–1.[18]

Table 28–1. **Radiographic Evaluations and Normal Values**

Patient Foot	1 R	1 L	2 R	2 L	3 R	3 L	4 L	5 R	6 R	6 L	7 L	8 R	8 L	9 L	10 L	Range	Average	Normal
Talor declination angle[1]																		
Preoperative	30	35	34	30	35	40	29	25	28	35	32	40	29	30	32	25–40	32	
Postoperative	20	26	23	22	16	23	17	19	23	30	26	14	24	25	25	16–30	22	21
Change	10	9	11	8	19	17	12	6	5	5	6	26	5	5	7	5–26	10	
Calcaneal inclination angle[1]																		
Preoperative	15	14	11	10	18	18	9	15	8	7	18	8	9	8	10	7–18	12	
Postoperative	24	18	16	21	26	26	14	20	16	15	25	18	17	12	16	12–26	19	18–22
Change	9	4	5	11	8	8	5	5	8	8	7	10	8	4	6	4–11	7	
Talo-first metatarsal angle[1] ***(Lateral)***																		
Preoperative	16	28	14	13	18	20	19	20	11	20	16	25	18	17	17	11–28	18	
Postoperative	4	6	0	0	4	2	3	0	6	15	5	3	5	9	10	0–15	5	<15
Change	12	22	14	13	14	18	16	20	5	5	11	22	13	8	7	5–22	13	
Talocalcaneal angle[1] ***(Anteroposterior)***																		
Preoperative	37	45	23	20	27	20	20	25	23	22	30	25	30	27	25	20–45	27	
Postoperative	29	37	20	10	20	16	14	18	15	15	21	18	25	16	20	10–37	20	17–21
Change	8	8	3	10	7	4	6	7	8	7	9	7	5	9	5	3–10	7	
Talonavicular joint congruity[2] ***(Anteroposterior)***																		
Preoperative	60	50	66	65	45	40	70	65	65	65	60	65	65	50	50	40–70	58	
Postoperative	90	70	75	80	65	60	85	85	80	80	65	80	80	75	75	60–90	76	>75
Change	30	20	15	15	20	20	15	20	15	15	5	15	15	25	25	5–30	18	

[1]Degrees
[2]Percent

DISCUSSION

Our experience with flatfoot reconstructive surgery has been favorable. The average case scenario was that of a 13-year-old child who experienced frequent pain resulting in avoidance of common activities. After attempts at conservative management failed, surgery resulted in a more active lifestyle with an occasional slight ache occurring only after heavy activities.

One patient was unsatisfied with the appearance of both feet postoperatively and stated that she would not have the surgery again. On the pain and activity level assessment, this patient improved from a severe preoperative level to a mild postoperative level, and her overall improvement was 80%. Radiographic improvement was also favorable in this case.

Radiographically, the average postoperative improvement in the talar declination angle of 10 degrees compares favorably with the 6-degree change reported by Marcinko[13] and the 4.2-degree change reported by Beck and McGlamry.[11] Postoperatively, our calcaneal inclination angle increased an average of 7 degrees, increasing from 12 to 19 degrees. Previous studies have reported average increases of 2 and 3.4 degrees.[11, 13] Bordelon[19] considers the lateral talo-first metatarsal angle to be the most significant radiographic indicator of flatfoot severity with mild being 1 to 15 degrees, moderate being 16 to 30 degrees, and severe being greater than 30 degrees. Our average decrease in this angle was 13 degrees with 18 degrees being the average preoperative measurement and 5 degrees the average postop measurement.

SUMMARY

Combined operative procedures that specifically address the individual components of the flexible flatfoot can yield a synergistic result by interrupting the pronatory cycle at multiple points. We advocate combining a varus-producing opening wedge calcaneal osteotomy with an anterior tibial tenosuspension and Achilles tendon lengthening. A long-term retrospective study of subjective and radiographic results has demonstrated a high level of patient and surgeon satisfaction.

References

1. Gleich A: Beitzag zur operativen Plattsfussbehandlung. Arch Klin Chir 1893; 46:358.
2. Lord JP: Correction of extreme flatfoot. JAMA 1923; 81:1502.
3. Lowman CL: An operative method for correction of certain forms of flatfoot. JAMA 1923; 81:1500.
4. Miller OL: A plastic flatfoot operation. J Bone Joint Surg 1927; 9:84–91.
5. Hoke M: An operation for the correction of extremely relaxed flatfeet. J Bone Joint Surg 1931; 13:773–783.
6. Young CS: Operative treatment of pes planus. Surg Gynecol Obstet 1939; 68:1099–1101.
7. Dwyer FC: Osteotomy of the calcaneum in the treatment of grossly everted feet with special reference to cerebral palsy. *In* Huitieme Congres Internationale de Chirurgie Orthopedique, New York, 1960. Bruxelies, Societé Internationale de Chirurgie Orthopedique de Fraumatologie 1960; p. 892.
8. Silver CM, Simons SD, Litchman HM: Calcaneal osteotomy for valgus and varus deformity of the foot in cerebral palsy. J Bone Joint Surg 1967; 49A:232–246.
9. Koutsogiannis E: Treatment of mobile flatfoot by displacement osteotomy of the calcaneous. J Bone Joint Surg 1971; 53B:96–100.
10. Silver CM, Simmons SD, Litchman HM: Long-term follow-up observations on calcaneal osteotomy. Clin Orthop 1974; 99:181–187.
11. Beck EL, McGlamry ED: Modified Young tenosuspension technique for flexible flatfoot. *In* McGlamry ED (ed): Reconstructive Surgery of the Foot and Leg. New York, Intercontinental Medical Book Corporation, pp. 293–325.
12. Jacobs AM, Oloff LM, Visser HJ: Calcaneal osteotomy in the management of flexible and nonflexible flatfoot deformity: A preliminary report. J Foot Surg 1981; 20:57–66.
13. Marcinko DE, Lazerson A, Elleby DH: Silver calcaneal osteotomy for flexible flatfoot: A retrospective preliminary report. J Foot Surg 1984; 23:191–198.
14. Jacobs AM, Oloff LM: Surgical management of forefoot supinatus in flexible flatfoot deformity. J Foot Surg 1984; 23:410–419.
15. Schwartz NH, Tursi FJ: A new technique for the treatment of pes planus deformity: A preliminary report. J Foot Surg 1987; 26:149–152.
16. Root M, Orien W, Week J: Normal and Abnormal Function of the Foot, Vol. 1. Los Angeles, Clinical Biomechanics Corporation, 1977.
17. Mahan KT, McGlamry ED, Green DR: Pesplano valgus deformity. *In* McGlamry ED (ed): Comprehensive Textbook of Foot Surgery. Baltimore, Williams & Wilkins, 1987, pp. 769–817.
18. Weissman SD: Biomechanically acquired foot types. *In* Weissman SD (ed): Radiology of the Foot. Baltimore, Williams & Wilkins, 1983, pp. 50–76.
19. Bordelon RL: Flatfoot in children and young adults. *In* Mann RD, Coughlin MJ (eds): Surgery of the Foot and Ankle. St. Louis, Mosby, 1992, pp. 717–756.

29

Cotton Osteotomy

J. Barry Johnson, D.P.M.

F. J. Cotton first described his dorsal open wedge osteotomy of the first cuneiform in 1935 to correct the elevatus deformity present in some hallux abducto valgus deformities.[1] In 1981 I first used the Cotton osteotomy to correct supinatus deformity of the first ray in flatfoot. A modification of the Hoke[2] procedure had been used to correct so-called midtarsal joint fault (naviculocuneiform breech or sag). However, it was thought that fusion of the naviculocuneiform joint would limit plantar flexion of the first ray during the propulsive phase of gait and limit first metatarsophalangeal (MTP) joint dorsiflexion. Fusion of the first ray (i.e., in the Lapidus procedure) reduces the functional range of first MTP joint motion.

INDICATIONS

The Cotton osteotomy has been used to correct elevatus deformity of the first ray in more than 150 cases of adolescent flatfoot along with procedures to correct other elements of this complex triplane deformity with remarkable results. Due to the excellent results achieved in adolescent flatfoot correction over a period of several years this osteotomy has in recent years been used in older patient populations to correct elevatus deformity in flatfoot and certain hallux limitus conditions. The first ray is hypermobile and ligamentous laxity usually coexists to some degree clinically. When not bearing weight the medial longitudinal arch may appear normal. On bearing weight dorsiflexion of the hallux[2] may produce a normal arch. In the great majority of cases a rearfoot varus deformity is present that compensates only to vertical, preventing unlocking of the midtarsal joint. Therefore, because of the hypermobility of the first ray the next bone to sublux owing to pronatory forces is the cuneiform at the naviculocuneiform joint.

For radiographic analysis weight-bearing angle and base of gait dorsal plantar and lateral radiographs are mandatory to evaluate the transverse plane deformity at the midtarsal joint and the sagittal plane deformity at the talonavicular and naviculocuneiform joints. A so-called "midtarsal" joint breech or sag is evident on the lateral view. This is seen when the dorsal cortical surface of the navicular and the medial cuneiform are convergent plantarly. The navicular width dorsally is less than its width plantarly. There may be evidence of irregularity of the dorsal area of the naviculocuneiform joint due to compressive and subluxatory forces. Superimposition of the navicular over the cuboid is evident with lowering of the medial longitudinal arch. In most cases talonavicular

joint sag is absent except in patients with valgus deformities of the rearfoot or oblique talar deformities or after significant sagittal plane subluxation requiring eversion of the calcaneus and unlocking of the subtalar joint. In most cases a coexisting transverse plane deformity of the midtarsal joint is evident on the dorsal plantar radiograph. To evaluate the transverse plane deformity at the midtarsal joint a line is drawn on the lateral border of the calcaneus and extended distally. If a significant portion of the cuboid is lateral to this line, abduction of the cuboid on the calcaneus is evident, and an Evans[4] osteotomy is also indicated. However, I have seen two cases in which only a sagittal plane breech of the naviculocuneiform joint was present, and in one of these patients no equinus was present. In a limited number of feet a coexisting plantar-flexed talus is seen, probably due to an oblique talus at birth. A significant plantar flexion deformity of the talus may require a Selakovich[5] osteotomy (sustentaculum tali osteotomy) to correct that element of the deformity.

The most common combination has proved to consist of tendo Achillis lengthening, Evans procedure, and Cotton procedure. In a very few cases the Cotton osteotomy alone is indicated to reduce the triplane flatfoot deformity. An equinus element is evident in almost every flatfoot deformity and must be addressed by tendo Achillis lengthening or gastrocnemius recession. I prefer to perform a percutaneous tendo Achillis lengthening with the patient in the prone position. Two stab incisions are made. The first is made over the posterior lateral aspect of the Achilles tendon just above the insertion into the calcaneus. A No. 15 blade is inserted through the Achilles tendon at this level from posterior lateral to anterior medial, and the anterior lateral half of the tendon is incised. Approximately 5 cm above the insertion and just medial to the tendon a second linear stab incision is made. With the tip of the blade picking up the paratenon and then rotated 90 degrees with the blade directed anteriorly, the medial half of the tendon is severed at this level along with the plantaris tendon if present. Care must be taken to cut only the medial one half of the tendon initially to prevent possible rupture. The position of the blade can be evaluated by pushing the point posteriorly. The end of the blade can then be palpated along with the lateral border of the tendon while the assistant dorsiflexes the foot. The subtalar joint is inverted and the knee is extended while the foot is forcefully dorsiflexed. If lengthening does not occur, a few additional tendon fibers at each level are severed, and the foot is forcefully dorsiflexed again. No more than two thirds of the tendon should be severed at each level before lengthening occurs.

In rare instances a very high degree of forefoot supinatus may be present, and the largest bone graft (1-cm based wedge) will not be enough to reduce the deformity. Other or additional medial column procedures such as transpositional or dorsal wedge osteotomies of the navicular or other plantar-flexory osteotomies of the first ray may be indicated in these cases.

EVANS OSTEOTOMY

The Evans open osteotomy on the lateral aspect of the calcaneus is performed just at the anterior edge of the floor of the sinus tarsi where the bone slopes upward. The bone can be measured on the dorsal plantar radiograph to estimate its width at the osteotomy site. The approximate width of the bone graft required to correct the transverse plane deformity can be ascertained in two different ways. The first way is to compare a second dorsal plantar radiograph with the foot held in a neutral subtalar joint position. The opening on the lateral aspect of the calcaneocuboid joint may be approximately the width of the wedge necessary to correct the deformity.

A second method is to construct a triangle from the apex of the osteotomy at the level of the beginning of the up-slope of the sinus tarsi as measured on the lateral radiograph. This anatomic position for the osteotomy is preferred to the prescribed measurement from the calcaneocuboid joint due to differences in length of individual calcanei, especially from the sinus tarsi to the anterior end of the bone. This distance varies depending on the length of the calcaneus. On the dorsal plantar radiograph a line is constructed on the lateral border of the calcaneus and extended distally. If a significant portion of the cuboid is not lateral to the line, excessive abduction of the midtarsal joint is not present and the Evans procedure is not indicated. The distal lateral aspect of the cuboid is marked, and a line is constructed from this point to the apex of the osteotomy near the medial cortical surface of the calcaneus. This distance is measured and transposed from the apex of the osteotomy to the lateral calcaneal line distally, creating a triangle. The width of the calcaneus at the level of the osteotomy is then measured down both sides of the triangle, the width of the base of the triangle at that level closely matches the size of the wedge of bone needed to correct the transverse plane abduction at the midtarsal joint.

These methods can assist in preoperative planning and precutting of the bone grafts but should not be assumed to be exact. Intraoperative measurements as well as the clinical alignment of the foot at the time of correction are required for the final assessment.

COTTON OSTEOTOMY

Preoperative Considerations

Age

The age of the patient is an important consideration. Although this procedure can be used in all age groups, the most appropriate ages for use of this as well as other osteotomies for correction of dysfunctional flatfoot appear to be 10 to 13 years. In younger children, depending on their osseous maturity, adequate correction of flatfoot deformities may be achieved with surgical tendo Achilles lengthening and good mechanical control with functional orthotics. Older teenagers may already show early evidence of arthritic changes that could have been prevented by earlier surgical intervention. Arthritic changes are usually minimal in the 10- to 13-year-age group and are certainly not a contraindication to osteotomy.

Radiographic Measurements

On the dorsal plantar view, the length of the first cuneiform is measured. On the lateral view the height at the middle of the first cuneiform is measured. These measurements are used intraoperatively to guide the position of the osteotomy on the dorsal surface and the depth of the osteotomy. Additionally, an isosceles triangle may be constructed from the apex of the osteotomy at the plantar cortex of the first cuneiform to the plantar aspect of the first metatarsal and a second line of equal length constructed from the apex to a desired distance beneath the first metatarsal (i.e., 1 cm) to reduce the forefoot supinatus. The height of the cuneiform is then transposed down both sides of the triangle from the apex; the distance between these points represents the width of the base of the wedge of bone needed to accomplish this change. Still, intraoperative measurements and clinical alignment are always the basis for the final assessment.

Procedure

A dorsal incision measuring approximately 3 cm is made from the base of the first metatarsal to the naviculocuneiform joint. This incision is deepened and the extensor hallucis longus tendon is reflected and retracted medially or laterally to expose the dorsal surface of the first cuneiform. The incision is carried down to the bone, and the subcutaneous tissues are reflected, taking care not to strip the periosteum. The cuneiform has a radiant blood supply by way of the periosteum. Identification of either the first metatarsocuneiform or naviculocuneiform joint is necessary to measure half the length of the bone to find its midpoint. The bone is then scored, and a thin-bladed oscillating bone saw is used to osteotomize the bone perpendicular to the dorsal surface. Approximately half the depth of the bone is cut with the bone saw. The osteotomy is then carefully deepened with a thin osteotome and mallet. The assistant's hands should be free of the forefoot because any plantar force could result in fracture of the plantar cortex. No prying of the osteotomy should be allowed until it has been deepened to at least two thirds to three fourths of the way into the bone. If prying is begun before the osteotomy is sufficiently deep, fracture may occur. Once the osteotomy is deep enough, a prying motion will open it dorsally, and plantar flexion of the medial column will be appreciated clinically.

With the foot held in a neutral subtalar joint position, the plane of the ball of the foot is observed. The forefoot varus or supinatus is reduced when the osteotomy is opened. Forefoot valgus should be avoided, but all of the varus should be reduced to a neutral position of the forefoot if possible. Sometimes this results in a plantar-flexed first metatarsal relative to the plane of the second through fifth metatarsals. Once the surgeon has determined the appropriate position by prying open the osteotomy, the dorsal opening is measured. A wedge-shaped cortical bone graft is then cut from freeze-dried femur. The piece of pie-shaped wedge should be narrower than the width of the cuneiform and shorter than the depth. The graft is fenestrated with multiple 2.0-mm drill holes to allow migration of capillary buds through the graft; however, its strength should not be compromised with too many holes. The graft is inserted and driven into the first cuneiform, using a bone tamp, until it is countersunk beneath the dorsal cortical surfaces. Countersinking of the graft below the cortical surfaces prevents extrusion postoperatively because it indents slightly. Due to this inherent stability no internal fixation is required. The wound is then closed in the usual manner (Figs. 29–1 and 29–2).

Postoperative Management

Adolescents make excellent patients and experience little or no postoperative discomfort, probably because they have no preconceived ideas of postoperative pain, although I still use a long-acting local anesthetic and soluble steroids following closure of the wounds.

Following application of the bandage, a below-the-knee (short leg) walking cast is applied with a pull-out under the first metatarsal head. I prefer to have the patient in a prone position during application of the cast. The knee is flexed to 90 degrees, thus relaxing the gastrocnemius muscle. The foot is aligned to the leg at 90 degrees with the subtalar joint in a neutral position. A ¼-inch thick by 1-inch wide piece of felt 6 to 8 inches long is placed under the stockinet on the plantar surface of the first ray and the first MTP joint and extending beyond the hallux distally. Webril is then applied; I prefer

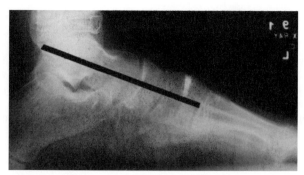

Figure 29–2. Insertion of graft in cuneiform, plantarflexing the first ray.

one 6-inch roll of plaster of Paris as the initial layer because of its superior conformity to the foot and lower leg. This layer should be well molded to the foot, especially over the dorsum of the first metatarsal. The remainder of the cast is fiberglass and consists of a posterior splint 4 inches × 30 inches and a 2-inch roll to anchor the walking heel covered with a 4-inch roll. Significant elevation is required for the first 12 to 24 hours. Crutches are used for bathroom privileges only for the first 3 days. Weight bearing may begin after 3 days, but elevation of the foot is encouraged while sitting or lying down. More aggressive ambulation is not allowed during the first several days. Three weeks postoperatively the cast is changed, the sutures are removed, the foot is redressed, and a new below-the-knee cast with a first ray pull-out is applied. Six weeks postoperatively the cast is removed, and impressions for Rohadur functional orthotics are made. A sock height Unna boot and first ray splint is then applied and used for at least 2 weeks or until the orthotics are ready. Elastic ankle braces are used for several weeks to prevent edema following removal of the Unna boot.

Even though orthotics may have been made for the patient prior to surgery, postoperatively new orthotics are mandatory because the foot is changed. My clinical experience has been that patients who lack this mechanical control postoperatively lose some correction. Because of the length of time (6 to 12 months) needed for incorporation of the bone grafts, control of the foot around a neutral subtalar joint with a rearfoot post that allows 4 to 6 degrees of motion is recommended.

References

1. Cotton FS: Foot statics and surgery. Trans New Engl Surg Soc 1935; 18:181–208.
2. Hoke M: An operation for the correction of extremely relaxed flat-feet. J Bone Joint Surg 1931; 13:773–783.
3. Jack EA: Naviculo-cuneiform fusion in the treatment of flatfoot. J Bone Joint Surg 1953; 35B:279.
4. Evans D: Calcaneo-valgus deformity. J Bone Joint Surg 1975; 57B (3):270–278.
5. Selakovich W: Medial arch support by operation: Sustentaculum tali procedure. Orthop Clin North Am 1973; 4:117–144.

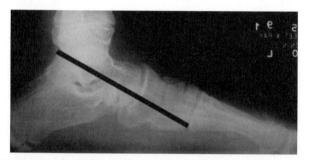

Figure 29–1. Limitation of dorsiflexion at the ankle joint induces a pronatory force at the naviculocuneiform joint and hypermobility of the first ray, resulting in forefoot supinatus as seen in this illustration.

30

Cavus Deformity

Richard M. Jay, D.P.M.

It is well documented that many forms of cavus deformity are associated with neuromuscular disease such as Charcot-Marie-Tooth syndrome, cerebral palsy, Friedreich's ataxia, and poliomyelitis. The incidence of association is reportedly as high as 65%[1] and could be as high as 95% if our methods of neurologic evaluation were more refined. Although a young child with a cavus foot still has a fairly flexible foot, it is not uncommon for this type of foot to become progressively more rigid and stiffer with time. This occurs whether spasticity secondary to hyperinnervation or contracture due to a mechanical advantage of one muscle over another is present.

MECHANICS

A tight Achilles tendon insertion medially on the posterior aspect of the calcaneus pulls the rearfoot into a varus attitude. As the heel becomes inverted, supinating the subtalar joint and locking the midtarsal joint, the plantar fascia tightens with weight bearing and plantar flexion. The stable lateral column enables the peroneus longus to gain a mechanical advantage and plantar-flex the first ray. This, in effect, brings the origin and insertion points of the plantar fascia closer together and further contributes to the contracture of this plantar structure (Fig. 30–1).

In the presence of a strong peroneus longus, the tibialis anterior becomes weaker, and the deformity continues to progress. The intrinsic forces plantar-flex the forefoot on the rearfoot. This in turn alters the function of the anterior extensors of the forefoot and produces a loss of dorsiflexory power to the metatarsals. Therefore, the stabilizing forces at the metatarsal phalangeal joints are unbalanced, and the digits become contracted by the extensors. A retrograde force from the contracted digits additionally pushes the metatarsal heads in a plantar direction. As the ankle dorsiflexes in an attempt to bring the forefoot up, the toes contract even more. This creates dorsal excrescences and painful plantar lesions, which may cause an awkward gait secondary to compensation. Depending on the degree of the deformity, these lesions may be present in children as young as 4 or 5 years of age; however, this is usually a late finding in children (Fig. 30–2).

It is evident that a single change in the position of the calcaneus or an increase in plantar flexion of the first ray has a domino effect on the entire cavus foot. These deformities can originate at various levels and may occur at different times during development in any of these locations. Because of the progressive nature of the cavus foot, the deformity and rigidity increase as the child ages.

AREA OF DEFORMITY

Sagittal Plane

In the anterior cavus foot (Fig. 30–3) the forefoot is plantar-flexed on the rearfoot either at Chopart's joint or

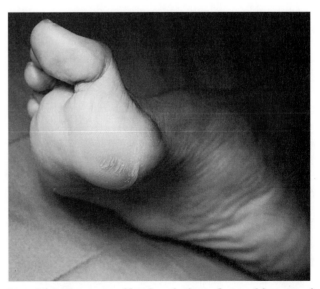

Figure 30–2. Sixteen-year-old male with plantar flexion of first ray and cocked-up hallux. Note the increase in callus formation on the plantar-flexed first metatarsal. This is secondary to the pull of the peroneus longus on the first ray.

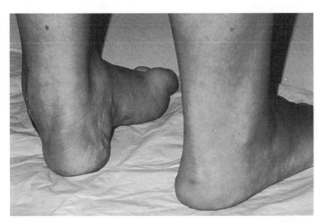

Figure 30–1. Left foot with marked heel varus and first ray plantar flexion. This cavus foot is rigid, and the child has lateral ankle instability.

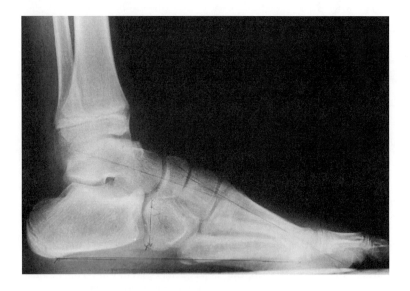

Figure 30–3. Anterior cavus deformity. Plantar flexion of the first metatarsal on the cuneiform with flat-top talus.

at Lisfranc's joint. These two types of anterior cavus exist with either the first ray alone plantar-flexed (an anterior local cavus) or all of the metatarsals plantar-flexed either at Chopart's or at Lisfranc's joint (a global deformity). The sagittal plane posterior cavus (Fig. 30–4) takes into consideration the angle of inclination of the calcaneus. When the angle is increased to more than 35 degrees from the plantar surface of the calcaneus to the supporting surface, a posterior cavus is present. It is not unusual for both deformities, anterior and posterior, to be present in one foot. This is known as a combined or two-island cavus foot type (Fig. 30–5).

Frontal Plane

In addition to the sagittal plane deformity, the foot may also have a deformity in the frontal plane. The calcaneus is either in varus or in valgus. The cavovarus foot with its subtalar varus and heel varus position has greater ankle instability and a greater degree of sagittal plane deformity (Fig. 30–6).

Transverse Plane

The cavoadductus foot has the most significant pathology. This is a rare finding in children and is usually seen in patients with longstanding rigid deformities. As stated earlier, most types of cavus deformities in children are flexible. The transverse plane deformity does not usually appear until marked osseous changes have developed over a number of years owing to the inverted and plantar-flexed position of the forefoot. A continuous internal driving force on this adducted foot type creates a rigid deformity that is usually manually irreducible and requires surgical intervention.

DEGREE OF DEFORMITY

The degree of deformity of the cavus foot in a young child can be divided into three categories: flexible, a mild deformity; semiflexible, a moderate deformity; and rigid, the most severe form.

Flexible Deformity

A flexible deformity is usually difficult to differentiate from the normal foot; on weight bearing, the child usually compresses the medial arch so that all of the digital contractures are reducible. The foot presents with plantar flexion of the first ray and slight inversion of the rearfoot during weight bearing. This type of deformity is therefore

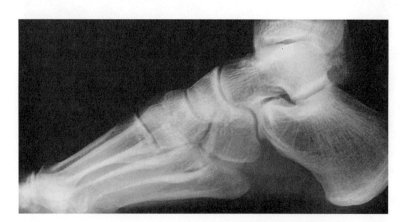

Figure 30–4. Posterior cavus with "pistol grip" calcaneus. Apparent flat-top talus secondary to marked adduction of the talus.

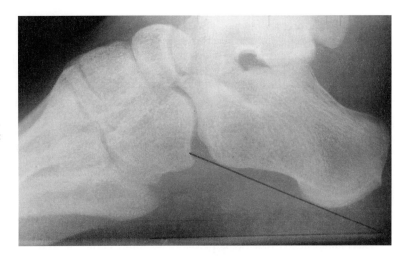

Figure 30–5. Posterior and anterior cavus. Marked increased calcaneal inclination with plantar flexion of first ray in relation to midtarsal and subtalar joints.

significant in that it is usually overlooked by the physician. This is especially important because one must always rule out a neurologic component with any cavus deformity. As stated earlier, at least 65% of cavus deformities are reported to have a neurologic origin.[1, 2]

In addition, the early stage is the best time for controlling this flexible foot. With proper mechanical control, the osseous changes taking place can be minimized by limiting the mechanical advantage of the peroneus longus tendon over the tibialis anterior tendon. With proper control one can see a gradual decrease in the degree of deformity of the cavus foot and prevent its vicious progression.

The last type of flexible cavus foot includes a forefoot valgus component that flattens significantly on weight bearing. This foot is very unstable and develops significant forefoot symptomatology, including severe hallux abducto valgus and submetatarsal lesion patterns. When the patient is nonweight bearing, the structural forefoot-to-rearfoot relationship is one of valgus, but when weight is introduced, the ground reactive forces cause the medial column to collapse. In gait, the medial column is not locked against the rearfoot and therefore is unstable. Early recognition of this foot type is necessary to prevent the development of severe hallux abductus and bunion deformity.

Semiflexible Deformity

This deformity does not completely reduce with weight bearing. Nonreducible contracted digits induce plantar submetatarsal keratomas as well as helomas dura on the interphalangeal joints dorsally. A cock-up hallux deformity occurs at the great toe interphalangeal joint and becomes rigid. Soft tissue contractures occur at all of the joints in the forefoot. Radiographic examination of the semiflexible cavus foot shows the development of osseous changes, with mild jamming of joints and resultant lipping on the dorsal surfaces of the articulating bones.

Rigid Deformity

This is the most severe cavus deformity and usually does not appear until late adolescence or early adulthood. These feet do not vary with weight bearing. Joint position is usually subluxed, and motion is limited or rigid. Gait is very awkward: There is an increase in lateral ankle instability, and all of the digits are flexed and contracted. Displacement of the anterior fat pad allows the metatarsal heads to protrude as large bony prominences on the plantar aspect of the forefoot, depending on the presence of anterior global or anterior local cavus. Shoe gear is very difficult to find for these young people; the foot is arched and inverted to such an extent that the patient rolls off the shoe and experiences maximum wear on the lateral surface of the heel area.

In rigid forefoot valgus there is an everted forefoot-to-rearfoot relationship in which the subtalar joint is in

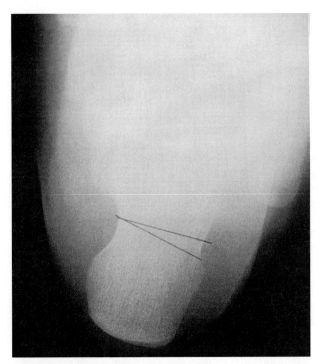

Figure 30–6. Zero-degree axial view of the calcaneus. The body of the calcaneus is actually torqued on the frontal plane. Markings note the wedge needed to reduce the inverted position.

neutral position and the midtarsal joint is maximally pronated and locked. The entire forefoot may be everted, or only metatarsals 1 and 5 may be everted to the rearfoot with metatarsals 2 through 4 either in a varus attitude or perpendicular to the bisection of the calcaneus.

Due to the everted position of the forefoot on the rearfoot when the forefoot strikes the ground (at about 10% to 15% of the stance phase of gait), the subtalar joint is rapidly supinated. This is known as a "supination rock," which immediately transfers weight laterally onto the fifth metatarsal head area.[3] At the same time, this rapid supination often causes subtalar and ankle joint instability with resultant inversion sprains. In addition, shoe gear friction contributes to a pump-bump and associated bursitis posterior to the Achilles insertion.

The plantar-flexed first ray is probably the most common type of forefoot valgus and is associated usually with uncompensated or partially compensated rearfoot varus or compensated or partially compensated forefoot varus. With the latter, the relationship of metatarsals 2 through 5, relative to the calcaneus, is a position of varus, but metatarsals 1 through 5 demonstrate a perpendicular relationship. It is believed that the first ray plantar-flexes because of the increased pull of the peroneus longus secondary to a stable cuboid/lateral column, which in effect increases the rearfoot varus and supinates the subtalar joint even more.

CONSERVATIVE CARE

Conservative management of cavus deformities has been a perplexing problem for as long as the deformity has been recognized. When considering orthotic control, it must be realized that periodic changes in the device corresponding to the altered structure and function of the foot are probably necessary. A rearfoot varus and a forefoot valgus are commonly associated with this deformity. The rearfoot varus may be primarily of an uncompensated or partially compensated nature; it causes a secondary forefoot valgus via plantar flexion of the first ray. On the other hand, the rearfoot varus may be secondary to a total forefoot valgus which causes a rapid supination of the subtalar joint in gait and the subsequent development of subtalar and ankle instability and an increasing position of varus in the subtalar joint.

Forefoot valgus is a common deformity that may be even more common than forefoot varus. Forefoot valgus develops secondary to an uncompensated or partially compensated forefoot varus, either as a primary deformity or associated with rearfoot varus. When a foot remains in a varus position, it has a greater tendency for lateral stability, which enhances the pull of the peroneus longus and results in plantar flexion of the first ray. Initially, the first ray may be hypermobile and lesion formation is evident more laterally, but in time the first ray becomes more rigid and the lesions are subtibial sesamoid and markedly intractable. As the first ray increases its plantar flexion, it raises the medial column and prevents subtalar pronation. Eventually, through a retrograde force, the plantar-flexed first ray increases the varus position of the subtalar joint.

Flexible Deformity

In a flexible deformity in which the medial column collapses and causes an unstable rearfoot, rigid orthoses stabilize the rearfoot and maintain the first ray and medial column in an everted position relative to the locked midtarsal joint. This is necessary for stable propulsion. Therefore, neutral position orthoses are used with a rearfoot varus post and a total forefoot valgus post for metatarsals 1 through 5. With this type of device, the forefoot symptomatology is greatly reduced.

Rigid Deformity

In the past, conservative treatment for patients with a rigid deformity included balanced padding, dancers' pads, semirigid orthoses, metatarsal bars, and lateral dutchmen's wedges as well as numerous shoe modifications. Many practitioners have questioned the use of rigid orthoses with these foot types and have erroneously shied away from using them.

It is commonly thought that since the orthosis is rigid and the foot is rigid, the orthosis will not be tolerated. In actuality, functional orthoses are intended to allow normal function of the foot and to eliminate abnormal compensatory movements. It may even be stated that a rigid orthosis may be the best form of control for symptoms such as ankle sprains associated with the supinatory rock of the contact phase. Following a biomechanical examination and neutral position casting, the problem is usually found to be a forefoot valgus and rearfoot varus deformity. The question of which deformity should be posted and how much must be addressed.

If the patient has a total forefoot valgus, the forefoot should be posted in valgus in the number of degrees measured, and the rearfoot should also be posted in the number of degrees measured. However, this should not exceed 7 degrees; contact phase instability may lead to ankle sprains. Commonly, the amount of rearfoot varus is equal to the amount of forefoot valgus; for example, for a 5-degree forefoot valgus post a 5-degree rearfoot varus post is added. This type of control eliminates the rapid subtalar resupination that occurs after the forefoot hits the ground because it equalizes the weight across all of the metatarsals. The retro-achilles irritation is also eliminated. In the forefoot, distribution of the weight across all metatarsal heads diminishes the concentrated pressure below metatarsals 1 and 5 (Figs. 30–7 and 30–8).

In the management of this rigid cavus foot type, a rearfoot post controls the rearfoot varus and a forefoot post is used beneath metatarsals 2 through 5 in the number of degrees of the forefoot-to-rearfoot relationship. The first ray is not posted on the medial border. The orthosis is in the first intermetatarsal space and is not intended to support the first ray; it allows the first ray to use its own range of motion.

It should be mentioned at this point that the first ray should not be casted. By dorsiflexing the first ray, the longitudinal axis of the midtarsal joint may be inverted as well, and this is undesirable. Furthermore, dorsiflexing the first ray creates a functional limit at the first metatar-

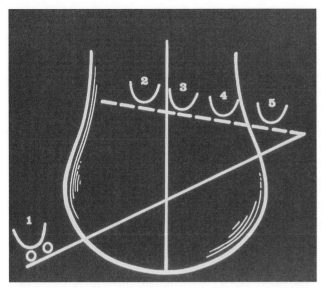

Figure 30–7. Frontal view of anterior cavus with metatarsals 1 through 5 in valgus and metatarsals 2 through 5 in varus.

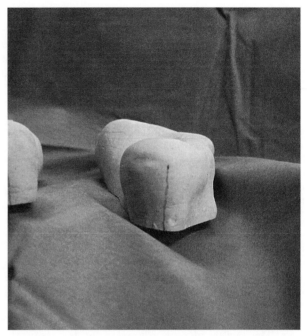

Figure 30–9. A neutral position cast of a child with plantar flexion of the first ray as in an anterior local cavus deformity. Posting of this child is done with a neutral rearfoot varus post and a forefoot valgus post of approximately 5 degrees.

sophalangeal joint that may lead to structural abnormalities. This type of forefoot valgus can also be posted in valgus in the forefoot if the relationship of the plane beneath the first and fifth metatarsals relative to the rearfoot is in valgus (Fig. 30–9).

General Considerations

Regardless of whether the foot type is associated with a neuromuscular disorder or a purely congenital mechanical abnormality, the deformity is progressive in nature; this makes all forms of mechanical control temporary and dynamic. Conservative management must be constantly reevaluated, and many alterations in treatment may be necessary. In some cases, additional neutral position casts

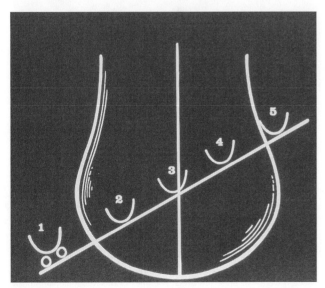

Figure 30–8. Rigid forefoot valgus as noted on frontal plane with metatarsals 1 through 5.

may be considered. As the deformity progresses, numerous mechanical and functional changes occur.

The key to the conservative treatment of congenital cavus is to stabilize the rearfoot and maintain an everted forefoot. With the midtarsal joint locked, stable propulsion is guaranteed. If the child presents with forefoot lesions, an extension can be incorporated into the orthosis to balance out the lesions. This is rare, however, in the young child because lesion patterns usually do not develop until the deformity is rigid and of long standing. Flexible sport orthotics with compressible posts are recommended. If a rigid orthosis is used, compressible posts are recommended to aid in shock absorption at the heel, which is under tension from the tendo Achillis and the plantar fascia. No matter what type of orthosis is used, one should maintain the heel in a deep heel seat to provide the best control.[3–5]

SURGERY

The decision to proceed with surgery in the pediatric patient is a complicated and controversial one. Many factors must be assessed including the severity of the deformity, the progression of the deformity, conservative attempts at treatment, and the overall physical and mental health of the child. Furthermore, parents must clearly understand the goals of any surgical procedure as well as the details of the preoperative and postoperative course.

Generally, it is believed that soft tissue procedures are better suited to pediatric patients than osteotomies. In children, the bones have not fully ossified and are more amenable to soft tissue procedures such as tendon transfers. However, it must be realized that a rigid cavus foot is unlikely to benefit from a soft tissue procedure. Furthermore, because the majority of cavus feet are associated with neurologic diseases, the problem is more likely to be progressive in nature. Therefore, a tendon transfer may be effective only temporarily before the deforming forces overcome it as well.

The location of the deformity in the cavus foot is of prime importance when considering surgery. Depending on the degree and location of the deformity, an osteotomy can be modified to address the plane in which the deformity exists. For example, a triplane calcaneal osteotomy is indicated for a cavovarus foot type. The osteotomy is performed by removing a wedge on the lateral aspect of the calcaneus just proximal to the peroneal tendons and parallel with these tendons as they pass across the calcaneus. The wedge is directed from the lateral to medial side but is modified so that it passes from dorsolateral to plantarmedial. The medial cortex is left intact as a hinge, and the osteotomy is closed laterally. By executing the procedure in this manner, the transverse deformity is reduced by being closed laterally, while the frontal plane is addressed by rotating and decreasing the amount of varus. The sagittal plane is addressed by decreasing the calcaneal inclination angle. As this osteotomy site is closed, a change of position occurs in all three body planes.

If the cavus deformity is isolated to the forefoot, the midtarsal area is the focus of surgery, as described by Japas.[6] The Cole modification is a navicular-cuneiform arthrodesis-transcuboidal osteotomy in which a dorsiflexory wedge is removed to realign the foot without jeopardizing the subtalar joint or midtarsal joint motion. Although the procedure was originally described as using one longitudinal incision, the two-incision approach is preferred because it allows better access to the cuboid. One longitudinal incision is placed medially along the dorsum of the foot, and a smaller one is placed over the cuboid. Using a power saw, a through-and-through dorsiflexory wedge is resected from the navicular-cuneiform articulation and cuboid. Fixation is achieved with crossed Kirschner wires or staples; screw fixation is generally not recommended because of the risk of violating the surrounding joints. In addition, tight plantar structures can be addressed through a Steindler stripping or plantar fasciotomy.

With plantar flexion of the forefoot at metatarsals 1 through 5, a rearfoot varus results; this is usually seen with a rigid forefoot valgus deformity. The metatarsals, predominantly metatarsals 1, 2, and 3, are plantar-flexed in relation to the lesser tarsus. Usually, on a lateral view, metatarsals 1 through 5 are in a plantar-flexed position; however, metatarsals 4 and 5 are essentially dorsiflexed compared to the midfoot and rearfoot. For this reason, the deformity must be addressed at the metatarsals thus affected. When addressing this deformity, the metatarsals must be dorsiflexed by performing osteotomies at the bases to raise the metatarsals' declination. Topographically, on a child, a dorsal prominence may be noted at the area of the first metatarsal cuneiform. The first metatarsal should be dorsiflexed to a position that lies perpendicular to the bisected calcaneal inversion axis. However, care must be taken to avoid damaging the epiphysis of the first metatarsal. Therefore, all osteotomy cuts and fixation

should be performed distal to the epiphysis at the base of the first metatarsal (Fig. 30–10).

If a calcaneal varus deformity is present, a Dwyer osteotomy is necessary to rotate the calcaneal inversion axis perpendicular to the supporting surface. In doing so, the forefoot is brought parallel to the ground. An absence of calcaneal varus obviates the need for a rearfoot osteotomy.

Once the deformity is present, regardless of the etiology, the condition is progressive. When the deformity is present during the early developmental years, the calcaneus starts to change its frontal plane alignment. The insertion of the tendo Achillis pulls on the medial side of the posterior surface, and the predominant origin of the plantar fascia is also on the medial inferior surface. The net effect is a continual deforming force on the calcaneus that creates a heel varus. When a decision is made to osteotomize the calcaneus to reduce the heel varus, correct placement of the osteotomy is essential. The lateral surface of the calcaneus is exposed, and the periosteum is incised parallel to and just under the peroneal tendons.[7] The osteotomy must be parallel to the peroneals if complete reduction is to occur. Often, because the cuts are made too perpendicular to the supporting surface, no change occurs in the frontal plane deformity but the posterior surface is rotated along the transverse plane.[8]

Fixation is required, and bone contact must be complete. The osteotomy is made to but not through the lateral cortex. The cortex is scored with an osteotome but not split, thus allowing the lateral cortex to bend and the medial cortex to close on the calcaneal body for proper fixation. The foot should be slowly dorsiflexed on the leg because the tension from the tendo Achillis helps to close the osteotomy site.

In correcting cavus deformities in children with neuromuscular disease, it is not uncommon for the deformity to recur. In these children adjunct procedures should be

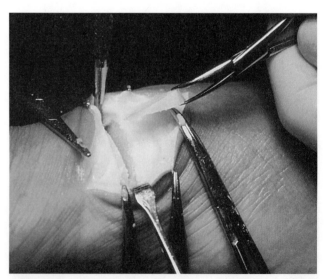

Figure 30–10.   Dorsiflexory wedge osteotomy of the first metatarsal with resected wedge of bone removed. The apex of the wedge is plantar, the base dorsal. The plantar cortex is kept intact, and the first ray is dorsiflexed and then secured with either wire, staple, or screw.

considered. A Steindler stripping, plantar fasciotomy, or tendo-Achillis lengthening may be necessary to remove the deforming force from the calcaneus. The bone will grow in the varus direction if the pull from the fascia and tendo Achillis are allowed to continue. Once the calcaneal varus position is reduced, the forefoot responds by unlocking because the power of the peroneus longus on the first ray is decreased secondary to the pronated rearfoot position. The cuboid is no longer stable enough to allow the peroneus longus to function. The forefoot abducts and dorsiflexes at the midtarsal joint, further reducing the cavus deformity.

Other osteotomies indicated for reduction of the rearfoot component in a cavus foot type include an opening wedge osteotomy with insertion of a bone graft. This serves the same purpose as a closing wedge osteotomy; however, the complexity of the procedure is greater when a medial approach is used to insert a bone graft. The Koutsogiannis displacement osteotomy also can be used to approach the foot from the lateral aspect of the calcaneus and is effective in correcting a true posterior cavus. An incision is made proximal and parallel to the peroneal tendons extending from the superior to the inferior margins of the calcaneus. In this case, a crescentic osteotomy is made from lateral to medial, and the cortex is not left intact. The osteotomy can thus be rotated in the sagittal plane and also reduced in the frontal plane. By shifting the weight-bearing surface to the medial axis of the calcaneus, the foot is moved into a more valgus position. Fixation is achieved through the use of one or two Steinmann nonthreaded pins, staples, or cancellous screws. Recently, the advent of the cannulated screw system has aided in achieving a more stable and effective osteotomy.

Techniques

Dwyer Osteotomy

Under pneumatic tourniquet control, a 6-cm curvilinear skin incision is made over the lateral aspect of the calcaneus 1.5 to 2.0 cm posterior and inferior to the peroneal tendons. Dissection through the subcutaneous tissues allows visualization of the many lateral calcaneal neurovascular structures as well as the sural nerve, which must be retracted dorsally. A periosteal incision is made on the calcaneus, and the periosteum is elevated with a key elevator to expose the superior and inferior borders. The longer 240 blade is used with the microsagittal saw to create a laterally based wedge of bone that is removed while the medial cortex is kept intact. The cut in the calcaneus should be parallel to the peroneal tendons. An osteotome and mallet can be used to finish the cuts if the saw fails to reach across the width of the calcaneus. In the young child, the cortex of the calcaneus is thin, and the osteotomy can be made simply by cutting it with a No. 10 blade. The width of the wedge removed should be consistent with the severity of the deformity.

The osteotomy site is then closed to reduce the varus deformity, the heel should be in 0 to 5 degrees of valgus. Closure of the osteotomy is performed by gently dor-

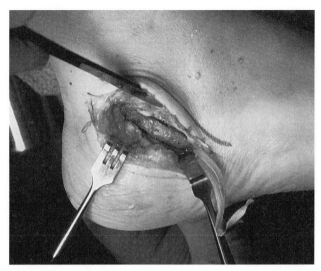
Figure 30–11. Two parallel cuts are made in the peroneal tendons. The base is lateral, and the apex is placed medially.

siflexing the foot (Figs. 30–11 and 30–12). Since the tendo Achillis inserts into the posterior aspect of the calcaneus, the force of dorsiflexion tightens the tendo Achillis and creates pressure to reduce the osteotomy site. The osteotomy can be fixed with staples, Steinmann pins, or a cancellous screw placed percutaneously from the posterior heel. A Kirschner wire (Micro-Aire, Valencia, CA) can be driven from the plantar aspect running proximally while the osteotomy is held closed. Pins used for fixation should not enter the subtalar or ankle joint. Staple fixation provides firm fixation; however, care must be taken not to strike the staples too hard because the lateral cortex could fracture, driving the posterior aspect of the calcaneus medially and creating an unstable fragment. The lateral surface of the calcaneus is held firmly by the assistant, and the staple is tapped in cautiously flush with the cortex. The tissues are closed in layers, and a closed suction drain is recommended. The patient is placed in a short leg nonweight-bearing cast for 6 to 8 weeks until

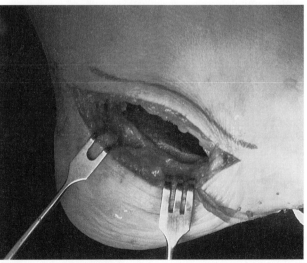
Figure 30–12. Wedge of bone removed and closed by gently dorsiflexing the foot. The medial cortex must remain intact.

healing is adequate. This procedure can be performed similarly on the medial side of the calcaneus by creating an opening wedge osteotomy with a bone graft inserted to swing the calcaneus out of varus.

Steindler Stripping

Under pneumatic tourniquet control, a 3.5-cm longitudinal skin incision is made on the medial aspect of the foot to provide adequate exposure of the plantar tuberosity of the calcaneus. After cutting through the subcutaneous tissues, blunt dissection can be used to separate the fat pad from the plantar fascia. The fascia is isolated by bluntly freeing it from the plantar intrinsic muscles all the way back to the insertion on the calcaneus. A Smiley knife or meniscotome can then be used to catch the plantar fascia between its prongs. It is sectioned off from its origin as the forefoot is dorsiflexed. The insertion of the abductor hallucis, flexor digitorum brevis, and abductor digiti quinti are isolated from the underlying quadratus plantae muscle and sharply dissected from the calcaneal tuberosity. Care must be taken to avoid the lateral plantar nerve and artery. The abductor hallucis should be resected right at the bony interface when releasing it to avoid neurovascular damage. Finally, the long plantar ligament is isolated under the quadratus plantae muscle belly and sharply released. The forefoot is then dorsiflexed on the rearfoot to assess reduction of the cavus deformity. The subcutaneous tissues are closed with absorbable suture, and the skin is closed with everted nylon sutures. After a sterile, mildly compressive dressing has been applied, a short leg fiberglass cast is applied with the forefoot maximally dorsiflexed on the rearfoot to maintain the reduced cavus deformity. It is advisable to encourage the parents to try to prevent the child from ambulating on the cast for at least 3 weeks; however, this is quite a feat in the youngster. If the child does bear weight it will not disrupt the separation but may slow healing of the incision. In children who I believe will walk no matter what we do, I fabricate the cast in a neutral position with a thickened flat-bottom fiberglass reinforcement.

Dorsiflexory Wedge Osteotomy—First Metatarsal and Lesser Metatarsals

In the rigid anterior cavus foot, osteotomies of the first or all metatarsals can be performed to dorsiflex and reduce the deformity. Proper evaluation of the radiograph is essential. If the procedure is isolated just to the forefoot, the rearfoot must not show any calcaneal elevation or inversion, and the talus must not show evidence of high elevation on the calcaneus. If these conditions are noted, a combined procedure of the forefoot with the rearfoot is indicated.

Three longitudinal incisions are made on the dorsum of the foot. The medial incision gaining access to the first metatarsal base is made directly over the first metatarsal. The other lateral incisions are made between the second and third metatarsals and between the fourth and fifth metatarsals. The incisions are deepened to gain visualization to the metatarsal base periosteum. A periosteal incision is made transversely, and the periosteum is reflected proximally and distally with the use of a Freer elevator. A sagittal saw is used to create an osteotomy wedge with the apex directed plantarly and the base dorsally. The plantar cortex must remain intact because it acts as a stabilizing hinge. If an adductus deformity of the metatarsals is present the base of the wedge is placed slightly lateral on the dorsal surface and the apex is directed plantar medially. When all osteotomies are complete the metatarsals are gently dorsiflexed and secured to the base. Screws, pins, wires, or small staples can be used to accomplish this reduction. The child is maintained in a cast for 6 weeks and should remain nonweight-bearing. A strong plantar plate should be considered if the child accidentally bears weight.

Dorsiflexory Wedge Osteotomy— Cole Procedure

In the cavus foot with no apparent rearfoot inversion component the Cole midfoot procedure can be used to reduce the arch elevation. It should be remembered, however, that the articular surfaces of the cuneiform-navicular joints are resected in this procedure. If the osseous structure of the foot is immature, the procedure is not indicated.

Under pneumatic tourniquet control, two longitudinal skin incisions are mapped out. A 5-cm medial incision is made over the navicular-cuneiform joint between the anterior and posterior tibial tendon insertions. The subcutaneous tissues are divided, taking care to avoid the vessels in this area. The tibialis anterior tendon is identified and retracted dorsomedially while the tibialis posterior is retracted plantarly. A periosteal incision is made on the navicular and medial cuneiform and elevated, preserving the talonavicular joint. Another dorsal linear skin incision is made over the medial aspect of the cuboid. The extensor brevis muscle belly is identified and retracted laterally, and the extensor longus tendons are retracted medially. A periosteal incision is made into the cuboid. A key elevator can be used to elevate all the soft tissue and neurovascular bundle dorsally. The medial and lateral surgical areas are now connected.

A malleable retractor is placed across the foot from medial to lateral underneath the soft tissue; this will protect the soft tissue from the osteotomies. The longer No. 240 blade is used with the microsagittal saw to perform a through-and-through osteotomy across the navicular and cuboid. An osteotome and mallet can be used to complete the cut if the sagittal saw fails to reach across the opposite cortex. A second osteotomy is then performed through the cuneiform bones to excise a dorsally based transverse wedge of bone. The width of the wedge of bone should coincide with the severity of the deformity. The forefoot is dorsiflexed on the rearfoot to close down the osteotomy site, thus reducing the cavus deformity.

It may be necessary to perform other procedures to release soft tissue contractures that may restrict full closure across the osteotomy site. Steinmann pins, staples, or cancellous screws can be used to fix the osteotomy. The tissue should be closed in layers, and a closed suction drain is recommended. The patient is immobilized in a nonweight-bearing short leg cast for at least 6 weeks. I prefer to use a walking brace for an additional 2 to 3 weeks until the child feels secure enough to walk unassisted and the fusion site is well coapted.

Jones Tenosuspension

Under pneumatic tourniquet control, a 5-cm dorsal linear skin incision is performed just medial to the extensor hallucis longus tendon beginning on the hallux just proximal to the proximal nail fold and extending onto the first metatarsal. Dissection through the subcutaneous tissues allows visualization of the extensor tendon, which is bluntly isolated. The extensor hallucis longus tendon is then transected at its distal insertion at the great toe, tagged, and freed up proximally. A periosteal incision is made on the first metatarsal, and the periosteum is elevated with a Freer elevator. A drill hole is made in the center of the first metatarsal on the medial aspect of the head. The hole travels from medial to lateral and is just large enough to allow passage of the extensor tendon. I prefer to use a power trephine because a core from the metatarsal head can be removed. The core is then replaced in the excavated hole bearing the tendon. The tendon may or may not occupy the entire hole, and the core can be modified to fit snugly and ensure tenodesis with the metatarsal. The tendon is looped through the drill hole from medial to lateral and sutured onto itself with the medial forefoot in dorsiflexion to reduce the plantar-flexed first metatarsal. A hallux interphalangeal joint fusion is recommended in conjunction with this procedure to prevent a cock-up hallux deformity. The tissue layers are closed anatomically. A short leg cast is applied with the foot in the corrected position. Weight bearing is discouraged; however, a reinforced plantar shelf on the cast can protect against the inevitable.

References

1. Dwyer FC: Osteotomy of the calcaneum for pes cavus. J Bone Joint Surg 1959; 41B:80.
2. Dwyer FC: The present status of the problem of pes cavus. Clin Orthop 1975; 106:254.
3. Jay RM, Schoenhaus HD: Cavus deformity—conservative management. J Am Podiatr Med Assoc 1980; 70(5):235–238.
4. Burns L, Burns MJ, Burns GA: A clinical application of biomechanics. J Am Podiatr Assoc 1973; 63:394–460.
5. Root ML, Orien JH, Weed JH: Biomechanical Examination of the Foot. Los Angeles, Clinical Biomechanics Corp., 1971.
6. Japas LM: Surgical Treatment of pes cavus by tarsal V osteotomy. J Bone Joint Surg 1968; 50A:927–944.
7. Krackow KJA, Hales D, Jones L: Preoperative planning and surgical technique for performing a Dwyer calcaneal osteotomy. J Pediatr Orthop 1985; 5:214–218.
8. Ayres MJ, Bakst RH, Baskwill DF, Pupp G: Dwyer osteotomy: A retrospective study. J Foot Surg 1987; 26:429–434.

31

Cole Midfoot Osteotomy

Bruce D. Harley, D.P.M.

PRINCIPLES

A dorsiflexory wedge osteotomy is placed through the lesser tarsus. The base of the wedge is dorsal and the apex is plantar. The Cole procedure[6] involves resection of the naviculocuneiform joints and an osteotomy of the cuboid. The procedure is used to correct sagittal plane lesser tarsal deformities in patients with pes cavus conditions. The navicular and the cuneiform bones are osteotomized through all cortices. The naviculocuneiform articulations are reinforced plantarly by strong ligaments. The plantar cortex of the cuboid is left intact to ensure sagittal plane stability.

The axis of the osteotomy is at the junction of the frontal and transverse planes, an orientation that maximizes sagittal plane correction. The apex is placed at the plantar cortex of the cuboid. The osteotomy extends from the medial to the lateral column and achieves equal angular correction of each column. Because greater osseous mass is resected from the medial column, a forefoot adductus may result.

Two modifications to correct cavoadductus deformity in the midfoot region may be made. Cavoadductus deformity is a two-component, sagittal plane plantar flexion deformity and a transverse plane adductus deformity of the midfoot region. The first modification involves changing the orientation of the osteotomy axis from a dorsomedial direction to a plantar lateral one. With this technique the mass of bone resected is more uniform from medial to lateral. Placement of the axis at this angle enables a combined correction of the sagittal and transverse plane deformity. The distal fragment is dorsiflexed and abducted into a rectus anatomic position.

The second modification involves a dorsiflexory naviculocuneiform joint resection of the medial column and a laterally based trapezoidal cuboid osteotomy of the lateral column. The dorsiflexory correction is directed primarily at the medial column because the sagittal plane pathology is more severe in this region.[11] Osteotomy correction of the medial column alone can result in exacerbation of forefoot adductus because of the osseous shortening. Resection of a laterally based trapezoid from the cuboid enables application of several geometrical principles. The trapezoidal cuboid osteotomy shortens the lateral column and allows transverse plane abduction of the forefoot. Transverse correction is achieved by rotating the forefoot about a relatively vertical axis located at the lateral aspect of the naviculocuneiform osteotomy-fusion. This centrally located axis increases the amount of abductory correction while minimizing the mass of osseous resection.

After gross anatomic correction has been achieved, the foot is carefully evaluated. The osteotomy is reciprocally planed to ensure flush apposition of the osteotomy-fusion site. Fixation devices are inserted at this time.

Another modification of the Cole procedure involves performing dorsiflexory wedge cuneiform osteotomies rather than naviculocuneiform fusion.[21] The naviculocuneiform joints are preserved by this technique. The disadvantage is that the amount of correction is limited by the small size of the cuneiforms. A pes cavus deformity that requires a midfoot osteotomy for correction is usually a severe deformity. A significant wedge should be resected to achieve adequate reduction. Fusion of the naviculocuneiform joint is generally the midfoot procedure of choice for correction of severe cavus deformities.

Fixation is usually achieved by using three dorsally placed barbed bone staples. The plantar ligamentous structures are very strong, so fixation is only required dorsally. Staples are the simplest and most effective form of fixation for this type of osteotomy.

INDICATIONS

The Cole midfoot osteotomy-fusion is performed to correct severe pes cavus conditions in patients who have a plantar-flexion deformity in the midfoot[6, 14] region (Fig. 31–1). Surgical correction is directed at the apex of the deformity. The deformity should be evaluated both clinically and radiographically. The neuromuscular status of the patient must be either normal or amenable to rebalancing by tendon transfer techniques.[2, 3, 7, 9, 17] Failure to rebalance the soft tissue apparatus will result in recurrence of the deformity.[3, 5, 9, 12, 15, 18, 19]

The Cole procedure is performed in combination with other pes cavus operations.[1, 3, 8, 13, 17] Correction of all aspects of the deformity is necessary to achieve a successful outcome.

CONTRAINDICATIONS

A neuromuscular imbalance of either central or peripheral origin that cannot be corrected by a rebalancing

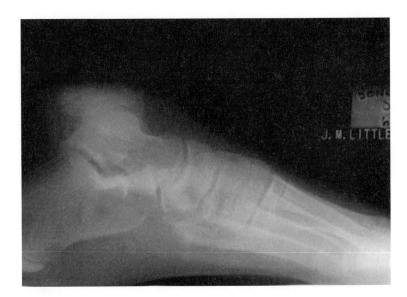

Figure 31–1. Pes cavus deformity. Lateral view of preoperative foot.

operation is a contraindication; failure to achieve neuromuscular balance by such procedures as tendon transfers or digital fusions will result in recurrence of the deformity.[2, 3, 7, 9, 17] When rebalancing is not possible, the osseous rearfoot correction should be achieved by triple arthrodesis, which results in correction and stability.[7]

The Cole procedure is not indicated when the apex of the deformity is in a location other than the midfoot.[6] A pes cavus condition with multiple deformities requires multiple procedures for corrrection.[17]

APPROACH AND SURGICAL DISSECTION

The Cole procedure has been performed using several different incisional techniques, including single, double, and three-incision approaches. The incisions are oriented in a linear fashion. Each approach has its advantages and disadvantages. The single-incision approach requires a longer incision and more forceful retraction. Wide exposure is achieved by the two-incision technique, which consists of linear medial and lateral incisions in the midfoot region. The medial incision is placed over the extensor hallucis longus tendon and is centered at the naviculocuneiform joint. The lateral incision is placed along the lateral border of the extensor digitorum brevis muscle belly and is centered over the cuboid. This is generally the most effective technique.

The three-incision approach includes the medial and lateral incisions of the double approach. A third incision is placed centrally. The advantages of the three-incision approach include wide exposure, ease in performing the osteotomy, and less forceful retraction. The three-incision approach provides excellent exposure and allows the use of a shorter saw blade. Shorter saw blades afford greater control and result in a more exact osteotomy. The disadvantage of this technique is that the excessive dissection can result in wound dehiscence and more swelling.

TECHNIQUE

The medial incision is placed over the extensor hallucis longus tendon and is centered over the naviculocuneiform joint. The incision is deepened through the superficial fascia to the capsuloperiosteal layer. Superficial bleeders are ligated or coagulated; ligation is preferred to electrocoagulation because of the proximity of the medial marginal vein. The extensor hallucis longus tendon is identified and retracted. The neurovascular bundle is then identified just lateral to the extensor hallucis longus. The capsuloperiosteal layer is incised in a linear fashion just medial to the dorsalis pedis artery. The osseous structures are exposed for osteotomy using a subperiosteal dissection technique.[20] A scalpel blade is the best instrument for dissection in the lesser tarsus because the cortical surface is generally rough. Subperiosteal dissection is carried laterally from the medial incision to preserve the neurovascular bundle. Direct handling of the artery and nerve should be avoided because it can lead to neurovascular damage.

The lateral incision is placed along the lateral border of the extensor digitorum brevis muscle belly. Dissection is carried directly through the superficial fascia and the capsuloperiosteal layer. The extensor digitorum brevis can be retracted medially to allow more medial placement of the capsuloperiosteal incision. Subperiosteal dissection is performed with a scalpel blade and a quarter-inch Key elevator to expose the osseous tissue sufficiently for the proposed osteotomy. The medial and lateral incisions should be joined subperiosteally to allow accurate visualization and performance of the midfoot osteotomy. Malleable retractors allow good visualization, reduce the number of hand rakes required, and require less assistance.

The osseous midfoot structures are carefully examined, and the osteotomy is marked on the dorsal cortex. The axis of the osteotomy is generally at the juncture of the transverse and frontal planes at the plantar cortex of the cuboid. In pes cavus conditions the naviculocuneiform region is located farther from this plantar axis. A greater

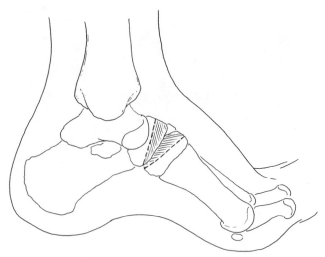

Figure 31–2. Wedge resection of the medial column. Planned resection of cuneiform–navicular joint.

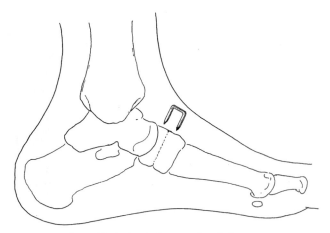

Figure 31–4. Staple fixation of medial aspect.

amount of bone must be removed medially to obtain a congruent medial to lateral wedge. The navicular is very narrow from anterior to posterior, so the majority of the wedge resection must come from the cuneiform bones.

The plane of the naviculocuneiform joint is visualized, and the navicular resection is wedged slightly dorsal.[20] The apex of the wedge should be located plantarly at the junction of the plantar and anterior navicular surfaces. The anterior portion of the wedge osteotomy is performed through the cuneiforms. Approximately 1 cm of bone is initially removed from the dorsum of the medial column. The cuboid osteotomy is made parallel with the navicular osteotomy from a lateral approach and is angled obliquely posteriorly as visualized from the dorsal point of view. The cuboid osteotomy converges at the plantar cortex of the cuboid, forming a wedge. The plantar cortex is left intact and serves as a fixation device. The strong plantar ligaments, the intrinsic musculature, and the plantar fascia provide plantar reinforcement for the medial column.

The osteotomy is closed by forced dorsiflexion of the forefoot on the rearfoot. The adequacy of correction is carefully evaluated, and further osseous resection is per-

formed when necessary. After the desired correction has been obtained, the high points of the osteotomy interface are reduced using a reciprocal planing technique. The osteotomy is then flushed with a saline or antibiotic solution.

Fixation is achieved using three barbed Blount bone staples. One staple holds the cuboid, one holds the navicular-first cuneiform fusion, and the third holds the navicular-third cuneiform fusion. Extrinsic and intrinsic compression is achieved by staple technique. Extrinsic compression is the manual compression obtained prior to the insertion of the staples and is maintained by the staples. Intrinsic compression refers to the compression obtained by divergent predrill technique. Divergent predrilling allows the achievement of compression as the staple is inserted. The angle of divergence is 5 degrees. Predrilling with a 5/64-inch Steinmann pin prevents fracture of the cortex.

The Cole procedure has now been completed. The malleable retractors are removed, and the wound is packed. All other pes cavus surgical procedures are completed, and closure of all incisions is achieved simultaneously. A closed suction drainage system is inserted subperiosteally prior to closure. Closure consists of 3–0 absorbable suture for the capsuloperiosteal layer, 4–0 absorbable suture for the subcutaneous tissue, and 4–0

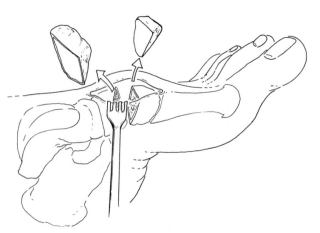

Figure 31–3. Resection of osteotomized cuneiform and navicular.

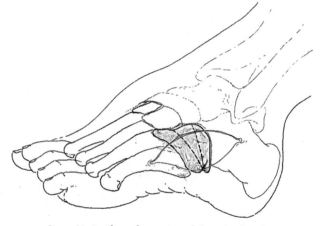

Figure 31–5. Planned resection of the cuboid wedge.

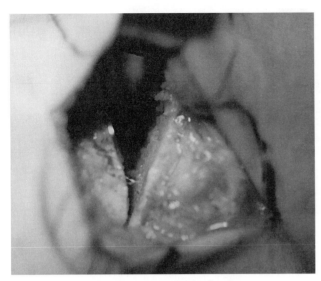

Figure 31–6. Resected cuboid wedge.

nylon for skin. Because swelling can be fairly significant in major reconstructive operations, larger gauge suture is recommended because it does not cut into the skin (Figs. 31–2 to 31–10).

A sterile dressing and a posterior splint are applied to the foot and leg at the completion of surgery. The initial dressing change is performed 2 to 3 days postoperatively.

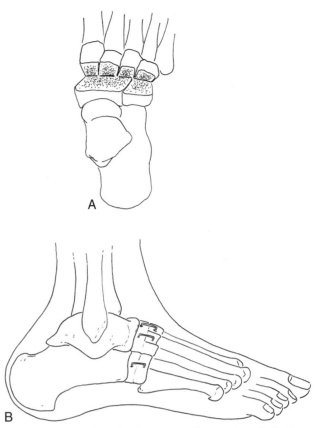

Figure 31–8. A and B, Closed osteotomized site with staple fixation.

The drains are removed, and a below-the-knee cast is applied at this time.

POSTOPERATIVE MANAGEMENT

A 5- to 6-week nonweight-bearing period is generally employed in the postoperative management of the Cole procedure. This nonweight-bearing period allows osseous union to proceed free of disruptive forces and is consis-

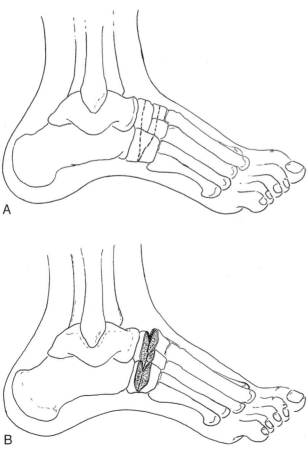

Figure 31–7. A, Total plan of resection. B, Total wedge resected.

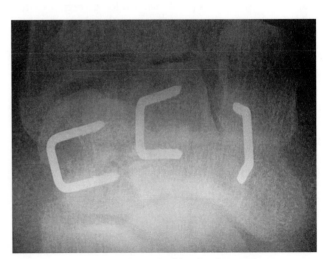

Figure 31–9. Radiograph of fused Cole procedure.

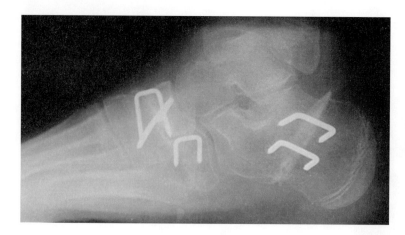

Figure 31–10. Postoperative radiograph of total reduction.

tent with current bone healing and bone fixation principles.

The plantar ligamentous and muscular structures are very strong. The plantar aspect of the osteotomy is under tension during weight bearing, and the tension is resisted by these structures. As long as plantar gapping is prevented, no disruption of the osteotomy site should occur. Individuals undergoing the Cole procedure, in the absence of unstable metatarsal base osteotomies, have traditionally been allowed to bear weight 2 to 3 weeks postoperatively after application of a below-the-knee weight-bearing cast.

COMPLICATIONS

Failure to address all components of the pes cavus foot will lead to inadequate correction of the deformity.[3, 10, 17] Failure to neutralize a neuromuscular imbalance by tendon transfer will lead to recurrence of the pes cavus deformity. When neuromuscular imbalances cannot be neutralized, major fusion techniques such as triple arthrodesis are indicated to prevent recurrence. Midfoot arthrosis is a rare complication of this procedure. Fixation device irritation may occur. Staples are easily removed after osseous union has been achieved. The amount of swelling and pain is similar to that reported with other major reconstructive operations. Undercorrection of the deformity may occur if wedge resection is inadequate. Delayed osseous union and nonunion are rare in the midfoot region.

SUMMARY

The Cole procedure is performed in combination with other osseous and soft tissue procedures. This multiprocedural approach to pes cavus correction is diagnostically and technically difficult. A detailed understanding of the relevant anatomy, biomechanical principles,[4, 12, 16] surgical dissection, tendon transfer techniques, and methods of internal fixation is necessary. The operative time is generally longer than that needed for triple arthrodesis.

References

1. Alvik I: Operative treatment of pes cavus. Acta Orthop Scand 1953; 23:137.
2. Basmajian JV, et al: The role of muscles in arch support of the foot. J Bone Joint Surg 1963; 45A:1181–1190.
3. Bradley GW, et al: Treatment of the calcaneocavus foot deformity. J Bone Joint Surg 1983; 63A:1159–1166.
4. Seibel MD: Foot Function. Baltimore, Williams & Wilkins, 1988, pp. 179–182, 202–205.
5. Chuinard EG, Baskins M: Clawfoot deformity. J Bone Joint Surg 1973; 55A:2.
6. Cole WH: The treatment of claw-foot. J Bone Joint Surg 1940; 23:4.
7. Coonrad RW, et al: The importance of plantar muscles in paralytic varus feet: The results of treatment by neurectomy and myotenotomy. J Bone Joint Surg 1956; 38A:563–566.
8. Dwyer FC: The present status of the problem of pes cavus. Clin Orthop 1975; 106:254.
9. Hibbs RA: An operation for "claw foot." JAMA 1919; 73:1583–1585.
10. Jahss MH: Tarsometatarsal truncated-wedge arthodesis for pes cavus and equinovarus deformity of the fore part of the foot. J Bone Joint Surg 1980; 62:713–722.
11. McElvenny RT, Caldwell GD: A new operation of correction of cavus foot: Fusion of first metatarsocuneiform navicular joints. Clin Orthop 1958; 11:85–92.
12. McGlamry ED, Kitting RW: Equinus foot—analysis of the etiology, pathology and treatment techniques. J Am Podiatry Assoc 1973; 63:164–184.
13. Mitchell GP: Posterior displacement osteotomy of the calcaneus. J Bone Joint Surg 1977; 59B:233.
14. Japas LM: Surgical treatment of pes cavus by tarsal vosteotomy. J Bone Joint Surg 1968; 50A:927–944.
15. Paulos L, et al: Pes cavovarus. J Bone Joint Surg 1980; 62(A):942.
16. Root ML, Orien WD, Weed JH: Normal and Abnormal Function of the Foot, vol. II. Los Angeles, Clinical Biomechanics Co, 1977, pp. 344–345.
17. Samilson RL, Dillin W: Cavus, cavovarus and calcaneocavus. Clin Orthop 1983; 177:125–132.
18. Steindler A: Operative treatment of pes cavus: Stripping of the os calcis. Surg Gynecol Obstet 1917; 24:612–615.
19. Steindler A: The treatment of pes cavus. Arch Surg 1921; 2:325.
20. Tachdjian MO: Pediatric Orthopedics, Vol. 2. Philadelphia, W. B. Saunders, 1972.
21. Wilcox PG, Weiner DS: The Akron midarsal dome osteotomy in the treatment of rigid pes cavus: A preliminary review. J Pediatr Orthop 1985; 5(3):333–338.

32

Tarsal Coalition

Stephen D. Lasday, D.P.M., and Nicholas Pachuda, D.P.M.

COALITIONS

In the young child it has been reported that the most common site of fibrocartilaginous unions is the posterior region of the subtalar joint. It is common practice for the coalesced joint to be mobilized rather than fused. Release of the fibrous tissue can restore motion to the rearfoot, but only when the foot matures (at 16 to 18 years of age) does one consider any type of single or multiple joint fusions.[1] Conservative treatment of calcaneonavicular bridges usually fails, and success is reported when this bridge is resected in the young active child. Subtalar fusion is not necessary even in the presence of talar beaking in a child who is first seen with calcaneonavicular coalition. However, in the adult, the prognosis is worse if talar beaking is present. Simple resection of the calcaneonavicular bar in the adult, replacing the bone with wax, silicone, or interposition of the belly of the extensor digitorum brevis, does not guarantee mobilization. The young child is more active, and it is possible that this activity level explains the higher success rate in children.[2]

The difficulty with coalitions and the usual complication that arises in young children who complain of pain in the rearfoot is the risk of misdiagnosis and inappropriate treatment. Without proper visualization of the rearfoot one cannot treat this condition. Computed tomography (CT) has certainly helped in the diagnosis of osseous or narrow coalitions, but with the aid of magnetic resonance imaging (MRI) one can isolate the exact position, thickness, and length of the fibrous bond in any of the joints.

When the subtalar joint is restricted and the midtarsal joint loses its gliding motion, the talus starts to override the navicular, and talar beaking results[3] (Figs. 32–1 and 32–2). When the coalition is present in the early development stages, adjacent joint changes also take place. In addition to the future arthritic changes and adaptive changes (lipping and jamming of joints) that occur, another phenomenon occurs at the ankle. The development of the ball and socket ankle is a compensatory response to the restricted motion of the subtalar joint[4] (Figs. 32–3 to 32–5). The tibial plafond becomes concave, and the dome appears to be convex and ball-shaped; the ankle joint then accepts a full range of motion in dorsiflexion, plantar flexion, inversion, and eversion. Ankle stability is at risk; however, since the foot is in a valgus position, and since after fusion this is the position one strives for, the instability is not pronounced. In the older child or the child who develops the coalition late, the result will not be a ball and socket ankle but an ankle with degenerative joint changes. This is the type of ankle that will eventually require pantalar fusions. As with many childhood conditions, early recognition reduces the need for future radical complication-prone procedures (Figs. 32–6 to 32–8).

Although tarsal coalitions have been a documented

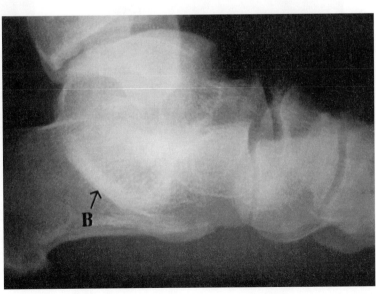

Figure 32–1. Subtalar coalition with beaking of the anterior process of the talus as well as navicular beaking. A full halo sign is marked (B).

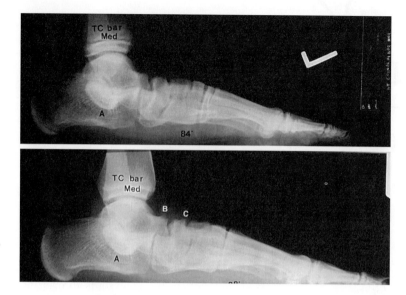

Figure 32–2. Four-year progression of talocalcaneal bar. Note loss of the subtalar joint at the middle facet and the increase in beaking noted at B and C in 1988.

clinical entity for hundreds of years, new ideas and approaches have surfaced in the last several years that warrant close scrutiny. This chapter will concentrates on talocalcaneal and calcaneonavicular coalitions. Other types of coalition in the rearfoot, midfoot, and forefoot are not often symptomatic and are almost always incidental findings. The surgical correction of tarsal coalition is reviewed giving some consideration to newer aspects of treatment. In addition, the concept of a subclinical calcaneonavicular bar, which we refer to as a "functional coalition," is presented, along with treatment options. Clinically useful diagnostic tools are also discussed.

Written documentation of the tarsal coalition as an anatomic entity extends back over two centuries, beginning with Buffon.[5] Other authors wrote various treatises on specific sites of coalition throughout the nineteenth century, including talocalcaneal, calcaneonavicular, and talonavicular[6] coalitions. The pathology was first seen ra-

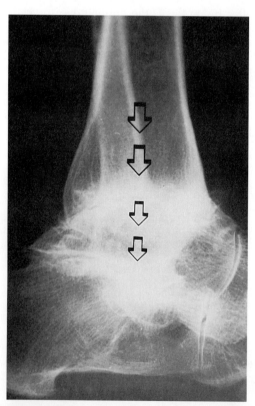

Figure 32–3. Traumatic pantalar coalition *(arrows)*. Direct compression after a fall in this 17-year-old eventually created fusion of the subtalar and ankle joint.

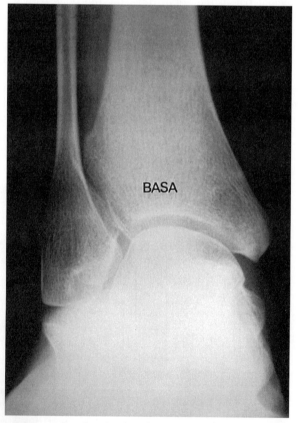

Figure 32–4. Ball and socket (BASA) joint secondary to early subtalar coalition. Note thickening of the fibular styloid process and rounding of the talar dome with joint adaptation of the tibia.

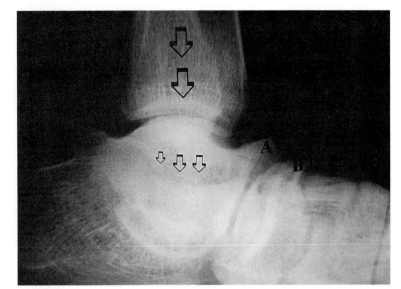

Figure 32–5. Subtalar coalition in a 16-year-old with compression of the talus on the calcaneus *(arrows)*; the result is marked beaking of the remaining talar head (A) along with beaking of the navicular (B). There is jamming at the cuneiform-navicular joint as well.

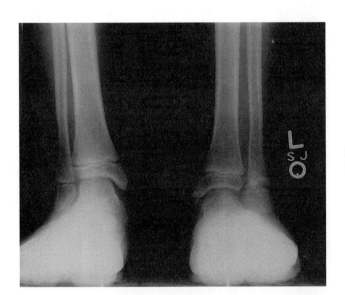

Figure 32–6. Left ball and socket ankle secondary to middle facet coalition in a 9-year-old. (Courtesy A. Saxena, D.P.M.)

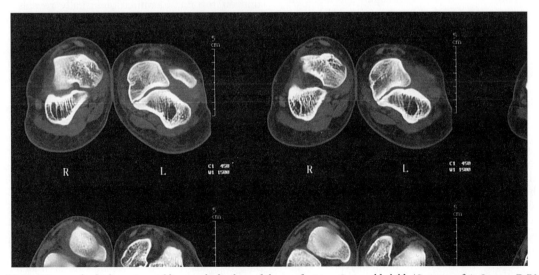

Figure 32–7. CT scan of subtalar union yielding marked valgus of the rearfoot in a 9-year-old child. (Courtesy of A. Saxena, D.P.M.)

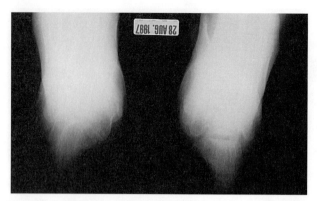

Figure 32–8. Harris-Beath view of middle facet union and drop of middle facet angle in a 9-year-old child. (Courtesy A. Saxena, D.P.M.)

diographically by Korvin in 1934,[7] and it was actually this technique that Harris and Beath refined and popularized in 1948.[8] In fact, in their 1948 paper, Harris and Beath discussed surgical techniques that offered new perspectives on the current treatment of the era, although they are most commonly remembered for their radiologic insights. Their work allowed visualization of the posterior and middle subtalar joint facets, and Isherwood described how to obtain a very technically difficult view of the anterior facet in 1961.[9] Other imaging techniques have gained and lost popularity in the last 30 years, ranging from scintigraphy[10] to arthrography.[11] CT scanning was the imaging technique of choice throughout the 1980s and probably still is the most common procedure ordered by foot and ankle specialists. Since Smith and Staple described this technique in 1983, it has become a widely accepted diagnostic tool for visualizing tarsal coalitions.[12–19]

MRI was mentioned in 1989 as a method of evaluating tarsal coalition,[20] and in 1990 Pachuda and colleagues[21] strongly suggested that MRI, not CT, should be the primary imaging technique used for understanding tarsal coalition because this abnormality involves a high prevalence of nonosseous coalitions, especially in skeletally immature patients. Fibrous and cartilaginous bridges are not clearly defined on CT, but they are on MRI, as is osseous tissue.

ETIOLOGY

Although many causes of tarsal coalition have been proposed,[6, 22–26] it is commonly accepted that an autosomal dominant gene, initially appearing as a mutant, causes the fetal mesenchyme to halt normal developmental differentiation. The clinical outcome is a fusion of two or more bones of the tarsus. Of course, coalitions are also acquired, either as a result of inciting trauma or as a chronic degenerative process. Enlightening new research from Japan even shows that tarsal coalitions can be induced during pregnancy by exposure to selected teratogenic agents.[27] An intra-articular joint depression type of calcaneal fracture is probably the most common type of traumatically induced subtalar coalition, whereas biomechanical arthrosis in the lesser tarsus is seen commonly in children with chronic pes planus. Other types of acquired fusion, including infectious and autoimmune arthropathies, are even less common, and these, owing to pain or patient disability, are most often seen clinically prior to complete fusion.

The incidence of tarsal fusion has always been reported to be predominantly male, but this information is skewed because early studies were performed on army recruits; the present reported frequency is 1% to 2%.[6, 28, 29] A number of studies performed in this decade have reported ratios that come close to sexual equality.[30, 31] Talocalcaneal and calcaneonavicular coalitions are by far the most common types, with combined rates approaching 90%. Talonavicular coalitions are a distant third and almost always involve complete osseous fusions that are asymptomatic.

CLINICAL FEATURES

The presence of rearfoot, midfoot, or ankle pain should always alert the practitioner to a possible coalition. Despite the low overall frequency quoted earlier, the frequency of this condition is higher in the patient population of the foot and ankle surgeon. These patients historically have been pediatric, but this fact is due to the higher demands usually made on children who participate in scholastic athletic programs. Our personal experience has demonstrated that coalitions first appear symptomatic in all age groups, with less selection to the pediatric population. In adults, the inciting problem is either injury or chronic untreated pes planus, which leads to biomechanical failure of the medial column over time, and the associated immobility of the rearfoot cannot keep up with the changing demands of the midfoot.

The pain is located in the tarsus, tarsal sinus, or ankle. Occasionally the arch is involved. There may or may not be a related report of a recent or past injury. The onset of symptoms is usually insidious. The discomfort may not always occur in the area of the coalition and is often referred pain. Pain increases with activity, especially on uneven terrain. Examination usually reveals stiffness in the affected joint, which has a severely decreased and painful range of motion.

Peroneal spasm is sometimes present, although this is more infrequent than originally believed. The Mayo Clinic reported that 2 of 60 patients with coalition actually had a real peroneal spasm.[32] We have seen spasm in talocalcaneal coalitions as often as in calcaneonavicular bars. Care must be taken to rule out tarsal fracture in patients with peroneal spasm, since any traumatic or inflammatory condition of the tarsus can cause spasm of any adjacent muscle group, including the peroneals. It is also noteworthy that spasm is often the result of functional shortening of the peroneus brevis due to prolonged muscle guarding. In these cases, any attempt at nerve block to relieve the spasm will be fruitless.[33] Nerve blocks are of some value in making the diagnosis in patients in whom the radiographs are equivocal. A calcaneonavicular bar responds very well to anesthesia injected into the tarsal sinus. Several minutes following the injection, the patient should be able to walk and run pain free in

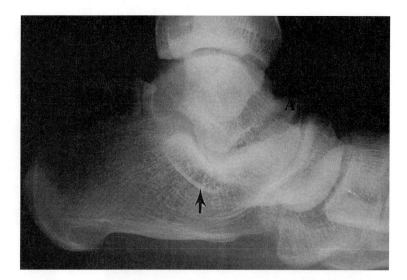

Figure 32–9. The halo sign, which is a sclerotic circle extending from the dome of the talus down below the sustentaculum tali. This is the result of trabecular realignment resulting from increased mechanical stresses. Talar or talonavicular beaking, rounding of the lateral process of the talus, and loss of the subtalar joint space are all signs of talocalcaneal coalition.

the office setting. While it is not pathognomonic, this procedure should place coalition high on the list of the differential diagnosis.

The general appearance of the foot is not always that of a rigid flatfoot. Cavus or rectus feet can also present with tarsal coalition, and the astute practitioner will not exclude a coalition from the differential diagnosis based on the absence of a clinically apparent "flatfoot." More important is the decreased range of motion or painful range of motion in the tarsus. Frontal plane testing should be performed for range of motion on the subtalar joint and Chopart's joint. Stuecker and Bennett reported several cases of subtalar coalition in cavus feet with no associated neuromuscular disease.[34]

IMAGING

Plain film radiographs should be obtained in the anteroposterior, lateral, and lateral oblique views. Classic signs to be observed on the lateral view include the halo sign, which is a sclerotic circle extending from the dome of the talus to below the sustentaculum tali (Fig. 32–9). This is

the result of trabecular realignment due to increased mechanical stresses. Talar or talonavicular beaking, rounding of the lateral process of the talus, and loss of the subtalar joint space are all signs of talocalcaneal coalition, although individually none of these signs confirm the diagnosis (Figs. 32–10 to 32–12). The calcaneonavicular bar appears best on the oblique view as an osseous connection between the calcaneus and the navicular (Fig. 32–13). Even if there is no visible osseous connection, the clinician must consider a fibrous or cartilaginous coalition or a functional coalition, in which there is no real coalition but a demonstrable decrease in functional range of motion. The lateral view of a suspected calcaneonavicular bar shows the anteater sign, which is the enlargement and extension of the anterior beak of the calcaneus.[35]

The next step in the algorithmic approach to radiologic diagnosis has historically been the Harris-Beath or Isherwood views or both. However, since these views are technically difficult to perform and offer absolutely nothing in the way of preoperative planning data, even if technically perfect, we suggest that these techniques be abandoned in favor of the various computed imaging techniques available. The cost of these studies, whether

Figure 32–10. Post-traumatic compression (B) of the posterior and middle facet talocalcaneal coalition. Note narrowing of joint space.

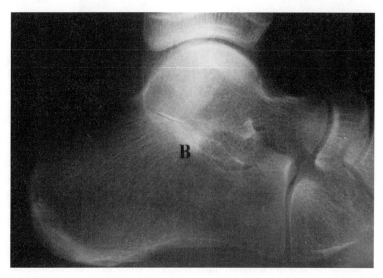

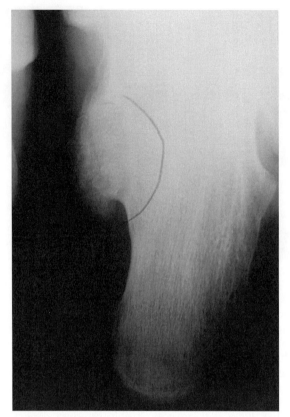

Figure 32–11. Axial radiograph of middle facet talocalcaneal coalition. Hypertrophy of sustentaculum tali is present.

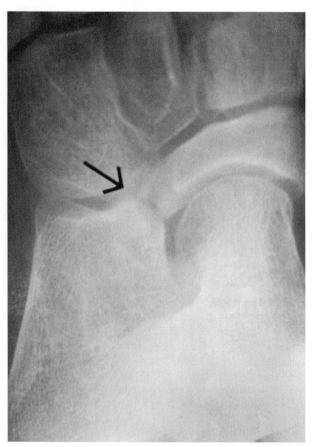

Figure 32–13. Calcaneonavicular coalition *(arrow)*. Oblique view.

MRI or CT, is more than made up by the clarity and wealth of dimensional information afforded by the newer technology.

CT scanners are generally more widely available than

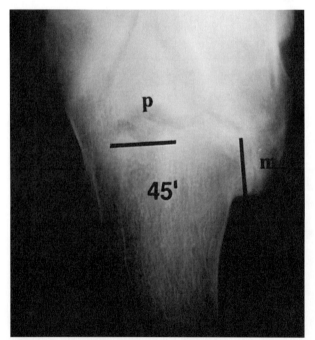

Figure 32–12. Middle facet talocalcaneal coalition. Note the vertical position of the joint in this Harris-Beath view (p, posterior facet; m, middle facet).

MRI equipment. Smaller hospitals are more apt to have a CT scanner than an MRI device. Many new companies own portable MRI units that make weekly rounds to smaller hospitals in a modified tractor trailer. Although these are convenient, they are usually low-powered magnets of 0.5 Tesla$_1$ and provide unacceptable clarity for foot and ankle imaging. When possible, it is well worth the time and effort to refer patients to a center that has a 1.5 Tesla$_1$ magnet and uses the latest software to run the unit. Also, one-on-one interaction with the radiologist is imperative to get the most from an MRI study. The radiologist finds it immensely helpful if the referring doctor includes the important clinical findings as well as the suspected pathology. A call or visit to the radiology department during hospital rounds will result in a more accurate reading of the MRI study as well as mutual education of the radiologist and the foot and ankle surgeon (Figs. 32–14 and 32–15).

CT imaging undeniably produces the best osseous resolution, but MRI technology provides for total visualization of all relevant structures involved in coalition pathology. Many coalitions are of the fibrous or cartilaginous type, and CT affords only incomplete visualization of the site of bridging. MRI, however, delineates the fibrous or cartilaginous soft tissue interface, showing the surgeon the length, width, and direction of the coalition and allowing better preoperative planning. A recent study in the Italian literature showed that MRI allowed more accurate evaluation of talocalcaneal coalition. MRI proved

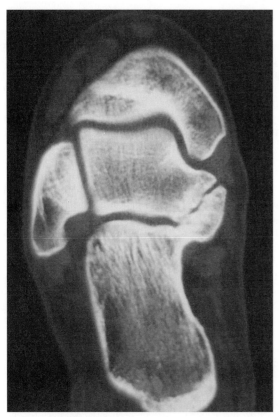

Figure 32–14. Middle facet talocalcaneal coalition is present in this unusual dorsally directed joint.

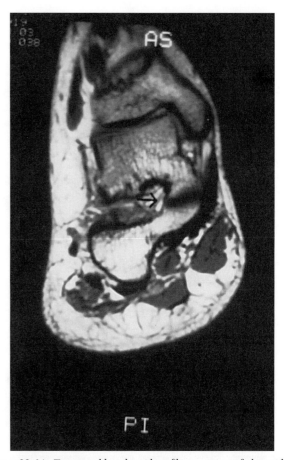

Figure 32–16. Ten-year-old male with a fibrous union of the middle facet of the subtalar joint as detected by MRI.

capable of showing subchondral ischemic disease in a patient with fibrocartilaginous coalition[36] (Fig. 32–16).

TREATMENT

Once the diagnosis has been made, treatment begins with thorough patient education. When the patient has been made aware of his or her condition, a serious estimate must be made of how much pain or disability the patient suffers. If the coalition causes only minor discomfort, it is possible that an orthotic designed to limit the painful motion will be helpful. However, an orthotic is likely to prove unfruitful if serious infirmity is caused by the coalition.

Conservative Management

If injury or overuse brought about the presenting complaint, casting and nonweight bearing for 6 weeks may bring relief of symptoms. However, the great majority of tarsal coalitions are surgical problems. Orthotics, rest, and casting prove useless. It is in the field of surgery that the informed clinician has the most options.

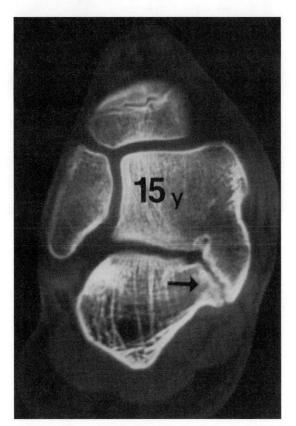

Figure 32–15. Fifteen-year-old with middle facet talocalcaneal coalition. Angular change noted with loss of joint space.

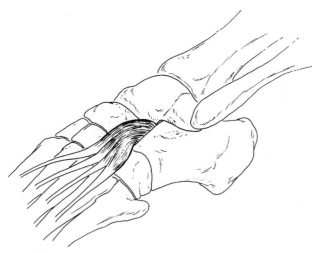

Figure 32–17. Extensor digitorum brevis imbedded in the calcaneus and separating from the navicular.

Surgery

Badgley Procedure

Surgical repair is the definitive treatment when conservative measures fail to bring relief of pain. Resection of the fusion site has been touted as the treatment of choice in children in whom there are no associated degenerative

changes. Badgley's resection has remained the gold standard for almost 60 years in the treatment of calcaneonavicular bar.[37] When performed properly, the procedure is curative. The dissection includes reflection of the extensor digitorum brevis muscle belly distally exposing the bar, although more extensive medial dissection may be needed to fully visualize the bar. The resection must be made in the shape of a plantar-based quadrangle to avoid bone contact plantarly and subsequent reossification. The original procedure included excision of the coalition followed by interposition of the extensor digitorum muscle belly (EDB) between the calcaneus and the navicular. This has the advantage of preventing both hematoma formation from exposed cancellous bone ends and bony regrowth. Modifications using bone wax, cautery of exposed bone, and interposition of adipose tissue[3, 33] can aid in bony regrowth. When passing the Keith needle through the plantar aspect of the foot to secure the EDB, care must be taken because the needle can cause unintended vascular or neurologic damage in the plantar vault of the foot.

New surgical instrumentation has made the Badgley procedure simpler than it was originally. Various soft tissue anchor devices have become available that allow attachment of the EDB between the calcaneus and the navicular. A screw-like device or small piton like those used in mountain climbing is driven into the bone, and the muscle is attached to this bone anchor by suture material of the surgeon's choice (Figs. 32–17 and 32–18).

This procedure also works well for patients who lack a

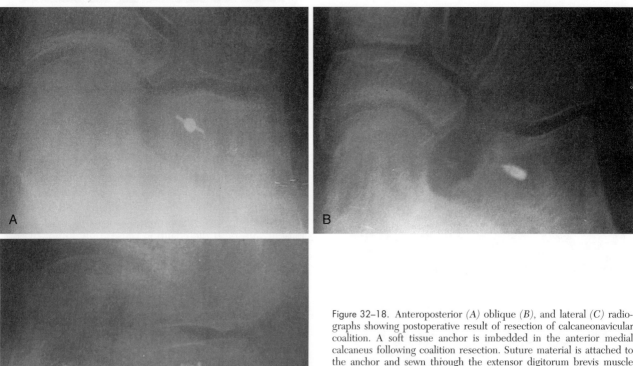

Figure 32–18. Anteroposterior *(A)* oblique *(B)*, and lateral *(C)* radiographs showing postoperative result of resection of calcaneonavicular coalition. A soft tissue anchor is imbedded in the anterior medial calcaneus following coalition resection. Suture material is attached to the anchor and sewn through the extensor digitorum brevis muscle belly. This avoids placement of a needle through the plantar vault, as is done in the traditional procedure.

real coalition but have what we call a functional coalition. We define this as a calcaneonavicular relationship wherein there is no coalition, not even a suspected fibrous coalition, but a functional decrease in range of motion within the tarsus. This clinical entity can be supported by what Harris referred to as a subclinical presentation due to variable genetic penetrance.[8] The radiographic sign of a functional coalition is an anterior beak of the calcaneus that is somewhat enlarged but not as much as in an anteater sign.[35] In such cases, we believe that the enlarged anterior beak of the calcaneus occupies the space between the talus and the cuboid and does not allow a full range of motion in the rearfoot (see Fig. 32–3). These patients also have significant pain in and around the tarsal sinus as well as referred pain to the subtalar and midtarsal complexes. Treatment parallels that used for a real coalition, and therapy should begin with a functional orthotic, but a modified Badgley procedure provides excellent results. Intraoperatively, a distinct space is found between the calcaneus and the navicular. Range of motion is limited because the calcaneal beak jams between the talus and the cuboid (see Fig. 32–4). The calcaneal beak is resected approximately 5 mm, and equal amount is resected from the lateral aspect of the navicular. This change produces an increase in range of motion in the subtalar and midtarsal complexes.

Resection

The painful talocalcaneal coalition is cured by means of the triple arthrodesis in most cases when degenerative changes in adjacent structures are present. Although conservative therapy for the talocalcaneal coalition is similar to that used for other coalitions, it rarely brings total relief of symptoms. Downey presented a classification system that attempts to summarize historical ideas on the subject as well as synthesize proved surgical treatments, and this articular classification is probably the soundest system that has been presented.[38]

Resection of the talocalcaneal coalition in an early stage before biomechanical degeneration has occurred is an acceptable approach. The purpose of resection is to retain the mobility of the rearfoot, especially in the developing foot of the child. Coalition resection has been reported as part of clubfoot repair by Spero and colleagues in 4 of 14 patients.[39] If sectional imaging shows that the coalition measures less than 50% of the involved facet, resection is likely to give acceptable long-term results. If the coalition involves more than 50% of the facet, fusion is the recommended approach.[40] The more the coalition involves the joint, the more narrowed, nonanatomic, nonfunctional joint exists, and therefore resection can be predicted to fail. When resection is chosen, the surgeon can choose to put a spacer in place of the resected coalition, as in the Badgley technique for calcaneonavicular coalition as previously mentioned. One should avoid exuberant resection that can inadvertently create an unstable collapsing subtalar complex. Collins uses a condylar cap that he believes increases postoperative subtalar motion.[41] Kumar and colleagues use a hemisection of the flexor hallucis longus tendon, which is inserted between

the talus and the calcaneus to prevent regrowth. He found that this worked better than interposed adipose tissue.[30]

Resection alone may leave the patient with a relatively rigid deformed foot that has resulted from many years of osseous adaptation to malposition. Some patients may improve after an isolated resection, although those with more serious problems may need flexible flatfoot type reconstructive procedures to correct concomitant deformities. These associated deformities may include sagittal deformities such as ankle equinus and medial column fault. Frontal plane deformities include calcaneal valgus and varus or valgus deformity of the forefoot. Transverse plane deformities usually involve abduction at Chopart's joint.

Arthrodesis

Fusion can produce a predictable result for symptomatic talocalcaneal coalition. There are two ways to approach a possible fusion. The subtalar complex alone can be fused, or a triple arthrodesis can be performed. When the pathology is limited to the subtalar joint and there is no osseous degeneration, an isolated subtalar fusion can be performed. If compensatory changes such as talonavicular beaking or calcaneocuboid spurring have already occurred, triple arthrodesis is the most popular surgical option (Fig. 32–19). However, subtalar fusion with resection of small talar beaks may be a viable alternative to triple arthrodesis (Fig. 32–20).

During surgical exposure of the subtalar joint for arthrodesis, an ancillary medial incision may be necessary to resect the osseous bridge to allow adequate removal of the joint surface through the lateral incision in preparation for fusion. The medial coalition does not allow the joint to be opened wide enough on the lateral aspect. In these cases, removal of the coalition provides some freedom within the subtalar complex to gain wide enough exposure to excise all of the facet cartilage for fusion.

In performing subtalar fusion in children, one must be careful to take into account the degree of osseous maturity that exists. Screw fixation in subtalar arthrodesis must

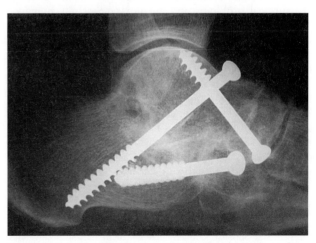

Figure 32–19. Triple arthrodesis in a 16-year-old with subtalar coalition.

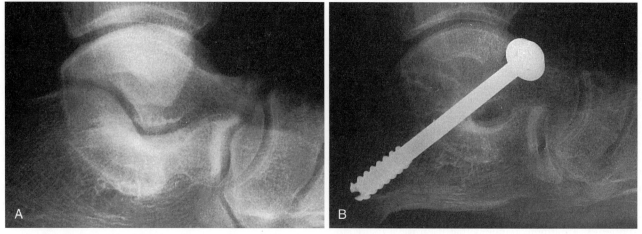

Figure 32–20. *A,* Talocalcaneal coalition in a 15-year-old girl. Note halo sign as well as a small talar beak. *B,* Subtalar fusion was performed because there was no articular damage or joint derangement in the midtarsal joints.

avoid the calcaneal apophysis if it is still open. The literature indicates that approximately 75% of subtalar fusions followed to skeletal maturity are successful. If there are associated deformities that are not addressed, the rate of success drops to 39%.[42]

SUMMARY

The diagnosis of tarsal coalition is simplified by a careful clinical examination followed by appropriate imaging techniques. We stress that coalitions, while historically considered a pediatric deformity, can present in any age group, including adults and the elderly. In addition, coalitions can present in any foot type, including a pes cavus foot. One should not suspect tarsal coalition only in the rigid pes valgus or spastic flatfoot. MRI is the best single technique for analyzing a suspected coalition, especially in the pediatric population, in whom a significant portion of the foot is not yet ossified. Coalitions may occur alone or with associated foot deformities that also must be addressed. The anterior beak of the calcaneus can inhibit full motion and function if it is enlarged and protrudes between the talus and cuboid. This can occur in the absence of an actual calcaneonavicular bar; we call this a functional coalition. The majority of tarsal coalitions are surgical problems and are not successfully managed with conservative therapy. Resection of the coalition is most appropriate in cases of a calcaneonavicular bar or subtalar coalition with no associated pathology. Subtalar fusion works well with talocalcaneal coalitions that are associated with no degeneration in adjacent joints. Talar beaking can be insignificant and does not represent real intra-articular derangement. Resection of the beak allows a successful subtalar fusion if little cartilaginous damage has occurred within the talonavicular joint. Triple arthrodesis provides acceptable results as well and should be reserved for adults with subtalar and midtarsal arthritis.

References

1. Lee MS: Subtalar joint coalition in children: New observations. Radiology 1989; 172:635–639.

2. O'Neill DB: Tarsal coalition: A follow-up of the adolescent athlete. Am J Sports Med 1989; 17:544–549.

3. Mosier KM: Tarsal coalitions and peroneal spastic flatfoot. J Bone Joint Surg 1984; 66A(7):976–983.

4. Takakura Y, Tamai S, Mashura K: Genesis of ball and socket ankle. J Bone Joint Surg 1986; 68B(5):834–837.

5. Buffon GLL: Histoire Naturelle Generale et Particuliere, Vol. 3. Paris, Panckouke, 1769.

6. Cruveilhier J: Anatomie Pathologique du Crops Humain, Vol. 1. Paris, J.B. Balliere, 1829.

7. Korvin H: Coalitio talocalcanea. Z Orthop Chir 1934; 60:105.

8. Harris RI, Beath T: Etiology of peroneal spastic flatfoot. J Bone Joint Surg [Br] 1948; 30(4):624–634.

9. Isherwood I: A radiological approach to the subtalar joint. J Bone Joint Surg [Br] 1961; 43(3):566–574.

10. Goldman AB, Pavlov H, Schneider R: Radionuclide bone scanning in subtalar coalitions: Differential considerations. AJR 1982; 138:427–432.

11. Resnick D: Radiology of the talocalcaneal articulation. Radiology 1974; 111:581–685.

12. Smith RW, Staple TW: Computerized tomography (CT) scanning technique for the hindfoot. Clin Orthop 1983; 177:34–38.

13. Marchisello PJ: The use of computerized axial tomography for the evaluation of talocalcaneal coalition: A case report. J Bone Joint Surg [Am] 1987; 69(4):609–611.

14. Pineda C, Resnick D, Greenway G: Diagnosis of tarsal coalition with computed tomography. Clin Orthop 1986; 208:282–288.

15. Herzenberg JE, Goldner JL, Martinez S, Silverman PM: Computerized tomography of talocalcaneal tarsal coalition: A clinical and anatomic study. Foot Ankle 1986; 6(6):273–288.

16. Migliori V, Pupp J, Kanat IO: Computerized tomography as a diagnostic aid in a middle facet talocalcaneal coalition. J Am Podiatr Med Assoc 1985; 75(8):406–410.

17. Sarno RC, Carter BL, Bankoff MS, Semine MC: Computed tomography in tarsal coalition. J Comput Tomog 1984; 8(6):1155–1160.

18. Stoskopf CA, Hernandez RJ, Kelikian A, Tachdjian MO, Dias LS: Evaluation of tarsal coalition by computed tomography. J Pediatr Orthop 1984; 4(3):365–369.

19. Martinez S, et al: Computed tomography of the hindfoot. Orthop Clin North Am 1985; 16(3):481–496.

20. Crimm JR, Cracchiolo A, Bassett LW, et al: Magnetic resonance imaging of the hindfoot, foot and ankle. 1989; 10(1):1–7.

21. Pachuda NM, Lasday SD, Jay RM: Tarsal coalition: Etiology, diagnosis, and treatment. J Foot Surg 1990; 29:474–488.

22. Outland T, Murphy ID: Relation of tarsal anomalies to spastic and rigid flatfeet. Clin Orthop 1953; 1:217–227.

23. Harris RI: Rigid valgus foot due to talocalcaneal bridge. J Bone Joint Surg 1955; 37A:169.

24. Wiles S, Pallidino SJ, Stavosky JW: Naviculocuneiform coalition. J Am Podiatr Med Assoc 1988; 78(7):355–360.

25. Leboucq H: De la soudure congenitale de certains os du tarse. Bull Acad R Med Belg 1890; 4:103–112.

26. Wray JB, Herndon CN: Hereditary transmission of congenital coalition of the calcaneus to the navicular. J Bone Joint Surg 1963; 45A:365–372.

27. Rahman ME, Ishikawa H, Watanabe Y, Endo A: Carpal and tarsal bone anomalies in mice induced by maternal treatment of Ara-C. Reprod Toxicol 1994; 8:41–47.

28. Vaughan WH, Segal G: Tarsal coalition, with special reference to roentgenographic interpretation. Radiology 1953; 60:855–863.

29. Ehrlich MG: Tarsal coalition. In Jahss MH (ed): Disorders of the Foot, Vol 1. Philadelphia, W.B. Saunders, 1982, pp. 521–538.

30. Kumar SJ, Guille JT, Lee MS, Couto JC: Osseous and non-osseous coalition of the middle facet of the talocalcaneal joint. J Bone Joint Surg 1992; 74A:529–535.

31. Gonzalez P, Kumar SJ: Calcaneonavicular coalition treated by resection and interposition of the extensor digitorum brevis muscle. J Bone Joint Surg 1990; 72A:71–77.

32. Stormont DM, Peterson HA: The relative incidence of tarsal coalition. Clin Orthop 1983; 181:28–36.

33. Downey MS: Tarsal coalition: Current clinical aspects with introduction of a surgical classification. In Mcglamry ED (ed): Reconstructive Surgery of the Foot and Leg—Update '89. Tucker, GA, Podiatry Institute, 1989.

34. Stuecker RD, Bennett JT: Tarsal coalition presenting as a pes cavovarus deformity. Foot Ankle 1993; 14:540–544.

35. Oestreich AE, Mize WA, Crawford AH, Morgan RC: The anteater nose sign: A direct sign of calcaneonavicular coalition on the lateral radiograph. J Pediatr Orthop 1987; 7(6):709–711.

36. Masciocchi C, D'Archivio C, Barile A, Fascetti E, Zobel BB, Galluci M, Passariello R: Talocalcanel coalition: Computed tomography and magnetic resonance imaging diagnosis. Eur J Radio 1992; 15:22–25.

37. Badgley CE: Coalition of the calcaneus and navicular. Arch Surg 1927; 15:75–88.

38. Downey MS: Tarsal coalition. In Mcglamry ED, Banks AS, Downey MS (eds): Comprehensive Textbook of Foot Surgery, 2nd ed. Baltimore, Williams & Wilkins, 1992, pp. 898–930.

39. Spero CR, Simon GS, Tornetta P: Clubfeet and tarsal coalition. J Pediatr Orthop 1994; 14:372–376.

40. Wilde PH, Torode IP, Dickens DR, Cole WG: Resection for symptomatic talocalcaneal coalition. J Bone Joint Surg [Br] 1994; 76B:797–801.

41. Collins B: Tarsal coalitions: A new surgical procedure. Clin Podiatr 1987; 4(1):75–98.

42. Scott SM, Janes PC, Stevens PM: Grice subtalar arthrodesis followed to skeletal maturity. J Pediatr Orthop 1988; 8(2):176–183.

33

Soft Tissue Calcaneonavicular Coalition

Richard M. Jay, D.P.M., Gary Feldman, D.P.M.,
and Diane Collier, D.P.M.

Tarsal coalition is an abnormal union between adjoining tarsal bones that causes restriction or absence of motion. The exact cause of tarsal coalitions is unclear, but most authors agree that they can be either congenital or acquired, with the congenital form being more frequently reported.[1] The intervening tissue involved in congenital tarsal coalitions is either fibrous, cartilaginous, or osseous, corresponding to the maturation level of the tissue involved; it is referred to as syndesmosis, synchondrosis, or synostosis, respectively.[2–4]

Talocalcaneal and calcaneonavicular coalitions are by far the most common types, comprising about 90% of all tarsal coalitions; the third most common is talonavicular coalition.[2] The onset of ossification and as the beginning of painful symptoms occur as follows: Talonavicular coalition ossifies between the ages of 3 and 5; calcaneonavicular coalition ossifies between the ages of 8 and 12, and talocalcaneal coalition ossifies between the ages of 12 and 16.[5] Other less commonly reported coalitions include calcaneocuboid, cuboidnavicular, naviculocuneiform, and various other combinations. Although the relative incidence of calcaneonavicular coalitions is high, there is a lack of information and reported cases of calcaneonavicular coalitions occurring in any foot type with a metadductus forefoot component.

CLINICAL, RADIOGRAPHIC, AND MRI FINDINGS

Pain is a common finding and usually begins insidiously following some recent activity or trauma. Limitation of subtalar and midtarsal joint motion is typically an obvious clinical finding. The subtalar joint is usually limited in the direction of inversion, with greater limitation if peroneal muscle spasm is present. Patients may present with a valgus deformity due to intense tonic peroneus brevis spasm, which is simply a reflex mechanism that limits painful inversion. Inversion and eversion of the midtarsal joint induce pain. With time, the valgus deformity becomes more rigid. There are, however, several reported cases of spasticity of muscles other than the peroneus

brevis and of a varus position of the heel in patients with calcaneonavicular coalitions.[6]

Pain is usually isolated to the midtarsal joint region, and when asked to locate the pain, the child points directly to the arc of the sinus tarsi. As midtarsal and subtalar joint motion becomes limited, the foot begins to compensate in the direction of abduction and eversion. The peroneals become shorter because of this compensated position. Any attempt to invert or plantar-flex the foot creates extreme pain. All too often a peroneal spastic flatfoot is diagnosed inappropriately.

Calcaneonavicular coalitions are usually identifiable on the medial oblique view. This type of coalition usually appears as a 1-cm wide bar that bridges the gap normally found between the calcaneus and the navicular.[7] A "pseudocoalition" due to bony overlap can create a false impression of a calcaneonavicular bar, making it necessary to obtain several medial oblique views at different angles to differentiate between positional artifact and true coalition.[8] In the case of a fibrous or cartilaginous calcaneonavicular coalition, the diagnosis will be more difficult. On the lateral view, an elongated anterosuperior process of the calcaneus, known as the anteater sign, may be seen. The calcaneus and navicular are closer than normal on the medial oblique view, and the bones appear flattened with irregular, indistinct cortical surfaces (Figs. 33–1 to 33–3).[9, 10]

However, with the advent of magnetic resonance imaging (MRI), the difficulty diagnosing the soft tissue was virtually eliminated. MRI provides the physician with an advantage when nonosseous coalitions are suspected. Although they are relatively invisible on conventional radiographs, fibrous or cartilaginous unions can be confirmed with the use of MRI.

TREATMENT

Conservative treatment is aimed at restricting subtalar and midtarsal joint motion, thereby reducing pain. This may be accomplished through the use of shoe modifications, orthoses, padding, or casting. Physical therapy, anti-inflammatory medications, and local steroid injections

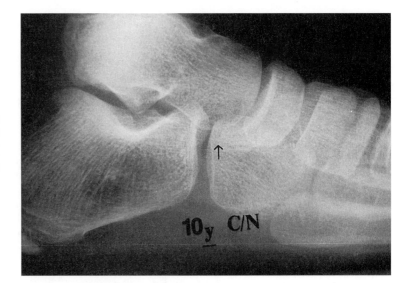

Figure 33–1. Lateral radiograph of the progression of a calcaneonavicular coalition. Talar beaking begins at age 13 with a narrowing between the calcaneus and the navicular. Eventual fragmentation of the navicular occurs secondary to the jamming effect. See also Figures 33–2 and 33–3.

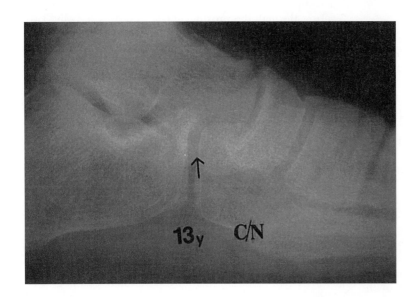

Figure 33–2. Calcaneonavicular coalition, lateral view.

Figure 33–3. Calcaneonavicular coalition, lateral view.

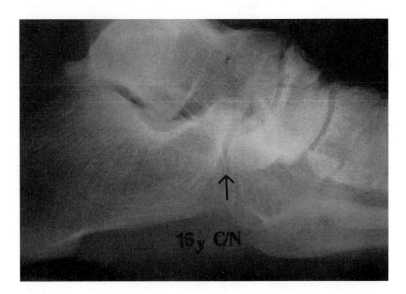

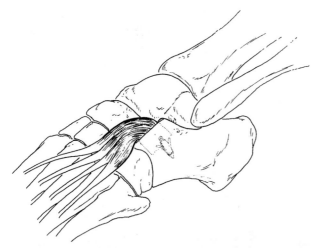

Figure 33–4. Drawing of a calcaneonavicular fusion. Extensor digitorum brevis securely placed within the newly created space between the calcaneus and the navicular. Anchor is placed deep in the calcaneus.

into the area of the coalition may be used as adjuncts. Although the symptoms may resolve for a while, they may recur at any time, requiring repeated casting or even surgical intervention.[6]

Surgical treatment of calcaneonavicular bars may involve resection of the fusion or a more radical operative procedure involving fusion of the midtarsal complexes.[11] When no secondary arthritic changes are present in the rearfoot, resection may be the most appropriate choice. The procedure, proposed in 1921 by Slomann[12] and performed in 1927 by Badgley,[13] involves excision of the coalition followed by interposition of the extensor digitorum brevis muscle belly between the calcaneus and the navicular to maintain space. This prevents both bony regrowth and hematoma. Other methods of inhibiting bone growth following resection may be used as an alternative.

Radiographically, intimate apposition of the anterior process of the calcaneus and the posterior aspect of the navicular is noted. There is no obvious evidence of bony contact. However, compared to earlier radiographs, a noticeable increase in bone and soft tissue density can be identified at this location.

As a result of the radiographic and clinical findings, a fibrous or cartilaginous coalition of the calcaneus and navicular is suggested. Treatment should start with a below-the-knee cast. The child is given a nonsteroidal anti-inflammatory drug and instructed in partial weight bearing with crutch assistance. At that time an MRI scan is ordered.

Positive MRI findings of the foot show increased signal intensity on STIR images of the distal aspect of the calcaneus and the posteromedial aspect of the navicular. The distal aspect of the calcaneus is in close proximity with the posteromedial aspect of the navicular. Increased signal intensity is also seen in both bones at this junction. Further examination reveals a difference in signal intensity between the body of the navicular and the tissue present at the pseudoarticular site. This is suggestive of tissue rather than bone at this location.

PROCEDURE

A curvilinear incision is made at the proximal aspect of the extensor digitorum brevis (EDB). The EDB is reflected off its osseous origin by cutting into the fibrous end of the proximal muscle belly. This incision is made through to the bone surface. With the use of a Key elevator the entire proximal muscle belly is released and reflected distally to give visualization of the fibrous coalition. The medial side of the navicular and the lateral side of the calcaneus are identified as they form the soft tissue bond. A rectangular block approximately 5 mm wide into each bone past the fibrous bond is resected. The block should be large enough to prevent reformation of the coalition; usually a total of 1.5 cm is sufficient. The articular surfaces of the talus and surrounding bone are protected with the use of a small flexible band retractor. The exposed bone surfaces can be covered with bone wax, or the EDB muscle belly can be interposed. This is accomplished by running a 2–0 Vicryl or any absorbable suture through the proximally resected muscle belly. Two Keith needles are placed on the suture, and the needles are passed through the plantar medial aspect of the foot. The suture is then tied over sterile felt and a button. In an alternative approach a bone anchor is driven into the calcaneus. In approximately 3 to 4 weeks the suture weakens by absorption and snaps, freeing the felt and the button. The EDB muscle belly is well seated by this time (Figs. 33–4 to 33–7). The child is maintained in a nonweight-bearing cast for 3 weeks. At the end of 3 weeks a walking cast or a Cam walker can be used for an additional 3 to 4 weeks. After this, the child should immediately be fitted with a neutral position orthosis, which will allow the foot to stay supinated rather than pronated. If the foot continues to pronate, the resected bone surfaces may reunite (Figs. 33–8 to 33–11).

Early intervention is essential. Young children who have talar beaking secondary to compensation respond

Text continued on page 243

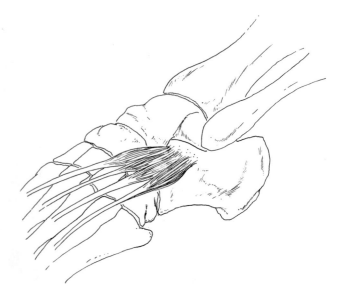

Figure 33–5. Origin of the extensor digitorum brevis muscle.

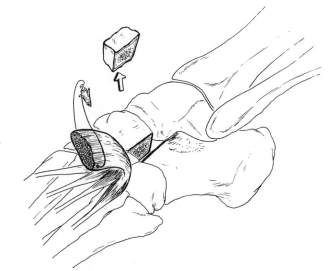

Figure 33–6. A rectangular section of bone resected from calcaneonavicular fusion site. Extensor digitorum brevis muscle with suture and bone anchor.

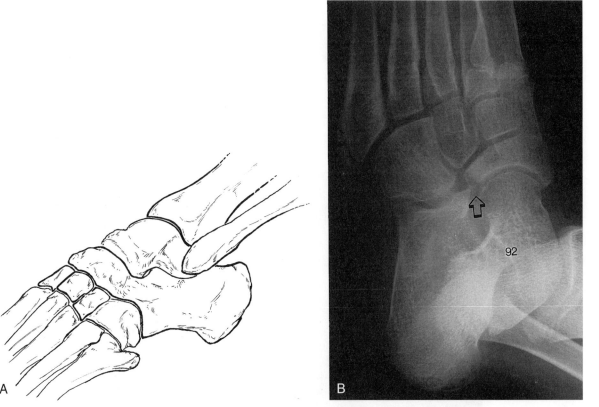

Figure 33–7. A and B, preoperative view of calcaneonavicular coalition (1992).

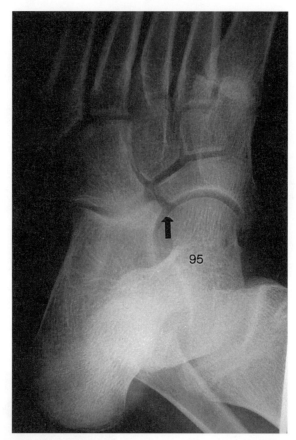

Figure 33–8. Resected calcaneonavicular coalition bar 3 years after surgery.

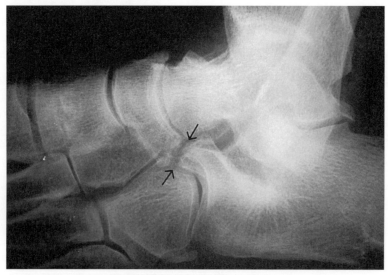

Figure 33–9. Isherwood view of calcaneonavicular fibrous coalition.

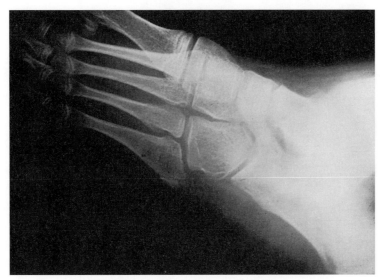

Figure 33–10. Isherwood view of calcaneonavicular osseous coalition.

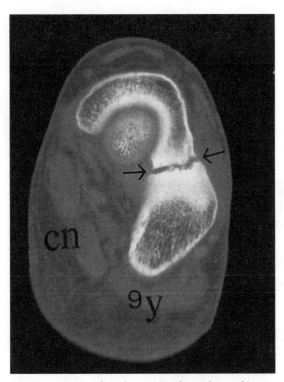

Figure 33–11. CT scan of a calcaneonavicular coalition of a 9-year-old male. Note the close proximity of the navicular to the calcaneus and the irregularity of the joint space.

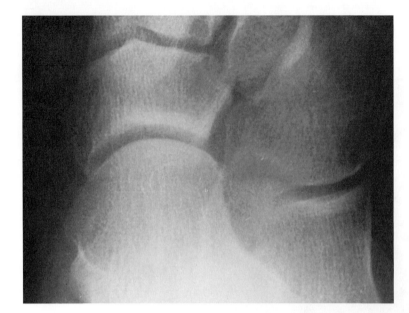

Figure 33–12. Fibrous coalition of calcaneonavicular site.

Figure 33–13. Resected fibrous coalition of calcaneonavicular site. Wedge of navicular and calcaneus resected.

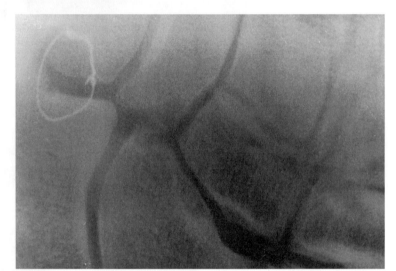

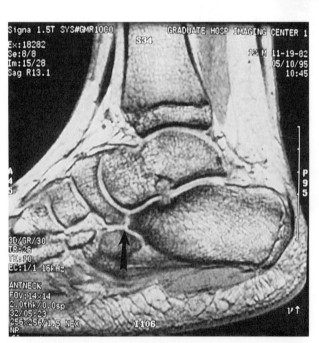

Figure 33–14. Calcaneonavicular fibrous coalition. Note separation of the area between the navicular and the calcaneus. Range of motion of the midtarsal joint was 0 degrees.

favorably to resection of the calcaneonavicular soft tissue coalition. When talar beaking is present in the older child or young adult, however, the response is less favorable and may result in the need for a triple arthrodesis.

Radiographs and CT scans have not proved reliable in the identification of fibrous tarsal coalitions (Figs. 33–12 to 33–14). MRI accurately and reliably indicates fibrous, cartilaginous, and osseous coalitions of the talocalcaneal and calcaneonavicular joints and is useful for detecting the presence of coexisting bars. MRI is recommended for patients with suspected tarsal coalitions when radiography and CT scans are negative.

References

1. Downey MS: Tarsal coalitions: A surgical classification. JAPMA 1991; 81:187.
2. Perlman MD, Wertheimer SJ: Tarsal coalitions. J Foot Surg 1986; 25:58–67.
3. Jacobs AM, Sollecito V, Oloff LM, Klein N: Tarsal coalitions: An instructional review. J Foot Surg 1981; 20(4):214–221.
4. Tachdjian M: Pediatric Orthopedics, 2nd ed. Philadelphia, W.B. Saunders, 1990, p. 1346.
5. Cowell JR: Talocalcaneal coalition and new causes of peroneal spastic flat foot. Clin Orthop 1972; 85:16–22.
6. Downey MS: Tarsal coalition. In Comprehensive Textbook of Foot Surgery, Vol. 1. Baltimore, Williams & Wilkins, 1992, pp. 898–930.
7. DeValentine SJ: Foot and Ankle Disorders in Children. New York, Churchill Livingstone, 1992, p. 199.
8. Vaughn WH, Segal CI: Tarsal coalition with special reference to roentgenographic interpretation. Radiology 1953; 60:855.
9. Jayakumar S, Cowell HR: Rigid flatfoot. Clin Orthop 1977; 122:77.
10. Cowell HR, Elener V: Rigid painful flatfoot secondary to tarsal coalition. Clin Orthop 1983; 177:54.
11. Pachuda NM, Lasday SD, Jay RM: Tarsal coalition: Etiology, diagnosis and treatment. J Foot Surg 1990; 29:474.
12. Slomann HC: On coalition calcaneo-navicularis. J Orthop Surg 1921; 3:586–602.
13. Badgley CE: Coalition of the calcaneus and navicular. Arch Surg 1927; 15:75–88.

34

Clubfoot

Mitchell Pokrassa, D.P.M., and Raymond K. Tsukuda, D.P.M.

Surgery for congenital talipes equinovarus (CTEV), commonly known as clubfoot, is an important component of the therapeutic continuum for this most challenging and difficult deformity. Central to the continuum are the principal components of etiology, physical examination, radiologic findings, neuromuscular examination pathoanatomy, conservative care, and follow-up care. Investigations of each of these components of CTEV continue to be reported throughout the worldwide podiatric and orthopedic literature. The focus of this chapter is on a sequential approach to the circumferential soft tissue release for CTEV as performed and modified over the past 20 years at the Baja Project for Crippled Children based in Mexicali, Mexico.

The collective term clubfoot denotes a multiplanar deformity of the foot and ankle in which the hindfoot is plantar-flexed below perpendicular with equinus contracture of the triceps surae, flexors, and posterior joint capsules.[2, 5, 9, 10] Varus deformity of the hindfoot as well as adduction and varus of the forefoot is also observed (Fig. 34–1). In more severe cases, subluxation of the talonavicular joint is present to the extent that the talus is laterally rotated in the mortise, the navicular slides medially, abutting the medial malleolus. Additionally, in these advanced deformities, the calcaneus is horizontally displaced 45 degrees so that the leading edge moves medially beneath the talar head and the posterior aspect moves laterally against the fibular malleolus. Clubfoot can be divided into congenital and acquired types; this chapter focuses on surgery for the congenital idiopathic type of clubfoot. CTEV can be further subdivided into rigid (intrinsic) and supple (extrinsic) deformities.[20, 21]

The intrinsic and extrinsic deformities are readily apparent on palpation and observation. Morphologically, the rigid CTEV demonstrates lower leg atrophy and wasting with marked diminution of heel size; deep-seated skin folds are manifest along the medial and posterior aspects of the foot and ankle. Traditional bony landmarks are obscured both medially and laterally with loss of the usually recognizable medial malleolus and talar head–navicular tuberosity–cuneiform sequence. The talar head is palpable laterally with loss of the lateral calcaneal profile as a result of subtalar adduction and varus. These same morphologic markers are consistently absent in the extrinsic clubfoot as well. The supple clubfoot is also readily responsive to manipulation, whereas the rigid deformity is not.[33, 34]

A certitude of clubfoot therapeutics is that prognosis and treatment guidelines correspond to clubfoot type; supple clubfeet normally respond to conservative, nonoperative care, whereas rigid deformities require surgical treatment.[38, 39, 40, 41] One should never ignore the basic tenets of continuity of care or serial follow-up even in patients with extrinsic (supple) deformities because these feet can progress to a rigid status in a relatively brief time frame if they are neglected or undertreated.

Etiologic theories of clubfoot are numerous.[12–20, 22, 23] Among all possible causes of acquired CTEV, the treating clinician must attempt to establish the presence (or absence) of any potential neuromuscular factors because these entities (e.g., spinal abnormalities, poliomyelitis, meningitis, cerebral palsy) are associated with an even more rigid deformity that influences both prognosis and treatment plans. A thorough neuromuscular examination as well as pediatric neurologic consultation is critical.

SURGICAL APPROACH

A thorough understanding of the pathoanatomy involved is central to surgical therapeutics. Clubfoot surgery is, in effect and practice, an anatomic dissection exercise in which nearly every soft tissue structure in and around the rearfoot, midfoot, and ankle is exposed and/or sectioned. Whether one views the distorted anatomy of clubfoot as a product of a primary germ plasm defect of the talus[20, 22] (Fig. 34–2) or as a function of secondary ligamentous, tendinous, and capsular contracture (Fig. 34–3), the surgical approach remains constant. Just as hallux valgus surgery is a balancing act between soft tissue release and structural repair, so is clubfoot surgery. Current technology including magnetic resonance imaging (MRI), computer modeling, and computed tomography (CT) has led to a greater understanding of the multiple axes of deformity in CTEV.[30–32] Evolving surgical technique for clubfoot repair has tended to move away from partial repair operations or "piecemeal surgery" to one-step operations in which the normal hindfoot relationships are restored with a single aggressive procedure. Subtotal corrections or piecemeal operations often ignore components of the deformity, leading to multiple serial procedures and abundant scar tissue accumulation. The single greatest failure of nonperitalar circumferential releasing operations in our series at the Baja Project for

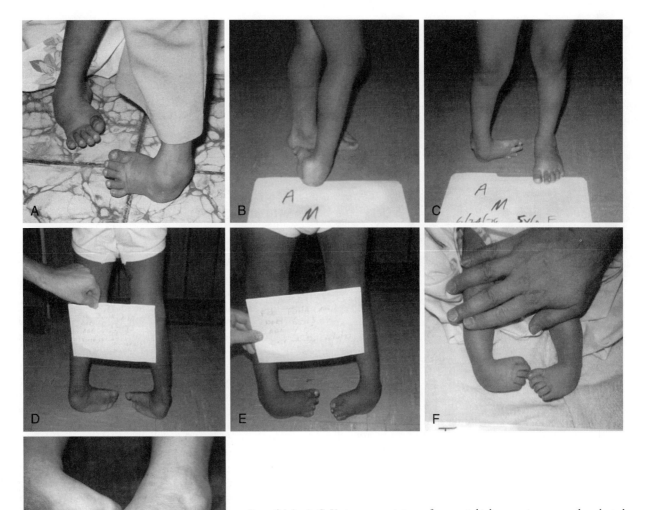

Figure 34–1. *A–G,* Various presentations of congenital talipes equinovarus and neglected adult clubfoot. *A–E,* Various presentations of clubfoot. *G,* Adventitious bursa over the base of the fifth metatarsal and cuboid resulting from weight bearing on the area as a sequela of the deformity.

Crippled Children has been a failure to restore talocalcaneal divergence or "opening of the closed scissors." Any incomplete operation that falls short of the goal of restoration inevitably results in spurious correction of the deformity.

The stated goals of hindfoot realignment must remain as follows: (1) Realignment of the talocalcaneal joint by medial, lateral, and plantar release around the talus with associated lateral and posterior release of the horizontally rotated calcaneus. (2) Restoration of normal talonavicular alignment with release of all tethering influences (i.e., spring ligament, posterior tibial tendon, tibionavicular component of the deltoid ligament, talonavicular joint capsule, and bifurcate ligament). Talar realignment in the transverse plane also reduces "medial spin" of the foot and posterior fibular displacement. (3) Calcaneocuboid repositioning, which is essential to bring the medially and plantarly deviated cuboid back in alignment with the leading edge of the calcaneus, allowing correction of the

forefoot and midfoot adducto varus and diminishing the medial tethering of the anterior calcaneus.

DIAGNOSIS

The diagnostic parameters encompass both clinical and radiographic findings, and evaluation for surgical intervention also draws from both entities. Recognition of clinically stiff and unyielding feet with fixed equinus, medially subluxed navicular, laterally rotated talus, and severely adducted and inverted heel to documents the need for surgical treatment. Similarly, radiographic interpretation of the complex hindfoot derangement allows further appreciation if the osseous pathology.

MRI and CT are excellent tools for diagnostic radiography. These modalities are an excellent adjunct to analytic radiography, providing additional information to the clinician. Yet the use of standardized postmanipulation,

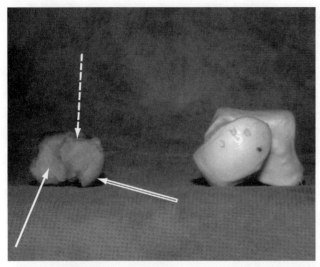

Figure 34–2. Comparative view of a normal talus versus a talus excised from 14-year-old male with neglected clubfoot. Note the decreased adaptive shortening of the head and neck of the talus as shown by arrows demonstrating the lateral process, neck, and articular portion of the head of a clubfoot talus. The broken arrow shows the talar neck, the solid arrow shows the lateral process of the talus, and the open arrow represents the medial and plantar deviated articular cartilage.

serially exposed radiographs (anteroposterior and lateral views) remains the diagnostic standard in clubfoot radiology. Although many methods exist for interpretation of clubfoot radiographs,[24] we have used Simons' methods[25–27] to assess forefoot adduction, hindfoot equinus and varus, and talonavicular subluxation (Fig. 34–4). The value of serially exposed, standardized postmanipulation films is critical to the surgeon for several reasons: (1) The clinical appearance of the foot is a relatively poor indicator of the success or progress of treatment. External morphology cannot address the presence of under- or overcorrection or spurious correction such as midtarsal breaching. (2)

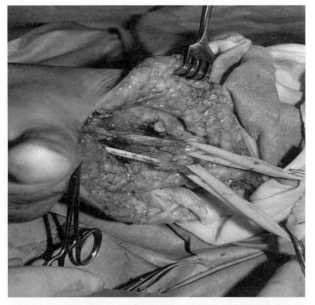

Figure 34–3. Anterior view of flexor digitorum longus (FDL) and tibialis posterior (TP) acting as a medical tether.

Serial films alert the practitioner to the presence of a treatment impasse in which the hindfoot angles resist correction. (3) Serial films can detect the severity of deformity with relative "hardness" or "softness." (4) The development of iatrogenic complications such as extensive compression forces used during manipulation and cast therapy can be evaluated. (5) The restoration of normal angular relationships is confirmed by serially exposed films, which monitor the success of conservative care or surgical intervention and postsurgical results.

BASIC SURGICAL PRINCIPLES

Manipulation and casting remain the standard of care for nonoperative treatment of CTEV.[34] However, in the presence of a treatment impasse (i.e., failure to correct the deformity of the talocalcaneonavicular complex clinically and/or radiographically), surgery is indicated. Our experience at the Baja Project has evolved in such a way that we now perform earlier and more aggressive soft tissue releases. Such early intervention precludes the adaptive osseous and soft tissue changes that occur if surgery is delayed. We have noted consistently better objective results in our Baja clinic series with early surgical intervention in children with severe deformities from CTEV. If treatment fails or reaches a plateau within the first 3 months of a child's life we advocate and perform extensive soft tissue releases using either a traditional hockey stick incision posterior to the medial malleolus or a Cincinnati circumferential release[46, 49] (Figs. 34–5 and 34–6). The transverse circumferential incision is preferred because, since the patient is prone, it allows increased visualization of the medial, plantar, posterior, and lateral structures. The incision allows simultaneous evaluation of the released structures in a sagittal, frontal, and transverse fashion. The lateral arm or extension of the incision allows clear access to the lateral structures (e.g., sural nerve, peroneal tendons, peroneal retinaculum, calcaneofibular ligament, origin of extensor digitorum brevis, lateral talocalcaneal ligament or joint capsule, bifurcate ligament, and dorsal calcaneocuboid ligament), which in the traditional medial hockey stick incision remain unexposed. These structures must be released to reverse the tethering of the posterior calcaneus to the fibula (i.e., horizontal calcaneal rotation) and to allow calcaneocuboid relocation to correct the midfoot and forefoot adduction and varus as well as talar relocation into the medial column.

The circumferential incision is not without its drawbacks. For example, it is difficult to expose the tendo Achillis high enough or proximal enough along its course to allow a generous and adequate Z-plasty. Additionally, it is occasionally necessary to leave the foot slightly plantar-flexed at the time of closure to allow adequate circulation to the flap created posteriorly (see Fig. 34–6). Clearly, the advantages of exposure combined with unobstructed access to all aspects of the deformity make the horizontal incision a viable alternative to other incisional approaches. The circumferential incision is detailed in sequence in Figures 34–7 to 34–29.

Prior to closure of the incision as shown in these

Text continued on page 258

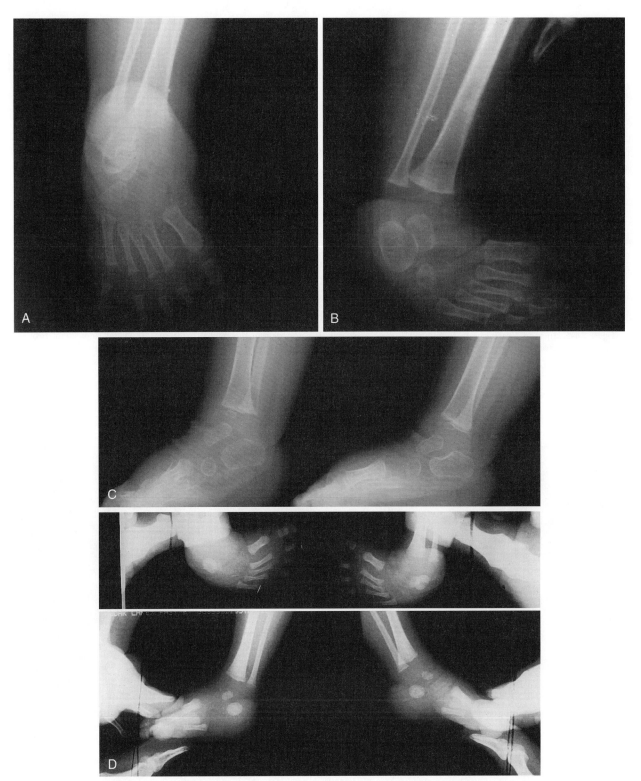

Figure 34–4. Radiographs. On the anteroposterior (AP) view (*A*), as the talocalcaneal angle approaches 0 degrees, the heel is in severe varus and inversion beneath the leading edge of the talus. On the lateral view (*C*), as the talocalcaneal angle approaches 0 degrees, varying degrees of equinus are reflected. *A,* Talonavicular subluxation is detectable in the presence of a radiographically silent navicular prior to navicular ossification by the presence of a talar-first metatarsal angle of more than 15 degrees with a concomitant talocalcaneal angle of less than 15 degrees. Simons[25–27] confirmed this by subsequent intraoperative findings in which the talonavicular joint was found to be subluxed with the navicular abutting against the medial malleolus. *B,* Parallelism of the talocalcaneal angle (Kite's angle) in the neonatal clubfoot in which the adduction of the leading edge of the calcaneus indicates severe varus deformity of the hindfoot. *C,* Lateral view of a pediatric clubfoot; note that the talocalcaneal angle approaches 0 degrees, indicating severe hindfoot equinus and varus of the calcaneus. *D,* Angular relationship of a premanipulated neonatal clubfoot in the upper radiograph compared with the same clubfoot after 15 minutes of manipulation in the radiograph below. Note the improvement in Kite's angle after manipulation. Such pre- and postmanipulative studies have significant diagnostic, prognostic, and therapeutic value.

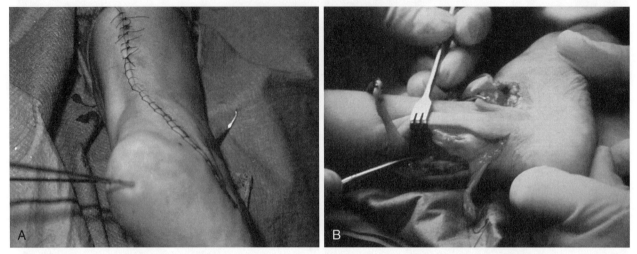

Figure 34–5. Incisional variants. *A,* Traditional "hockey stick" incision posterior to the medial malleolus. *B,* Medial and lateral two-incisional approach.

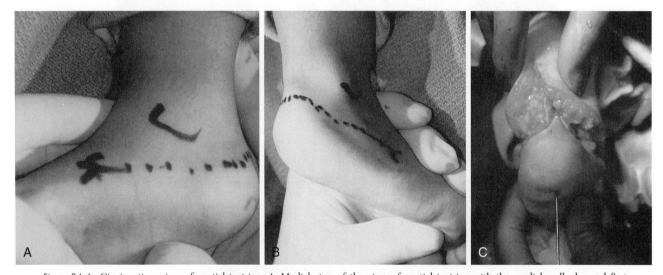

Figure 34–6. Cincinnati or circumferential incision. *A,* Medial view of the circumferential incision with the medial malleolus and first metatarsal-cuneiform joint as marked landmarks. *B,* Lateral view of the circumferential incision with the fibular malleolus and fifth metatarsal base as landmarks. *C,* Posterior view of the circumferential incision. Note the proximally based angular flap, which is a modification of the original horizontal incision. This modification is used to provide proximal exposure for the Achilles release as well as to preclude the need for posterior skin grafting or leaving the foot in an equinus position because the closure was performed under tension due to the equinus correction. A frequent point of dehiscence occurs at the apex of this flap in much the same way as wound dehiscence occurs at the apex of a hockey stick incision beneath the medial malleolus as a result of tension at closure. Fortunately, the elastic nature of pediatric skin is such that minimal scarring occurs in this area.

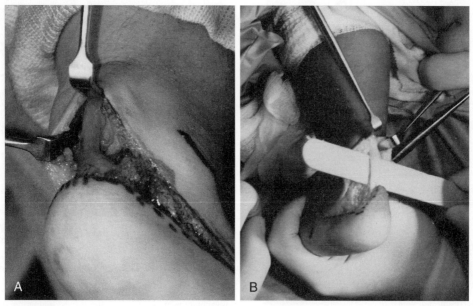

Figure 34–7. Posterior release. *A*, Circumferential soft tissue release as performed in a sequential fashion from posterior to medial to plantar to lateral. Initially the Achilles tendon is exposed; proximal exposure to the triceps tendon is achieved based on proximal retraction, dorsiflexion of the foot, and modification of the skin incision as described in Figure 34–6C. As a result of the severe hindfoot equinus, a generous Z-plasty lengthening is necessary. The Z-plasty should be made long enough so that with dorsiflexion the respective proximal and distal ends of the Z-plasty do not pull apart forming a large unbridgeable gap. Care must be taken to preserve the Achilles tendon sheath for subsequent repair. Note that a tongue blade or No. 3 handle may be used on the underside of all tendons that are to be lengthened during the circumferential release. The use of these instruments provides counter pressure for the sectioning as well as protection of the deeper structures. *B*, Protection of the Achilles tendon using a tongue blade.

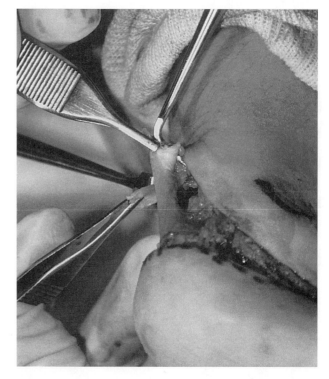

Figure 34–8. Tendo Achillis lengthening. This procedure may be performed either sagittally from medial to lateral, or coronally from anterior to posterior. As with all tendon lengthening procedures in clubfoot surgery, the Z-plasty should remain absolutely midline to avoid fraying the two wings of the Z-plasty. The distal portion of the Z should be medial to release the medial tethering of the deformity. After lengthening the Achilles tendon, the plantaris tendon is located and sectioned. After each step in the release, one should stop and check the correction or increase in the amount of dorsiflexion obtained with each maneuver.

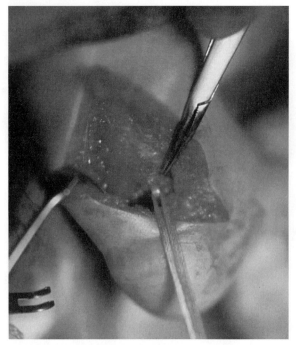

Figure 34–9. Delivery of flexor hallucis longus (FHL). After sectioning the Achilles tendon and before entering the deep posterior compartment of the ankle, the FHL is located as it traverses the posterior aspect of the lower leg from its lateral origin to its course in the groove of the Stieda process. The surgeon's finger is introduced into the posterior compartment, and the great toe is manipulated to facilitate this maneuver. It should be kept in mind that the posterior tibial nerve and vasculature are immediately against the FHL tendon. If one does not initially locate and dissect the FHL at this time, it can easily be transected during the posterior joint capsulotomy as part of the operation. Thus, the surgeon may choose to perform Z-plasty of the FHL at this time or merely retract it and lengthen it during the medial release portion of the surgery.

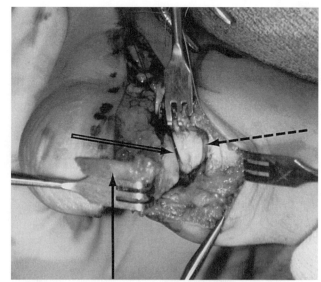

Figure 34–10. Posterior release: Sectioning of the posterior ankle joint (AJ) and posterior facet of the subtalar joint (STJ). Sequential sectioning of the AJ and STJ are carried out by introducing the surgeon's finger and dorsiflexing and plantar-flexing the foot to detect a puckering or invagination at the level of the AJ. By palpating the AJ and carefully sectioning the posterior tibiotalar ligament, one avoids potential damage to the distal tibial epiphysis. Location of the STJ, which in a neonate is usually several millimeters inferior to the AJ, is challenging. In order to facilitate location of the posterior facet of the STJ, one should incise the joint capsule longitudinally from superior to inferior so that it is identifiable without blindly sectioning the posterior STJ ligaments. In a neonate or young child, it is extremely easy to "create your own joint space" by sharply incising the cartilaginous precursors with a surgical blade. Again, after each joint capsule is excised, the surgeon checks for sagittal plane correction. (Broken arrow, trochlear surface of the talus; open arrow, posterior facet of the STJ; solid arrow, reflected distal portion after Z-plasty of the Achilles tendon.)

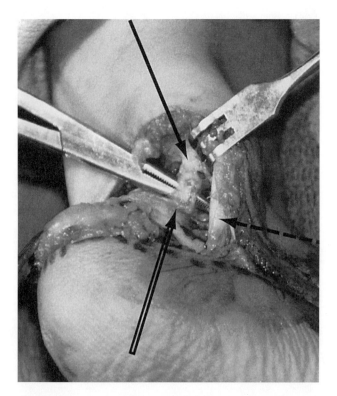

Figure 34–11. Release of calcaneofibular (CF) ligament. The exposure and release of the CF ligament is central to both posterior release and lateral release as the ligament restricts both dorsiflexion of the foot on the ankle and medial rotation of the posterior calcaneus. The ligament is sectioned at this point. After the initial four maneuvers of the posterior release have been performed, if adequate dorsiflexion is not present an additional step is undertaken (see Fig. 34–12). (Solid arrow, fibular attachment of the CF ligament; open arrow, calcaneal attachment of the CF ligament; broken arrow, peroneal tendons.) The hemostat is under the central portion of the CF ligament.

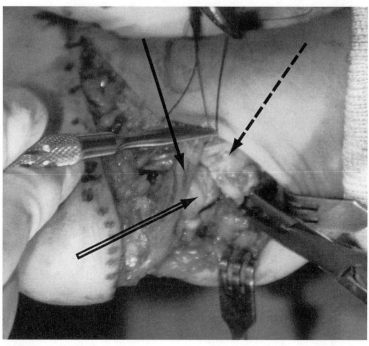

Figure 34–12. Syndesmosis release. As Coleman[11] has advocated, if inadequate dorsiflexion persists, the surgeon may choose to section the syndesmotic ligament longitudinally between the posterior tibia and the fibula. By sectioning this ligament, the wider anterior trochlear surface of the talus may rock further back in the ankle mortise. *Note:* The syndesmosis should be sectioned lateral of the midline to avoid the neurovascular bundle. (Broken arrow, tibia; open arrow, trochlear surface of the talus; solid arrow, Achilles tendon.) The hemostat exposes the syndesmosis.

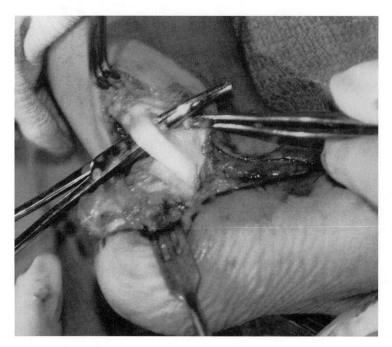

Figure 34–13. Medial release. The initial step in the medial release is to open the posterior compartment behind the medial malleolus and sequentially expose the tibialis posterior (TP) tendon, the flexor digitorum longus (FDL) tendon, neuromuscular bundle, and the flexor hallucis longus (FHL) tendon if it has not been previously lengthened posteriorly. The TP is exposed, and Z-plasty is sectioned proximally and posterior to the medial malleolus. The distal portion of the tendon is subsequently used as a guide to the sectioning of the laciniate ligament and the location of the navicular tuberosity. *Note:* As each medial tendon is lengthened by Z-plasty, each tendon component should be tagged with a separate identifiable colored suture so that during the "confusion of closure," as the tendons are reapproximated, the surgeon can attach the correct proximal tendon to the correct distal tendon. The hemostat denotes the TP tendon. The Brown-Adson is grasping the laciniate ligament.

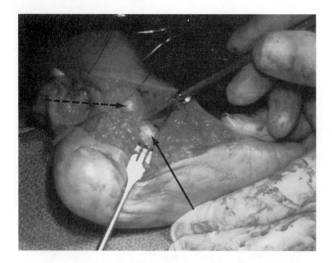

Figure 34–14. Medial column pathology. This figure demonstrates talonavicular subluxation. The solid arrow points to the navicular; broken arrow points to the medial malleolus. Note that the navicular articulates directly with the medial malleolus. The talus is nowhere to be found. Upon dissection it is often noted that an actual articular facet forms between the navicular and the medial malleolus.

Figure 34–15. Mobilization of the neurovascular bundle. In order to expose the flexor hallucis longus (FHL) tendon as well as the medial subtalar joint (STJ) ligaments, the neurovascular bundle is carefully dissected free and mobilized to allow adequate medial exposure. *Note:* The neurovascular bundle as well as the tibiotalar components of the deep deltoid ligament are two of the few structures that are left intact in a clubfoot release. The bundle should be dissected proximally from the lower third of the leg to its distal entry into the abductor canal. By tracing the bundle into the abductor canal, the master knot of Henry can be identified and released. The hemostat is under the bundle, and the Brown-Adson is oriented toward the abductor canal. Also note the use of sutures serving as tags.

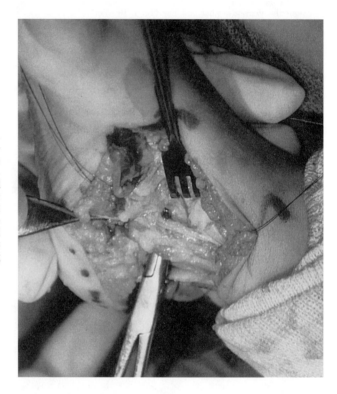

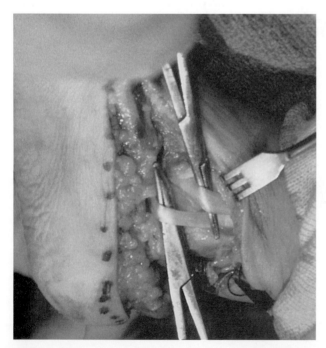

Figure 34–16. Harvesting of medial tendons. As the flexor digitorum longus and flexor hallucis longus tendons are fully exposed, the surgeon should always consider lengthening the digital flexors if flexion or clawing of the respective digits occurs when the ankle is dorsiflexed past the perpendicular.

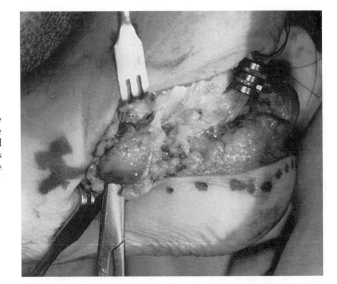

Figure 34–17. Abductor hallucis brevis (AHB) release. At this point in the operation, the AHB tendon is identified medially, and a section of the myotendinous junction is excised. Care should be taken to retract and protect the neurovascular bundle during this maneuver. The hemostat is under the AHB tendon, and the Senn retractor is carefully reflecting the neurovascular bundle.

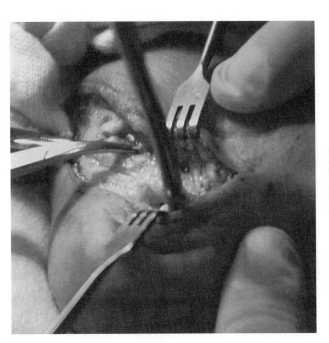

Figure 34–18. Plantar release. The operating scissors are releasing the plantar aponeurosis and intrinsic musculature attachments from their calcaneal origin. Once again, the neurovascular bundle is identified and retracted prior to this maneuver. *Note:* On release of the aponeurosis and intrinsic musculature, the long and short plantar ligaments are released simultaneously to alleviate forefoot adduction and equinus forces cumulatively.

Figure 34–19. Continuation of medial release. The medial ligamentous and capsular attachments along the dorsal, medial, and plantar aspects of the talonavicular, naviculocuneiform, and first metatarsal-cuneiform articulations are serially exposed and sectioned. *Note:* Extra care must be used when excising the thickened tissue that fills the void over the talonavicular articulation because the laterally rotated talar head is readily incised during dissection of the joint. The surgical assistant should gently distract the navicular distally during this maneuver. Similar care should be taken to not avulse the tibialis anterior tendon at its insertion at the first metatarsal-cuneiform articulation. Once again, to facilitate location of these often obscure joint spaces, a horizontal incision is recommended preliminarily while the assistant abducts the forefoot to place these vertically oriented joints under tension. The left Senn retractor is distracting the navicular; the right Senn retractor reflects the neurovascular bundle; and the inferior Senn retractor retracts the anterior aspect of the subtalar joint, exposing the interosseous ligament. (Broken arrow, intact interosseous talocalcaneal ligament; solid arrow, middle facet of subtalar joint.)

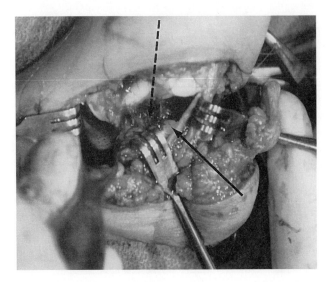

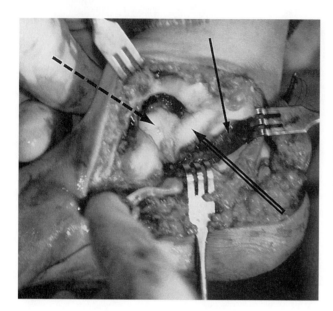

Figure 34–20. Medial subtalar joint (STJ) release. After sectioning the superficial deltoid ligament (i.e., tibiocalcaneal component), the medial aspect of the talocalcaneal ligament or joint capsule is sectioned. Note the carefully preserved deep deltoid ligament. (Solid arrow, sectioned medial capsule of STJ; broken arrow, articular portion of talar head; open arrow, preserved tibiotalar component of the deep deltoid ligament.)

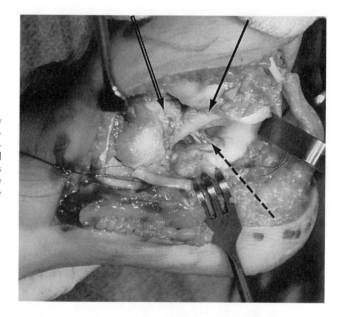

Figure 34–21. Talocalcaneal interosseous ligament. The broken arrow points to the interosseous ligament prior to sectioning. Ideally, this ligament is left intact; however, in the resistant talipes equinovarus, a horizontal deformity of the calcaneus remains uncorrected in which the distal aspect of the calcaneus remains medially displaced while the calcaneus is tethered posteriorly to the fibula. In this case, the ligament must be released. (Open arrow, articular portion of the talar head; solid arrow, the neck of talus.)

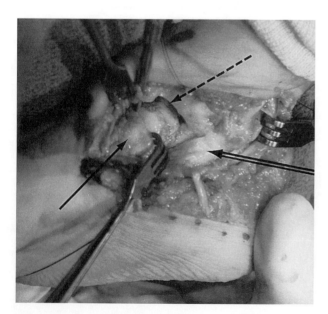

Figure 34–22. Anterior ankle capsulotomy. To facilitate transverse plane relocation of the talus into the medial column, it is often necessary to section the anterior talotibial ligament. Anterior migration of up to 30% of the talus out of the ankle mortise is noted in conjunction with the lateral rotational deformity of the talus. (Broken arrow, anterior ankle capsulotomy; solid arrow, navicular; open arrow, intact deep deltoid ligament.) The Senn retractor distally distracts the navicular from the laterally rotated talus. The articular portion of the talar head is visible above the Senn retractor.

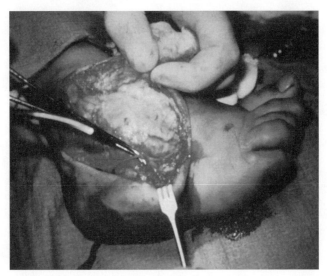

Figure 34–23. Exposure for lateral release. The initial maneuver along the lateral aspect of the circumferential incision is made to identify and retract the sural nerve as demonstrated by the hemostat.

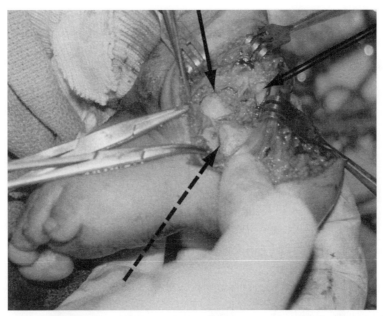

Figure 34–24. Further rationale for lateral exposure and release. This intraoperative photograph demonstrates the lateral rotation of the talus within the ankle mortise. The solid arrow identifies the laterally rotated head of the talus immediately superior to the calcaneocuboid articulation marked by the broken arrow. The open arrow points to the lateral malleolus. The Senn retractor reflects the peroneal tendons.

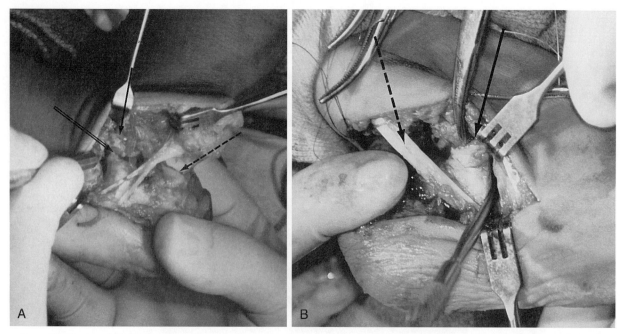

Figure 34–25. *A* and *B*, Continuation of lateral release. To release the posterolateral tethering of the calcaneus, the peroneal sheaths and retinaculum are sectioned and dissected free. The bifurcate ligament is also released along with the dorsal calcaneocuboid ligament and the origin of the extensor digitorum brevis (EDB) to allow lateral relocation of the anterior calcaneus and realignment of the calcaneocuboid joint. Lateral talonavicular joint capsulotomy is performed as well. *A*, The open arrow shows the location of the origin of the EDB, the dorsal calcaneocuboid ligament, and the bifurcate ligament. The solid arrow denotes the laterally rotated talar head abutting the anterior process of the calcaneus. The broken arrow is at the posterior facet of the subtalar joint. Also note that the peroneal retinaculum and peroneal tendon sheaths are freed from the peroneal tuberosity. *B*, The elevator is in the calcaneocuboid joint. The solid arrow indicates the origin of the EDB, the bifurcate ligament, and the dorsal calcaneocuboid ligament. The broken arrow shows the peroneal tendon sheath.

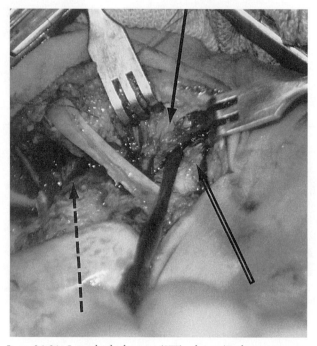

Figure 34–26. Lateral subtalar joint (STJ) release. (Broken arrow, superior surface of posterior aspect of calcaneus; solid arrow, cervical ligament; open arrow, anterior process and calcaneocuboid joint.) The elevator demonstrates longitudinal sectioning of the talocalcaneal ligaments and joint capsule, which further advances medial talar relocation and calcaneal repositioning.

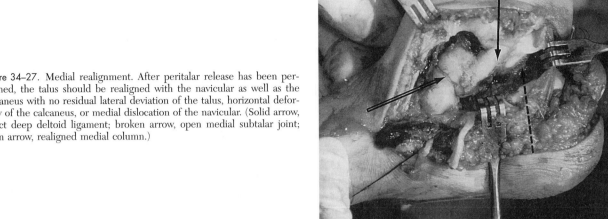

Figure 34–27. Medial realignment. After peritalar release has been performed, the talus should be realigned with the navicular as well as the calcaneus with no residual lateral deviation of the talus, horizontal deformity of the calcaneus, or medial dislocation of the navicular. (Solid arrow, intact deep deltoid ligament; broken arrow, open medial subtalar joint; open arrow, realigned medial column.)

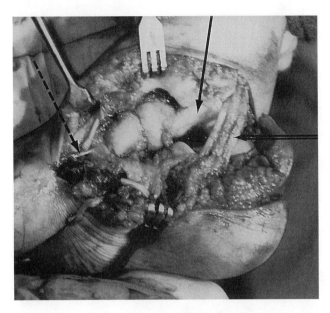

Figure 34–28. Fixated medial column. Note the K-wire traversing the talonavicular, naviculocuneiform, and first metatarsal-cuneiform articulations (*broken arrow*). The K-wire is introduced in a retrograde fashion from the posterior aspect of the talus distally. (Open arrow, intact neurovascular bundle; solid arrow, deep deltoid ligament.)

Figure 34–29. Lateral column shortening. In patients in whom talonavicular subluxation persists after soft tissue release, a lateral closing wedge osteotomy may be performed to induce lateral navicular rotation and shortening of the elongated lateral column. This maneuver may be performed using a sharp No. 15 blade. Rarely is a saw required in a neonate or young child. Fixation is readily achieved with K-wires. The Brown-Adson is grasping the wedge of bone removed from the lateral column.

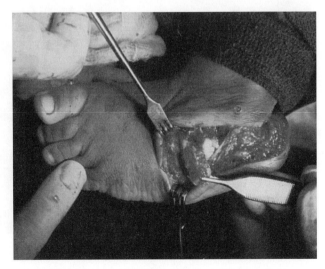

figures, several goals must have been achieved to prevent incomplete or spurious correction:

- Adequate sagittal motion of the ankle; ideally 10 to 15 degrees of dorsiflexion should be present with the knee extended and the knee flexed with no abduction of the foot with dorsal motion, which, if it occurs, may indicate persistent lateral rotation of the talus.
- Release of the adducted forefoot by virtue of medial soft tissue sectioning and lateral calcaneocuboid realignment.
- Lateral repositioning of the anterior calcaneus combined with medial relocation of the posterior calcaneus.
- Relocation of the medially displaced navicular.
- Reversal of the anterior subluxation and lateral rotation of the talus within the mortise.

- Reversal of posterior fibular displacement with restoration of normal bimalleolar axis (the critical angle formed by the long bisection of the rearfoot and the bimalleolar plane).
- Restoration of a supple, plantargrade foot
- Exposure of intra-operative AP and lateral radiographs to confirm restoration of normal hindfoot relationships prior to closure.

After release of the tourniquet, normal neurovascular return should be observed; a well-padded dressing protecting the K-wires is then applied (Fig. 34–30) followed by an above-knee (AK) cast with the knee flexed 90 degrees and the foot corrected in all three planes (Fig. 34–31). If vascular congestion becomes apparent, the cast may be valved at anytime from immediately postopera-

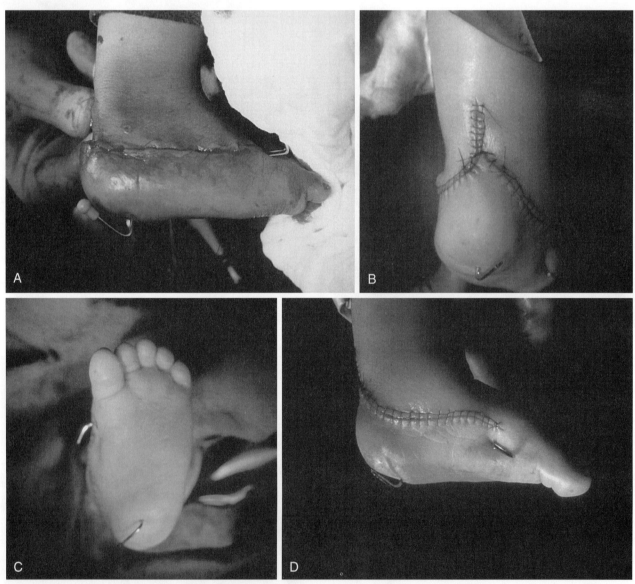

Figure 34–30. Meticulous closure of all tendon sheaths and retinaculum are performed using adipose and deep fascial tissue over all joint spaces. This is critical to avoid adhesion, capsulodesis, and restricted range of motion postoperatively. Release of the tourniquet prior to closure is performed to control bleeding and ensure maximum hemostasis in children. Subcutaneous tissue and skin are carefully closed. *A,* Lateral view demonstrating correct K-wire placement and closure of skin. *B,* Closure of the apex of the posterior aspect of the circumferential incision. *C,* Plantar view showing correction of heel varus and forefoot adduction along with skin closure. *D,* Medial view of skin closure and K-wire placement.

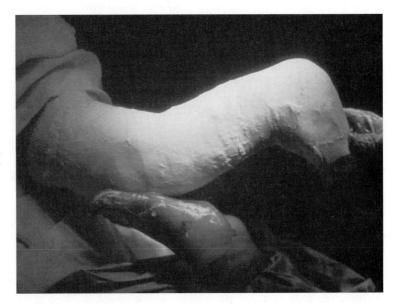

Figure 34–31. Above-knee (AK) cast application. A well-padded AK cast is applied from the tips of the child's toes to the groin area with flexion of the knee. Digital color should be checked frequently after cast application.

tively to the same evening of surgery. The initial AK cast should be maintained for at least 1 month, windowing it only for suture removal and inspection of the incision. The cast may then be changed at weekly intervals with maintenance of all planes of correction. Kirschner wires may be removed at the 6 to 8-week interval; in the final 2 to 4 weeks of cast immobilization the cast may be a below-knee (BK) cast. After 10 to 12 weeks of immobilization the cast is bivalved and the posterior portion is maintained as a night splint or retention splint that can be used around the clock except for bathing and range-of-motion exercises. The nonambulatory child is then fitted with Denis Browne splints or any of the Denis Browne clones. The ambulatory child is fitted additionally for single or double upright splinting or ankle-foot orthotics (AFOs) with dorsiflexory assistance and a valgus T strap. A straight-last or reverse-last shoe with a valgus heel wedge and sub-fifth metatarsal or outer sole wedge may then be employed. Semi-annual follow-up visits including serial radiographs and clinical examination are recommended until the child reaches skeletal maturity.

SUMMARY

Traditionally, it has been a given that a child born with CTEV will never have a normal functional appendage. The most likely reason for this tenet of clubfoot therapeutics is the results achieved with incomplete or partial correction, which is followed by late relapse of several or multiple components of the original deformity. The decades of the 1980s and 1990s have seen major therapeutic advances in the treatment of clubfoot. Diagnostic imaging, analytic radiology, computer modeling, and enhanced understanding of pathologic anatomy have significantly advanced the diagnostic and prognostic considerations in clubfoot care. Circumferential release and early osteotomy have resulted in significant therapeutic advances. As the tide ebbs on the twentieth century, the approach to clubfoot therapeutics used in the coming century will reverse the long-held tenet that children

born with this deformity will never have normally functioning feet.

References

1. Pokrassa MA: Clubfoot. *In* McGlamry ED, Banks AS, Downey MS (eds): Comprehensive Textbook of Foot Surgery, 2nd ed. Baltimore, Williams & Wilkins, 1992, pp. 853–875.
2. Robertson WW Jr., Corbett D: Congenital clubfoot. Clin Orthop 1997; 338:14.
3. Miyagi N, Iisaka H, Yasuda K, et al: Onset of ossification of the tarsal bones in congenital clubfoot. J Pediatr Orthop 1997; 17:36.
4. Diepstraten AFM: Congenital clubfoot, how do I do it. Acta Orthop Scand 1996; 67(3):305.
5. Fukuhara K, Schollmeier G, Uhtoff HK: The pathogenesis of clubfoot. J Bone Joint Surg [Br] 1994; 76(B):450.
6. Scarpa A: A memoir on the congenital clubfeet of children, and the mode of correcting that deformity. Clin Orthop 1994; 308:4.
7. Spero CR, Simon GS, Tornetta III P: Clubfeet and tarsal coalition. J Pediatr Orthop 1994; 14:372.
8. Westin GW: Clubfoot: Where to stop the wheel. Contemp Orthop 1989; 19(3):235.
9. Pokrassa MA, Rodgveller B: Talipes equinovarus. J Am Podiatr Med Assoc 1981; 71(9):472.
10. Rodgveller B: Talipes equinovarus. Clin Podiatr 1984; 1(3):477.
11. Coleman SS: Complex Foot Deformities in Children. Philadelphia, Lea & Febiger, 1983.
12. Gomez VR: Clubfeet in congenital annular constricting bands. Clin Orthop 1996; 323:155.
13. Weinberg CR, Skjaerven R, Wilcox AJ: Statistical evidence for shared transient causes of anatomically distinct birth defects. Stat Med 1996; 15:2029.
14. Kohn G, Malinger G, El Shawwa R, et al: Bilateral ulnar hypoplasia, clubfeet, and mental retardation: A new mesomelic syndrome. Am J Med Genet 1995; 56:132.
15. Feldbrin Z, Gilai AN, Ezra E, et al: Muscle imbalance in the aetiology of idiopathic clubfoot. J Bone Joint Surg [Br] 1995; 77B:596.
16. Muir L, Laliotis N, Kutty S, et al: Absence of dorsalis pedis pulse in the parents of children with clubfoot. J Bone Joint Surg [Br] 1995; 77B(1):114.
17. Miller PR, Kuo KN, Lubicky JP: Clubfoot deformity in Down's syndrome. Orthopedics 1995; 18(7):611.
18. Sodergard J, Ryoppy S: Foot deformities in arthrogryphosis multiplex congenita. J Pediatr Orthop 1994; 14:768.
19. Sirca A, Erzen I, Pecak F: Histochemistry of abductor hallucis muscle in children with idiopathic clubfoot and in controls. J Pediatr Orthop 1990; 10:477.

20. Kawashima T, Uhthoff HK: Development of foot in prenatal life in relation to idiopathic clubfoot. J Pediatr Orthop 1990; 10:232.

21. Hersh A: The role of surgery in the treatment of clubfeet. J Bone Joint Surg [Am] 1967; 41:1684.

22. Wang J, Palmer RM, Chung CS: The role of major genes in clubfoot. Am J Hum Genet 1988; 42:772.

23. Sodre A, Bruschini S, Mestriner LA, et al: Arterial abnormalities in talipes equinovarus as assessed by angiography and the Doppler technique. J Pediatr Orthop 1990; 10:101.

24. Blakeslee TJ: Comparative radiographic analysis of congenital talipes equinovarus in infancy: A retrospective study. J Foot Surg 1988; 27(3):188.

25. Simons GW: Analytical radiography and the progressive approach in talipes equinovarus. Orthop Clin North Am 1978; 9:187.

26. Simons GW: A standardized method for the radiographic evaluation of clubfeet. Clin Orthop 1978; 135:107.

27. Simons GW: The diagnosis and treatment of deformity combinations in clubfeet. Clin Orthop 1980; 150:229.

28. Napiontek M: Clinical and radiographic appearance of congenital talipes equinovarus after successful nonoperative treatment. J Pediatr Orthop 1996; 16:67.

29. Miller JH, Bernstein SM: The roentgenographic appearance of the "corrected clubfoot." Foot Ankle 1986; 6(4):177.

30. Zimny ML, Willig SJ, Robets JM, et al: An electron microscopic study of the fascia from medial and lateral sides of clubfoot. J Pediatr Orthop 1985; 5:577.

31. Chami M, Daoud A, Maestro M, et al: Ultrasound contribution in the analysis of the newborn and infant normal and clubfoot: A preliminary study. Pediatr Radiol 1996; 26:298.

32. Pagnotta G, Maffulli N, Aureli S, et al: Antenatal sonographic diagnosis of clubfoot: A six-year experience. J Foot Ankle Surg 1996; 35(1):67.

33. Ganley JV: Corrective casting in infants. Clin Podiatr 1984; 1(3):501.

34. Karski T, Wosko I: Experience in the conservative treatment of congenital clubfoot in newborns and infants. J Pediatr Orthop 1989; 9:134.

35. Fagan JP: The four quadrant approach to clubfoot surgery. Clin Podiatr Med Surg 1987; 4(1):233.

36. Lawrence SJ, Botte MJ: Management of adult, spastic, equinovarus foot deformity. Foot Ankle Int 1994; 15(6):340.

37. Brand PW: A personal revolution in the development of clubfoot correction. Clin Podiatr Med Surg 1997; 14(1):1.

38. Cooper DM, Dietz FR: Treatment of idiopathic clubfoot. J Bone Joint Surg [Am] 1995; 77A:1477.

39. Harrold AJ, Walker CJ: Treatment and prognosis in congenital clubfoot. J Bone Joint Surg [Br] 1983; 65B:8.

40. Nather A, Bose K: Conservative and surgical treatment of clubfoot. J Pediatr Orthop 1987; 7:42.

41. Magone JB, Torch MA, Clark RN, et al: Comparative review of surgical treatment of the idiopathic clubfoot by three different procedures at Columbus Children's Hospital. J Pediatr Orthop 1989; 9:49.

42. Ryoppy S, Sairanen H: Neonatal operative treatment of clubfoot. J Bone Joint Surg [Br] 1983; 65B(3):320.

43. Porter RW: Congenital talipes equinovarus: A staged method of surgery. J Bone Joint Surg [Br] 1987; 69B(5):826.

44. Cummings RJ, Lovell WW: Operative treatment of congenital idiopathic clubfoot. J Bone Joint Surg [Am] 1988; 70A(7):1108.

45. McKay DW: New concept of and approach to clubfoot treatment: Sections I and II. J Pediatr Orthop 1982; 2:347.

46. Brougham DI, Nicol RO: Use of the Cincinnati incision in congenital talipes equinovarus. J Pediatr Orthop 1988; 8:696.

47. Esser RD: The medial sagittal approach in the treatment of congenital clubfoot. Clin Orthop 1994; 302:156.

48. Pandey S, Pandey AK: Soft tissue release in clubfoot by double incision. J Foot Ankle Surg 1995; 34(2):163.

49. Napiontek M: Transposed skin graft for wound closure after Cincinnati incision. Acta Orthop Scand 1996; 67(3):280.

50. Bensahel H, Csukonyi Z, Desgrippes Y, et al: Surgery in residual clubfoot: One-stage medioposterior release "a la carte." J Pediatr Orthop 1987; 7(2):145.

51. Yamamoto H, Furuya K: One-stage posteromedial release of congenital clubfoot. J Pediatr Orthop 1988; 8:590.

52. Yngve DA, Gross RH, Sullivan JA: Clubfoot release without wide subtalar release. J Pediatr Orthop 1990; 10:473.

53. Otremski I, Salama R, Khermosh O, et al: An analysis of the results of a modified one-stage posteromedial release (turco operation) for the treatment of clubfoot. J Pediatr Orthop 1987; 7(2):149.

54. Hudson I, Catterall A: Posterolateral release for resistant clubfoot. J Bone Joint Surg [Br] 1994; 76B(2):281.

55. Yamamoto Y, Muneta T, Ishibashi T, et al: Posteromedial release of congenital clubfoot in children over five years of age. J Bone Joint Surg [Br] 1994; 76B(4):555.

56. Lindell EB, Carroll NC: Longitudinal tendon splitting: A simple technique. J Pediatr Orthop 1994; 14:385.

57. Haasbeek JF, Wright JG: A comparison of long-term results of posterior and comprehensive release in treatment of clubfoot. J Pediatr Orthop 1997; 17:29.

58. Maffulli N, Kenward MG, Irwin AS, et al: Assessment of late results of surgery in talipes equinovarus: A reliability study. Eur J Pediatr 1997; 156:317.

59. Widhe T: Foot deformities at birth: A longitudinal prospective study over a 16-year period. J Pediatr Orthop 1997; 17:20.

60. Yamamoto H, Muneta T, Furuya K: Cause of toe-in gait after posteromedial release for congenital clubfoot. J Pediatr Orthop 1994; 14:369.

61. Otremski I, Salama R, Khermosh O, et al: Residual adduction of the forefoot. J Bone Joint Surg [Br] 1987; 69B(5):832.

62. Ghali NN, Smith RB, Clayden AD, et al: The results of pantalar reduction in the management of congenital talipes equinovarus. J Bone Joint Surg [Br] 1983; 65B(1):1.

35

Internal Tibial Torsion

Richard M. Jay, D.P.M.

The most common cause of tocing in, estimated to occur in 5% to 10% of children who have an in-toe, is internal or medial tibial torsion. During the development of the fetus, the lower limb buds rotate externally along the axial plane. Tibial torsion at birth has been estimated at 0 degrees. During the child's development, the tibia normally torques laterally to approximately 23 degrees external. This gradual unwinding of the bone in a lateral direction takes place over the course of 18 years, increasing external torque by 1 to 1.5 degrees per year.[1]

Various studies of this outward growth of the tibia have been performed. Arkin[2] demonstrated a plasticity of the bone under direct perpendicular stress to the epiphyseal plate that always allows an outward or inward spiraling effect to occur. This stress causes newly formed bone to change its position either internally or externally. Similar studies have been performed by Wilkinson,[3] Salter,[4] Brookes and Wardle,[5] and Moreland.[6] Their studies on the hip, femoral, and leg segments substantiated the original premise by Hueter[7] and Volkmann[8] in 1862, otherwise known as the Hueter-Volkmann law, that increased pressure inhibits growth and decreased pressure accelerates growth at the epiphyseal growth center. In 1980, Moreland[6] conducted an experiment on the tibias of live rabbits in which he applied an external rotatory force through the long axis of the bone. After a period of torque to the bone, the animals were sacrificed, and longitudinal sections were taken from the proximal tibial epiphysis. An angled primary trabecula was noted, as well an angulated hypertrophic cell between the cartilaginous struts of the layers of the provisional calcification. Moreland determined that an external spiraling effect of the newly laid-down bone occurred in the direction of torque applied to the bone.

ETIOLOGY

These findings provided insight into the cause of medial tibial torsion. A rapidly growing fetus can be subject to extrinsic constraining forces that mold the fetal tissues into certain positions according to the laws of bone growth. These congenital forces may also be present with intrauterine constraint. They are more likely to occur with first-borns, when the mother has tight uterine musculature, with a large fetus, or in multiple-fetus pregnancies. In the presence of uterine fibroids or a paucity of amniotic fluid, the fetus cannot develop or continue to progress through a normal ontogeny. Constrained by these underlying problems, extrauterine compression can prevent normal lateral unwinding of the tibial segment. A tight abdominal muscle in a woman with a small pelvis or a prominent lumbar spine can also inhibit the natural lateral twisting of the tibial segment. The vertex position maximizes uterine space and allows the fetus to go through its normal stretch and rotation of the limb buds. The breach position or a transverse lie further constrains the fetus and prevents normal ontogeny.

DIAGNOSIS

The diagnosis of tibial torsion is simple to make. In a clinical assessment the child is placed in a seated position with the legs dangling over the tabletop and the knees parallel to the frontal plane. In younger children, this position can be difficult in that the femoral segment is in an external position while the hip is normally in an abducted position; in such children the hips are drawn together and abducted in the seated position. This brings the legs closer together and the knees parallel to the frontal plane. The malleoli are examined. When the foot and leg are in a normal position in the developing child the tibial malleolus faces forward, and the lateral malleolus lies posterior to the medial malleolus (Figs. 35–1 to 35–4). Jakob,[9] in 1980, found that a relationship exists between tibial torsion and the transmalleolar axis. This transmalleolar axis is the angle between the distal tips of the tibial and fibular malleolus in the frontal plane. Jakob determined that a line drawn from the tip of the medial malleolus to the tip of the lateral malleolus on the frontal plane should be approximately 27 degrees in the adult. Jakob's values, determined by computed tomography (CT), showed that the transmalleolar axis is normally 5 to 7 degrees greater than the tibial torsion angle. Earlier studies by La Damany[1] and Elftman[10] noted a normal tibial torsion angle at birth of 0 degrees. Thus, a newborn should have 0 degrees of tibial torsion and a 5- to 7-degree lateral transmalleolar axis. Due to the normal unwinding of the tibial segment during growth, the transmalleolar axis increases 1 to 1.5 degrees per year. It is thus a simple matter to compute the appropriate normal axis for a given age. A child of 10 years, for example, should have a transmalleolar axis of approximately 15 degrees. Keeping in mind that tibial torsion is normally 5 degrees less than the transmalleolar axis, the normal tibial

261

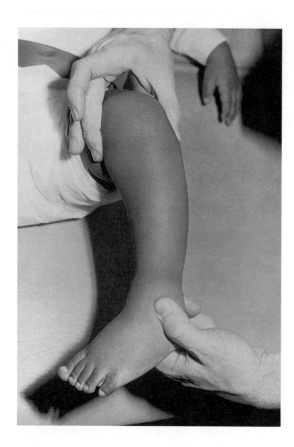

Figure 35–1. Internal tibial torsion of the left leg as shown by the knee resting on the frontal plane when the lateral malleolar is palpated by the thumb directly anterior. The medial malleolus is placed markedly posteriorly.

Figure 35–2. A 13-month-old child with internal tibial torsion and genu varum. When the tibial segment is internally rotated, the lateral aspect of the gastrocnemius muscle becomes increasingly apparent. This rotation produces a visible increase in the genu varum.

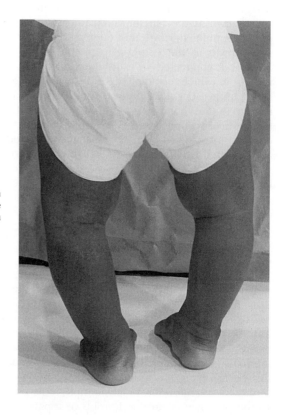

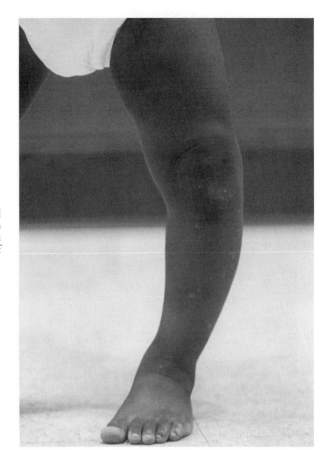

Figure 35–3. Internal tibial torsion with genu varum. The internal tibial torque is evident by the position of the medial and lateral malleoli, which rest parallel to the frontal plane when the foot is internally positioned. In isolated genu varum the curvature at the knee is present, but the foot itself is positioned in a more external angle.

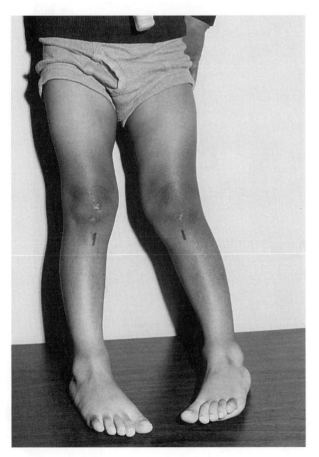

Figure 35–4. Six-year-old child with internal femoral segment and internal tibial torsion. Note the internal position of the patella as well as the anterior position of the lateral malleoli in relation to the posteriorly placed medial malleolus.

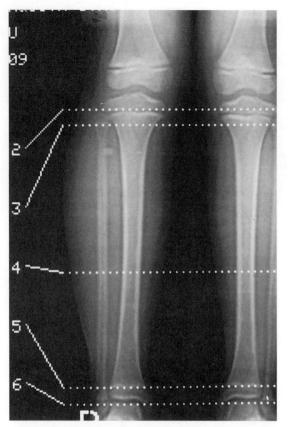

Figure 35–5. Frontal plane CT scan with markers. Measurements were taken at the proximal popliteal surface (marked 3) and the distal syndesmosis (marked 5).

were performed. In both methods tibiofibular torsion is determined by the deviation of the axes as seen in the proximal and distal cuts. The mean value of lateral torsion was 14.3 degrees (0 to 27 degrees) with MRI and 13.6 degrees (4 to 25 degrees) with anatomic measurements, whereas the difference between the two techniques averaged 4.1 degrees (0 to 15 degrees). MRI showed that the most marked increase in lateral torsion was localized to the upper part of the tibia, with a decrease in the supramalleolar segment. This finding differed from the classical ideas of Le Damany,[1] who had used the tibia alone in his studies. The clear lateral torsion of the tibiofibular unit at birth can help in understanding foot function with regard to its internal or external position and the resultant pronatory changes. On the other hand the MRI studies showed very interesting results in analyzing limb torsion in infants because allowed they visualization of the cartilage epiphysis.[13]

Another method of computing a more precise angle is to measure the distance between the medial malleolus and the lateral malleolus, project their positions onto the frontal plane, and determine the angle by the law of tangent—that is, the opposite side over the adjacent side equals the tangential angle of the transmalleolar axis. Keeping in mind that the transmalleolar axis is greater than the tibial torsion angle, one can determine the prognosis and the form of therapy needed to correct the deformity.

torsion angle can be extrapolated by subtracting 5 degrees from the transmalleolar axis.

More involved studies can be performed to determine the degree of tibial torsion precisely. Until recently, the standard methods used by Rosen and Sandick[11] and Hutter and Scott[12] were difficult to repeat, and the findings in these values were inconsistent. Now, with the use of CT, a child can be placed in a CT scanner the absolute torque of the tibia and the position of the transmalleolar axis. Correlation is made between the distal tibiofibular syndesmotic surface and the proximal posterior surface of the tibia in the area of the insertion of the popliteus (Figs. 35–5 to 35–7).

The torsion of the tibiofibular functional unit corresponds to the angle between the transverse axis of the proximal tibial epiphyseal plateau and the axis through the middle of both malleoli. A recent anatomic study demonstrated that clear lateral tibiofibular torsion exists from the beginning of the fetal period with a positive gradient at birth.[13] A comparative imaging and anatomic study using magnetic resonance imaging (MRI) was performed to control the previous results. Both legs of 10 aborted fetuses, free of malformation and ranging in age from 27 to 39 weeks, were used. All calculations were based on cross-sections, which were taken at multiple levels along the tibial and fibular segments. MRI analysis was performed first, using a 0.5-Tesla resistive MRI unit and a 30/1200 spin echo pulse sequence. Data were collected on a 256/256 matrix. Then anatomic sections

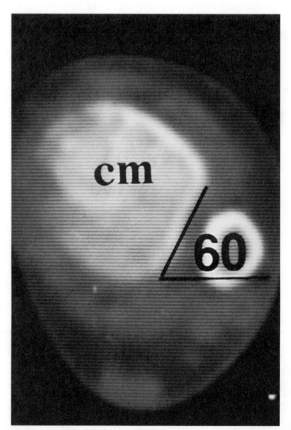

Figure 35–6. CT scan of leg, distal segment. Measurement of flat surface of syndesmosis on tibial surface in relation to the resting frontal plane, in this case, 60 degrees.

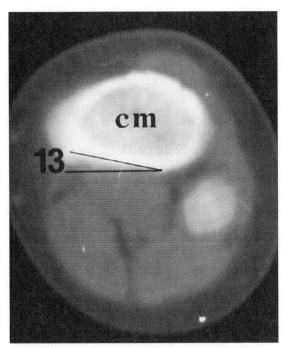

Figure 35–7. CT scan of tibia, proximal segment. Measurement of the flattened popliteal surface in relation to the resting frontal plane, in this case, 13 degrees.

SEQUELAE OF UNTREATED TIBIAL TORSION

Bone in the living body is subject to a variety of forces such as gravity, muscle activity, and the dynamic support system and bends and twists in response to these forces. The tensile and compressive forces that act upon this rapidly growing bone eventually become permanently fixed. It is for this reason that early diagnosis and treatment are of paramount concern. Unfortunately, children are not usually brought into the physician's office for this complaint until it is too late. Once the bone has formed

in this inward fashion and has not progressed through its external spiral torque, certain sequelae occur. These can include apparent bowing of the lower leg or an increased tendency to trip as the foot becomes locked in the ankle joint in an inward position. An unlocking mechanism can occur in which the leg is twisted and driven internally while the foot is locked and positioned on the ground and then starts to abduct at the subtalar joint through the reactive force of gravity, (Fig. 35–8). The midtarsal joint along the transverse plane also abducts, dorsiflexes, and pronates. The result is a flatfoot deformity secondary to the reaction of the internal drive of the tibia. As the child develops, the in-toe appears to be reduced. As the leg unscrews the talus downward and the midtarsal joint unlocks, the appearance of an externally positioned foot is gained at the cost of abduction and pronation of the foot (Fig. 35–9). When seen by the parent or the untrained eye, the answer is simple—the child outgrew the deformity. Unfortunately, the child did not actually outgrow the deformity; rather, a new flatfoot abducted deformity has now replaced the intoe[14] (Fig. 35–10).

TREATMENT

Let's consider the younger child between the ages of 6 months and 1 year who has just started to stand. It is at this age parents notice that the legs are bent and the feet are turned inward. If the physician is fortunate enough to see children at this age, he or she can undo any constraining factors and use to the child's advantage the laws that promote outward bone growth. Merely by understanding that the tibia normally goes through a process of increasing external torque, and then by taking away all constraining internal factors, the physician can promote the external rotation of the tibia. This can be achieved simply by placing the tibia in an outward position and maintaining it in that position for a period of time. There is much disagreement about whether to treat medial tibial torsion or not.

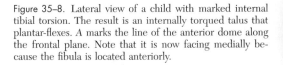

Figure 35–8. Lateral view of a child with marked internal tibial torsion. The result is an internally torqued talus that plantar-flexes. A marks the line of the anterior dome along the frontal plane. Note that it is now facing medially because the fibula is located anteriorly.

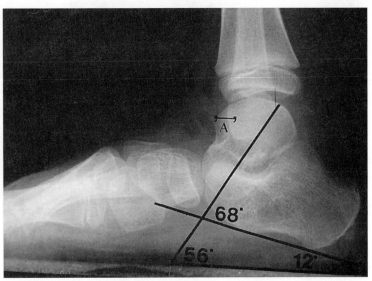

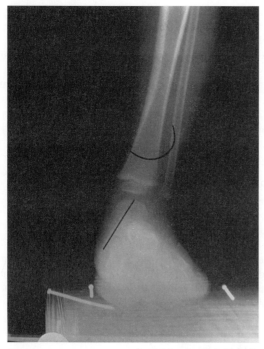

Figure 35–9. Anteroposterior view of a child with internal tibial torsion. Note the direction of motion on the tibial and fibular unit as it is driving medially. The talus is locked in the ankle mortise, thus increasing internal transverse plane motion as it follows the direction of the tibia and fibula.

Cast Treatment

One method of treatment is to use a long leg, externally twisted cast. The net result is an externally and laterally rotated leg that is locked at the knee and ankle joints. This cast is maintained for a period of 3 to 4 weeks (Figs. 35–11 and 35–12), during which time the outer roll of Scotchrap (3M Health Care Products, St. Paul, MN) is removed, allowing further rotation of the lower cast on the upper cast. The lower segment is then twisted again externally approximately 2 cm, and another roll of Scotchrap is applied to secure the twisted position. Locking around the foot is necessary to prevent the cast from creating a cylinder effect. At the end of the fourth week the cast is removed. Three rolls of 2-inch or 3-inch Scotchrap are used depending on the child's size. The first roll extends from the toes to the proximal tibia, and the second roll extends from the proximal tibia to the proximal thigh with a 1-cm separation between the first and second rolls at the level just below the knee. While laterally twisting the lower leg on the thigh, the third roll is applied over the entire cast and locked over the foot to maintain an external lateral torque. Casting is recommended before the child becomes ambulatory, and the foot need not he dorsiflexed. If the older child is already ambulating, the foot must be dorsiflexed and held in a neutral position. With the knee flexed approximately 25 degrees, the foot must also be flexed; otherwise the child

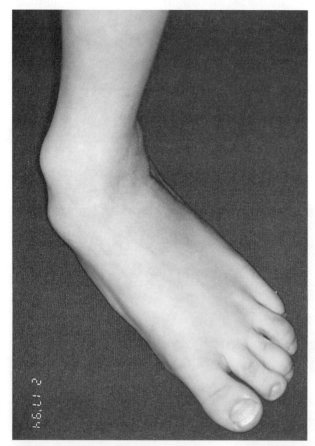

Figure 35–10. Marked transverse plane deformity secondary to internal tibial torsion. Note the medial bulge of the talus as it protrudes on an even parallel plane with the tibia. The foot is markedly abducted.

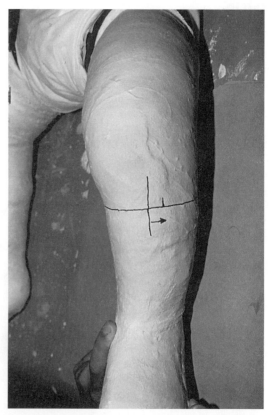

Figure 35–11. Circumferential marker placed along the proximal aspect of the leg just distal to the knee joint. The two proximal markings demonstrate the amount of motion needed to rotate the lower segment of the cast on the upper segment. This usually equals approximately 2 cm during each visit. These visits continue for no more than 3 weeks.

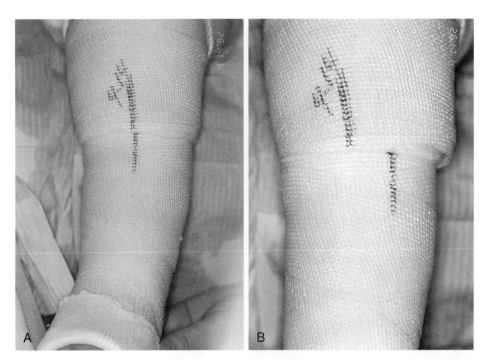

Figure 35–12. *A,* A circumferential separation is present between the proximal and distal portions of the cast. The lower segment will be externally torqued to reduce the internal tibial torsion deformity. *B,* Distal segment of cast being rotated externally to reduce internal tibial torque.

will not be able to stand flat on the cast's end and walk properly. Plantar flexion of the cast must be avoided in the ambulating child to prevent the precaution of pressure sores (blisters) on the dorsal surface of the toes.

After Cast Treatment

After removal of the cast, the foot and leg must be maintained in the new laterally twisted position. If they are not, the deformity may recur. Arkin[2] described how a torque in the long bone produces a spiraling of the growth cells in the direction of the applied torque. However, he also noted that when the torque was released, the spiraling effect' ceased as growth returned to the original columnar position. To apply the principles of the dynamic system that causes bone growth, an externally placed splint or bracing system should be applied. The use of a Counter Rotational System (CRS) (Langer Laboratories, Deer Park, NY) is recommended because it not only places the transverse plane of the leg in an external position but also allows normal muscular development and normal motion in the knee and hip.

It must be noted here that bars, splints, and braces do not obtain correction of any torque or rotatory changes in the bone. They do, however, maintain the desired position and eliminate any extrinsic internally directed forces. When using a device such as a CRS, Fillauer (Durr-Flower Medical Inc., Orthopedic Division, Chattanooga, TN), Denis Browne bar (Durr-Flower Medical Inc., Orthopedic Division, Chattanooga, TN), or Unibar (Spectra Industries Corp., Yeadon, PA), the position of the foot should not exceed 15 to 25 degrees external, and the rearfoot must be maintained in approximately 5 to 7 degrees varus. This is accomplished by bending the bar of the Denis Browne bar or the Fillauer in the center. The rearfoot will then be positioned in an inverted varus attitude. The Unibar has a universal joint that should also be set in varus beneath each shoe plate. The CRS already has a built-in 5- to 7-degree rearfoot varus position. An excessive external position of the shoe plates does not produce the desired effect on the leg but rather forces the foot to abduct and pronate the talocalcaneal joint. The talocalcaneal joint angle increases as the talus unlocks in the ankle mortise. The result is that the foot (calcaneus) then abducts under the talus.

In the child over 18 months of age, casting for an in-toe deformity is quite difficult. The child is more active and has more motion in the lower extremity and more awareness of being constrained by a cast. A cast makes it more difficult for the child to crawl, stand, and walk. In these children it is especially important to remove the constraining factors that continually inhibit the leg from unwinding inward. The leg may not go through its normal ontogenous external rotation in the axial segment because its position during either sitting or sleeping gently twists and maintains the leg inwardly. For example, some children sit in a reverse tailor position (Fig. 35–13) or sleep with their legs tucked up toward their buttocks. Removing constraining positions and maintaining an external attitude at this stage requires a bar, splint, or other system that maintains correction. Again, it most be stressed that these devices should be used only to maintain position, not to obtain correction.

In the child who is older than 6 years and still has an inward tibial torsion, the deformity probably will not decrease, and the sequelae of a flatfoot will increase. A flatfoot that is secondary to a transverse plane abnormality can become a fixed rigid flatfoot. A simple orthosis is recommended for these children. By maintaining the rearfoot in a subtalar neutral position, one can prevent the internal driving forces through the midtarsal and subtalar joints that create a flatfoot. It is often asked whether, since the subtalar and midtarsal joints are sup-

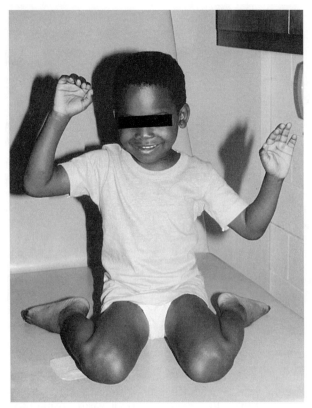

Figure 35–13. Reverse talar position. Note the internally torqued femoral segments. The tibial segment is being held externally, and both feet are forced into abduction. This is also known as a W sitting position. During gait the child still has a rectus position because the femoral segment is internally positioned and the tibial segment is externally positioned. The net effect is a rectus gait with flattening of the foot.

on the tibia (Figs. 35–14 to 35–19), which is part of the normal development of the child. Any delay in treatment will result in a permanently positioned in-toe or a compensated transverse plane flatfoot deformity (Fig. 35–20). Operative correction of tibial torsion should be delayed until after age 9 when tibial torsion has been stabilized and post-healing changes are unlikely to occur. Rotational tibial osteotomies can safely be performed at either the proximal or distal level, but fewer serious complications occur with distal osteotomies.

Bremer Tibial Transformer, Wheaton Splint, and Ipos Anti-adductus Devices

The Bremer Tibial Transformer, Wheaton splint (Wheaton Brace Co., Coral Stream, IL), and the Ipos Anti-adductus (Ipos USA, Niagara Falls, NY) device provide similar degrees of external torque to maintain tibial torsion. These devices have been marketed as primary reducing products; however, if they are used as a form of adjunctive treatment after cast reduction, the results are good. The splints address the deformity directly and can be used primarily if the parents use them continually. Once the splints are removed the potential for loss of correction is high. Cast treatment guarantees compliance. I personally apply a cast if the child is young enough and follow this with one of these splints. If the child is over the age of 18 months cast treatment is too restrictive, some compromise is needed. The Bremer Tibial Transformer, Wheaton splint, or Ipos Anti-adductus device provide external torque during nap and sleep time. If

ported in a supinated position, won't this accentuate the toe-in? It will, but the support is needed to maintain a corrected position of the foot to prevent creation of another problem as the child grows older. This should be explained to the parent before initiating treatment with an orthosis. The child is still encouraged to remove all internal medial forces that are twisting the leg. When these forces are removed, the leg will go through its normal ontogenous process of external lateral growth.

Alternative treatments consisting of gait plates or wedged shoes have also been recommended for the treatment of tibial torsion causing a resultant toe-in. These must maintain a subtalar neutral position. However, these devices actually allow the foot to pronate through the gait cycle and abduct the midtarsal joint. This gives an illusion of an abducted foot position and a reduction of the toe-in deformity. It must be kept in mind that gait plates should be used only for children who have a toe-in problem consisting of tripping only. These devices do not directly reduce internal tibial torsion.

The basic concern with a child with an in-toe problem secondary to medial tibial torsion is early recognition and treatment. Treatment before the age of ambulation is of prime importance. It is at this age that the deformity can be reduced by taking away the constraining factors and promoting normal external bone growth. Whether this treatment is accomplished by casting or maintenance with the CRS, splints, or bars, the result is an external torque

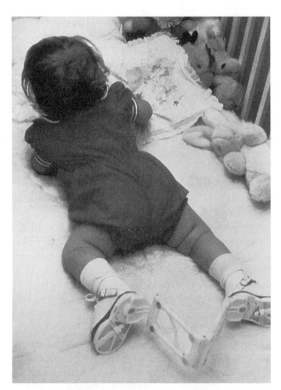

Figure 35–14. A child with a counter rotational splint (CRS) system, which is used to maintain an external axial segment by allowing the child to move freely.

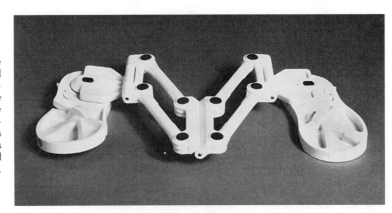

Figure 35–15. Counter rotational splint. Two foot plates are glued to the inferior surface of a pair of leather-bottomed flat shoes. The rearfoot is automatically held in approximately a 5-degree inverted position by the angle to the longitudinal bars. The external or internal rotation of the plate is adjusted by unscrewing the plate from the stationary bar. The plate is set to the required number of degrees as marked on the inferior portion. The flexible bar allows for motion of the device in a parallelogram fashion and maintains the position of both feet in the correct alignment.

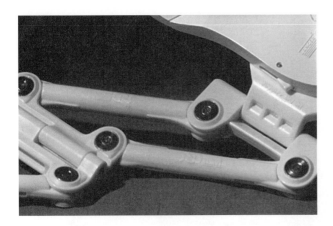

Figure 35–16. Counter rotational system parallelogram splint allows motion while maintaining the footplate in the direction in which it was set. Motion is allowed as the child crawls.

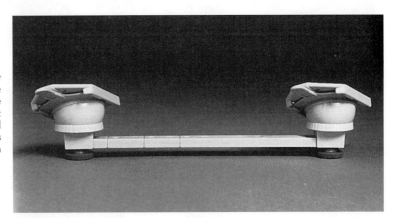

Figure 35–17. A Uni-Bar. The Uni-Bar is held together by a transverse bar set to a specified distance between the anterior iliac spines. In the infant 6 to 18 months old, the distance is approximately 6 inches. The rearfoot plate is set in 5 degrees varus, which is maintained by the universal joint connecting to the transverse bar. The foot plate is removable. This allows the child to be placed gradually in the splint and minimizes its disturbing effect during sleep.

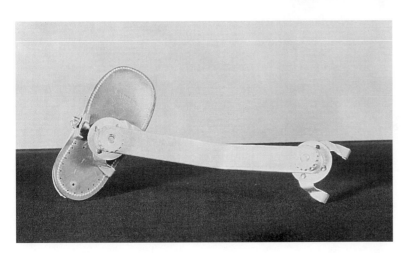

Figure 35–18. A Fillauer splint. The Fillauer splint is bent in the center to prevent pronatory changes. A bend of approximately 5 to 10 degrees is placed in the longitudinal bar, yielding a rearfoot varus. The foot plate is then positioned to reduce the internal or external tibial component. The splint is used only during rest and at night.

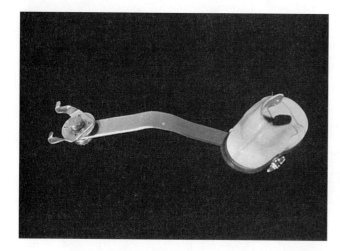

Figure 35–19. The Fillauer bar is bent in the center to yield 5 to 10 degrees of heel varus to minimize the pronatory effect of externally torquing the foot plate.

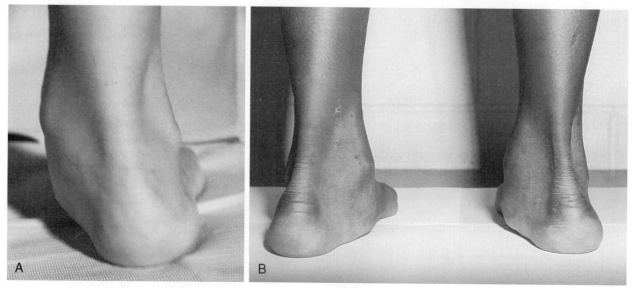

Figure 35–20. *A*, Increase in transverse plane motion secondary to internal drive of tibial torsion. *B*, Iatrogenically induced flatfoot. Note the loss of the medial column arch with a continuation of an internal tibial position. The medial malleoli are posteriorly placed in relation to the lateral malleoli. This child was held in excessive external torque using a Denis Browne bar.

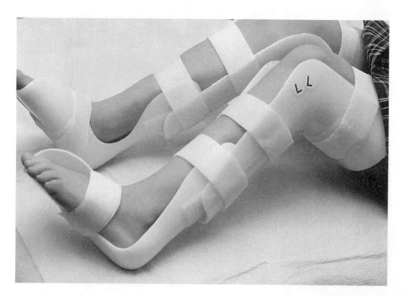

Figure 35–21. Bilateral Wheaton splints being used to externally torque the tibial segment and abduct the metatarsals in a child with metatarsus adductus.

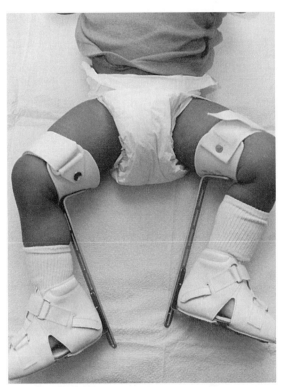

Figure 35–22. Bilateral IPOS anti-adductus splint maintains the child in external tibial torsion to reduce an internal tibial deformity.

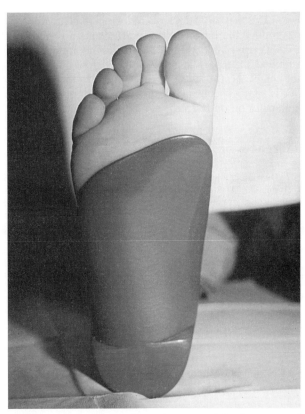

Figure 35–24. Gait plate used to induce internal forefoot position by exerting pressure beneath the first metatarsal head. Discomfort results because the child must force the foot to supinate, putting pressure on the lateral distal aspect of the fifth metatarsal. The end result is a toe-in position.

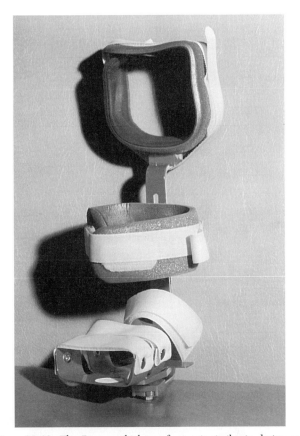

Figure 35–23. The Bremer tibial transformer is similar in design and function to the IPOS splint; however, a shoe is placed on the child first, and this is placed in the shoe plate of the device. The foot is then angled externally or internally to obtain reduction of the tibial component.

the child is cooperative, the parents should certainly be encouraged to use the splints throughout the day.

The lower foot-leg segment should be twisted externally at least 25 degrees; any greater degrees increases the chance of creating knee pathology. A long sock or stocking should be used under the splint because the splint conforms to the leg, and irritation can result if some protection is not used. If the child resists the use of splints, they can be discontinued. When used after cast therapy, splint therapy should be encouraged for 3 to 6 months. The older the child the more difficult compliance becomes (Figs. 35–21 to 35–23).

University of California Biomechanic Laboratory, Dynamic Stabilizing Innersole System (DSIS), and Roberts Plate Orthotics

The child over 2 years of age with internal tibial torsion is prone to a torque that drives the foot into a pronated position. An attempt should be made to prevent this internal drive. The standard orthotic device with a rearfoot varus position supinates and locks the subtalar and midtarsal joints. The frontal plane motion on the calcaneus creates an external rotatory force on the talus that results in the entire lower extremity rotating on the axial plane. This has no effect on reducing tibial torsion but does reduce the internal drive on the talus. Prevention of the talus from adducting on the calcaneus minimizes the likelihood of a permanently flattened foot. Augmenting the height of the orthotic with a high medial flange affords greater control of the talus and prevents talar plantar flexion on the sagittal plane[15-17] (Fig. 35–24).

References

1. LaDamany PLa torsion du tibia. J L Anat Physiol 1909; 45:598–615.
2. Arkin AM: The effects of pressure on epiphyseal growth: The mechanism of plasticity of growing bone. J Bone Joint Surg 1956; 38A:1056–1076.
3. Wilkinson JA: Femoral anteversion in the rabbit. J Bone Joint Surg 1962; 44B:386.
4. Salter R: The present state of innominate osteotomy in congenital dislocation of the hip. J Bone Joint Surg 1966; 48B:853.
5. Brookes M, Wardle EN: Muscle action and the shape of the femur. J Bone Joint Surg 1962; 44B:398.
6. Moreland MS: Morphological effects of torsion applied to growing bone. J Bone Joint Surg 1980; 62B(2):230–237.
7. Hueter C: Anatomische Studien an den Extremita tengelenhen Neugeborener und erwach Sener. Virchows Arch 1862; 25:572.
8. Volkmann R: Chirurgische Erfahrungan über Knochenverbiegurgen. Arch Pathol Anat 1862; 24:512.
9. Jakob RP: Tibial torsion calculated by computerized tomography and compared to other methods of measurement. J Bone Joint Surg 1980; 62B:238–242.
10. Elftman H: Torsion of lower extremity. Am J Physiol Anthropol 1945; 3:255–265.
11. Rosen H, Sandick H: The measurement of tibiofibular torsion. J Bone Joint Surg 1955; 37A:847–855.
12. Hutter CG, Scott W: Tibial torsion. J Bone Joint Surg 1949; 31A:511–518.
13. Badelon O, Perraudin JE: Comparison of MRI and anatomic cuts in measurement of tibiofibular torsion in fetus. J Bone Joint Surg Orthop Trans 1991; 15(1):136.
14. Jay RM: In-toe secondary to medial tibial torsion. Curr Podiatr Med 1990; 39:9–13.
15. Jay RM, Schoenhaus HD: Hyperpronation control with a Dynamic Stabilizing Innersole System. J Am Podiatr Med Assoc 1992; 82:140–153.
16. Jay RM, Schoenhaus HD: The Dynamic Stabilizing Innersole System (DSIS): The management of hyperpronation in children. J Foot Ankle Surg 1995; 34:124–131.
17. Jay RM: Pediatric orthoses. Biomechanics 1995; 2:51–54.

Four

Equinus

36

Equinus

Richard M. Jay, D.P.M.

Equinus deformity develops when an imbalance exists between the anterior dorsiflexors (L4–L5) and the posterior plantar flexors (L4,L5,SI) (Table 36–1). Equinus is a limitation of dorsiflexion of the foot on the leg. When this limit is present for a prolonged period of time, the foot responds by compensating for the limitation of dorsiflexion at the ankle. Ten degrees of dorsiflexion is needed at the ankle joint when the knee is extended fully and the subtalar joint is in its neutral position. The 10 degrees is needed because at 50% to 60% of the gait cycle the thigh is extended 10 degrees on the torso. The knee is extended and locked, the subtalar joint is in neutral position, and the midtarsal joint is locked and ready for propulsion. A child with an equinus deformity is a midstance pronator.[1]

UNCOMPENSATED EQUINUS

Toe-Walking

Uncompensated equinus presents without dorsiflexion at the ankle joint, midtarsal joint, or subtalar joint. These children appear to walk on the metatarsal heads with the toes maximally dorsiflexed at the metatarsophalangeal joints. No heel contact is made during the gait cycle or stance. The foot is plantar-flexed during the majority of the gait cycle.

The young healthy child who toe-walks usually walks in this position from habit rather than in response to any overt spasticity of the posterior group of muscles. The child's foot that appears to be in equinus at stance can easily be diagnosed by allowing the child to stand still. In stance the heels eventually drop to the ground with no recurvatum at the knee. If the same child is told to run, the heels immediately rise or appear to bounce off the supporting surface too early. The deep tendon reflexes are usually intact, and the foot can be actively dorsiflexed

to a right angle. This should be considered a normal variation of gait.[2,3]

UNCOMPENSATED WITH SPASTICITY

The most commonly reported cause of toe walking is secondary to a type of spasticity as seen in cerebral palsy. In considering equinus in patients with spastic cerebral palsy, it is important to understand the cause of the condition. Spastic equinus results from a neurologic condition that causes a spastic plantar-flexed position of the foot on the ankle. The deformity may be caused by one of several interactions. The gastrocnemius-soleus complex may be partially or entirely spastic, or weakness of the anterior muscles may result in relative overpowering of the posterior group.

Spastic equinus is nonprogressive and may be caused by a variety of problems. Prenatal anoxia, drug reactions with the mother, fetal alcohol syndrome, birth trauma, meningitis, and cerebral injury are a few of the common causes of cerebral palsy. The neurologic impairment is static, but the effect of the condition is progressive. As the child grows the spastic tendon maintains its contracted tensive state on the bone and joint. Eventually, the tension is too great, and the flexible undeformed young foot begins to contract; eventually it becomes rigid. The motor involvement may be that of hypotonia, but the result is the same as that previously mentioned. If the anterior group is hypotonic, the normally innervated posterior group will eventually overpower it, resulting in an equinus foot.

If the anterior and posterior muscles in a normal child's gait pattern are compared, it is apparent that the triceps surae start to function soon after heel contact. The soleus becomes active when the leg moves forward. This causes a stabilizing plantar-flexory force. As the forward movement of the leg continues, it promotes a stretch reflex in the gastrocnemius muscle. The gastrocnemius then fires, transmitting a force that plantar-flexes the foot at the ankle joint. This continues through toe-off.[1] The anterior muscles are mainly active during the swing phase.

It must be remembered that in normal gait, the dorsiflexors are not antagonists to the gastrocnemius-soleus complex, since they do not function during the same interval of the gait cycle.[4,5] This is not true in the presence of spastic equinus. The gastrocnemius-soleus complex is spastic throughout the gait cycle. The gait is no longer

Table 36–1. **Normal Ankle Dorsiflexion Sequence**

1. Subtalar joint is in its neutral position.
2. The midtarsal joint is maximally pronated and locked due to the reactive force of gravity from the ground (reactive ground force).
3. The thigh is extended 10 degrees to the pelvis.
4. The knee joint is fully extended.
5. The ankle joint dorsiflexes 10 degrees to compensate for thigh extension.

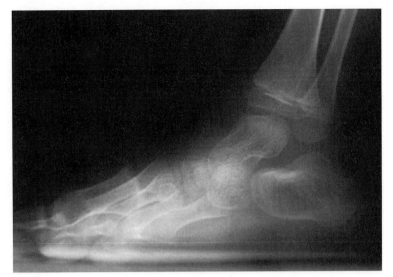

Figure 36–1. The leg is positioned approximately 15 degrees from the vertical neutral position, yielding a plantar-flexed talus in relation to the leg; the heel is elevated off the ground. There is an unequal balance between the flexors and the extensors. The gastrocnemius-soleus complex is spastic throughout the gait cycle. The gait is no longer heel-toe; the pattern is one of toe-toe, and the spastic condition of the triceps surae is so tight that even the child's weight cannot force the rearfoot down.

heel-toe; the pattern becomes one of toe-toe, with the spastic condition of the triceps surae so tight that even the child's weight cannot force the rearfoot down. If the triceps surae spasticity is less tense, the heel may come down after the toe touches, or the entire foot may strike in a plantar-grade fashion. All of this contact depends on the degree of spasticity of the gastrocnemius-soleus complex in relation to the function of the anterior muscles.[6] In light of these facts, it is evident that the primary cause of the equinus deformity is the unequal balance between the flexors and the extensors. To reduce the equinus, the function of the gastrocnemius-soleus complex must be diminished (see Fig. 36–1).

COMPENSATED EQUINUS

Compensated with Spasticity

The most interesting phenomenon in cerebral palsy children is that the equinus or toe-toe gait can disappear and is replaced by a severely pronated valgus foot. The same mechanism of compensatory pronatory changes occurs in the spastic condition as in children with a congenitally shortened tendo Achillis. The foot compensates before the talar head flattens. In the presence of this limitation of motion at the ankle joint, dorsiflexion occurs the foot at the midtarsal joint. This is the type of foot that must be addressed with more than just a tendo-Achillis lengthening. Additional procedures are required, consisting of either arthrodesis, arthroereisis, or tendon transfers. Unfortunately, delay in treatment is common, and this results in permanent osseous changes and a need for more aggressive procedures.[7]

The spasm acts as a strong deforming force on the foot. Subtalar malposition causes midtarsal instability, which promotes increased subtalar pronation as compensation for the lack of dorsiflexion that is necessary for adequate propulsion. Pronation subsequently creates a flexible flatfoot deformity. In many patients with spastic equinus, prevention of compensatory pronation is of paramount importance in achieving an adequate functional gait (Fig. 36–2).

If the equinus is not reduced, mechanical compression

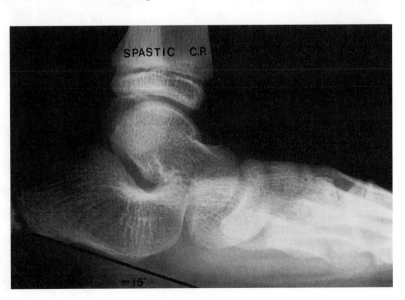

Figure 36–2. The spasm acts as a strong deforming force on the foot. Subtalar malposition causes midtarsal instability, which promotes increased subtalar pronation as compensation for the lack of dorsiflexion that is necessary for adequate propulsion. Pronation subsequently creates a flexible flatfoot deformity. The heel elevates and the forefoot dorsiflexes at the midtarsal joint.

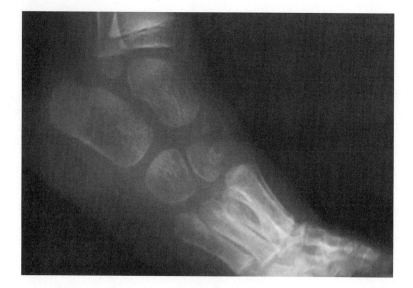

Figure 36–3. Flattening of the dome of the talus. The talus abuts against the anterior aspect of the tibia and becomes locked, preventing dorsiflexion. With increased weight bearing, the dorsiflexion increases compression of the foot through the talus on the leg. The result is compression on the osteochondral surface, where an ischemic necrosis occurs. This process continues until there is a total loss of motion within the ankle.

occurs on the talar dome, causing a decrease in endochondral bone growth and creating the flat-top talus. The flattening of the talar dome prevents ankle dorsiflexion owing to the osseous block. Dorsiflexion is not possible, even with future lengthening of the tendo Achillis. This is an unstable foot that does not allow the child to ambulate in an acceptable position. The child walks high on the toes as if walking on stilts, thus increasing compression on the talar head.

Flat-top Talus

In the presence of true flattening of the dome of the talus a posterior glide does not occur in the direction of

dorsiflexion. The talus abuts against the anterior aspect of the tibia and becomes locked, preventing dorsiflexion. With increased weight bearing, as in a child who is growing, dorsiflexion increases compression of the foot through the talus on the leg. The result is compression on the osteochondral surface, which can lead to ischemic necrosis. This process continues until a total loss of motion occurs in the ankle (Figs. 36–3 and 36–4).

When reviewing a suspected flat-top talus in a patient with either a cavus or equinus deformity, a radiograph of the foot in a normal weight-bearing lateral projection is recommended. Another weight-bearing lateral view is taken with the leg slightly adducted or internally rotated to approximately 20 degrees. With a supinated foot, the

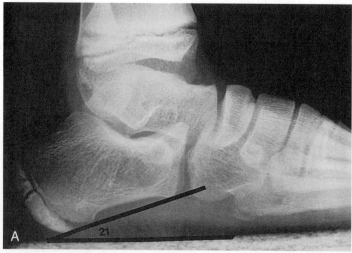
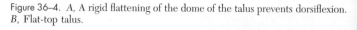

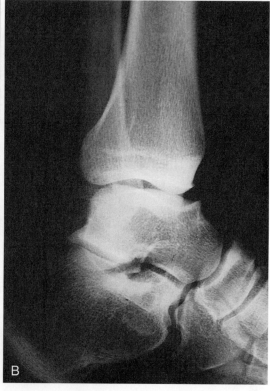

Figure 36–4. A, A rigid flattening of the dome of the talus prevents dorsiflexion. B, Flat-top talus.

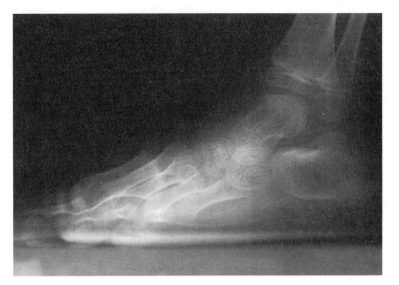

Figure 36–5. The talus rides high on the calcaneus, and the superior condyles or dome of the talus appear to be superimposed, thus flattened. This is not a true flattening of the talus but rather a radiographic finding.

talus rides high on the calcaneus, and the superior condyles or dome of the talus gives the appearance of being superimposed and thus flattened. This is therefore not a true flattening of the talus but rather a radiographic finding. When the leg is internally rotating 20 degrees the talar dome is positioned more internally, and the true appearance of the rounded dome is appreciated (Figs. 36–5 and 36–6).

Mechanisms of Compensated Equinus

If there is a limitation of dorsiflexion at the ankle when the knee joint is fully extended, dorsiflexion must be gained somewhere. Compensation is gained by dorsiflexing the subtalar joint and, more important, the midtarsal joint. Abduction and dorsiflexion increase at the midtarsal joint, causing significant changes over time. Here, dorsiflexion comprises the majority of triplane motion. When it is of a congenital or primary nature, equinus is a severe pronatory force. Primary gastrocnemius equinus, probably the strongest of all pronatory forces, produces pronation

in the foot equalled only by internal torque. The subtalar joint does not have a wide dorsiflexory range of motion, while in the midtarsal joint dorsiflexion around the oblique axis and abduction are the major components of its range of motion (Figs. 36–7 and 36–8).

In partially compensated equinus, the heel approaches the ground through midtarsal joint and subtalar joint pronation. These children exhibit a bouncing gait and early heel-off. Calcaneal apophysitis is a common finding in these children.

Children with fully compensated equinus have abnormal subtalar joint and midtarsal joint pronation that allows the foot to attain the necessary 10 degrees of dorsiflexion. Pronation at the midtarsal and subtalar joints is the severe deforming force in foot function.

CLINICAL DIAGNOSIS

The child is placed in a supine position with the leg extended and the toes hanging over the edge of the examination table. The examiner's hand is placed under

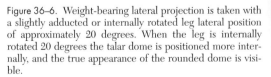

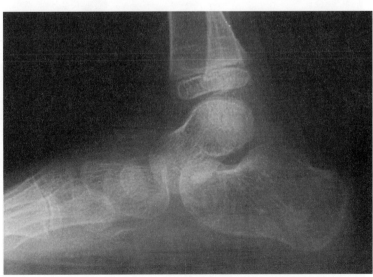

Figure 36–6. Weight-bearing lateral projection is taken with a slightly adducted or internally rotated leg lateral position of approximately 20 degrees. When the leg is internally rotated 20 degrees the talar dome is positioned more internally, and the true appearance of the rounded dome is visible.

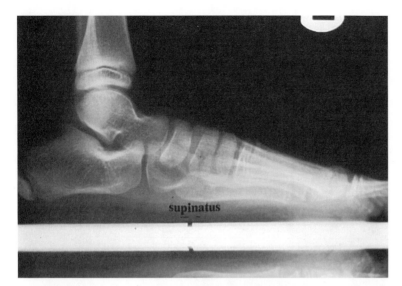

Figure 36–7. With dorsiflexion limited at the ankle joint, the foot compensates for the lack of dorsiflexion at the midtarsal and subtalar joints. The calcaneal inclination decreases, and the forefoot supinates at the midtarsal joint, increasing dorsiflexion in the foot.

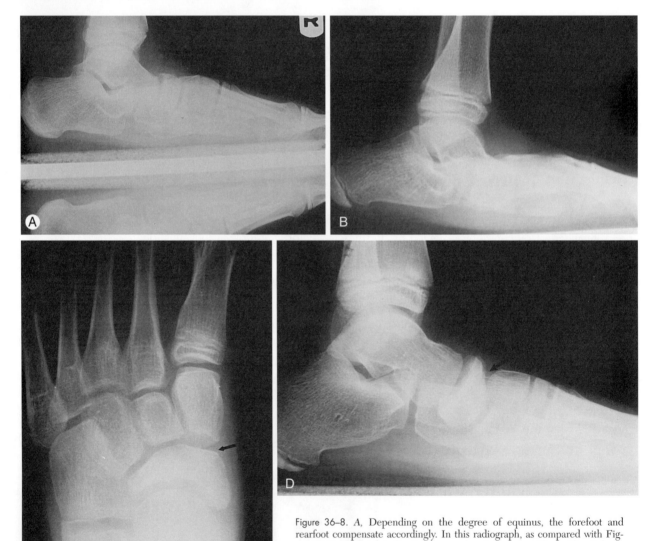

Figure 36–8. *A,* Depending on the degree of equinus, the forefoot and rearfoot compensate accordingly. In this radiograph, as compared with Figure 36–7, calcaneal inclination approaches 0 degrees with significant dorsiflexion at the midtarsal joint. *B,* With increased tightness at the posterior group, the deformity increases compared with the situation shown in *A* and Fig. 36–7. *C,* Distal flattening of the medial aspect of the cuneiform-navicular articulation. This is secondary to equinus and produces limited ankle dorsiflexion and increased dorsiflexion at the cuneiform-navicular joint. *D,* Child presenting with gastrocnemius-soleus equinus. A lack of dorsiflexion at the ankle joint results in dorsiflexion at the cuneiform-navicular joint. This 12-year-old child now demonstrates a wedging of the distal aspect of the navicular. Dorsiflexion is occurring at the cuneiform-navicular articulation as marked by the arrow.

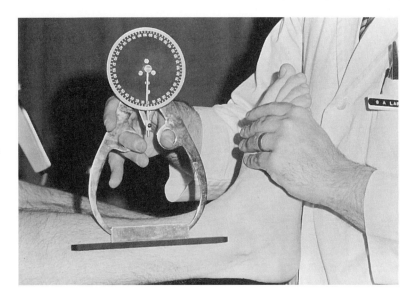

Figure 36–9. The foot is held in neutral position with the leg positioned parallel to the supporting surface.

the leg distally, raising it slightly to bring the leg parallel to the table surface. The opposite hand grasps the forefoot while the, examiner visualizes the lateral border of the calcaneus as it runs just proximal to the fifth metatarsal base and cuboid. The foot is dorsiflexed until it is parallel with the tibia. The forefoot is neither abducted nor adducted to this plane of the tibia. With abduction of the foot (pronation), dorsiflexion appears to be increased. This is midtarsal joint oblique axis dorsiflexion, not ankle joint dorsiflexion. An angle is then observed between the leg and the lateral calcaneal border. Dorsiflexion of the foot is repeated with the knee flexed; the angle should increase as the gastrocnemius muscle becomes lax. A gastrocnemius equinus from a gastrocnemius-soleus equinus can now be diagnosed (Figs. 36–9 to 36–11).

With limitation of dorsiflexion, it is not uncommon for a child to complain of pain in the posterior calf area. The intensity of the discomfort depends on the tightness of the gastrocnemius-soleus complex and on the activities of the child. On examination, the child displays a markedly abducted foot in stance with an obvious break laterally in the direction of abduction at the calcaneal cuboid joint

(Figs. 36–12 and 36–13). The forefoot demonstrates a high degree of soft tissue varus deformity, otherwise known as a forefoot supinatus (Fig. 36–14). The supinatus is secondary to midtarsal joint pronation. With a gastrocnemius equinus, the posterior calf also loses its definition, and the muscle appears to run directly into the distal leg. Normally, one can visually define the gastrocnemius heads proximally. The nonweight-bearing foot shows no arch definition, and there is no apparent plantar flexion of the first ray.

One must be cautious in recommending control of equinus by an orthotic device; since the dorsiflexory component of gait occurs at the midtarsal joint, the foot will pronate with great impact into the medial surface of the orthosis, causing discomfort to the child. If no dorsiflexion is available at midstance, the orthosis will probably fail. This is the child who is most likely to be a candidate for a lengthening procedure. If, however, at least 5 degrees of dorsiflexion are available at the ankle joint, an orthosis will control the problem. The orthosis could be casted with the child's foot in a slightly pronated position to eliminate the possibility of medial arch fatigue and allow

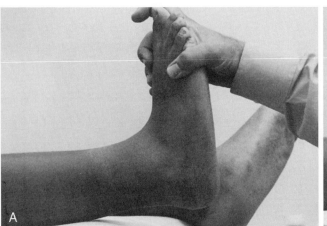
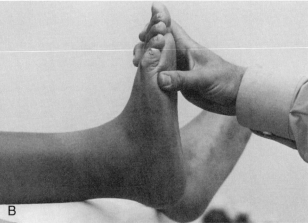

Figure 36–10. A, The foot is dorsiflexed with the knee extended while the neutral position of the foot is maintained the entire time. B, One should avoid dorsiflexing the foot on the lateral side or forcing the foot into abduction because this will only produce dorsiflexion of the ankle at the cost of midtarsal and subtalar pronation.

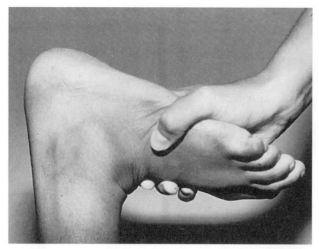

Figure 36–11. Dorsiflexion of the foot is repeated as in Figure. 36–10A with the knee flexed.

the foot to pronate through gait while the orthosis blocks end-range pronation. This allows dorsiflexion to occur at the midtarsal joint to a lesser degree.

During the time the child is wearing a fully posted orthosis (rearfoot and forefoot post), gastrocnemius-soleus stretching exercises are encouraged. If length increases in the gastrocnemius-soleus complex, the pronation that would have been taken up by the subtalar and midtarsal joints now takes place, as it should, at the ankle joint. The subtalar and midtarsal joints remain in neutral position; the cuboid remains stable and allows the peroneus longus to plantar-flex the first ray. When this occurs, the forefoot posting should be reduced gradually. It is easier to reduce an extrinsic forefoot varus post than an intrinsically posted forefoot. Every month the forefoot post is ground down approximately 1 to 2 degrees. If this posting is not reduced, a first ray elevatus develops. Some practitioners believe that it is necessary to completely recast the child at 2-month intervals to capture the changing forefoot. If cost is not a factor, this would be the best approach. Otherwise, gradual reduction of the forefoot extrinsic post is usually sufficient.

If there is concern about midtarsal joint breakdown creating pain at the orthosis medially, one might consider

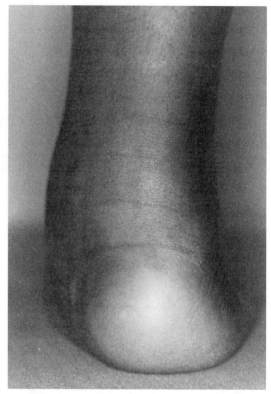

Figure 36–13. Collapse of medial arch with abduction at the calcaneocuboid articulation along with heel eversion.

using a more flexible sport orthotic device. The addition of compressible posts also allows some "give" in the orthotic in the direction of pronation. It should be remembered that an orthotic device does not correct anything if the cause of the problem is not addressed. In this case, the gastrocnemius-soleus complex must be lengthened either by stretching or by a surgical lengthening procedure.

MODIFIED GASTROCNEMIUS LENGTHENING PROCEDURE

Equinus is a severe pronatory force, especially when it is of a primary or congenital nature. It creates a compen-

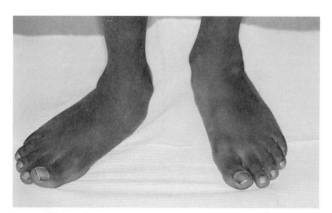

Figure 36–12. Right foot with severe equinus is maximally abducted with loss of medial arch.

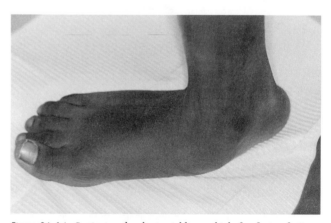

Figure 36–14. Supinatus develops, yielding a high forefoot soft tissue varus component.

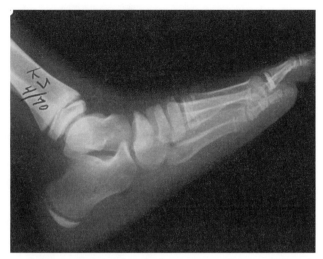

Figure 36–15. Note dorsal wedged appearance of the navicular. The cuneiform has a dorsiflexed position on the navicular during weight bearing, resulting in flattening of the dorsal aspect of the navicular.

satory pronated foot that is most difficult to control, and surgical attention is required. If the problem is left unaddressed, osseous adaptation occurs in the midtarsal joint. With the severe loss of dorsiflexion that occurs at the ankle, osseous changes will occur anywhere that dorsiflexion can be attained (Figs. 36–15 and 36–16). All too often in patients with compensated equinus, a standard tendo Achillis lengthening is performed when in fact the deformity does not lie in the gastrocnemius-soleus complex but rather is isolated to the gastrocnemius muscle.[6] The complication or result of this inappropriate lengthening is an instability at the knee joint with possible development of a genu recurvatum because of the loss of stability about the knee. In addition, because the amount of dorsiflexion has been increased at the expense of power for propulsion, an apropulsive gait can result. Weakness is easily demonstrated by the child's inability to stand on his toes. The isolated gastrocnemius recession or lengthening allows an increase in dorsiflexion at 50% to 60% of

the midstance in the gait cycle and reduces the resultant and compensated dorsiflexion at the midtarsal joint.[1,3,8,9] The power to plantar-flex at this segment of gait is not reduced, and propulsion is not reduced either as it is with the complete tendo Achillis lengthening.

In the modified gastrocnemius lengthening procedure,[1] a linear incision is approximated over the lower to middle third of the leg; this extends for approximately 5 cm. Once the incision is deepened by both sharp and blunt dissection, avoiding the short saphenous vein and the sural nerve, the fascia overlying the tendon of the gastrocnemius can be visualized. A curved hemostat is placed in the lateral border of the gastrocnemius, taking care to preserve the peritenon; the No. 11 blade is used to incise the peritenon and fascia, and the hemostat is inserted, extending from the lateral to medial border. This procedure is performed at the proximal and distal ends of the incision. The hemostat separates the myotendinous junction of the gastrocnemius from the soleal fibers. A cut is made in the gastrocnemius tendon from medial to lateral at the proximal end of the incision, and from lateral to medial in the distal segment of the incision. Entrance is gained to the tendon by gently lifting the peritenon. Both of the cuts should extend just past the midline. This approach cuts all of the fibers and is essential in allowing the tendon to glide upon itself. The partial transverse cuts of the gastrocnemius tendon are completed. The foot is then actively dorsiflexed while the knee is held in full extension. Approximately 1 to 1.5 cm of additional length is noted in both the distal and proximal segments (Figs. 36–17 to 36–19). The small cut to the peritenon that was made with the No. 11 blade is closed with 4–10 Dexon suture. Finally, skin is approximated with subcuticular absorbable 4–10 Dexon.

The child is placed in a below-the-knee cast with the foot held in a neutral position. If this is a bilateral procedure, the child may ambulate in bilateral casts. After 3 to 4 weeks, the cast is removed, and an orthosis that had been constructed prior to the surgery is immediately applied. This orthosis is the same device with a gradual

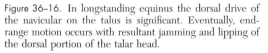
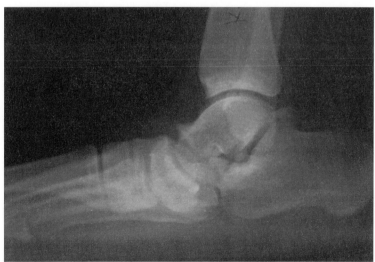

Figure 36–16. In longstanding equinus the dorsal drive of the navicular on the talus is significant. Eventually, end-range motion occurs with resultant jamming and lipping of the dorsal portion of the talar head.

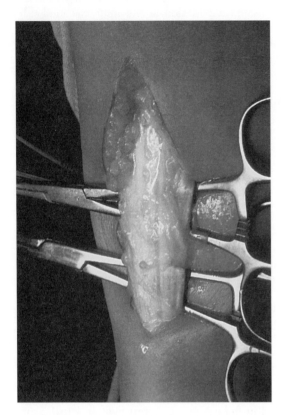

Figure 36–17. The cut is performed at the proximal and distal ends of the incision. The hemostat separates the myotendinous junction of the gastrocnemius from the soleal fibers.

Figure 36–18. A cut is made in the gastrocnemius tendon from medial to lateral at the proximal end of the incision, and from lateral to medial in the distal segment of the incision. Entrance is gained to the tendon by gently lifting the peritenon. Both cuts should extend just past the midline. This approach cuts all of the fibers and is essential in allowing the tendon to glide on itself.

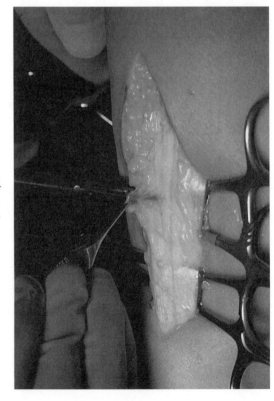

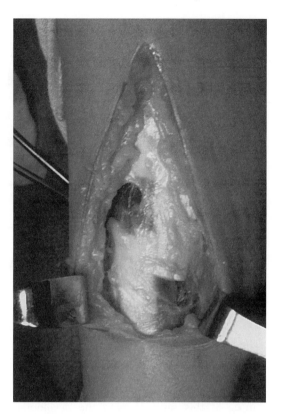

Figure 36–19. The partial transverse cut of the gastrocnemius tendon is complete. The foot is actively dorsiflexed while the knee is held in full extension. Approximately 1 to 15 centimeters of additional length are noted in both the distal and proximal segments.

reduction of the forefoot posting that was described earlier.

References

1. Schoenhaus HD, Jay RM: Modified gastrocnemius lengthening. J. Am Podiatr Med Assoc 1978; 68:31–37.
2. Griffin PP, Wheelhouse W, Shiavi R, Bass W: Treatment of toewalking: Habitual toewalkers. J Bone Joint Surg 1977; 59(A):97–101.
3. Illingworth RS: General articles on toewalking of unknown etiology. *In* Common Symptoms of Disease in Childhood. Oxford, Blackwell Scientific Publications, 1979, pp. 237–238.
4. Root ML, Orein WP, Weed JH: Normal and abnormal function of the foot. Clin Biomecha, 1977; 2: 127.
5. Sgarlato TE: A Compendium of Podiatric Biomechanics, California College of Podiatric Medicine, San Francisco, 1972.
6. Perry J, Hoffer MM: Preoperative and postoperative dynamic electromyography as an aid in planning tendon transfers in children with cerebral palsy. J Bone Joint Surg 1977; 59A:531.
7. Schwartz JR, Carr W, Basset FH: Lessons learned in the treatment of equinus deformity in ambulatory cerebral palsy. Orthop Trans 1977; 1:84.
8. Jay RM, Schoenhaus HD: Anterior advancement of the tendo Achille—Further insights. J Am Podiatr Med Assoc 1981; 71(2):73–76.
9. Blockey NJ: Children's Orthopedics—Practical Problems. London, Butterworths, 1975, pp. 2–4.

37

An Approach to Toe-Walking: Appropriate Decision Making

Edwin J. Harris, D.P.M.

The normal adult pattern of the stance phase of gait is characterized by distinct heel contact, followed by a clear period of midstance and a recognizable toe-off. Beginning walkers do not show heel contact at the initiation of stance. At this same time in the development of the mature gait pattern, a very small number of infants may transiently toe-walk for a few months. However, persistent toe-walking during this time is not considered normal. By the age of 2 years, most children have developed the heel-toe pattern that typifies mature gait.[7, 8, 11, 28, 35, 36]

Abnormality of the first component of stance produces an equinus gait pattern or toe-walking. Toe-walking and equinus gait are terms that are frequently used interchangeably, but not all equinus gait patterns produce recognizable toe-walking. There are mechanisms that can partly or completely compensate for equinus. Compensatory mechanisms allow heel contact as the form of stance phase initiation.

Persistent toe-walking in infancy is significant because there is no period in the normal evolution of gait during which toe-walking can be considered a developmentally acceptable finding.[18] Some investigators[33] have quoted Hall and colleagues,[20] Katz and Mubarak,[23] and Burnett and Johnson[7, 8] as saying that toe-walking is a developmentally normal pattern. Careful review of these articles shows no such statements. Therefore, persistent toe-walking must be considered a pathologic gait pattern. Although many children prove to be neurologically normal after investigation, others toe-walk because of neuromuscular pathology.[10, 18] Failure to appreciate the significance of this gait disturbance often leads to a delay of several years in making the correct diagnosis and initiating treatment for these serious problems.[31]

When the infant first begins to walk at around 12 months of age, the stance pattern is full flat toe-off.[35] There is relative foot drop along with exaggerated knee and hip flexion during the swing phase of gait. It is important to understand that this is not pathologic. In addition, this pattern should not be confused with toe-walking. A distinction between the two must be made so

that normal and abnormal gait patterns can be recognized during gait evaluation.

FORMS OF EQUINUS

Toe-walking is only one clinical expression of equinus. Although the term equinus is used in the context of gait evaluation to describe abnormal initiation of stance phase, it is also used to describe both abnormal ankle joint motion and abnormal movement of the foot as a unit independent of the kinetics of the ankle joint. Therefore, equinus may describe an abnormality of early stance phase, restriction of available ankle dorsiflexion, and an inability to dorsiflex the foot adequately above a right angle to the long axis of the leg. Although all three of these appear to be the same, there are some very important differences among them. These distinctions are etiology dependent and also have major therapeutic and prognostic implications.

Abnormal Stance Phase Patterns

Pattern I

In the simplest form of equinus gait, stance phase begins with heel contact. Stance phase is then abbreviated by premature heel-off. Since heel contact initiates stance, it can be presumed that there are at least 10 degrees of foot dorsiflexion. Without 10 degrees of motion, it is difficult to initiate a distinct heel contact.

Pattern II

In a slightly more complicated pattern, stance phase begins in midstance (full-flat). This is followed by toe-off. Since there is no heel contact, this pattern should not be confused with premature heel-off.

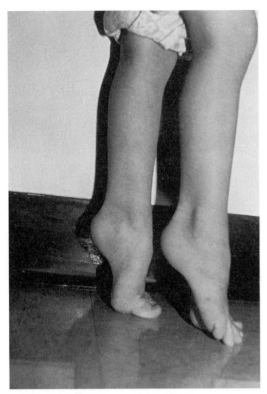

Figure 37–1. A 3-year-old female who has the diagnoses of Charcot-Marie-Tooth syndrome and nemaline rod myopathy. She has marked cavus deformity as well as severe posterior muscular contracture. She is an obligate toe-walker and cannot assume an ankle neutral position.

Pattern III

The toe-heel pattern is characterized by the initiation of stance phase by toe contact. This is followed immediately by heel contact. This pattern can occur with or without deceleration of the limb through use of the muscles of the leg. In most cases, this pattern results from the inability of the anterior compartment muscles to dorsiflex the foot enough during swing phase to allow it to clear the floor. Careful gait analysis usually shows that there is excessive hip and knee flexion during swing. This

is an attempt to compensate for the anterior compartment abnormality by raising the foot high enough above the weight-bearing surface to allow it to clear.

Pattern IV

Finally, the heels may not come down to the ground. Stance phase begins with toe contact, and the child remains in equinus. This pattern may be associated with contracture of the posterior compartment muscles (myostatic contracture), or it may occur in the presence of a full potential range of ankle dorsiflexion (dynamic contracture) (Fig. 37–1).

Inability to Adequately Dorsiflex the Foot

There are four factors that can restrict adequate dorsiflexion of the foot. The first of these is inability to dorsiflex the foot adequately even in the presence of enough ankle joint motion. This is usually caused by some contracture of soft tissue in the posterior compartment of the ankle. The second is muscular limitation of ankle motion in the absence of contracture. This is a neurologic event and is almost always associated with hypertonia and spasticity. If this is left unchecked, the ankle will become rigid over time as myostatic contracture develops. The third factor is bony block of the ankle resulting from some deformity in the shape of the talus or the tibia. This is very uncommon in pediatric practice. The fourth factor is some structural deformity within the foot. Abnormal anatomy either plantar-flexes the distal portion of the foot or causes the anterior margin of the tibia to abut against the superior surface of the talar neck before the foot can move above a right angle to the long axis of the leg. In many cases, fixed subtalar supination is the cause (Fig. 37–2). In other cases, cavoid deformity alone is the cause (Fig. 37–3).

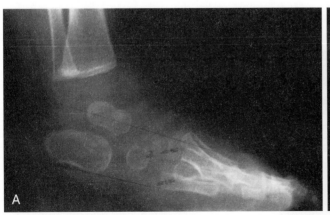
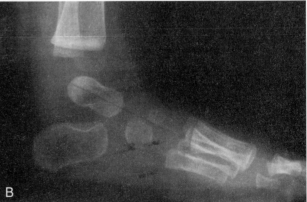

Figure 37–2. A, Unilateral talipes equinovarus. The lateral talocalcaneal angle is almost zero. The subtalar joint remains in fixed supination. The heel is not in contact with the weight-bearing plane. In this case, equinus is the sum of ankle joint equinus and subtalar "equinus." B, For comparison, the normal foot of the infant shown in A.

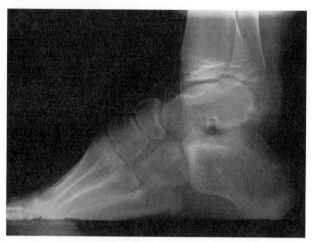

Figure 37–3. A 13-year-old male who has a diagnosis of Charcot-Marie-Tooth syndrome. The talus is almost maximally dorsiflexed in the ankle mortise. There is marked subtalar supination. The medial column is abnormally plantar-flexed (anterior equinus).

Abnormal Motion of the Ankle Joint

In some pathologic states, ankle joint motion may not allow the foot to come to neutral. In this condition, there is insufficient ankle dorsiflexion to allow the heel to come to the ground. This is a true equinus deformity. In other cases, the ankle joint motion may actually be greater than neutral, but the amount of motion is insufficient to either allow adequate heel contact or to prevent early heel-off (abbreviated stance phase). In yet other situations, an adequate range of ankle motion is available, but inappropriate muscle action produces an equinus gait. This is referred to as functional or dynamic equinus.

Clinically, range of ankle motion is determined by measuring the angle formed by the long axis of the leg and the plantar surface of the foot (Fig. 37–4). Soft tissue limitation of ankle joint motion is caused by contracture of muscle, ligaments, and capsule. To meet the criteria for soft tissue limitation, some ankle joint range of motion must be available.

Equinus of the Foot

If ankle dorsiflexion is insufficient, it might be presumed that the ankle joint is in equinus and that there is some soft tissue impediment to additional ankle motion. This often is an unwarranted assumption. Cavus deformity in the sagittal plane is a good example (see Fig. 37–3). In severe deformity, there may be insufficient motion to allow the foot to dorsiflex above the neutral position. In maximal dorsiflexion, the ankle is anatomically in the calcaneus position. The anterior tibial margin abuts against the dorsal talar neck before the angle formed by the plantar surface of the foot and the long axis of the leg reaches 90 degrees.

Supination of the subtalar joint plantar-flexes the distal segment of the foot against the rearfoot. This abnormal position adds another dimension to equinus occurring distal to the ankle joint. The equinus deformity associated with talipes equinovarus illustrates this point well (see Fig. 37–2). The overall equinus position of the foot is the sum of the fixed ankle equinus plus the component of equinus produced by the fixed heel varus (subtalar joint complex supination).

EQUINUS TYPES

There are five types of equinus. Uncompensated equinus occurs when the subtalar joint is in fixed supination and cannot allow pronation as a mechanism for adding apparent foot dorsiflexion. Partially compensated equinus occurs when the sum of inadequate ankle dorsiflexion plus subtalar compensation allows heel contact at the beginning of stance phase (Fig. 37–5). However, there is not enough overall dorsiflexion to allow a normal stance phase of gait. Early heel elevation during stance is the characteristic gait disturbance in this form. Fully compensated equinus is characterized by extreme pronation. The resulting motion is usually sufficient to allow a normal stance phase sequence. Pseudoequinus is a term applied to patients with anterior forefoot cavus (Fig. 37–6). Osseous equinus describes abnormal ankle joint morphology that develops over time as the result of pathologic function of the foot and ankle in equinus. This usually takes the form of flattening of the talar dome.

Diagnosis of Underlying Causes of Equinus

It is important for the surgeon to keep in mind that all forms of equinus gait are symptoms of disease. Equi-

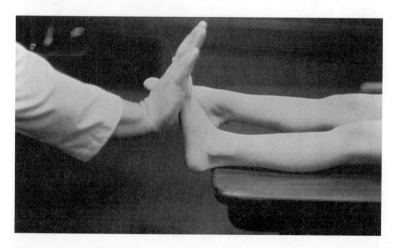

Figure 37–4. The child's knee is in full extension. Dorsiflexion of the foot at the ankle with the subtalar joint in neutral position fails to move the plantar surface of the foot to a right angle position with the leg. By definition, the foot is in equinus. Although the amount of dorsiflexion of the foot with the knee in extension approximates the range during much of the gait cycle, this method of testing ankle range of motion gives very little information about cause.

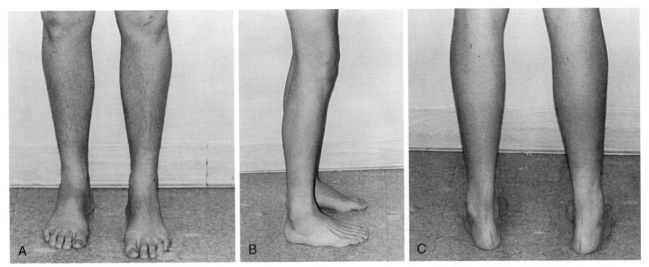

Figure 37–5. *A,* This 13-year-old male with a diagnosis of Charcot-Marie-Tooth syndrome began some toe-walking about 6 months before these photographs were taken. Foot dorsiflexion on the leg was limited to 5 degrees below neutral. There is bilateral fixed heel varus on both sides. *B,* Same child as shown in A. When seen from the side, the heels just touch the weight-bearing surface. Of interest, the patient flexes his knees slightly to accomplish this. *C,* Same child as in A and B. From the back, both heels are in varus. This position represents the maximum heel eversion available.

nus gait is not a disease in itself. It is critical to make an appropriate diagnosis because both the prognosis and the treatment of equinus are dictated by the underlying cause of this symptom. A careful history and physical examination are the first steps toward identifying the cause of equinus.

A careful history will usually reveal clues to underlying disorders. The history begins with clarification of the nature of the symptom. The chronology of the complaint is helpful. Toe-walking that begins after the child has established a normal walking pattern is more likely to be caused by serious and progressive disease than toe-walking that exists from the time the child first begins to walk. Circumstances that aggravate toe-walking should be identified. Information about previous medical evaluation and interventions should be carefully documented. This is especially true when there has been intervention that may change the clinical presentation.

The past medical history must include a developmental review. This begins with the prenatal period and should include the age of the parents and their general health at the time of conception. A history of fetal exposure to teratogens, environmental toxins, therapeutic medications, ethanol, nicotine, and recreational drugs should be obtained. Fetal recreational drug and alcohol exposures are endemic problems in today's society. There are no educational, economic, or social bounds. Fetopathy as the result of these exposures is becoming more and more common. The physician should maintain a high index of suspicion about the possibility of exposure even if there is parental denial.

The developmental history should include specific questions about each of the trimesters of pregnancy. Bleeding in any trimester means fetal distress. Premature onset of labor has the same significance. Preterm labor, premature amniotic rupture, meconium staining, induction of labor, and nonelective caesarean section correlate with development of movement disorders secondary to static encephalopathy. Prolonged and difficult labor, low Apgar scores, low birth weight, and need for resuscitation are additional risk factors for neurologic injury.

A delay in acquisition of major motor landmarks also

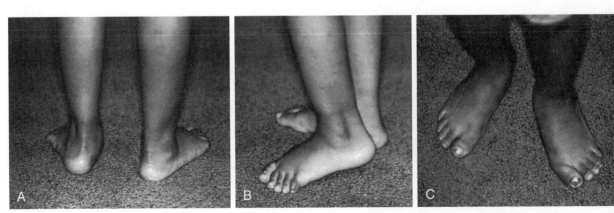

Figure 37–6. *A,* A 5-year-old girl with left equinus deformity fully compensated by severe pronation of the subtalar joint. From the back, the left calcaneus is everted. The heel is on the weight-bearing surface. *B,* Same child as shown in A. There is severe compensatory pronation for the equinus deformity. Much of the compensation is occurring through the midtarsal joint complex. *C,* Same child as in A and B. Severe forefoot abduction results from the attempt to compensate for equinus.

suggests underlying pathology. Rolling over from the prone to supine position and from supine to prone, independent sitting, crawling, cruising, independent standing, independent walking, toilet training, and development of hand preference are early motor milestones that parents tend to remember. They can be used as rough gauges of neurologic maturation.

A family history of toe-walking suggests the possibility of a hereditary neuropathy or myopathy. Although parents often take comfort in the fact that there are other toe-walking family members, the genetic significance of this familial history should not be missed. Additional questioning about a family history of muscle and neurologic disease may reveal other family members with known neuromuscular diagnoses.

A careful systems review may turn up co-morbidities (such as bowel and bladder dysfunction). These additional symptoms support the existence of an underlying pathology.

The Work-Up

The physical examination is extremely important. It should begin with a careful general physical examination. Evaluation of the skin may reveal lesions specific for neurocutaneous disease (Fig. 37–7). The café-au-lait spots of neurofibromatosis, hyperpigmented nevi of Proteus syndrome, hemangiomas of the Sturge-Weber syndrome, and the midline skin changes on the back associated with spinal dysraphisms are all examples. Examination of the face, head, neck, upper extremities, chest, and abdomen

is important but is unfortunately frequently omitted during work-up.

The most important component of the physical examination is the neurologic examination. It should begin with an examination of gait. This gives the examiner the opportunity to verify the symptom of the presenting complaint. Gait evaluation also allows the examiner to assess gross motor skills and muscle strength. In addition to the obvious gait findings, the examiner should look for evidence of hyperlordosis, a positive Gowers' sign, and a Trendelenburg waddle. All of these findings suggest girdle weakness.

The neurologic examination should include a sensory evaluation, which should include testing of vibratory and position sense. A detailed sensory evaluation is usually not possible in the office or clinic setting. However, evaluation of vibration and sharp-dull sensation is the most important aspect of the sensory evaluation, and since these tests require very little equipment, they are easy to perform in the offices.

The examination continues with cranial nerve testing, deep tendon and superficial reflexes, and formal evaluation of muscle strength. Since so many of the disorders associated with equinus begin proximally, specific evaluation of upper and lower girdle function is necessary. Muscles are evaluated for bulk appropriate to the age and build of the individual. Muscle strength can be manually evaluated using the Medical Research Council muscle-grading scale. The results are more useful if the evaluation is performed by a pediatric physical therapist. The resting muscle tone is assessed at the same time. Deep tendon reflexes should be evaluated in all cases. The upper and lower reflexes should be tested and compared. Superficial reflexes are usually limited to the abdominal skin reflex, cremasteric reflex (in boys), and the plantar reflex.

Musculoskeletal Evaluation

Examination of range of motion must include evaluation of the hip, knee and ankle. Since equinus gait is very often associated with knee and hip flexion contracture, it is important to regard these three joints as a functional unit. Many surgical judgmental errors are caused by failure to consider the interaction of all three of these joints.

Ankle dorsiflexion must be measured with the subtalar joint stabilized so that its effect on total foot dorsiflexion and plantar flexion does not confuse the picture. Ankle dorsiflexion should be measured first with the knee extended and then again with the knee flexed. This technique is referred to as Silfverskiold's test (Fig. 37–8). Its purpose is to isolate the individual effects of the soleus and the gastrocnemius on ankle range of motion.[16]

Knee range of motion should be evaluated for total range and evidence of flexion contracture. The popliteal angle should be measured with the thigh flexed at right angles to the trunk (Fig. 37–9).

Evaluation of hip range of motion includes internal and external rotation, flexion and extension, and adduction and abduction. The perineal angle should be measured in thigh flexion. Ely's test identifies quadriceps contracture (Fig. 37–10). Stability of the hips should be

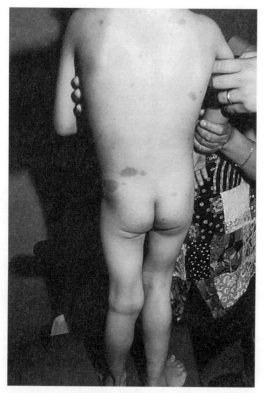

Figure 37–7. Multiple café-au-lait spots in a 4-year-old male with neurofibromatosis and a large plexiform neuroma in the right foot and leg.

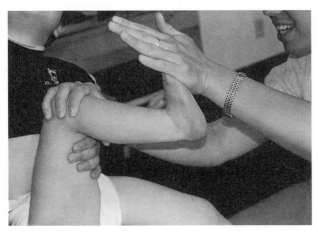

Figure 37–8. The knee is flexed, and dorsiflexion is attempted. In this case, there is additional dorsiflexion. It may be inferred that the additional dorsiflexion is caused by flexing the knee, which removes the gastrocnemius component. This is a valid presumption in children who are neurologically intact. In children who are not neurologically intact, there may be some inadvertent active hip flexion in this position. This may trigger a confusion reaction that may not be appreciated by the examiner.

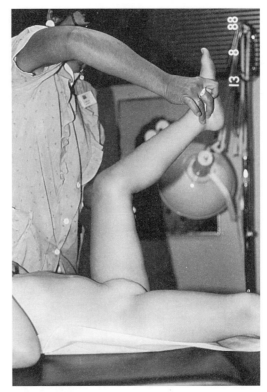

Figure 37–9. The popliteal angle is measured by placing the child supine, flexing the thigh at right angles to the trunk, and attempting to extend the knee. The popliteal angle is measured as the number of degrees the knee fails to meet full extension.

tested. Hip flexion contracture is evaluated by the Thomas test (Fig. 37–11) and the Staheli modification (Fig. 37–12). The limbs should be examined for length difference.

Appropriate weight-bearing radiographs of the foot should be taken. These include weight-bearing antero-posterior (AP) and lateral radiographs of the feet. AP radiographs of the ankles may be helpful. Stress dorsiflex-ion lateral x-ray films may identify a bony impediment to adequate ankle dorsiflexion. In addition to the position of the talus in the ankle mortise, the status of the subtalar joint is evaluated for evidence of abnormal supination. Subtalar joint supination plantar-flexes the foot distal to the talocalcaneal joint. This produces a true subtalar joint equinus that is independent of equinus at the ankle joint.

Other Investigations

Following the neurologic examination, all toe-walkers without an immediate explanation of the disorder should undergo some additional baseline work-up. This should include a complete blood count and differential, erythro-cyte sedimentation rate, electrolytes, creatine phosphoki-nase, and aldolase.[12] Additionally, a radiograph of the spine should be obtained even if there are no objective findings on inspection of the back. If there is any suspi-cion, magnetic resonance imaging (MRI) of the brain and spine should be performed. If the surgeon has any ques-tion about the diagnosis, consultation with an experienced pediatric neurologist is recommended.

DIVISION BY ETIOLOGY

Patients with equinus gait can be broadly categorized into two groups: those with underlying muscular and

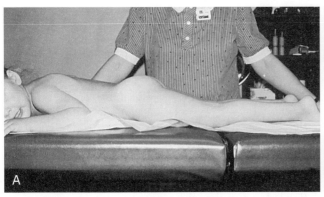
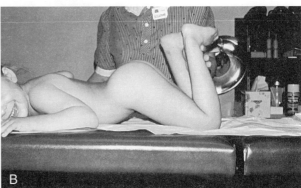

Figure 37–10. A, Ely's test. The child is placed prone with the chest on the examining table and the head to one side. The knees and hips are allowed to extend. B, The examiner flexes the knees (ideally, one at a time). Abnormal quadriceps tone or shortening causes increased lordosis and elevation of the buttocks.

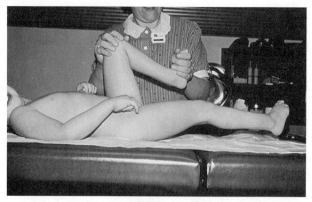

Figure 37–11. The Thomas test is performed by placing the child supine with the hips and knees in extension. The thighs and knees are flexed, and then each leg is allowed to resume extension while the other remains flexed. Iliopsoas contracture prevents full hip extension.

neurologic disease and those who are neurologically normal. The purpose of the initial work-up is to seek data to help the surgeon decide into which category to place a given child with equinus.

THE NEUROLOGICALLY NORMAL CHILD

Absence of neuromuscular disease is determined by careful history and physical examination and appropriate investigation. It is never presumed. It is the surgeon's responsibility to rule out latent neuropathy or myopathy before proceeding to treatment. It is not always easy to do this. The surgeon must remain open to the possibility that there may be some low-level dysfunction that is not identifiable when he first evaluates the child. Repeat examinations over time may eventually uncover pathology.

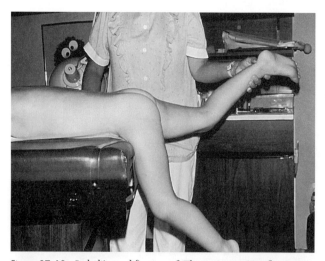

Figure 37–12. Staheli's modification of Thomas' test. Hip flexion may produce significant lumbar hyperlordosis. This may make Thomas' test difficult to interpret. To circumvent lumbar hyperlordosis, the child is placed prone, and the legs are allowed to dangle over the edge of the examining table. An assistant holds the child's shoulders for stability. This position flattens out the lordosis. The examiner then attempts to extend the hip. True limitation of full hip extension can be measured.

Idiopathic (Habitual) Toe-Walking

Idiopathic (habitual) toe-walking syndrome is a term used to describe a subset of toe-walkers who have no apparent disease but continue to walk in equinus. This gait pattern is not a habit. The term idiopathic toe-walking syndrome is more appropriate. The diagnosis should be one of exclusion and should not be considered until the child has been thoroughly investigated for possible neurologic or muscular causes. It is quite probable that some of these children actually do have undetectable neurologic or muscular pathology that remains unidentified even after a thorough work-up and a consultation with a pediatric neurologist.

These children have a history of persistent toe-walking from the time they became independent ambulators. This is such an important feature that the onset of toe-walking after a period of normal gait should raise questions about the diagnosis. Most idiopathic toe-walkers prefer a toe-toe gait pattern. They are capable of good balance and can walk forward and backward with equal ease while remaining on their toes. Older children may walk with a heel-toe pattern on command. They revert to a toe-toe pattern when distracted. In early childhood, physical examination usually demonstrates a full range of ankle motion that allows the foot to dorsiflex well above a right angle to the long axis of the leg. If the condition is left untreated, these children develop myostatic contracture and eventually lose the range of ankle joint motion. This loss of motion is usually gradual and may not occur until the child is 5 or 6 years of age. Additionally, a significant number of these children have a familial history of toe-walking. This has led some investigators to propose a hereditary cause.[20, 23, 24]

Boys and girls are affected equally. However, in a young boy the condition is particularly worrisome because of the possibility of the X-linked recessive muscular dystrophies. Duchenne's and Becker's muscular dystrophies very frequently begin with toe-walking.[6] The treatment of equinus deformity in children with X-linked forms of muscular dystrophy is so radically different from that of other causes of toe-walking and the prognosis is so different that correct diagnosis is mandatory.

Congenital Short Tendo Achillis

This condition was first described by Hall and colleagues in 1967.[20] They based the diagnosis on the absence of underlying disease, persistence of toe-walking from an early age, and the presence of triceps contracture. By definition, these children are neurologically normal and have no evidence of muscular disease. It is a diagnosis based on exclusion of other pathology. All of the original 20 children in Hall's series were treated with tendo-Achillis lengthening.

It is unclear whether congenital contracture of the triceps should be classified as a variant of habitual toe-walking syndrome. Furrer and Deonna make a distinction.[18] Many authors have noted that ankle range of motion in young idiopathic toe-walkers is normal or near normal at the onset of walking. In Furrer and Deonna's experience, congenital triceps surae contracture is a very uncommon finding. To accept the diagnosis of congenital contracture of the triceps, there must be irrefutable evidence that the equinus existed from birth, and in most cases, there are no early examination data available at the time of assessment to substantiate this.

Congenital contracture of the triceps is presumed to be an autosomal dominant trait. The tendo Achillis is anatomically short, and the muscle fibers extend much more distally than normal.[20, 23, 24] Levine described a sibship of three children with persistent toe-walking from infancy. All had fixed equinus deformity.[24]

I find it advantageous to group idiopathic toe-walkers into three classes. The first class contains those with a normal range of motion who preferentially walk in equinus. The second class comprises those who originally had adequate range of motion but lost it with time. The third class includes those who have always had fixed equinus. Unfortunately, the members of this latter group can only be confirmed by physical examination at a young age. In many cases, the children were never examined at the critical time.

Problems Associated with Idiopathic Toe-Walking

Idiopathic toe-walking has been associated with speech delay.[1, 2] It may also be associated with behavior disorders, attention deficit disorders, and hyperactivity states. I have encountered learning disability, attention deficits, and hyperactivity more frequently in toe-walkers than in any other pediatric population with foot and ankle disorders. These observations are supported in the literature.[18, 22, 26]

Toe-walking in these children may represent fixation in a transient pattern of motor activity from early infancy, although this concept requires acceptance of toe-walking as a developmentally normal stage at some point in the development of gait. This runs contrary to the current knowledge of gait development.

To qualify for the diagnosis, the child must be neurologically intact, have negative results of radiographic and clinical laboratory studies, have a negative family history for hereditary neuromuscular disease, and have no risk factors for acquired static encephalopathy. If these criteria are met, the surgeon can continue with symptomatic therapy of toe-walking.

Differential Diagnosis

Diastematomyelia, tethered cord, muscular dystrophy, myotonic dystrophy, cerebral palsy, and peripheral neuropathy must be excluded. Ruling out these diagnoses may be very difficult.[26] The most common differential diagnosis is between idiopathic toe-walking and mild spastic diplegia. Children with diplegia characteristically lack controlled plantar flexion following heel contact and decreased plantar flexion at toe-off. Children with idiopathic toe-walking begin stance in plantar flexion, whereas those with diplegic toe-walking enter stance with a flexed knee due to hamstring dysfunction. The walking pattern in diplegia is regular, whereas the idiopathic toe-walking pattern is irregular.

Work-up of habitual toe-walking by some investigators includes electromyography (EMG). EMG gives some insight into the muscle dynamics of the syndrome. Papariello and Skinner evaluated this condition with dynamic electromyography by sampling the gastrocnemius, soleus, tibialis anterior and posterior, peroneus longus and brevis, flexor hallucis longus and flexor digitorum longus.[26] Two of the four cases described had electrodiagnostic patterns more consistent with cerebral palsy.

Treatment for Idiopathic Toe-Walking

Initial management for this condition begins with an assessment and therapy program under the supervision of an experienced pediatric physical therapist. The program should include evaluation of muscle strengths and ranges of motion.[6] For children who have an adequate ankle range of motion, the therapist's role is assessment. For children who lack an acceptable range of motion, the therapist is responsible in addition for providing hands-on stretching therapy and supervising a home program that is administered by the parents.

Some of these children may require serial stretching casts to achieve a useful range of motion. Once an adequate range of ankle motion can be achieved, the child is ready to be fitted for ankle-foot orthotics. The goals of bracing are to teach a heel-toe gait pattern and to prevent the development of myostatic contracture by keeping the child out of the equinus position. Most children tolerate ankle-foot orthotics better if their first braces are solid ankle types. Subsequent orthotics can be articulated. These are designed to allow unrestricted ankle dorsiflexion, but they also prevent plantar flexion below the ankle neutral position. Ankle motion can be free or restrained to allow only a portion of the range of ankle dorsiflexion. An unrestrained ankle-foot orthotic can be used as a dynamic stretching modality when the child walks and navigates stairs.

In spite of these efforts, some of these children develop fixed equinus that cannot be managed by physical therapy and bracing alone. It is worth an attempt to try stretching casts.[30] Griffin and colleagues believe that casting not only increases the range of motion but also changes the muscle synergy pattern from abnormal to normal.[19] Despite these measures, many of these patients require tendo-Achillis lengthening (Fig. 37–13).

NEUROMUSCULAR DISEASES ASSOCIATED WITH EQUINUS

X-Linked Muscular Dystrophies

The two most important diseases in this group are Duchenne's pseudohypertrophic muscular dystrophy and Becker's muscular dystrophy. The primary pathophysiology in both conditions is noninflammatory degeneration of muscle with an attempt at repair. Both Duchenne's and Becker's muscular dystrophies are inherited as X-linked

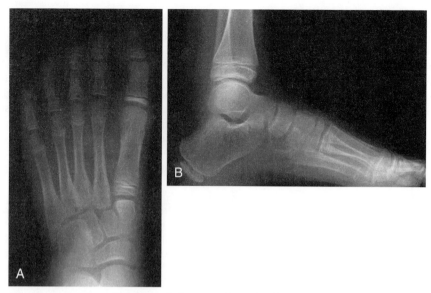

Figure 37–13. *A* and *B*, Anteroposterior and lateral weight-bearing radiographs of a 7-year-old girl who had a diagnosis of habitual toe-walking syndrome. After appropriate stretching, she was able to achieve dorsiflexion of the ankles only to neutral. Flexing the knees did not alter the ankle range of motion. She persisted in equinus gait and underwent heel cord lengthening in continuity. She wore articulated ankle-foot orthotics for 1 year and has remained down off her toes since then. Her radiographs show the paradox of subtalar pronation and mild cavus change. Despite the cavoid changes, no underlying neurologic disease was identified.

recessive traits. The genetic aberration is at the Xp21.2 site. A family history cannot always be obtained because there is a high degree of spontaneous mutation in these two diseases.

The biochemical error in both of these diseases is an abnormality in the production of dystrophin. Duchenne's muscular dystrophy is characterized by absence of dystrophin. Becker's variant results from a decrease in the amount of dystrophin or from dystrophin of abnormal molecular size.

Clinical Findings

Initial clinical signs of Duchenne's and Becker's muscular dystrophies include girdle weakness, delay in acquisition of ambulatory skills, clumsiness, and toe-walking. It is worth noting that some boys are presented early for evaluation of severe pes planus and lack of endurance. The age of onset, severity, and progression help to distinguish the two diseases.

Decreased strength in the hip extensors and abductors results in lordosis and Trendelenburg's gait. Hyperlordosis allows the child to keep his center of gravity posterior to the hip joints. This results in a compensatory mechanism for loss of active hip extension strength. With time, the quadriceps becomes weak, causing difficulty in maintaining the knee in extension. This problem can be compensated for by walking in equinus (Fig. 38–14).

Falling occurs frequently. As the disease progresses, the child has more difficulty in getting back up. The pattern of rising from the floor is very distinctive and is called Gowers' sign.

Investigations

Diagnosis is based on the sex of the patient, the pattern of limb and girdle weakness, pseudohypertrophy, absence of sensory abnormalities, and decreased or absent deep

tendon reflexes. Creatine phosphokinase and aldolase levels are dramatically increased. The EMG is myopathic. The muscle biopsy is highly suggestive. Stains for the presence or absence of dystrophin can confirm the biochemical abnormality. DNA analysis is highly specific and confirmatory.

Treatment

The diseases themselves are not treatable. The goals for management of children with Duchenne's and Beck-

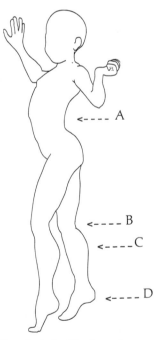

Figure 37–14. *A*, Hyperlordosis of lumbar spine to compensate for hip extensor weakness. *B*, Knee flexion resulting from quadriceps weakness. *C*, Calf pseudohypertrophy. *D*, Equinovarus feet.

er's muscular dystrophies are to maintain ambulation as long as possible and to prevent formation of contracture detrimental to function. Stretching exercises serve two purposes. First, they help to prevent the development of contracture, and second, they help maintain strength. As a consequence of the natural history of the disease, strength deteriorates with time. Immobilization resulting from trauma, major illness, and surgery causes acceleration of the weakness. Exercise and activity carried to excess can actually prove harmful.

Equinus becomes a therapeutic concern. To some extent, equinus can be advantageous. It acts as a compensatory mechanism to allow continued ambulation. Stretching therapy and serial casts are indicated as contracture of the tendo-Achillis develops. Daytime bracing may be a problem for the child because of the weight of the apparatus, but ankle-foot orthotics worn at night are useful adjuncts to help prevent the development of triceps contracture.

Early surgical intervention for equinus is not indicated because it produces additional triceps weakness. If the quadriceps are very weak, the result is an uncontrollable crouch that is very difficult to manage by any means. This results in complete loss of ambulation and wheelchair confinement.

As the child reaches 9 to 12 years of age, muscle weakness and contracture at all three lower extremity levels develops. Particularly, equinovarus deformity jeopardizes standing and walking. Surgical release of contractures may help, but long leg braces after surgery are necessary.

Walking and standing become more difficult as equinovarus deformity of the feet develops. There comes a time when although walking is extremely limited, the ability to stand is still desirable. Percutaneous lengthening of the tendo-Achillis will correct the equinus deformity. It is very unusual for the posterior ankle capsule to be contracted unless the deformity is of long standing. The tibialis posterior is usually contracted and is lengthened in the same operation. This surgery usually prolongs some useful standing ability, but meaningful walking is very limited. An additional disadvantage for the child is that long leg braces must follow the ankle release.

Eventually, the child becomes chairbound. Continued stretching therapy is needed to keep the feet supple, maintain the ability to keep the feet plantigrade on the wheelchair platforms, and allow shoe fitting during the time spent outdoors. If the deformity becomes fixed, the components of equinovarus are treated with simple tenotomy of the tendo Achillis and tibialis posterior. The plantar fascia is also released.

Cerebral Palsy

It is difficult to develop a good comprehensive definition of cerebral palsy. Cerebral palsy is caused by an insult to the immature central nervous system. Arbitrarily, 2 years has been selected as the upper age limit. Classically, the insult was presumed to occur in the immediate perinatal period. The list of potential causes has been broadened to include genetic disease, central nervous system infection, fetal exposure to toxins, exposure to legitimate and recreational drugs, prematurity, trauma, central nervous system malformations, and some metabolic disorders.

All of these potential causes are capable of producing a constellation of symptoms that can affect all levels of central nervous system function. From the orthopedic perspective, the two most important aspects of the disease are the movement disorders and the contracture states that may develop. Because of their causal interrelationship, the two cannot be separated.

The surgeon's initial responsibility is to confirm the diagnosis. In most cases, the presence of perinatal risk factors, the natural history, and the physical examination leave little room for doubt. However, it is important to bear in mind that there are a number of conditions that can mimic cerebral palsy. In doubtful cases, consultation with a pediatric neurologist is in order.

The movement disorders in cerebral palsy produce toe-walking by interfering with the phasic activity of the individual muscle groups. This, in turn, leads to abnormal positioning of the extremities during gait and at rest. If the muscles are not continually stretched to their maximum length, they fail to keep up in linear length as the bones grow. The effect is restriction of joint excursion.

It is not appropriate to view ankle function in isolation. The motions at the hip, knee, and ankle are so interdependent that contractures are likely to affect all three areas at the same time. An examination of the hip must include a number of tests to evaluate sagittal motion and contracture states. Thomas' test identifies iliopsoas contractures (see Fig. 37–11) but may fail to detect flexion contracture if there is significant lumbar hyperlordosis. Staheli is credited with a modification to isolate hip flexion contracture by neutralizing lordosis (see Fig. 37–12). The Ely test is used to identify contracture of the rectus femoris. (see Fig. 37–10). Knee flexion contracture is identified by attempting to fully extend the knee. The effect of the hamstrings on knee extension can be evaluated by measuring the popliteal angle (see Fig. 37–9).

Ankle range of motion is evaluated first with the knee extended and again with the knee flexed according to the technique of Silverskiold (see Fig. 37–8). Since the gastrocnemius is a triarticular muscle (crossing the knee, ankle, and subtalar joints), flexing the knee effectively lengthens the gastrocnemius and reduces its influence on restriction of ankle joint motion.

The confusion test is another evaluation tool. The child may be unable to volitionally dorsiflex the foot as an independent motion but can dorsiflex the foot as a part of a movement pattern when asked to flex the hip against resistance. It is thought that the confusion test is an expression of a normal patterned response that is modified by development and central nervous system maturation.[13] The examiner must be careful not to inadvertently elicit a confusion test while attempting to perform Silverskiold's test. Misinterpretation can lead to an error in surgical decision making if the surgeon decides to lengthen only the gastrocnemius when both gastrocnemius and soleus are dysfunctional in the position of knee extension.

Treatment for toe-walking in cerebral palsy is similar to

that for idiopathic toe-walking. It is important to involve physical and occupational therapists early in the course of the management. The initial therapeutic goals are prevention of contracture and improvement of fine and gross motor skills.

Triceps contractures in this patient population may be myostatic (permanently shortened) or dynamic (motion restricted by high resting tone and inappropriate contraction). Obviously, the latter is not really a contracture. It is appropriate to consider dynamic contracture a precontracture state.

Parental home stretching programs under the supervision of a physical therapist are started as soon as the diagnosis is made. As the child gains trunk stability, equinus deformity of the ankles interferes with efforts to begin independent standing and eventual walking. If the ankle is capable of dorsiflexing to neutral, ankle-foot orthotics with the ankle joint at neutral are indicated. They allow the child to stand upright. In many cases, the child walks independently soon after he or she starts to wear ankle-foot orthotics.

Serial stretching casts may be necessary in some cases. These are a logical step in children who are being considered for tendo-Achillis lengthening. The purpose of the casts is to gain ankle motion (Fig. 37–15). They are not to be confused with tonal inhibition casting techniques[30] (Fig. 37–16).

Tonal inhibitory casting has enjoyed several waves of popularity during the last 20 years. The results tend to be unpredictable. These casts are very difficult to apply, and the technique is very unforgiving for even minor errors in application. There are no data verifying any long-term benefits.

More recently, purified botulinum A toxin has been used both for presurgical testing and for augmentation during nonoperative therapy. Children who do not respond to botulinum A toxin are more likely to be candidates for surgical lengthening of tendons.

Transcutaneous electrical stimulation is currently being investigated to determine its role in the management of cerebral palsy in general and the prevention and treatment of contracture in particular. The response among physical therapists has been enthusiastic, but carefully controlled studies must be continued for some time before the indications for patient selection, realizable goals, and end-points in therapy can be identified.

Equinus Surgery in Cerebral Palsy

Careful surgical planning is the key to a successful outcome. A great deal of preoperative information is needed. The limitations of physical examination are well known, especially for interpretations that depend on observation. It is advisable for these children to undergo formal gait analysis, which should include appropriate videotaping and analysis as well as surface recorded electromyography. This is especially valuable if there is a possibility that hip and knee surgery may be performed in the same operation.

Patients with unyielding triceps contractures are surgical candidates for lengthening of the triceps mechanism.

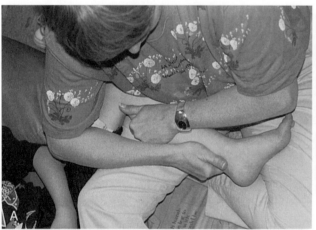
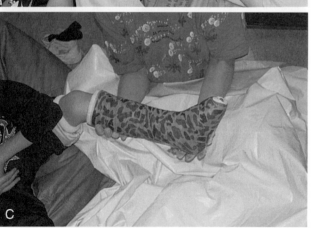
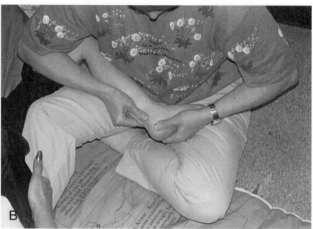

Figure 37–15. *A* and *B*, Stretch casting for children with cerebral palsy is best done in conjunction with the child's physical therapist. The application of the cast is preceded by stretching techniques performed by the therapist. The child is usually more comfortable in the presence of his or her own therapist. Since this is a two-person operation, the therapist can also assist in positioning the foot and ankle. *C*, Correct application of serial stretching casts is technically difficult. Problems with the skin are common, and meticulous attention to casting detail is critical to the success of the casting. Growth plate and metaphyseal fractures can result from poor technique. Malpositioning can result in failure of correction or correction at the wrong joint level. The surgeon should apply the cast and maintain position. This is not a task that should be delegated to a cast technician or other personnel.

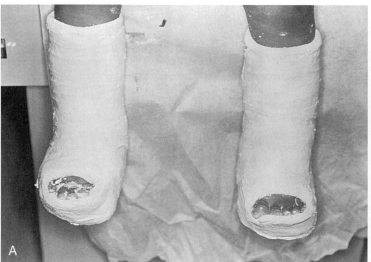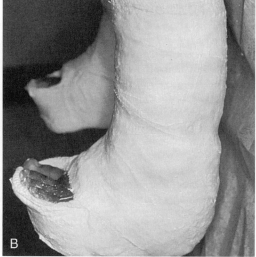

Figure 37–16. *A* and *B*, Tonal inhibition casting is based on the theory that positioning with hyperextension of the toes, ankles neutral, heels vertical, and a wide base of support will decrease tone in the proximal parts of the lower extremities as well as the trunk. These casts are very difficult to apply, and many children cannot tolerate them.

This surgery has two prerequisites. First, the surgeon must be certain that any flexion contractures of the hip and knee have been identified because they will have to be treated in the same operative setting. Failure to take this precaution results in development of crouch gait and leads to multiple operations. Second, the surgeon must determine whether surgical intervention must include all or only part of the triceps mechanism. If only the gastrocnemius is producing the limitation of joint excursion, this muscle can be selectively lengthened. If the gastrocnemius and the soleus are both involved, the lengthening must be done at the level of the tendo Achillis.

Neuronal Disease

The anterior horn cell is the final common pathway leaving the spinal cord to innervate the muscle. Anterior horn cell dysfunction is the major pathophysiology in many acute and chronic diseases. There are both acquired and hereditary diseases under this heading. They may affect the anterior horn cell alone or the sensory nerves in addition. They may be peripheral, central, or both.

Spinal Muscular Atrophy

Spinal muscular atrophy comprises a group of diseases distinguished by degeneration of spinal and bulbar anterior horn cells. This results in weakness, hypotonia, and respiratory insufficiency. There are three pathologies included under this heading. Type I (Werdnig-Hoffmann disease) is an autosomal recessive condition in which the symptoms begin between birth and 6 months of age. These infants quickly deteriorate. Most expire before the age of 2. They have severe generalized weakness and never become strong enough to sit. They have no ambulatory potential, and there is no role for rehabilitative limb surgery in this group.

Type II (intermediate severity spinal muscular atrophy) begins with symmetrical weakness that starts after the first 6 months of life. The proximal portions of the extremities are more involved than the distal segments. Most of these children will develop the ability to sit. Although they never stand independently, they do develop lower extremity contractures and scoliosis. Hip and knee flexion contractures are usually tolerated well because these are compatible with sitting. Equinovarus deformities cause problems in maintaining the feet plantigrade on the wheelchair platforms. Occasionally, palliative procedures are needed to correct undesirable foot postures. These are best managed by simple release tenotomies. If the contractures are of long standing, posterior ankle capsulotomy may also be necessary. As with many other equinus deformity patterns, prevention is most important. The use of lightweight plastic ankle-foot orthotics will help prevent this destructive equinovarus.

Type III (Kugelberg-Welander disease) usually presents after the child begins to walk. Independent walking usually begins on time, although there may be very slight delay. The child then develops girdle weakness with a waddling gait, Gowers' sign, and climbing difficulties. It is interesting that many of these children have pronated feet. Unlike boys with Duchenne's muscular dystrophy, they do not toe-walk early in the course of the disease. In fact, very few develop equinus unless they stop walking. As they reach 10 to 12 years of age, they may begin to lose function. If they must undergo surgery or suffer trauma or illness that confines them to bed, they may permanently lose the ability to walk independently.

A waddling gait with hyperlordosis in the absence of toe-walking suggests a diagnosis of type III spinal muscular atrophy. Some of these children initially present for evaluation for surgery to correct pronation. There are not enough data to draw conclusions about the necessity of or benefits to be derived from flatfoot surgery in this group. Before considering surgery, the diagnosis should be confirmed. CPK is usually normal in this group. It may be modestly elevated in the milder forms. Electromyography shows neurogenic muscle atrophy with evidence of degenerative motor neuron pathology. Muscle biopsy helps confirm the diagnosis.

As in other neuromuscular diseases, the first treatment is directed toward the prevention of contractures. Ambulatory patients rarely have contractures of the foot and ankle. The few children who become chairbound develop equinovarus deformity after they lose the ability to walk. The main therapeutic goal is to minimize contractures. In severe cases release of the contractures by tenotomy may be necessary if there are problems with positioning the feet in braces or on wheelchair platforms. Pain and difficulty with shoe wear are also indications for surgery.

Charcot-Marie-Tooth Disease

Advances in investigational techniques during the last few years have led to reclassification of the hereditary sensorimotor neuropathies. There are three main divisions of this group that are of interest to the foot surgeon because of their association with gait disturbances and foot deformity.

Type I hereditary sensorimotor neuropathy is a hypertrophic demyelinating peripheral neuropathy that has five subsets. Studies of the genetics of this condition have identified three dominant forms, one autosomal recessive trait, and one X-linked form.[14, 25] These variations most closely resemble the classic descriptions of Charcot-Marie-Tooth syndrome. Type IA is an autosomal dominant form. The location of the abnormality is on the short arm of chromosome 17. It is probably the most common form. Type IB is inherited as an autosomal recessive trait. As with most recessive traits, it is uncommon. The abnormality is on the long arm of chromosome 1. It may be linked to the presence of the Duffy factor. Onset is early, and it may present with equinus gait. Type IC is not well reported in the literature. It is thought to be an autosomal dominant trait, but its locus has not yet been determined. Two variations of X-linked forms have been identified. One is X-linked dominant, and the other is X-linked recessive.

The initial symptoms in type I disease are almost always first noted in the feet. They usually begin in the first decade of life. The first findings are most likely to be hammering of the toes and cavus deformity. Occasionally, the child will be presented because of falling and clumsy gait. Anterior compartment weakness leads to foot drop during swing phase. Excessive knee and hip flexion occurs during swing phase to compensate for the foot drop. Balance becomes difficult because of the anterior and lateral compartment weakness. Progressive muscle imbalance leads to the development of pes cavus and cavo-adductus deformity.

Careful evaluation will demonstrate weakness in the anterolateral compartment of the leg. Early in the course, an off-weight bearing cavus deformity that disappears on weight bearing may be present (Fig. 37–17). The intrinsic muscles in the foot are involved as well, but they are hard to evaluate. There may be an obvious decrease in bulk of the intrinsic muscles. The hands are similarly involved. Tremors of the hands due to fatigue should not be mistaken for rest tremors.

Neurologic changes include a decrease or absence of the deep tendon reflexes and a decrease in vibratory sensation. Occasionally there is muscle pain and tremors due to weakness following overuse. Peripheral nerves may be hypertrophied. Muscle wasting is usually mild in type I disease. Nerve conduction velocity is delayed or slowed. Nerve biopsy shows hypertrophic neuropathy with decreased myelin.

Type II hereditary sensorimotor neuropathy is an autosomal dominant hypertrophic neuropathy that superficially resembles the classic form of Charcot-Marie-Tooth syndrome. There are some electrodiagnostic differences. Type II disease has a later onset of symptoms and does not have hypertrophic neuropathy. There is less hand weakness, more plantar flexor foot weakness, and much more muscle atrophy. Nerve conduction velocity is almost normal. Pes cavus and leg atrophy are seen. Upper deep tendon reflexes are usually normal.

Type III hereditary sensorimotor neuropathy (Dejerine-Sottas disease) is an autosomal recessive form. Type III begins in infancy with delays in motor milestones. Walking skill may not be acquired until 3 or 4 years of age. The child progresses for a period of time but then loses function with age. Hand weakness is a prominent finding. Weakness in the upper and lower extremities begins distally and spreads proximally.

Treatment of Charcot-Marie-Tooth Disease. Appropriate use of ankle-foot orthotics is valuable when anterior compartment weakness causes a gait disturbance in swing phase. An ankle-foot orthotic helps prevent the development of contractures. It also converts most patients from a toe-heel pattern to a heel-toe pattern as long as they have an adequate ankle range of motion. The presence of fixed equinus contraindicates the use of an ankle-foot orthotic to improve swing phase function.

The equinus component of Charcot-Marie-Tooth syndrome is the consequence of cavo-varus deformity and dropfoot resulting from anterior compartment weakness. Lengthening of the tendo Achillis to improve the ankle dorsiflexion is contraindicated. This procedure will actually worsen the equinus by increasing the cavus component of the deformity. Correct surgical planning requires evaluation of the components of the cavus deformity. Plantar release, calcaneal osteotomy, first metatarsal osteotomy, and tibialis posterior transfer are the procedures performed most commonly for cavus deformities associated with the hereditary sensorimotor neuropathies. For extremely rigid midfoot deformities, midtarsal wedge procedures (Cole and Japas procedures) are indicated.

Additional Causes of Toe-Walking

Although the diseases discussed above are the most common causes of equinus, most of the neuromuscular diseases of childhood are capable of causing toe-walking. Tethering of the spinal cord and diastematomyelia may produce gait symptoms. There are also a few non-neurologic causes of toe-walking. Problems such as short limb, developmental hip dislocation, and untreated clubfoot can also produce equinus gait.

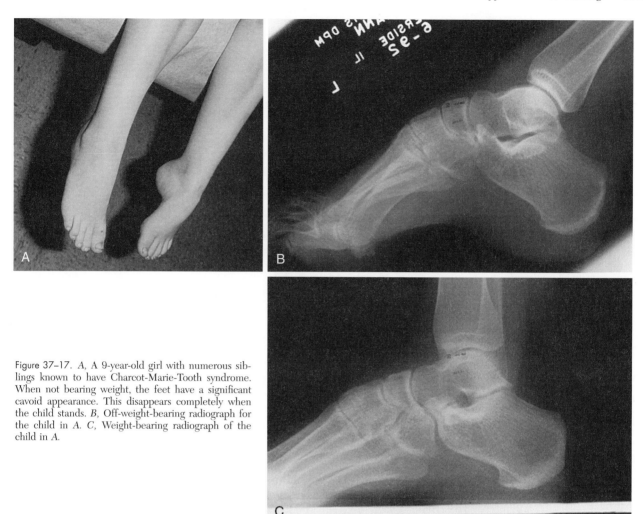

Figure 37–17. *A,* A 9-year-old girl with numerous siblings known to have Charcot-Marie-Tooth syndrome. When not bearing weight, the feet have a significant cavoid appearance. This disappears completely when the child stands. *B,* Off-weight-bearing radiograph for the child in *A. C,* Weight-bearing radiograph of the child in *A.*

MANAGEMENT OF CONTRACTURES

Once a muscle undergoes myostatic contracture, the joints controlled by that muscle become fixed in nonphysiologic positions. The treatment aim is to improve the range of motion of the joint. The therapeutic goals for equinus deformity of the ankle are the same as for any other contracture. The first intent is to prevent formation of contracture. Each cause has its own predictable natural history. With knowledge of this history, early intervention to prevent or minimize the development of contracture is possible; this is why early and correct diagnosis is so important.

The deformity may be reversible in the beginning stages of contracture development. This attempt usually requires the combined efforts of the physical therapist and the surgeon. Initially, supervised stretching may prove beneficial. Neuromuscular blockade technique with botulinum A toxin may facilitate stretching programs. Stretching casts can also be used to assist in achieving a useful range of motion. Bracing may be the initial option if range of motion is near normal. Appropriate use of bracing is always indicated when motion has been improved by physical therapy or casting.

Surgery for Contractures

There is a point at which a useful range of motion cannot be achieved through any of these nonoperative techniques. Some form of surgical intervention then becomes necessary. Surgical techniques may be grouped according to the physiologic goal.

Afferent and Efferent Denervation for Spasticity

Denervation of the muscle is one of the most direct forms of treatment. It can be accomplished in one of two ways. First, the dorsal roots may be sectioned (rhizotomy). This is a neurosurgical technique performed under intraoperative electromyographic control. Rhizotomy has been practiced for years but has fallen into some disuse because of its complications and disadvantages. It is now enjoying some degree of resurgence in popularity. The disadvantage is that the muscle loses some of its afferent innervation. Once this happens, significant strength is lost. This in turn requires a great deal of physical therapy for rehabilitation. The results are also unpredictable, since sectioning roots is imprecise.

The second method of denervation is to destroy the motor branches to the muscles surgically or chemically. This has the same local result as rhizotomy because the innervation to the muscle is destroyed, producing permanent weakness of the involved muscle. At the current time, this is not a very popular form of surgery.

Proximal Selective Gastrocnemius Release

Release of the gastrocnemius proximal to the knee joint converts it from a triarticular muscle to a biarticular muscle. Silverskiold popularized a method of proximal release and distal transfer of the heads of the gastrocnemius for equinus deformity caused purely by gastrocnemius contracture.[32] This form of proximal release may be modified by detaching the heads without transferring them distally. The heads are simply allowed to retract distally. At the current time, proximal release of the gastrocnemius heads is rarely performed. It is never indicated for ankle equinus unless it is part of knee release surgery.

Distal Selective Gastrocnemius Lengthening

A number of distal procedures are performed at the gastrocnemius aponeurosis of insertion. These are designed to lengthen the gastrocnemius alone. Vulpius and Stoffel described a transverse (Fig. 37–18) (later modified to an inverted V (Fig. 37–19) incision through the aponeurosis of insertion. The gastrocnemius was allowed to retract proximally, and there was no attempt to fixate the distal gastrocnemius.[37] Strayer modified the Vulpius-Stoffel procedure by suturing the gastrocnemius to the underlying soleus[34] (Fig. 37–20).

Baker described a tongue-in-groove procedure with the tongue based distally and the free end pointing proxi-

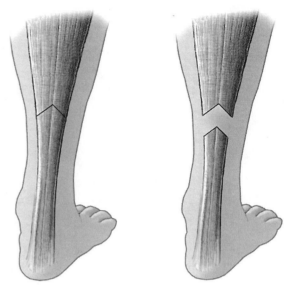

Figure 37–19. Vulpius-Stoffel procedure. The inverted V incisional approach.

mally[3] (Fig. 37–21). This procedure was modified by Fulp and McGlamry by reversing the cuts[17] (Fig. 37–22).

Tendo-Achillis Lengthening in Continuity

Controlled lengthening of the tendo Achillis can be performed by allowing the sectioned segments of the tendon to slide in side-to-side fashion without completely separating them. A number of these variations have been described. The two operations most frequently performed are the White procedure and the Hoke procedure. Both can be performed either by percutaneous or open approach. The choice of open or closed tendo-Achillis lengthening in continuity is determined by the surgeon's judgment about the status of the ankle joint. If the contracture of the triceps is longstanding, it is probable that posterior capsulotomy and flexor hallucis longus lengthening will be needed.[15] Deep contractures cannot be addressed during percutaneous lengthening of the tendo-Achillis.

White described a procedure for lengthening the tendo Achillis in continuity. This involves sectioning the anterior two thirds of the tendo Achillis just above the insertion on the calcaneus and the medial two thirds of the tendon about 5 to 6 cm proximal to the first incision. Passive dorsiflexion lengthens the tendon appropriately while the ends remain in side-to-side continuity.[38]

Numerous researchers[5, 21] have credited Hoke with a similar procedure. The medial half of the tendo Achillis is incised just proximal to the insertion of the tendon into the calcaneus. A second incision is made proximally on the medial side of the tendon just distal to the aponeurosis of the gastrocnemius insertion. A third incision is made in the lateral part of the tendon midway between the first two incisions. The foot is dorsiflexed at the ankle, and the tendon is lengthened appropriately so that there are no

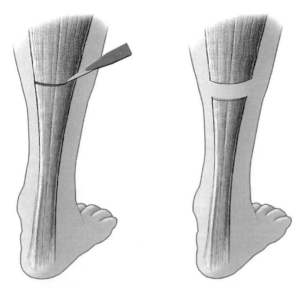

Figure 37–18. Vulpius-Stoffel procedure. The original transverse incisional approach.

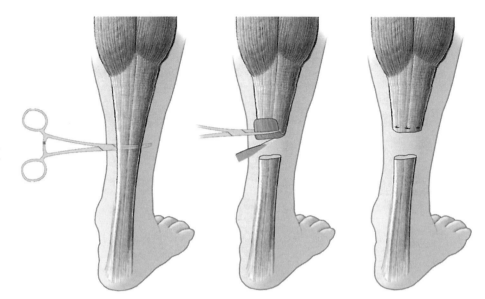

Figure 37–20. The Strayer procedure. The gastrocnemius aponeurosis is sutured to the soleus.

more than 10 degrees of dorsiflexion above the ankle neutral position (Fig. 37–23).

Tendo-Achillis lengthening in continuity is especially useful in children with cerebral palsy. There are three advantages. First, there is a decreased likelihood of overlengthening. Second, there is less spasm of the calves after surgery. Third, the procedure is easily performed in the outpatient operating room.

Z-Plasty of the Tendo Achillis

Z-plasty can be performed in either the sagittal or coronal plane; it is usually done through an open incision. The tendon is repaired at the appropriate length (Fig. 37–24).

Lever Arm Alteration

Shortening of the lever arm can be performed using Murphy's technique. The tendo Achillis is rerouted and implanted on the dorsum of the calcaneus anterior to its original insertion. It is routed from the medial side and directed anterior to the flexor hallucis longus tendon. It is sutured to the superior surface of the calcaneus proximal to its original insertion.[27]

Tenotomy

In some patients, muscle function is no longer an issue. For example, it is not important to maintain triceps function in nonambulators with equinovarus deformity. Simple tenotomy allows correction of the deformity with minimal morbidity. Additionally, sectioning of the tendon helps prevent recurrence.

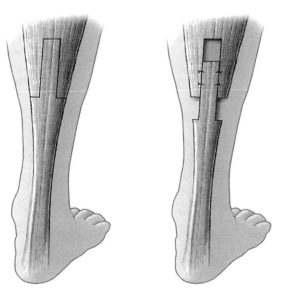

Figure 37–21. The Baker procedure.

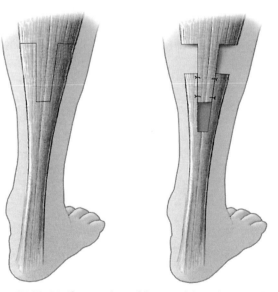

Figure 37–22. McGlamry-Fulp modification of the Baker procedure.

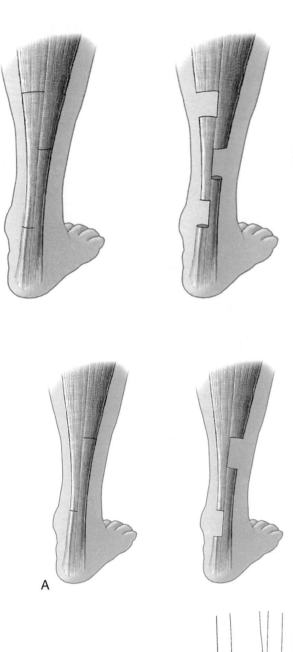

Figure 37–23. The Hoke percutaneous tendo-Achillis lengthening. This can also be performed in open fashion.

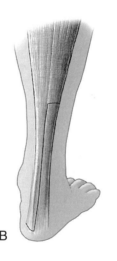

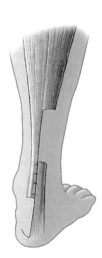

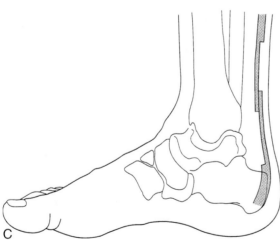

Figure 37–24. *A,* Percutaneous Z-plasty. Since it is a closed procedure, the tendon is not repaired by suture. *B,* Open Z-plasty of tendo Achillis in the sagittal plane. The lengthening is repaired with sutures. *C,* Z-plasty of the tendo Achillis in the coronal plane.

Possible Complications

The most common complications are overlengthening, recurrence of equinus, and failure to achieve an adequate range of motion.[29] Overlengthening is more likely to occur after Z-plasty. The result of overlengthening is calcaneocavus deformity. The ankle joint is in calcaneus, and the talus is maximally dorsiflexed in the ankle mortise. The calcaneal inclination angle becomes very high. Triceps strength is lost, as are propulsion and tibial stability. It is almost impossible to repair the consequences of overlengthening (Fig. 37–25). The best management is avoidance of the complication.

It is possible for the tendon to rupture in the healing phase. This occurs even if the tendon segments have been sutured. The effect may be similar to that seen with overlengthening. Appropriate casting after surgery is helpful in preventing this complication. It may also be reasonable to use an ankle-foot orthotic as additional protection after the postoperative casting period.

Only a finite amount of lengthening can be achieved. Open Z-plasty accomplishes a greater amount of lengthening than slide procedures. Careful preoperative assessment will determine the amount of lengthening needed, and the surgeon can select the technique that will allow the appropriate amount.

Another potential complication results from an erroneous interpretation of the amount of equinus deformity produced by the soleus. If the contribution of this muscle is misjudged, lengthening of the gastrocnemius alone will fail to produce an adequate excursion of joint motion.

Percutaneous lengthening of the tendo-Achillis may result in inadvertent tenotomy because of loss of side-to-side continuity during the slide. If this happens, the surgeon can perform an open repair. Berg reviewed a series of his own cases in which continuity of the tendo Achillis was lost. Static encephalopathy was present in all of the cases. He concluded that it is unnecessary to repair this condition as long as adequate postoperative immobilization is maintained.[4]

Recurrence may be the result of the natural history of the underlying disease. This is out of the surgeon's control. It may also result from insufficient lengthening, and this complication can only be avoided by experience and judgment. Timing of the index procedure is also very important. Lengthening performed in children under 5 years of age may have to be repeated later in childhood.

Failure to achieve an adequate range of joint motion is usually associated with deep posterior joint contracture. This can be avoided by being prepared to perform the tendon lengthening in an open fashion so that deep contractures can be released through the same incision.

Complications Secondary to the Etiology

Children with muscle disease are at greater risk for malignant hyperthermia. This is characterized by tachycardia, tachypnea, muscle fasciculation, rigor, hyperpyrexia, metabolic acidosis, myoglobinurea, renal failure, and cardiac arrest. Patients with congenital myopathy, muscular dystrophies, osteogenesis imperfecta, and myelomeningocele are particularly at risk. Succinylcholine and halothane are the two most common triggering anesthetic agents.

Children with myelomeningocele must be regarded as latex allergic. This sensitivity comes about through exposure to latex products through multiple surgeries, repeat catheterizations, fecal disimpaction, and other exposures to latex gloves. The risk is fatal anaphylaxis. Any surgery must be conducted in a latex-free environment.

SOME PERSONAL OBSERVATIONS ON EQUINUS AND ITS TREATMENT

Toe-walking is a common presenting complaint. Many of these children have been followed by pediatricians and other primary care physicians for years. The parents have been told that their children will outgrow this gait pattern. Most of these children have never been appropriately evaluated for underlying disease, a situation due to the widely held belief in the pediatric literature that toe-walking is a part of the normal maturation of the infant's gait. Since it is untrue, this belief must be changed

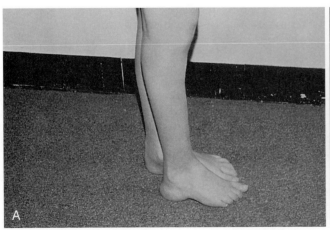
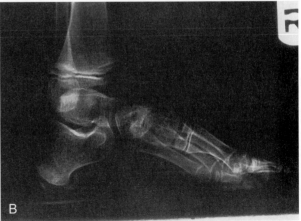

Figure 37–25. *A*, A 7-year-old boy had tendo-Achillis lengthening done elsewhere for equinus associated with cavus deformity. He lost all triceps function, and his cavus deformity became worse. *B*, Weight-bearing lateral radiograph of the child in *A*.

through education of pediatricians and family practice physicians.

This chapter has attempted to review some of the more common causes of toe-walking. It must be kept in mind that toe-walking is a symptom of pathology. It is not a distinct pathology in its own right. The foot and ankle surgeon must identify a causative etiology whenever it is possible to do so. Failure in this regard leads to inappropriate initial treatment and delay in identification of the true disease.

The Team Concept

The surgeon must keep in mind that management of equinus in childhood is a multidisciplinary team effort. The surgeon, pediatrician, pediatric neurologist, pediatric physical therapist, orthotist, and parents must all work together to manage toe-walking. Each member of the team must understand the benefits and limitations of his or her contribution to the effort.

Idiopathic Toe-walking

Idiopathic toe-walking is the most difficult of all equinus deformities to manage. The initial problem is the diagnosis. It is one of exclusion, and it is made only after a team effort to uncover a cause.

The initial goal is to prevent a contracture if one does not yet exist. This is accomplished by the early intervention of the physical therapist. It is the therapist's responsibility to assess, provide direct therapy, and supervise a home program. Since it is neither practical nor beneficial to rely solely on the therapy performed in clinical sessions, the parents must assume a major role in the daily management of the child.

Bracing is started once the range of ankle motion is adequate. Bracing has two goals. The first is to prevent loss of motion, and the second is to teach heel-to-toe gait through use of the braces as a training instrument.

Unfortunately, an inability to achieve an adequate range of ankle motion is regarded as a therapeutic failure by some members of the team. It would be better if all team members recognized that there are some children who simply cannot achieve an acceptable range of motion because of the underlying condition. It is at this point that the team goes on to the next step in attempting to achieve ankle dorsiflexion, which is the use of stretching casts. Many children fail to respond to casting, but again, this must not be regarded as a therapeutic failure. The next logical step is tendon lengthening to improve the range of joint motion.

Muscular Dystrophy

Equinus gait is actually beneficial in maintaining the ability to walk during a part of the natural history of the muscular dystrophies. Since loss of ambulation marks the beginning of the downward course toward wheelchair confinement, spine deformity, cardiopulmonary compro-

mise, and eventual death, every effort is made to keep these children walking as long as possible. Therefore, equinus can be tolerated until the child can no longer stand. At that time, tendo-Achillis lengthening will allow standing with the assistance of a long leg brace.

When the child becomes wheelchair-bound, equinus and equinovarus foot positions interfere with proper seating. At this time, simple tenotomy corrects these problems with a minimum of morbidity. Correct foot positioning with ankle-foot orthotics is still necessary.

Cerebral Palsy

Most cerebral palsy therapy is directed toward preventing contractures and managing them when they do occur. It is important to involve the physical therapist as soon as the diagnosis is made. Appropriate bracing of the lower extremities is part of the initial therapy. If contractures do develop, they may be reversible through the use of stretching casts, but this does not always happen. When there is no improvement, range of motion can be obtained only with surgery.

Before surgery, patients must be divided into two groups. The first group is composed of children who need hip, knee, and ankle surgery in the same operative setting. This requires the addition of a pediatric orthopedic surgeon to the team. In the second group are those children whose deformity is isolated to the ankle.

This second group has its own set of problems, most of which are associated with procedure selection. The surgeon must decide which triceps components must be addressed. The need for deep posterior release must also be considered. These decisions determine the selection of the appropriate procedures. Sometimes this determination is changed when the child is under anesthesia. Appropriate postoperative casting and bracing are as important to the outcome as the surgery itself.

All members of the team must be constantly reminded that they cannot successfully treat certain movement disorders, and that children with these disorders will never become normal. One must never lose sight of the fact that ataxia and athetosis are not responsive to bracing and are not operable.

Charcot-Marie-Tooth Syndrome

Although children with Charcot-Marie-Tooth syndrome have equinus, it results in part from cavus and its variants as well as from muscle weakness. Lengthening of the tendo Achillis alone in these children produces a very destructive calcaneocavus deformity. Careful evaluation of the cavus components allows the surgeon to select dorsiflexing metatarsal osteotomies, calcaneal osteotomy, anterior compartment tendon transfers, and tibialis posterior transfer in an anatomic and logical way.

References

1. Accardo P, Morrow J, Heaney MS, Whitman B, Tomazic T: Toe walking and language development. Clin Pediatr 1992; 31:158–160.

2. Accardo P, Whitman B: Toe walking. A marker for language disorders in the developmentally disabled. Clin Pediatr 1989; 28:347–350.

3. Baker LD: A rational approach to the surgical needs of the cerebral palsy patient. J Bone Joint Surg 1956; 38A:313–323.

4. Berg EE: Percutaneous achilles tendon lengthening complicated by inadvertent tenotomy. J Pediatr Orthop 1992; 12:341–343.

5. Bleck EE: Orthopaedic Management in Cerebral Palsy, 2nd ed. London, MacKeith Press, 1987, pp. 249–251.

6. Bowen JR, MacEwen GD: Muscle and nerve disorders in children. In Chapman MW, Madison M (eds): Operative Orthopaedics, 2nd ed. Philadelphia, J.B. Lippincott, 1993, pp. 3277–3310.

7. Burnett CN, Johnson EW: Development of gait in childhood. Part I: Method. Dev Med Child Neurol 1971; 13:196–206.

8. Burnett CN, Johnson EW: Development of gait in childhood: Part II: Dev Med Child Neurol 1971; 13:207–215.

9. Carmick J: Managing equinus in children with cerebral palsy: Electrical stimulation to strengthen the triceps surae muscle. Dev Med Child Neurol 1995; 37:965–975.

10. Caselli MA, Rzonca EC, Lue BY: Habitual toe-walking: Evaluation and approach to treatment. Clin Podiatr Med Surg 1988; 5:547–559.

11. Cioni G, Duchini F, Milianti B, Paolicelli PB, Sicola E, Boldrini A, Ferrari A: Differences and variations in the patterns of early independent walking. Early Hum Dev 1993; 35:193–205.

12. Cohen-Sobol E, Darmochwal V, Caselli M, Najjar S, Lambert C: Atypical case of Becker's muscular dystrophy. J Am Podiatr Med Assoc 1994; 84:181–188.

13. Davids JR, Holland WC, Sutherland DH: Significance of the confusion test in cerebral palsy. J Pediatr Orthop 1993; 13:717–721.

14. Dubowitz V: Muscle Disorders In Childhood. London, W.B. Saunders, 1995, p. 513.

15. Elstrom JA, Pankovick AM: Muscle and tendon surgery of the leg. In Evarts CM (ed): Surgery of the Musculoskeletal System. New York, Churchill Livingstone, 1990.

16. Feehery RV: Surgery of the achilles tendon and posterior muscle group. Clin Podiatr Med Surg 1991; 8:513–542.

17. Fulp MJ, McGlamry ED: Gastrocnemius tendon recession: Tongue-in-groove procedure to lengthen gastrocnemius tendon. J Am Podiatr Assoc 1974; 64:163–171.

18. Furrer FD, Deonna T: Persistent toe walking in children. Helv Paediatr Act 1982; 37:301–316.

19. Griffin PP, Wheelhouse WW, Shiavi R, Bass W: Habitual toe-walkers. J Bone Joint Surg 1977; 59A:97–101.

20. Hall JE, Salter RB, Bhalla SK: Congenital short tendo calcaneus. J Bone Joint Surg 1967; 49B:695–697.

21. Hatt RN, Lamphier TA: Triple hemisection: A simplified procedure for lengthening the Achillis tendon. N Engl J Med 1947; 236:166–169.

22. Hicks R, Durinick N, Gage JR: Differentiation of idiopathic toe-walking and cerebral palsy. J Pediatr Orthop 1988; 8:160–163.

23. Katz MM, Mubarak SJ: Hereditary tendo achilles contractures. J Pediatr Orthop 1984; 4:711–714.

24. Levine MS: Congenital short tendo calcaneus. Am J Dis Child 1973; 125:858–860.

25. Njegovan ME, Leonard EI, Joseph FB: Rehabilitation medicine approach to Charcot-Marie-Tooth disease. Clin Podiatr Med Surg 1997; 14:99–116.

26. Papariello SG, Skinner SR: Dynamic electromyography analysis of habitual toe-walkers. J Pediatr Orthop 1985; 5:171–175.

27. Pierrot AH, Murphy OB: Heel cord advancement: A new approach to the spastic equinus deformity. Orthop Clin North Am 1974; 5:117–126.

28. Rang M: Toeing in and toeing out: Gait disorders. In Wenger DR, Rang M (eds): The Art and Practice of Children's Orthopaedics. New York, Raven Press, 1993, pp. 58–59.

29. Rinsky LA: Surgery of the lower extremity in cerebral palsy. In Chapman MW, Madison M (eds): Operative Orthopaedics, 2nd ed. Philadelphia, J.B. Lippincott, 1993, pp. 3263–3266.

30. Selby L: Remediation of toe-walking behavior with neutral-position, serial-inhibitory casts. A case report. Phys Ther 1988; 68:1921–1923.

31. Shield LK: Toe walking and neuromuscular disease. Arch Dis Child (Correspondence) 1984; 59:1003.

32. Silfverskiold N: Reduction of the uncrossed two-joints muscles of the leg to one-joint muscles in spastic conditions. Acta Chir Scand 1924; 56:315–330.

33. Sobel E, Caselli MA, Velez Z: Effects of persistent toe walking on ankle equinus. Analysis of 60 idiopathic toe walkers. J Am Podiatr Med Assoc 1997; 87:17–22.

34. Strayer LM: Recession of the gastrocnemius. An operation to release spastic contracture of the calf muscles. J Bone Joint Surg 1950, 32A:671–676.

35. Sutherland DH: Gait Disorders in Childhood and Adolescence. Baltimore, Williams & Wilkins, 1984.

36. Sutherland DH, Olshen R, Cooper L, Woo SLY: The development of mature gait. J Bone Joint Surg 1980; 62A:336–353.

37. Vulpius O, Stoffel A: Orthopadische Operationslehre, 2nd ed Stuttgart, Ferdinand Enke, 1920, pp. 18–19.

38. White JW: Torsion of the Achillis tendon: Its surgical significance. Arch Surg 1943; 46:784–787.

38

Correction of Spastic Equinus

Renato J. Giorgini, D.P.M., and Ellen Sobel, D.P.M., Ph.D

Equinus is the most common foot deformity in children with spastic cerebral palsy. Surgical correction generally involves weakening the gastrocnemius and soleus muscle by one of three methods: (1) tendo-Achillis lengthening (TAL), (2) lengthening or recessing either the gastrocnemius alone or the gastrocnemius in combination with the soleus muscle, and (3) anterior transposition of the Achilles tendon insertion to change its lever arm (the Murphy procedure). A detailed description of each of these surgical techniques, postoperative management, advantages, disadvantages, and complications is provided here. Factors influencing the surgical outcome including the relative effectiveness of these surgical procedures, age at time of surgery, the amount of tendon lengthened, and postoperative management along with our personal experience and preferences are also considered.

Spastic equinus is the most common foot deformity in patients with cerebral palsy.[1-11] The primary cause of equinus arises from the unbalanced action of the extensor and flexor muscles with premature or prolonged activity of the gastrocnemius and/or soleus muscle.[12] When equinus has been present for a long period of time, adaptive shortening of the gastrocnemius and soleus muscle in conjunction with contraction of the posterior capsule of the ankle and subtalar joint and thickening of the neck of the talus create a fixed deformity,[11] and these problems must be dealt with surgically at the time of tendon lengthening.

The method of correcting spastic equinus deformity remains operative.[13] However, before surgery is performed and prior to the age of 3,[14] conservative therapy is instituted. This consists of passive mobilization of the hindfoot into maximum dorsiflexion and strengthening with active resistance performed several times daily. The foot and ankle are maintained in the proper position with prolonged continuous passive muscle stretching in well-padded splints, bivalved casts, or molded ankle-foot orthoses. However, once shortening of the tendo Achillis prevents ankle dorsiflexion to the neutral position, conservative measures will not prevent further deformity,[15] and surgical correction is necessary for improvement of function.[8]

Surgical correction of spastic equinus is performed in one of three general ways: (1) tendo-Achillis lengthening

using either the closed percutaneous or the open procedure; (2) lengthening or recessing of either the gastrocnemius alone or the gastrocnemius and the soleus; (3) anterior transposition of the Achilles tendon insertion to change its lever arm (the Murphy procedure). Elongation of the tendo Achillis or gastrocnemius recession reduces plantar flexion muscle power by one to two grades,[15] sufficiently weakening the strong gastrocnemius-soleus muscle complex to improve its balance with its weaker and less active antagonists.[8, 15] Antagonist function was improved more than 200% 14 months postoperatively when spasticity in the agonist was reduced by tendon lengthening.[16]

GOALS

The goal of surgery for the spastic equinus foot is to correct equinus and reduce spasticity, resulting in an efficient gait with relatively normal function of the ankle.[8, 17] In the ambulating patient, the goal of surgery is to improve gait and either obviate the need for an orthosis or improve the fit of an orthosis.[18] In the nonambulating patient surgical correction should improve standing and weight bearing, allow plantigrade foot position on the wheelchair footrest, and minimize or prevent the formation of skin calluses and pressure sores.

A full range of ankle extension is not the goal of surgery in spastic equinus. A small amount of residual equinus at follow-up is well tolerated and may even be an advantage in hemiplegics because it balances out limb length.[19, 20] It is preferable to a calcaneus gait, which is a worse deformity in terms of function.[17] Five degrees of postoperative equinus is considered acceptable.[21]

INDICATIONS

Surgery is indicated in patients with persistent or progressive equinus deformity that does not allow the foot to be passively dorsiflexed to the neutral position while being held in supination with the knee extended[22] and does not respond to conservative measures.[11, 14, 23] Surgery is also indicated to prevent the development of compensatory deformities such as genu recurvatum or rocker-bottom flatfoot.[14, 23, 24] If spastic activity of the gastrocnemius and soleus muscle causes persistent toe-walking, heel cord lengthening is indicated even if the foot can be passively dorsiflexed to the neutral position after a round of conservative therapy has failed.[14] In patients who are ambulatory, surgery is indicated for spastic equinus that interferes with walking and has not responded to conservative treatment. These children persistently walk on their toes, which results in a precarious balance with frequent tripping or falling. Surgical correction is also necessary for the nonambulatory child with a spastic equinus foot type that substantially interferes with foot positioning in a wheelchair. Twenty degrees or more of rigid equinus in wheelchair-confined individuals prevent proper foot positioning in a wheelchair.[25]

In patients with the severe equinovarus foot type Achilles tendon lengthening can be done in conjunction with other surgical procedures such as tibialis posterior tendon lengthening,[26] split posterior tibial tendon transfers,[27] and anterior transfer of the long toe flexors.[4] However, in one study it was noted that in more than half of cerebral palsy patients with the equinovarus foot type tendo-Achillis lengthening alone was adequate in correcting the spastic equinovarus foot.[26]

TENDON LENGTH

Questions often arise about how much to lengthen the Achilles tendon during surgery. Garbarino and Clancy[28] analyzed the Achilles tendon in terms of lever arms from the ankle joint to the Achilles tendon and from the ankle joint to the head of the first metatarsal (Fig. 38–1A). They thought that the amount of lengthening needed was half the distance from the plantar aspect of the heel to the plantar aspect of the distal aspect of the foot (see Fig. 38–1A–B). They reported excellent results with no recurrence or calcaneal gait using this calculation.[28] Others set the ankle in the neutral position in mild cases of spastic equinus, in 10 degrees in moderate cases, and in 20 degrees in severe cases.[8] We have found most commonly that passively extending the foot slightly beyond

the neutral position to about 5 degrees of dorsiflexion is adequate to obtain a plantigrade foot without recurrence of equinus or calcaneus.

PERCUTANEOUS TENDO-ACHILLIS LENGTHENING

Percutaneous tendo-Achillis lengthening involves the distal release of half of the lateral aspect of the tendo Achillis and proximal release of the medial half. The procedure involves a sliding process of lengthening that can be accomplished with two or three cuts in the tendon made with a small, specially shaped knife called a tenotomy knife. Its blade is not as sharp as the surgical knife, and it may be less likely to cut the skin. Wounds are cleaned, Steri-Strips are applied, and the wounds are then dressed. The surgery generally takes about 15 minutes to perform and is done on an outpatient basis. Mild nonnarcotic analgesics such as elixir of Tylenol or Motrin, or intramuscular meperidine (Demerol) or morphine can be used for control of pain during the first night.

Indications for percutaneous tendo Achillis lengthening include mild spastic ankle equinus deformity as part of the surgical correction for clubfoot deformity and severe flatfoot deformity.[29] This procedure is especially well adapted to outpatient surgery.[30] The results of Achilles tendon lengthening procedures, including percutaneous lengthening, are presented in Table 38–1.

Surgical Technique

With the patient under a general anesthetic and in the supine position, the knee is extended and the foot is inverted to maximum dorsiflexion. No tourniquet is required. A No. 15 surgical knife is used. Two small stab incisions approximately 1 cm long on the posterior aspect of the tendo Achillis are made. The distal stab incision is made 1 cm proximal to the insertion of the Achilles tendon from a lateral to medial direction to free up and section the anterior two thirds of the Achilles tendon (Fig. 38–2). A No. 15 disposable surgical blade is pushed

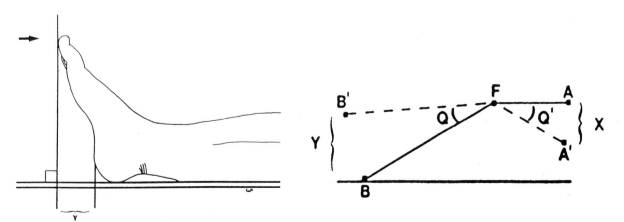

Figure 38–1. A, The lever arm approach in determining how much to lengthen the Achilles tendon. B, Diagrammatic representation of rigid ankle equinus. The amount needed for lengthening is half of Y. (A and B from Garbarino JL, Clancy M: A geometric method of calculating tendo-Achillis lengthening. J Pediatr Orthop 1985; 5:573–576.)

Table 38–1. **Results of Achilles Tendon Lengthening Procedures**

Study and Reference	Age at Time of Surgery (years)	Follow-up (years)	Surgical Procedure	Gait/Dorsiflexion	Recurrence	Calcaneus Deformity	Postoperative Course
Rattey et al (1993)[31]	5.4 (1–14)	10	77 Z-plasty heel cord lengthenings	Not reported	26%	4.5%	Length of time in cast did not matter: 3-week period and 6-week period gave equally good results; bracing not necessary
Cherg and So (1993)[1]	5.7 (3–9)	3	71 percutaneous tendo-Achillis lengthenings	Significant improvement in walking in 89%; 100% had plantigrade foot	6%	1%	Long leg fiberglass cast first 2 weeks, then BK cast. Immediate walking in cast PO. AFO worn by those who did not have active dorsiflexion
Graham and Fixsen (1988)[32]	6 (3–15)	13	35 sliding heel cord lengthenings (White)	Majority achieved heel-toe gait. Plantar flexion strength 4/5 in all. 6% had toe-heel gait	17%	None	Weight bearing in plaster cast 2–3 days after surgery. Plastic molded night splint used for 6 months. Physical therapy for those without active DF who showed signs of recurrence
Moreau and Lake (1987)[25]	5.6 (17 months–16 years)	1	9 percutaneous tendo-Achillis lengthenings;	97% improved in gait	6.7%	None	No AFO necessary; no physical therapy required
Garbarino and Clancy (1985)[28]	8.6 (4–17.5)	3.1	26 Z-lengthenings	All walked plantigrade: 17.5 degrees dorsiflexion preoperatively, 2.5 degrees DF postoperatively	0%	None	Long leg cast, knee flexed 60–90 degrees. AFO 6 months. Night splints worn to skeletal maturity
Grant et al (1985)[21]	5.4 (2–9)	4	40 open TALs; 22 Z-lengthenings; 12 White procedures; 6 Hoke procedures	85% heel-toe gait 80% active DF	15%	None	PO cast for 6 weeks. Night splinting essential. AFO used until active DF during gait or for 1 year
Gaines and Ford (1984)[8]	5.6 (3–20)	3.5	68 Z-plasty heel cord lengthenings	71% plantigrade feet 71% could walk on toes	4%	None	Not described
Banks and Green (1958)[33]			162 heel cord lengthenings (sliding lengthening and Z-plasty)	69.5% excellent or good results	29.6%	5%	Exercises 1 week PO. Long leg cast extended knee and foot 90 degrees. Weight bearing 6–8 weeks PO. Night splinting at least until growth is completed

TAL, tendo-Achillis lengthening; DF, dorsiflexion; PO, postoperative; AFO, ankle-foot orthosis; BK, below-knee

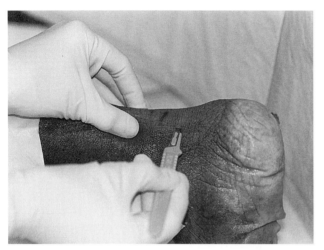

Figure 38–2. Percutaneous tendo-Achillis Lengthening. Distal stab incision shown with patient in prone position.

directly through the skin and the tendon, keeping it oriented longitudinally with the tendon. The blade of the knife is rotated 90 degrees toward the part of the tendon that is to be divided. The surgeon drops the hand to bring the blade of the knife under the tendon that is to be cut and, using a sawing motion, cuts two thirds of the tendon. Approximately 3 cm proximal to the first incision, on the midline of the tendo Achillis, the medial half of the tendon is dissected through a small stab incision. The foot is then placed in marked dorsiflexion (Fig. 38–3) and is elongated to 5 to 10 degrees of dorsiflexion, lengthening the Achilles tendon in a closed tendon-slide Z-plasty tendo-Achillis lengthening fashion.

Once this is accomplished the superficial skin incisions are closed using three 4–0 simple interrupted nylon sutures at the proximal and distal incisions on the posterior aspect of the foot. A dry sterile dressing is applied to the wound. The wound is clean, and there are no drains.

Postoperative Care

A below-knee cast with the foot in 5 to 10 degrees of dorsiflexion is applied and is reinforced with a single layer of fiberglass. The foot should be kept elevated with ice packs applied for the first 24 to 48 hours. The cast is left in place for 4 to 6 weeks with no weight bearing. At this time the patient can be placed in a bivalved plaster cast, and partial weight bearing is allowed. Physical therapy consisting of passive and active range of motion exercises of the ankle is begun and continues for 4 to 6 weeks. At the end of this period, if the child is walking very well and has 10 degrees or more of active ankle dorsiflexion, an ankle-foot orthosis is not required. Because spasticity is generally milder in patients selected for the percutaneous Achilles tendon lengthening procedure, postoperative treatment is generally shorter (Fig. 38–4).

Advantages

Percutaneous tendo-Achillis lengthening has been reported to have results that are as good as those achieved with the open procedure[23] (see Tables 38–1 and 38–2). Compared to the open Z-plasty tendon lengthening procedure, the closed tendo-Achillis lengthening is technically easier to perform, can be done on a child of any age, requires a shorter amount of time to perform and a shorter hospital stay, results in fewer surgical complications, is relatively more cost effective, and can easily be done after an open operation or as a repeat lengthening

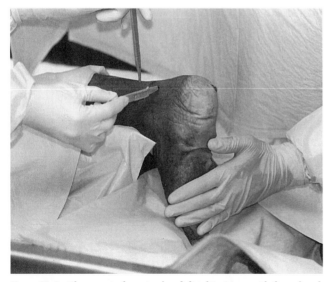

Figure 38–3. Placement of proximal and distal incisions with foot placed in dorsiflexion.

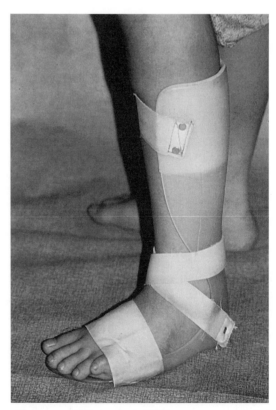

Figure 38–4. An ankle foot orthosis (AFO) worn postoperatively during the day.

Table 38-2. **Comparative Effectiveness of Surgical Procedures**

Study and Reference	Age at Time of Surgery (years)	Follow-up (years)	Surgical Procedures	Results	Recurrence
Yngve and Chambers (1996)[17]	9 years	1 year	27 Z-lengthenings 22 Vulpius muscle recessions	No significant difference between procedures; both gave satisfactory results	Not reported
Entyre et al (1993)[34]	7 years	1 year	12 Z-lengthenings 26 Vulpius muscle lengthenings	No difference between two procedures in ankle motion plots and EMG	12%
Deluca et al (1988)[35]			18 Z-lengthenings 22 muscle recessions	Both procedures effective in restoring normal stance phase motion. Baker procedure provided better push-off	Not reported
Lee and Bleck (1980)[36]	6.5 years	3 years	71 Hoke TAL 51 Strayer-Baker	Recurrence greater with muscle recession. 9% recurrence with TAL; 29% recurrence with Strayer-Baker procedure	9% TAL 29% muscle recession
Sharrard and Bernstein (1972)[15]	7 years	9 years	77 TAL 53 gastrocnemius recessions	Both procedures equally satisfactory. Prefer TAL for hemiplegia, gastrocnemius recession for paraplegia	20%
Conrad and Frost (1969)[23]	11 years (open) 9 years (closed)	3 years	87 TAL (open) 112 TAL (closed)	Closed TAL quicker, easier, better tolerated with less anesthetic, and surgical morbidity. Both procedures corrected deformities equally well	25%

TAL, tendo-Achillis lengthening; EMG, electromyography.

procedure.[23] This operation is particularly suitable as an outpatient procedure.[25, 30]

Disadvantages

The main disadvantage of percutaneous Achilles tendon lengthening is the problem of controlling the degree of lengthening.[14, 18] Inadequate lengthening, rupture, and overlengthening[5, 33, 37–40] have all been reported. Overlengthening of the Achilles tendon can be prevented by not stretching the ankle beyond the plantigrade position intraoperatively.[1]

Complications

Complications of the closed TAL procedure include calcaneus deformity and nonunion of the tendon,[41] bulky scar formation, bone formation in the tendon, adherence of scar to surrounding soft tissue,[23] superficial wound infection, sural nerve paresthesia, and wound hematoma.[25]

OPEN TENDO-ACHILLIS LENGTHENING Z-PLASTY TECHNIQUE

The tendo-Achillis sliding lengthening procedure is the easiest way to lengthen the Achilles tendon. The step-cut lengthening is a more difficult technique and is not required unless the posterior ankle or subtalar joint must also be released. The open tendo-Achillis sliding lengthening involves resecting the anterior two thirds of the Achilles tendon distally right above its insertion into the calcaneus; the medial two thirds is divided at the proximal aspect of the tendon. The proximal cut is as great a distance from the distal cut as possible while still remaining in the purely tendinous part of the tendon. The two bundles of fibers slide past each other as the foot is passively dorsiflexed leaving the fibers in continuity.[42] An open Z-plasty tendo-Achillis lengthening takes about 45 minutes to perform. The procedure can be performed on an outpatient basis, but more commonly the patient stays overnight in the hospital. Patients undergoing the open Achilles tendon lengthening generally have a severe equinus that is resistant to passive dorsiflexion (Figs. 38–5 and 38–6). See Table 38–1 for the results of studies involving Achilles tendon lengthening procedures.

Surgical Technique

General anesthesia is used, and the child is placed in the supine position. A tourniquet is used, and a 15-cm incision is made on the medial aspect of the inner border parallel to the tendo Achillis. The wound margins are deepened by sharp and blunt dissection. The tendo Achillis is identified, and the subcutaneous tissue is then separated. Using umbilical tape, the tendon is freed along

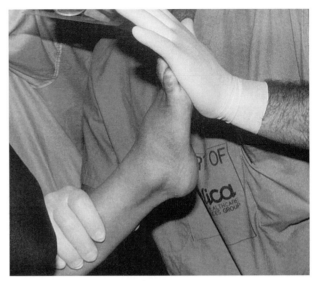

Figure 38–5. Preoperative passive dorsiflexion does not correct deformity.

its course from the musculocutaneous junction to its insertion in the posterior aspect of the calcaneus.

The tendon is then split, leaving the medial half. A Z-plasty technique is performed on the distal lateral half until the foot is brought into marked dorsiflexion of at least 5 degrees and maintained in the neutral position with approximately 5 degrees of dorsiflexion. End-to-end anastomosis of the Achilles tendon is accomplished with Bunnell-type suture using 2–0 Dexon. The deep structures are closed with 3–0 Dexon subcutaneous and 4–0

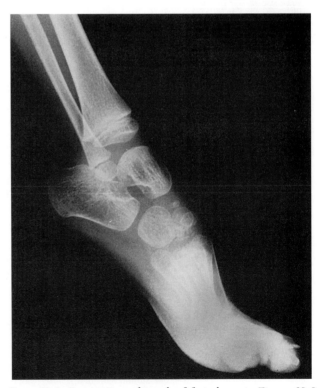

Figure 38–6. Preoperative radiograph of foot shown in Figures 38–8 and 38–9.

nylon subcuticular sutures. A compression dressing is applied. The wound is clean, and there is no drain.

Postoperative Course

A below-knee nonweight-bearing cast in the neutral position is applied for a period of 4 to 6 weeks. A second bivalved cast is applied during the next 4- to 6-week period with partial weight bearing. At this time active and passive dorsiflexion exercises are begun, and physical therapy is continued for another 6 months. At the end of this period the child is placed in an ankle-foot orthosis (Fig. 38–7), which is discontinued at the end of the next 4 to 6 weeks if the child is able to walk as well or better without it. Night splinting is used to prevent contractures from recurring during the remainder of the child's growth.

Advantages

Achilles tendon lengthening[22] has provided better surgical results than gastrocnemius aponeurotic lengthening and neurectomy[22] with a lower recurrence rate (Table 38–3; see Tables 38–1 and 38–2). The open posteromedial approach is more accurate than the percutaneous Achilles tendon lengthening.[44] Tendo-Achillis lengthening involves the common tendon of both the gastrocnemius and the soleus muscles. Electromyography has shown that both the gastrocnemius and soleus muscles are spastic in children with cerebral palsy.[45] Muscle recession techniques often involve the gastrocnemius muscle only.

The Achilles tendon lengthening procedure requires a smaller incision, less exposure and dissection, and less postoperative discomfort compared to more proximal muscle recession procedures.[18] Open Z-plasty lengthening

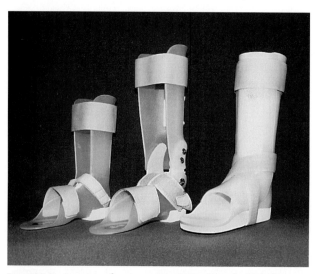

Figure 38–7. A variety of postoperative AFOs. Note the high flanges on the foot plates of all three devices; such flanges are tone reducing. The central AFO has an articulated ankle, which can be set with a 90-degree plantar flexion stop to allow free dorsiflexion and limit spastic plantar flexion. The right AFO has a pretibial shell, which is another tone-reducing feature.

can be used in the patient who has recurrent deformity following previous Achilles tendon lengthening.[18]

Disadvantages and Complications

Complications of the open tendo-Achillis lengthening procedure include painful scarring,[15, 23, 33] blistering, skin necrosis, cast ulcer, keloid formation, infection, postoperative swelling, and overcorrection or calcaneal gait.[15]

MURPHY'S PROCEDURE (MODIFIED)

The modified Murphy procedure for anterior advancement of the tendo Achillis is performed to reduce spastic equinus of the foot.[46] The Murphy procedure involves transplanting the insertion of the tendo Achillis to the dorsum of the calcaneus (Fig. 38–8). Theoretically, anterior advancement shortens the lever arm of the gastrocnemius-soleus complex about the ankle joint fulcrum and weakens its pull by approximately 48%.[10] However, during push-off, the fulcrum is shifted to the first metatarsal head, and the triceps surae function is altered by only 15% (Fig. 38–9). Therefore, equinus is reduced, and the ability to push off is retained. This result is notable compared to heel cord lengthening procedures, which weaken both forces equally. The result is that the patient does not walk with a calcaneus gait. See Table 38–4 for the results of studies of the Murphy procedure.

Technique

General anesthesia is used, with the child placed in the prone position. A tourniquet is used. Using posterior medial approach overlying the tendo Achillis (Fig. 38–10), an incision approximately 15 cm long is made. Wound margins are deepened by blunt and sharp dissection. The tendo Achillis is then identified and freed along its course both proximally and distally. It is detached at its posterior and inferior surfaces from the posterior aspect of the calcaneus, care being taken to avoid injury to the calcaneal apophysis. Ten percent of the lateral portion of the tendo Achillis is left attached to the calcaneus (Fig. 38–11). Wound margins are deepened by blunt and sharp dissection. The flexor hallucis longus tendon is then identified. The tendo Achillis is placed in front and anterior to the course of the flexor hallucis longus tendon and then secured in a large drill hole in the body of the calcaneus, which is deepened and sutured with through-and-through 1–0 and 2–0 sutures in a crisscross fashion. After curettage of the calcaneus, the end of the tendon is sutured into the body of the calcaneus. Once this is accomplished, the deep structures are closed using 2–0 and 3–0 sutures, and skin closure is accomplished using 4–0 nylon subcuticularly. A compression dressing is applied. There are no postoperative drains.

Postoperative Management

An above-knee non-weight-bearing cast is applied with the foot in neutral position for the first 2 postoperative

Table 39–3. **Results of Studies of Muscle Recession**

Study and Reference	Age at Time of Surgery (years)	Follow-up (years)	Surgical Procedure	Recurrence	Calcaneus Deformity	Postoperative Course
Onley et al (1988)[5]	6 (2–10)	7 yr, 7 mo	219 gastrocnemius aponeurosis lengthening (leaving soleus largely intact)	48%	None	Length of PO immobilization did not affect recurrence. Night bracing not used; perceived to be ineffective because spasticity disappears at night
Javors and Klaaren (1987)[43]	6 yr, 8 mo (2–14 yr)	5 yr, 7 mo	79 Vulpius procedures	4%	4%	Casts applied 4 weeks with foot in neutral position. Patients allowed to walk in these casts. If voluntary ankle dorsiflexion present postoperatively, no further bracing or splinting used. If no active dorsiflexion, AFOs used throughout growth
Craig and Johannesburg (1976)[24]	5 (4–14)	6	100 gastrocnemius recessions (Strayer) coupled with TAL	9%	3%	Lower extremity immobilized in full-length plaster cast with knee fully extended and foot and toes in 40 degrees dorsiflexion for 3 weeks. Second cast is BK or AK walking cast with 40 degrees dorsiflexion for another 3 weeks. Bracing afterwards plus quadriceps and free and resisted ankle dorsiflexion for another 3 weeks

TAL, tendo-Achillis lengthening; PO, postoperative; AFOs, ankle-foot orthoses; BK, below-knee; AK, above-knee.

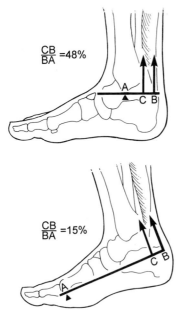

Figure 38–8. Murphy's Procedure. Diagrammatic representation of the modified Murphy procedure, showing the thin lateral portion of the tendo Achillis remaining attached to the calcaneus. (From Giorgini TL, Giorgini RJ, Cohen-Sobel E: Treatment of spastic equinus by heel cord advancement. Lower Extrem 1995; 2:41–45.)

weeks. A below-knee non-weight-bearing cast is maintained for the next 4 weeks, and a short leg weight-bearing cast is used for the final 2 weeks of postoperative casting. An ankle-foot orthosis (AFO) with a 90-degree plantar flexion stop is worn for the next 3 to 6 months. Night splinting is used if necessary to maintain correction. An AFO may be worn for an additional 3 to 6 months if necessary. Figures 38–12 through 38–15 show the modified Murphy procedure being performed on a 9-year-old boy with left spastic equinus as a result of varicella encephalitis that was a complication of chicken pox when he was 10 months old. Figure 38–16 shows the patient at the time of 2-year follow-up.

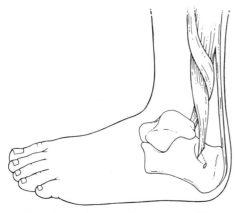

Figure 38–9. Murphy's Procedure. The biomechanics of the Murphy procedure. The lever arm of the calcaneus is shortened, reducing the muscle force of the gastrocnemius-soleus complex by 48% but altering it only 15% during push-off due to the shifting of the fulcrum to the metatarsophalangeal joint. (From Downey MS, McGlamry ED: Anterior advancement of the tendo Achillis. J Am Podiatr Med Assoc 1987; 77:117–122.)

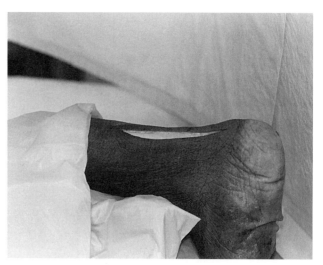

Figure 38–10. Murphy's Procedure. Posterior medial incision.

Advantages, Disadvantages, Complications

The reported advantages for this procedure include no loss of push-off, a very low recurrence rate during the longitudinal growth of the child, and no need for night bracing during the growth period.[2] Complications include the tendon pulling out of bone, breakage of wire fixation, and recurrence of equinus.[2]

MUSCLE RECESSION TECHNIQUE

General anesthesia is used, and the child is placed in the prone position. A tourniquet is used. A straight longitudinal incision is made 10 to 15 cm long over the lower third of the calf (Fig. 38–17). The sural nerve is identified and retracted laterally (Fig. 38–18), and the fascia overlying the triceps surae is split in line with the skin incision for later closure and exposure of the

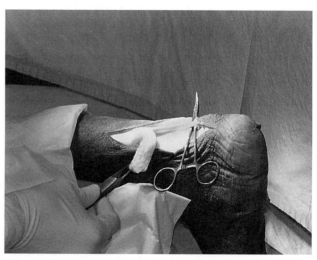

Figure 38–11. Murphy's Procedure. Ninety percent of the Achilles tendon is resected (*left*) from insertion, leaving a thin lateral slip of Achilles tendon (*right*).

Table 38–4. Results of Anterior Transposition of Achilles Tendon (Murphy's Procedure)

Study and References	Age at Time of Surgery (years)	Follow-up (years)	Surgical Procedure	Results	Recurrence	Calcaneus Deformity	Postoperative Course
Strecker et al (1990)[2]	6.5 (1–10)	4.5	161 anterior transpositions of Achilles tendon (Vulpius procedure sometimes added at time of surgery)	61% heel-toe gait. 37% flatfoot strike with or without push-off; 79% independent ambulators postoperatively versus 37% preoperatively	None	None	Short leg weight-bearing cast 6 weeks. AFO worn 3 months. Night splints worn next 3 months. Daily stretching and strengthening exercises.
Fernandez-Palazzi et al (1988)[3]	8.5	1.75	76 transfers of half of calcaneal tendon to dorsum of foot. Sometimes TAL procedure added at time of surgery	69% gait improved with no orthosis necessary	31%	Not reported	Below-knee cast with foot in 10–15 degrees dorsiflexion for 3 weeks, then posterior splint and exercises
Throop et al (1988)[10]	Not given	1–4	79 anterior transpositions of Achilles tendon	18% heel-toe gait with good push-off; 72% flatfoot strike with or without push-off	Not reported	Not reported	Short leg cast 6 months, AFO 6 months
Pierrot and Murphy (1972)[6]	7	6	32 anterior transpositions of Achilles tendon	9% heel-toe gait with good push-off; 66% flatfoot strike with or without push-off	Not reported	12.50%	Long leg cast with foot in 15 degrees plantar flexion; cast and sutures removed in 6 weeks. Physical therapy begun

TAL, tendo-Achillis lengthening; AFO, ankle-foot orthosis.

313

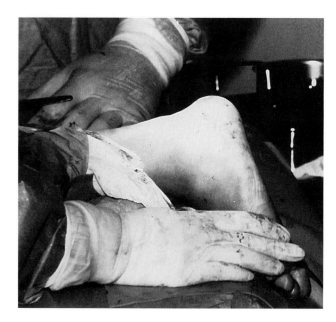

Figure 38–12. Murphy's Procedure. Preoperative equinus deformity with patient placed in prone position. (From Giorgini TL, Giorgini RJ, Cohen-Sobel E: Treatment of spastic equinus by heel cord advancement. Lower Extrem 1995; 2:41–45.)

Figure 38–13. Murphy's Procedure. Posterior medial incision is made, exposing the Achilles tendon. (From Giorgini TL, Giorgini RJ, Cohen-Sobel E: Treatment of spastic equinus by heel cord advancement. Lower Extrem 1995; 2:41–45.)

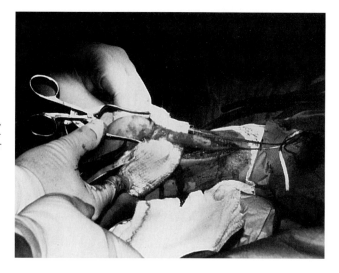

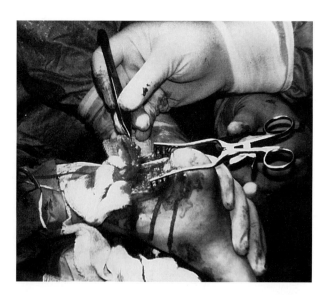

Figure 38–14. Murphy's Procedure. Ninety percent of the Achilles tendon is resected from the insertion at the posterior inferior aspect of the calcaneus. (From Giorgini TL, Giorgini RJ, Cohen-Sobel E: Treatment of spastic equinus by heel cord advancement. Lower Extrem 1995; 2:41–45.)

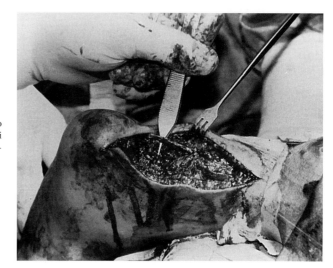

Figure 38–15. Murphy's Procedure. The thin lateral portion of the tendo Achillis remains attached to the calcaneus. (From Giorgini TL, Giorgini RJ, Cohen-Sobel E: Treatment of spastic equinus by heel cord advancement. Lower Extrem 1995; 2:41–45.)

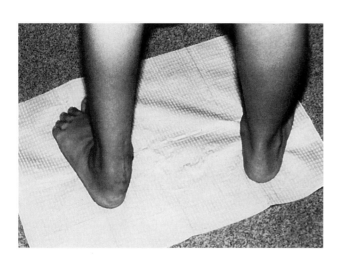

Figure 38–16. Murphy's Procedure. Two-year follow-up clinical photo of patient shown in Figures 38–25 to 38–28. The patient was a 9-year-old boy who had had a left spastic equinus resulting from varicella encephalitis, which he had contracted as a complication of chicken pox at the age of 10 months. (From Giorgini TL, Giorgini RJ, Cohen-Sobel E: Treatment of spastic equinus by heel cord advancement. Lower Extrem 1995; 2:41–45.)

Figure 38–17. Muscle Recession. Longitudinal incision over lower third of the calf.

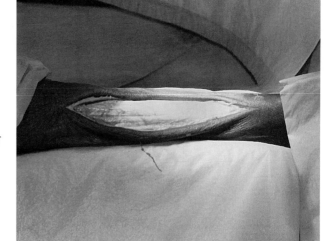

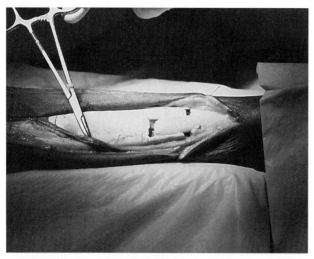

Figure 38–18. Muscle Recession. Hemostat demonstrates retraction of sural nerve and saphenous vein away from operative field.

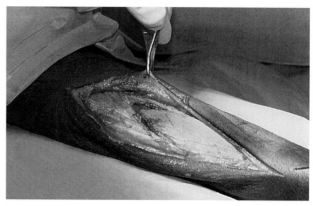

Figure 38–20. Muscle Recession. Vulpius procedure completed, showing inverted V cut in aponeurosis of the gastrocnemius.

gastrocnemius muscle. Using blunt dissection, the muscle is separated from the underlying soleus distally to the point where its aponeurotic tendon joins that of the soleus to form the tendo Achillis. A probe is inserted or a clamp is used deep to the gastrocnemius. Then the two muscle bellies are dissected from their medial and lateral attachments to the deep fascia proximally into the popliteal fossa, and a finger is passed from side to side beneath the muscle to separate it completely from the soleus. The proximal portion of the aponeurotic tendon is then sutured to the underlying soleus with an absorbable suture at a level at least 2.5 cm above its original attachment. The gastrocnemius muscle is lengthened either with an inverted V cut through the fascia (Figs. 38–19 and 38–20) or with a tongue-in-groove method (Fig. 38–21).

Postoperative Management

An above-knee non-weight-bearing cast is applied with the foot in neutral position for the first 2 postoperative weeks. A below-knee non-weight-bearing cast is maintained for the next 4 weeks, and a short leg weight-bearing cast is used for the final 2 weeks of postoperative casting. Active dorsiflexion and plantar flexion exercises are begun as soon as the cast is removed. Night splinting is particularly important until the child reaches skeletal maturity because there tends to be a high rate of recurrence. An ankle-foot orthosis with a 90-degree plantar flexion stop is worn for the next 3 to 6 months if needed. Table 38–3 describes the results of studies of the muscle recession technique used to correct spastic equinus surgically.

Advantages, Disadvantages, Complications

The procedure is simple and has a negligible complication rate, an excellent outcome in regard to scarring, and very little risk of overlengthening.[5] The main disadvantage is that it seems to result more frequently in recurrence than other techniques.[13, 36, 40, 45, 47] It may be that muscle

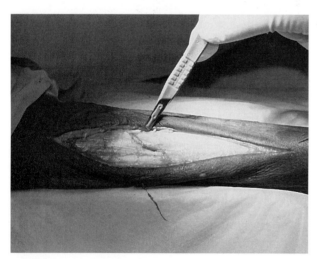

Figure 38–19. Muscle Recession. Lengthening of the gastrocnemius muscle by the Vulpius technique. The aponeurosis of the gastrocnemius is identified and cut by sharp dissection in an inverted V shape.

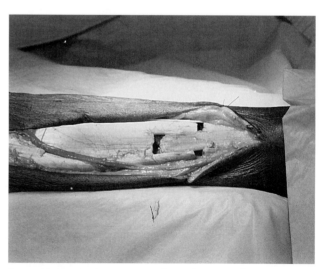

Figure 38–21. Muscle Recession. The Baker procedure. Tongue-in-groove lengthening of gastrocnemius aponeurosis with inverted U incision; underlying soleus is left intact.

recession induces more postoperative scar contracture because it involves more extensive dissection than that needed for tendo-Achillis lengthening.[36]

GENERAL CONSIDERATIONS

Age

Tendo-Achillis lengthening should not be performed in a child under 2 years of age,[14] since at this age the gastrocnemius-soleus muscle is not strong enough, and a calcaneus deformity is more likely to develop after surgery.[14] Children who underwent surgery earlier than age 5[36] or age 4[31] were more likely to have a recurrence of equinus deformity. In contrast, no child had a recurrence of equinus deformity when surgery was performed after the age of 6.[31] Consequently, several investigators recommend delaying surgery until after age 4 or 5, when a mature gait pattern is achieved,[44] or when ambulation is optimal between ages 8 and 12.[48] It is also thought that children are first able to cooperate during the postoperative period beginning at about age 4 to 6; this cooperation is critical to the outcome of surgery.[18] Prior to the age of 3, physical therapy, tone-reducing casts, or orthoses should be attempted.

COMPARISON OF SURGICAL PROCEDURES

No significant differences were observed in a number of studies between the postoperative results of tendinous and muscular surgical methods using a variety of criteria.[15, 17, 35, 36] See Table 38–2 for a comparison of surgical techniques. However, as previously stated, the muscle recession technique seems to result more frequently in a higher recurrence rate,[13, 36, 40, 45, 47] possibly because more postoperative scar contracture is present due to the more extensive dissection required compared to the tendo-Achillis lengthening procedure.[36] The tendo-Achillis lengthening technique has been preferred over muscle recession for correction of severe equinus,[17] correction of fixed equinus,[49] and in children with hemiplegia.[15] Finally, others have found that both tendo-Achillis lengthening and gastrocnemius recession performed together are necessary to prevent recurrence.[24]

Overlengthening, leading to calcaneus deformity with crouch gait, which is more disabling than equinus, can be prevented by correcting hip or knee flexion deformity prior to Achilles tendon lengthening, lengthening the gastrocnemius-soleus only when motor strength is 4 or 5, and providing adequate postoperative bracing.[18]

POSTOPERATIVE MANAGEMENT

Recurrence has been considered the most common problem in surgical correction for spastic equinus.[33, 49, 50] Banks[9] considered the postoperative regimen more important than the type of surgical procedure in preventing recurrence and believed that bracing, night splinting, and

heel cord stretching to develop balanced muscles was mandatory during the growth period.[33] Others have taken the opposite view that postoperative night splints, bracing, heel cord stretching, and special shoes are all unnecessary.[36]

The type of postoperative routine prescribed varies and includes many factors such as the type of cast and how long it is left on, the type and length of physical therapy, the need for night splinting, and bracing during the day. Long leg casts are preferred by some.[9, 21, 28, 36] Garbarino and Clancy[28] used long leg casts in 60 to 90 degrees of knee flexion. Although the fact that the gastrocnemius muscle crosses the knee joint could call for a long leg cast, this is rarely necessary.[51] A short leg cast applied with the foot in the desired position is almost always satisfactory.[15, 31, 36, 51] Sharrard and Bernstein[15] recommended immobilization postoperatively in a below-knee plaster or fiberglass cast for 3 to 6 weeks. A shorter period of postoperative immobilization seems to be as effective as longer periods of casting for both tendo-Achillis lengthening and muscle recession procedures. Three weeks of postoperative casting after a tendo-Achillis lengthening was as effective as 6 weeks.[31] Similarly, postoperative casting of either 3 to 4 weeks or 5 to 6 weeks did not affect the rate of recurrence for the aponeurosis lengthening procedure.[5]

Many surgeons recommend night splinting after surgery for correction of equinus contracture for anywhere from 6 months until completion of growth.[9, 10, 21, 31–33, 48, 52–55] Grant and colleagues[21] found that night splinting was a significant factor in decreasing the recurrence rate in children with spastic equinus. Night splinting is continued throughout the growth period and during the day if there are signs of recurrence.[9, 21] In contrast, a number of studies have found that night splints are ineffective in preventing recurrence.[6, 8, 15, 23, 36, 43, 47, 55, 56] Javors and Klaaren[43] reported only three recurrences of equinus among 79 procedures without night splinting and subsequently believed that if voluntary active dorsiflexion is present postoperatively, no further night splints or bracing are needed.[43]

An ankle-foot orthosis in the postoperative regimen is used when the anterior tibial muscle is weak to obtain ground clearance during the swing phase of gait, to generally improve the patient's gait, and to prevent recurrence.[21, 36, 43, 44] Grant and colleagues[21] used an ankle-foot orthosis postoperatively during the day for 6 months; if no voluntary control was obtained, they continued the bracing for another 6 months. However, a substantial number of surgeons consider day bracing unnecessary after surgery[9, 15, 31, 36, 57] and report that postoperative bracing does not diminish the recurrence rate.[15]

Although some claim that postoperative physical therapy, mainly in the form of heel cord stretching, is unnecessary,[31, 36] many consider it a critical part of the postoperative period as a way of developing balanced muscles.[21, 33] Conrad and Frost[23] caution that 3 months should elapse before passive daily heel cord stretches are begun.

SUMMARY

Tendo-Achillis lengthening, muscle recession, and anterior transposition of the Achilles tendon insertion have all been successfully employed in the surgical correction of the spastic equinus foot. Percutaneous Achilles tendon lengthening is a simple effective procedure that can be done on an outpatient basis. Open Achilles tendon lengthening performed in a sliding Z-plasty fashion is generally performed for patients with a more severe spastic equinus deformity or as a repeat surgery. The modified Murphy procedure can be performed in children with particularly severe equinus. Finally, muscle recession offers the advantage of the least reported amount of overlengthening but seem to have the highest degree of recurrence of equinus. Surgery is generally postponed until after age 4 or 5, when the child has attained a mature pattern of gait and can cooperate with a postoperative routine. It is important for the child to stand and walk as soon as possible after surgery to prevent muscle weakness and loss of function. Postoperative management generally involves an off-weight-bearing plaster cast for the first 4 weeks, which is then altered to a weight-bearing cast for the next 4 weeks. Night splinting is recommended until bone growth is complete, and day bracing is used when the ankle dorsiflexor muscles are weak to attain ground clearance during swing phase of gait and to prevent recurrence. Physical therapy in the form of passive and active range of motion exercises is used as early as possible and continued for variable periods of time.

References

1. Cheng JCY, So WS: Percutaneous elongation of the Achilles tendon in children with cerebral palsy. Int Orthop 1993; 17:162–165.
2. Strecker WB, Via MW, Oliver SK, Schoenecker PL: Heel cord advancement for treatment of equinus deformity in cerebral palsy. J Pediatr Orthop 1990; 10:105–108.
3. Fernandez-Palazzi F, Medina JR, Marcan N: Transfer of half the calcaneal tendon to the dorsum of the foot for paralytic equinus deformity. Int Orthop 1988; 12:57–59.
4. Hiroshima K, Hamada S, Shimizu N, Ohshita S, Ono K: Anterior transfer of the long toe flexors for the treatment of spastic equinovarus and equinus foot in cerebral palsy. J Pediatr Orthop 1988; 8:164–168.
5. Onley BW, Williams PF, Menelaus MB: Treatment of spastic equinus by aponeurosis lengthening. J Pediatr Orthop 1988; 8:422–425.
6. Pierrot AH, Murphy OB: Heel cord advancement: A new approach to the spastic equinus deformity. Orthop Clin North Am 1988; 5:117–125.
7. Downey MS, McGlamry ED: Anterior advancement of the tendo Achilles. J Am Podiatr Med Assoc 1987; 77:117–122.
8. Gaines RW, Ford TB: A systematic approach to the amount of Achilles tendon lengthening in cerebral palsy. J Pediatr Orthop 1984; 4:448–451.
9. Banks HH: The management of spastic deformities of the foot and ankle. Clin Orthop 1977; 122:70–76.
10. Throop FB, DeRosa GP, Reech C, Waterman S: Correction of equinus in cerebral palsy by the Murphy procedure of tendo-calcaneus advancement: A preliminary communication. Dev Med Child Neurol 1975; 17:182–185.
11. Pollock GA: Surgical treatment of cerebral palsy. J Bone Joint Surg 1962; 44B:68–81.
12. Hoffer MM, Perry J: Pathodynamics of gait alterations in cerebral palsy and the significance of kinetic electromyography in evaluating foot and ankle problems. Foot Ankle 1983; 4:128.
13. Bleck EE: Management of the lower extremities in children who have cerebral palsy. J Bone Joint Dis 1990; 72A:140–144.
14. Tachdjian MO: Pediatric Orthopedics, Vol. 3, 2nd ed. Philadelphia, W.B. Saunders, 1990, p. 1601–1705.
15. Sharrard WJW, Bernstein S: Equinus deformity in cerebral palsy. J Bone Joint Surg 1972; 54B:272–276.
16. Reimers J: Functional changes in the antagonists after lengthening the agonists in cerebral palsy. 1990; 253:30–34.
17. Yngve DA, Chambers C: Vulpius and Z-lengthening. J Pediatr Orthop 1996; 16:759–764.
18. Lutter LD, Mizel MS, Pfeffer GB: Orthopaedic Knowledge Update: Foot and Ankle. Rosement, IL, American Academy of Orthopaedic Surgeons, 1994, pp. 101–122.
19. Banks HJ, Panagako P: Orthopaedic evaluation of the lower extremity in cerebral palsy. Clin Orthop 1966; 47:117–125.
20. Staheli LT, Duncan WR, Schaefer E: Growth alterations in the hemiplegic child. Clin Orthop 1968; 60:205.
21. Grant AD, Feldman R, Lehman WB: Equinus deformity in cerebral palsy: A retrospective analysis of treatment and function in 39 cases. J Pediatr Orthop 1985; 5:678–681.
22. Jones ET, Knapp R: Assessment and management of the lower extremity in cerebral palsy. Orthop Clin 1987; 18:725–738.
23. Conrad JA, Frost HM: Evaluation of subcutaneous heel-cord lengthening. Clin Orthop 1969; 64:121–127.
24. Craig JJ, van Vuren Johannesburg J: The importance of gastrocnemius recession in the correction of equinus deformity in cerebral palsy. J Bone Joint Surg 1976; 58B:84–88.
25. Moreau MF, Lake DM: Outpatient percutaneous heel cord lengthening in children. J Pediatr Orthop 1987; 7:253–255.
26. Uyttendaele D, Burssens P, Pollefliet A, Claessens H: Simultaneous Achilles and tibialis posterior tendon lengthening in cerebral palsy. Acta Orthop Belg 1989; 55:62–66.
27. Kling TF, Kaufer H, Hensinger RN: Split posterior tibial-tendon transfers in children with cerebral spastic paralysis and equinovarus deformity. J Bone Joint Surg 1985; 67A:186–194.
28. Garbarino JL, Clancy M: A geometric method of calculating tendo-Achillis lengthening. J Pediatr Orthop 1985; 5:573–576.
29. Cohen-Sobel E, Giorgini R, Velez Z: Combined technique for surgical correction of pediatric severe flexible flatfoot. J Foot Ankle Surg 1995; 34:183–194.
30. Greene WB: Achilles tendon lengthening in cerebral palsy: Comparison of inpatient versus ambulatory surgery. J Pediatr Orthop 1987; 7:256–258.
31. Rattey TE, Leahey L, Hyndman J, Brown DCS, Gross M: Recurrence after Achilles tendon lengthening in cerebral palsy. J Pediatr Orthop 1993; 13:184–187.
32. Graham HK, Fixsen JA: Lengthening of the calcaneal tendon in spastic hemiplegia by the White slide technique. J Bone Joint Surg 1988; 70B:472–475.
33. Banks HH, Green WT: The correction of equinus deformity in cerebral palsy. J Bone Joint Surg 1958; 40A:1359–1379.
34. Etnyre B, Chambers CS, Scarborough NH, Cain TE: Preoperative and postoperative assessment of surgical intervention for equinus gait in children with cerebral palsy. J Pediatr Orthop 1993; 13:24–31.
35. Deluca PA, Giachetto J, Gage JR: Gait lab analysis of spastic equinus deformities: A new system of standardized assessment. Dev Med Child Neurol 1988; 57:16–17.
36. Lee CL, Bleck EE: Surgical correction of equinus deformity in cerebral palsy. Dev Med Child Neurol 1980; 22:287–292.
37. Bleck E: Orthopaedic Management of Cerebral Palsy. Philadelphia, McKeith Press, J.B. Lippincott, 1987, pp. 240–251.
38. Fulford GE: Surgical management of ankle and foot deformities in cerebral palsy. Clin Orthop 1990; 253:55–61.
39. O'Dwyer NJ, Nelson PD, Nash J: Mechanism of muscle growth related to muscle contracture in cerebral palsy. Dev Med Child Neurol 1989; 31:543–552.
40. Schwartz R, Carr W, Bosset PH, Conrad RW: Lessons learned in treatment of equinus deformity in ambulatory spastic cerebral palsy. Orthop Trans 1977; 1:84.
41. McCarroll HR, Schwartzman JR: Spastic paralysis and allied disorders. J Bone J Surg 1943; 25:745–767.
42. White WJ: Torsion of the Achilles tendon: Its surgical significance. Arch Surg (Am) 1943; 46:684.
43. Javors JR, Klaaren HE: The Vulpius procedure for correction of equinus deformity in cerebral palsy. J Pediatr Orthop 1987; 7:191–193.
44. Renshaw TS, Green NE, Griffin PP, Root L: Cerebral palsy: Orthopaedic management. Instr Course Lect 1996; 45:475–490.
45. Perry J, Hoffer MM, Gioven P, Antunelli D, Greenburg R: Gait

analysis of the triceps surae in cerebral palsy. A pre-operative clinical and electromyographic study. J Bone Joint Surg [Am] 1974; 56:511–520.

46. Giorgini TL, Giorgini RJ, Cohen-Sobel E: Treatment of spastic equinus by heel cord advancement. Lower Extrem 1995; 2:41–45.

47. Lemperg R, Hagbert B, Lundbert A: Achilles tenoplasty for correction of equinus deformity in spastic syndromes of cerebral palsy. Acta Orthop Scand 1969; 40:507–519.

48. Smith SJ: Pediatric spastic equinus deformity. *In* Camasta CA, Vickers NS, Ruch JA: Reconstructive Surgery of the Foot and Leg: Update '94. Tucker, GA, Podiatry Institute, 1994, pp. 21–26.

49. Banks HH: Equinus and cerebral palsy—Its management. Foot Ankle 1983; 4:149–159.

50. Shapiro A, Susak Z, Malkin C, Mizrahi J: Preoperative and postoperative gait evaluation in cerebral palsy. Arch Phys Med Rehabil 1990; 71:236–240.

51. Morrissy RT: Atlas of Pediatric Orthopaedic Surgery, 2nd ed. Philadelphia, Lippincott-Raven, 1996.

52. Feyen J, Libbracht P, Fabry G: Adductor myotomy, hamstring lengthening and Achilles tendon lengthening in cerebral palsy. Acta Orthop Belg 1984; 50:180–189.

53. Grabe RP, Thompson P: Lengthening of the Achilles tendon in cerebral paresis. S Afr Med J 1979; 56:993–996.

54. Greene WT, McDermott LJ: Operative treatment of cerebral palsy of spastic type. JAMA 1941; 118:434–440.

55. Strayer LM: Recession of the gastrocnemius. J Bone Joint Surg [Am] 1950; 32:671–676.

56. Frost HM: Surgical treatment of spastic equinus in cerebral palsy. Arch Phys Med Rehabil 1971; 52:270–275.

57. Truscelli D, Lespargot A, Tardieu G: Variation in the long-term results of elongation of the tendo Achillis in children with cerebral palsy. J Bone Joint Surg 1979; 61B:466–469.

39

Equinus: Anterior Advancement of the Tendo Achillis

Richard M. Jay, D.P.M.

In considering correction of equinus in spastic, cerebral palsy patients, it is important to understand the etiology of the condition. Spastic equinus results from a neurologic condition that causes a spastic plantar-flexed position of the foot at the ankle. The deformity may be caused by one of several interactions. The gastrocnemius-soleus complex can be partially or entirely spastic, or weakness of the anterior muscles can result in relative overpowering by the posterior muscles. In comparing the anterior and posterior muscles in a normal gait pattern, one sees that the triceps surae start to function soon after heel contact. The soleus itself becomes active when the leg moves forward. This causes a stabilizing plantar-flexory force. As the forward movement of the leg continues, it prompts a stretch reflex in the gastrocnemius muscle. The gastrocnemius muscle fires, transmitting a force that plantar-flexes the foot at the ankle joint. This continues through toe-off.[1] The anterior muscles are active mainly during the swing phase of gait. It must be remembered that in normal gait, dorsiflexors are not antagonists to the gastrocnemius-soleus complex, since they do not function during the same interval of the gait cycle.[2, 3] This, however, is not true in the presence of a spastic equinus. The gastrocnemius-soleus complex is spastic throughout the gait cycle. The gait is no longer that of heel-toe; the pattern becomes one of toe-toe, and the spastic condition of the triceps surae is so tight that not even the child's weight can force the rearfoot down. If the triceps' spasticity is less severe, the heel may come down after the toe touches, or the entire foot may strike in a plantargrade fashion. All of this contact depends on the degree of spasticity of the gastrocnemius-soleus complex in relation to the function of the anterior muscles.[4–8]

Considering this explanation, it is evident that the primary cause of the equinus deformity is the unequal balance between the flexor and extensor muscles. To reduce the equinus, the function of the gastrocnemius-soleus complex must be diminished. Numerous procedures have been performed to reduce its power, either by lengthening it or by neurectomy. The tendo Achillis is an alternative, positive approach to the correction of equinus deformity in the spastic cerebral palsy patient.

THEORY

By advancing the tendo Achillis on the dorsum of the calcaneus, the leverage of the gastrocnemius-soleus complex is decreased. This is accomplished by shortening the lever arm at the ankle joint by approximately 50%. Subsequently, the gastrocnemius-soleus complex is 50% weaker; thus, the dorsiflexors can function, and true heel strike is accomplished. During stance and forward propulsion of the body, the gastrocnemius-soleus becomes active, and the fulcrum, no longer at the ankle joint, moves to a distal position at the head of the first metatarsal, where push-off is about to occur. In examining the relationship of the anterior placement of the tendo Achillis to the push-off fulcrum, it can be seen that the plantar-flexory power of the gastrocnemius-soleus has been reduced by only approximately 15%.[9–11] In contrast, tendo-Achillis lengthening decreases power at both fulcrums.

Another consideration is the fact that the gastrocnemius-soleus complex passes over four growth areas: (1) the distal femur, (2) the proximal tibia, (3) the distal tibia, and (4) the calcaneal apophysis.[12] During the development of the child between the ages of 6 and 12, bone growth is rapid and can add contractures to the already spastic muscles. This creates more equinus deformity because of the increased tension in the spastic muscle. However, with the anterior placement of the tendo Achillis, one of the growth centers, the calcaneal apophysis, is bypassed. We must keep in mind that, if the insertion of the tendo Achillis remains on the posterior aspect of the calcaneus, it will continue to be a deforming force with growth. For example, posterior growth of the calcaneus lengthens the lever arm, thus increasing mechanical advantage. This, in turn, gives greater plantar-flexory power to the gastrocnemius-soleus complex. With the advancement procedure, we not only decrease the mechanical advantage of the gastrocnemius-soleus, we also reduce the rate of progression of the equinus deformity.

TECHNIQUE

The patient is placed in a prone position under general anesthesia. After sterile preparation and draping, a pneumatic cuff is inflated to 350 mm Hg. A 4-cm lazy S incision, which minimizes scar contracture, is made over the area of the tendo Achillis posteriorly. This extends to the more distal portion of the posterior aspect of the calcaneus. The incision is deepened, and the subcutaneous tissues are retracted medially and laterally; the sheath of the tendo Achillis is identified. The tendon is then followed down to its most distal insertion on the calcaneus and removed by sharp dissection without harm to the apophysis. With a small curved osteotome and mallet, a small wedge is taken from the superior surface of the calcaneus anterior to the insertion of the tendo Achillis. The wedge approximates the size of the distal cut end of the tendo Achillis. At that time, the foot is dorsiflexed on the leg to a neutral position. The free end of the tendo Achillis should be approximated into the wedge on the superior aspect of the calcaneus.

If the tendo Achillis is excessively long, it should be resected to allow for physiologic tension. With the use of 0-Dexon, a Bunnell suture is placed through the tendon distally. Using Keith needles, the two sutures are then passed through the superior surface of the calcaneus and out the plantar. The sutures are tied over a sterile piece of orthopedic felt and a large button on the plantar aspect of the foot.

By using 0-Dexon sutures, the possibility of pressure necrosis is eliminated on the plantar aspect of the heel because in approximately 20 days the tension on the suture is too great to be held, and the suture itself snaps. An alternative way to secure the tendon to the calcaneus is to use a bone anchor. Caution is in order, however, because the cancellous bone in children is quite soft. The bone anchor, even one as large as 4.5 mm, will pull out. I have personally found that the suture exiting through the plantar aspect of the foot is the best way to secure the tendon to the bone. Deep tissue is closed with single interrupted 3–0 Dexon, subcutaneous tissue with single interrupted 3–0 Dexon, and skin with single interrupted nylon. A sterile Adaptic dressing and Kling bandage are applied. The pneumatic cuff is dropped, and an above-knee cast in a neutral position is applied. The cast is windowed posteriorly in 1 week, and the wound site is inspected. In the sixth postoperative week, the above-knee cast is reduced to a below-knee cast for 2 to 3 weeks.

DISCUSSION

When considering any type of surgery for the correction of equinus caused by a spastic condition, the surgeon must not only be aware of the various surgical techniques available, he or she must also be able to explain to the patient and parents the reason for the correction. They must be made to realize that the equinus deformity can delay walking, that it gives the child the effect of walking on stilts, and that it causes a tendency to fall. The child tires easily and continues to fall after he has learned to walk. The result of this change is the shortening of the triceps and lengthening of the dorsiflexors. In time, mechanical compression decreases endochondral bone growth and leads to a flat-top talus. Eventually, the patient is left with a rigid foot, which will be subject to pressure sores and pain. The surgeon's only recourse at that time is a radical osseous procedure.

Early anterior advancement of the tendo Achillis does have certain advantages. It renders splints, braces, and stretching exercises unnecessary to control the progression of the equinus.[13, 14] The anterior advancement is permanent, and the equinus correction is maintained.

Complications, however, may occur. One of these is overlengthening. If too much length is allowed when the tendon is inserted into the calcaneus or if it is placed too far anteriorly, excessive weakening of the gastrocnemius-soleus occurs. If hip and knee contractures exist, a dorsiflexed foot would have to be maintained, resulting in a calcaneovalgus foot type. The heels would be down, but the child would walk with an appropulsive gait. Hip and knee contractures are therefore contraindications for this procedure.

SUMMARY

Anterior advancement of the tendo Achillis is recommended for only spastic equinus. By weakening its power during contact phase, we enable the heel to approach the supporting surface. As the child enters the propulsive phase, the tendon complex and force of propulsion are weakened by approximately 15%. Anterior advancement procedure make use of sound properties of physics to overcome the deforming forces of muscle tendon imbalances.

References

1. Schoenhaus HD, Jay RM: A modified gastrocnemius lengthening. J Am Podiatr Assoc 1978; 68:31.
2. Root ML, Orien WP, Weed JH: Normal and abnormal function of the foot. Clinical Biomechanics Inc., Vol. 2. Los Angeles, CA, 1977, p. 127.
3. Sgarlato TE: A Compendium of Podiatric Biomechanics. San Francisco, California College of Podiatric Medicine, 1971.
4. Schnieder M, Balon K: Lengthening of Achilles tendon for spastic equinus varus. Clin Orthop 1977; 125:11:3.
5. Hatt RN, Lamphier TA: Triple hemisection: A simplified procedure for lengthening the Achilles tendon. N Engl J Med 1947; 236:166.
6. Cummins EJ, Anson BJ, Carr BW, et al: The structure of calcaneal tendon in relation to orthopedic sorgery. Surg Gynecol Obstet 1946; 83:107.
7. White JW: Torsion of the Achilles tendon: Its surgical significance. Arch Surg 1943; 46:784.
8. McGlamry ED, Kitting RW: Equinus foot—an analysis of the etiology, pathology, and treatment techniques. J Am Podiatr Assoc 1973; 63:165.
9. Pierrot AH, Murphy OB: Heel cord advancement. Orthop Clin North Am 1974; 5:117.
10. Throop FB: Correction of equinus in cerebral palsy by the Murphy procedure of tendo calcaneus advancement. Dev Med Child Neurol 1975; 17:182.
11. Weil LS, Smith SD: Anterior advancement of the tendo Achillis for spastic equinus deformity. J Am Podiatr Assoc 1974; 64:1016.
12. Crenshaw AH: Campbell's Operative Orthopedics. St. Louis, C.V. Mosby, 1971.
13. Phelps WM: Braces—lower extremity—cerebral palsies. Instr Course Lect 1953; 10:303–306.
14. Stamp WC: Bracing in cerebral palsy. J Bone Joint Surg 1962; 44A:1457.

Five

Bone Pathology

40

Juvenile Fracture of Tillaux: A Distal Tibial Epiphyseal Fracture

William H. Simon, D.P.M.

In adolescents the distal tibial epiphysis can be injured, producing an isolated intra-articular vertical fracture that exits laterally through the epiphyseal plate. Sir Astley Cooper,[1] in 1882, was the first to describe the adult counterpart, an avulsion fracture of the anterior distal tubercle (tubercle of Chaput). Tillaux,[2] in 1892, performed experiments on adult cadavers and found that the anteroinferior tibiofibular ligament could produce an avulsion fracture of the anterior distal tubercle. However, it was not until 1964 that Kleiger and Mankin[3] reported a similar injury involving the anterolateral aspect of the distal tibial epiphysis. They suggested that this injury might be regarded as the adolescent counterpart of the Tillaux fracture. Avulsion fracture of the anterolateral distal tibial epiphysis is now commonly referred to as the juvenile fracture of Tillaux.[4–6]

INCIDENCE

The highest incidence of injury occurs in the distal physis of the extremities. Peterson and Peterson[7] reviewed the literature involving 330 epiphyseal injuries over a 20-year period and found that the male-female ratio was 2.7:1 and the distal tibial epiphysis was second to the distal radius in frequency of injury. In Rogers's[8] review of 118 epiphyseal injuries there was a 25% incidence of injuries involving the distal tibial or fibular physis.

The peak incidence of epiphyseal injuries as reported by Peterson and Peterson[7] occurred in boys between 12 and 16 years of age and girls between 8 and 13 years old. The age of the child at the time of injury is important because of the possibility of growth arrest or angular deformity. Knowledge of the mechanism of injury and the child's age and potential for healing is important in determining the appropriate course of treatment.

HISTOPATHOLOGY

There are two types of epiphysis. Traction epiphyses (e.g., calcaneal apophysis, styloid process of the fifth metatarsal) occur at sites of tendon attachment. Pressure epiphyses occur at the ends of long bones (e.g., the distal tibia and fibula). These epiphyses histologically have four zones of growth. Starting at the metaphysis and progressing distally to the epiphysis these are the zone of provisional calcification, the hypertrophic cartilage zone, the proliferating zone, and the resting zone.[8, 9] In the zone of hypertrophy there are chondrocytes that reach four to five times their normal size. Their presence reduces the amount of longitudinally oriented collagen fibers and chondroitin sulfate matrix, making the zone of hypertrophy weaker and more susceptible to fracture.[9] Harsh[10] reported that the epiphysis is two to five times weaker than the surrounding ligaments, so fractures of the physis occur more frequently. Therefore, the fracture pattern and classification must take into account the age of the growth plate, the type of force applied, and the surrounding ligamentous structures.

CLASSIFICATION

Ankle fractures in children are usually caused by indirect (shearing) or direct (crushing) trauma to the open physis. Lauge-Hansen,[11] in a study using cadaveric ankle specimens and clinical experience, developed a classification of adult ankle fractures based on three important elements: axial load, position of the foot at the time of injury, and direction of the injuring force. In 1963 Salter and Harris[9] developed a classification of epiphyseal growth plate injuries. Their classification is based on the fracture line to the germinal layer of the physis and the prognosis for disturbance of growth. Dias and Tachdjian[12] in 1978 developed a classification of ankle physeal injuries in children that combined the Salter-Harris classification of epiphyseal plate injuries with Lauge-Hansen classification criteria of foot position and direction of the injuring force. The juvenile fracture of Tillaux was not classified under their four main categories but was listed separately under miscellaneous fractures.

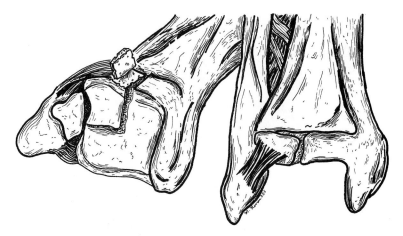

Figure 40–1. The juvenile fracture of Tillaux (Salter-Harris type 3) is produced by the pull of the anteroinferior tibiofibular ligament. An intra-articular vertical fracture through the epiphysis to the physis then exits laterally through the open physis, producing a fracture fragment that is quadrilateral. Note that the medial portion of the distal tibial physis is closed.

The juvenile fracture of Tillaux is best described by the Salter-Harris classification of epiphyseal growth plate injuries. This fracture is a Salter-Harris type 3 fracture: an intra-articular vertical fracture through the epiphysis of the distal tibia extending to the open physis and then exiting laterally through the open physis (Fig. 40–1).

MECHANISM OF INJURY

The juvenile fracture of Tillaux is an avulsion fracture of the anterolateral section of the distal tibial epiphysis. This area has been shown to be the last part of the physis to fuse (Fig. 40–2). Kleiger and Mankin[3] noted that the distal tibial epiphyseal growth plate fused in an asymmetrical manner, beginning in the middle of the physis and progressing first medially and then reaching the lateral aspect of the tibia. In 1982, MacNealy and colleagues demonstrated radiographically that the distal tibial physis fused asymmetrically, the anterolateral aspect being the last portion to fuse.[13] Closure usually is completed by 14 years of age but is earlier in girls than in boys; it takes about 1½ years for the anterolateral portion of the physis to fuse. Kleiger and Mankin[3] noted both radiographically and on gross dissection an elevation or hump in the medial aspect of the epiphyseal plate 1 cm from the

medial margin. They believed that this hump prevented displacement of the medial portion of the epiphysis in cases of ankle injury. Because of the zone of hypertrophy, the epiphyseal plate is weaker than the surrounding ligaments and joint capsule, causing adolescents to be more susceptible to the juvenile fracture of Tillaux.[8, 9]

The mechanism of the juvenile fracture of Tillaux is either a lateral rotation of the foot (abduction) or a medial rotation of the leg on the fixed foot. Kleiger and Mankin[3] were the first to show intraoperatively that separation of the avulsed fragment by the intact anteroinferior tibiofibular ligament could be reproduced by an external rotational force applied to the foot and could be reduced by the opposite mechanism. The fracture fragment produced is roughly quadrilateral because the fracture line runs vertically to the physis and exits anterolaterally, producing a Salter-Harris type 3 fracture (Figs. 40–3 and 40–4). The adult counterpart is more triangular because the physis is closed and is a true avulsion fracture of the tubercle of Chaput.[2, 3, 6]

TREATMENT

Initial treatment of a nondisplaced or mildly displaced juvenile fracture of Tillaux should consist of an attempt

Figure 40–2. Growth plate closure in the distal tibia. Fusion begins central-medial (A), progresses posteriorly B, then ends anterolaterally (C). It is at this time in growth that the physis is susceptible to a juvenile fracture of Tillaux. D, final physeal closure. (Redrawn from MacNealy GA, Rogers LF, Hernandez R, Pozanski AK: Injuries of the distal tibial epiphysis: Systematic radiographic evaluation. AJR Am J Roentgenol 1982; 138, 683.)

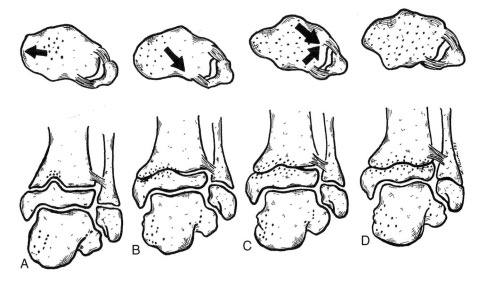

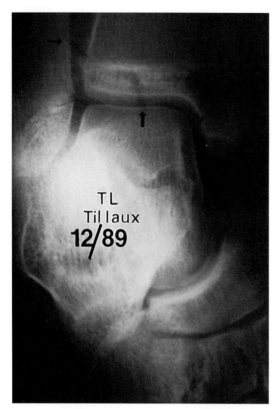

Figure 40–3. Anteroposterior view of ankle with a displaced intra-articular fracture of the anterolateral portion of the distal tibial epiphysis.

at closed reduction and placement of a below-knee cast with the foot in internal rotation. In patients with an acute injury a hematoma block with aspiration of the ankle joint is performed after appropriate skin preparation. The foot is placed in full dorsiflexion and abducted. The mechanism of injury is then reversed, with the clinician's contralateral thumb applying pressure to the anterolateral tibial physis and fracture fragment. Axial traction should be maintained while the foot on the leg is internally rotated. Anatomic reduction of the fracture fragment is mandatory. If the fracture is displaced more than 2 mm, open reduction and internal fixation should be performed. When the fracture fragment is rotated, closed reduction can be difficult owing to the interposition of the periosteum and ankle joint capsule.

Surgical reduction requires an anterolateral approach to the ankle joint between and parallel to the extensor digitorum longus tendon and the fibula. Special care should be taken to identify and avoid injury to the lateral cutaneous branch of the superficial peroneal nerve. The superior extensor retinaculum is the first dense structure encountered. When the peroneus tertius is present, the same surgical interval can be used with medial retraction of the tendon. Usually the anterolateral ankle joint capsule is found to be torn along with the syndesmosis, which can lead to instability between the distal tibia and fibula. The ankle joint is inspected to remove any debris, and the integrity of the dome of the talus is checked.

In open anatomic reduction of the articular surface, internal fixation is used to maintain correction. Most researchers recommend placing the internal fixation parallel

to the physeal plate, but if it is necessary to cross the physis, smooth Kirschner wires are advised (Figs. 40–5 and 40–6). Stefanich and Lozman[6] reported the use of cancellous bone screws across the physis with excellent functional results and no cases of early physeal arrest (Figs. 40–7 and 40–8). Once the fracture fragment has been fixated, the integrity of the syndesmosis is checked with a bone hook. If instability is present, an additional Kirschner wire is placed through the fibula, transfixing it to the tibia to ensure syndesmotic healing.[16] The leg is immobilized in a below-knee cast for 6 weeks with no weight bearing. Internal fixation is then removed, and protected weight bearing is prescribed for 2 weeks.

A new technique of arthroscopic-assisted surgery for treatment of acute fractures has been tried in limited numbers of patients.[17] Indications for treatment with this technique may vary from minimally to mildly displaced fractures in which debris and hematoma can be removed from the joint with irrigation and curettage. The fracture is then reduced under direct arthroscopic visualization and then fixated percutaneously. Although not reported to date, this technique could be very promising in treating the juvenile fracture of Tillaux.

PROGNOSIS

Prognosis for the juvenile fracture of Tillaux is good because the injury occurs in an older adolescent age group that is nearing skeletal maturity. Dias and Giegerich[14] advocated closed reduction and reported good results in five of nine patients who at follow-up examination were free of pain and had normal ankle motion. Kleiger

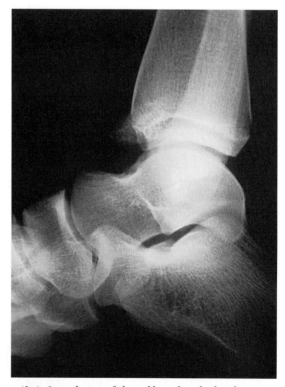

Figure 40–4. Lateral view of the ankle with a displaced intra-articular fracture of the anterolateral portion of the distal tibial epiphysis.

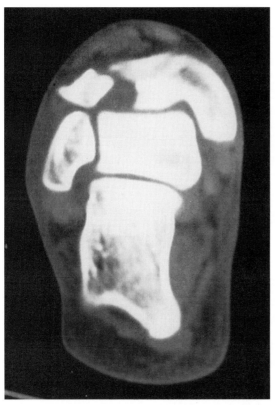

Figure 40–5. Preoperative computed tomography shows a quadrilateral fracture that is intra-articular, displaced, and rotated 90 degrees.

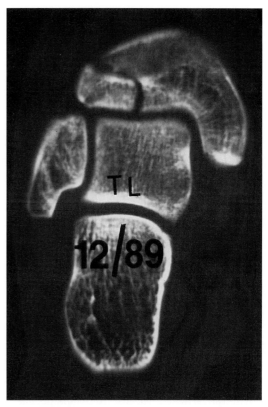

Figure 40–7. Preoperative computed tomography of fracture of Tillaux with laterally displaced fragment.

and Mankin[3] also reported good results in three of five patients. The largest series of juvenile fractures of Tillaux to date was reported by Rang,[18] who treated 30 patients by closed reduction and casting. However, at follow-up examination, eight patients had residual pain and stiffness with no gross deformity of the distal tibial plafond. This was thought to result from inadequate reduction of the articular surface.

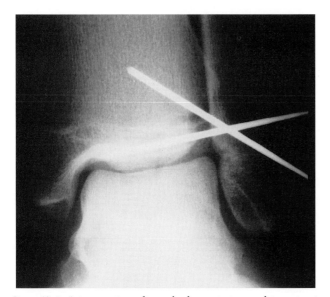

Figure 40–6. Intraoperative radiographs demonstrate complete anatomic reduction with two 0.062 smooth Kirschner wires.

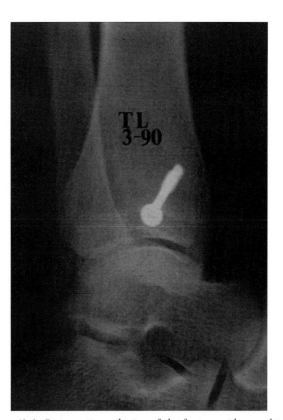

Figure 40–8. Postoperative reduction of the fracture with cannulated, cancellous lag screw.

Most researchers report that when closed anatomic reduction fails, open reduction with internal fixation produces excellent results.[3, 6, 7, 14] Dias and Giegerich[14] reported four patients treated with open reduction who at an average follow-up of 24 months had full pain-free ankle joint motion. Stefanich and Lozman[6] also reported four patients treated with open reduction; with an average of 5 years of follow-up they demonstrated complete anatomic healing and normal ankle joint motion. Dingman and Shaver[15] treated five patients with open reduction and internal fixation. At follow-up 11 months later they showed anatomic healing and symmetrical pain-free ankle motion and strength.

SUMMARY

The juvenile fracture of Tillaux is a Salter-Harris type 3 fracture of the distal tibial epiphysis. The mechanism of injury is an external rotational force of the foot in relation to the lower leg. The fracture fragment is avulsed from the anterolateral aspect of the distal tibial epiphysis by the anteroinferior tibiofibular ligament. Treatment is based on the amount of displacement of the articular surface after closed reduction has been attempted. If more than 2 mm of separation is present, arthroscopic-assisted or open reduction with internal fixation is recommended.[17] The prognosis is usually good if anatomic reduction of the articular surface is obtained. The most serious complications reported have been pain and stiffness secondary to articular joint incongruity following inadequate closed reduction.

References

1. Cooper AH: A Treatise on Dislocations and Fractures of the Joints. London, E Cox & Sons, 1882.
2. Tillaux PJ: Trate' d'Anatomie Topographique avec Applications a' la Chirurgie. Paris, Asselin et Hozeau, 1892.
3. Kleiger B, Mankin HJ: Fracture of the lateral portion of the distal tibial epiphysis. J Bone Joint Surg 1964; 46A:25.
4. Molster A, Soreide O, Solhaug JH, et al: Fractures of the lateral part of the distal tibial epiphysis (Tillaux or Kleiger fracture). Injury 1977; 8:260.
5. Simon WH, Floros R, Schoenhaus H, Jay RM: Juvenile fracture of Tillaux: A distal tibial epiphyseal fracture. J Am Podiatr Med Assoc 1989; 79:295.
6. Stefanich RJ, Lozman J: The juvenile fracture of Tillaux. Clin Orthop 1986; 210:219.
7. Peterson CA, Peterson HA: Analysis of the incidence of injuries to the epiphyseal growth plate. J Trauma 1972; 12:275.
8. Rogers LF: The radiography of epiphyseal injuries. Radiology 1970; 96:289.
9. Salter RB, Harris WR: Injuries involving the epiphyseal plate. J Bone Joint Surg 1963; 45A:587.
10. Harsh WN: Effects of trauma upon epiphysis. Clin Orthop 1957; 10:140.
11. Lauge-Hansen N: Fractures of the ankle. Combined experimental-surgical and experimental-roentgenologic investigations. Arch Surg 1963; 60:957.
12. Dias LS, Tachdjian MO: Physeal injuries of the ankle in children. Clin Orthop 1978; 136:230.
13. MacNealy GA, Rogers LF, Hernandez R, Pozanski AK: Injuries of the distal tibial epiphysis: Systematic radiographic evaluation. AJR Am J Roentgenol 1982; 138:683.
14. Dias LS, Giegerich CR: Fractures of the distal tibial epiphysis in adolescence. J Bone Joint Surg 1983; 65A:438.
15. Dingman RD, Shaver GB: Operative treatment of displaced Salter-Harris III distal tibial fractures. Clin Orthop 1978; 135:101.
16. Spinella AJ, Turco VJ: Avulsion fracture of the distal tibial epiphysis in skeletally immature athletes (juvenile Tillaux fracture). Orthop Rev 1988; 12:1245.
17. Guhl JL: Foot and Ankle Arthroscopy, 2nd ed. Thorofare, NJ, Slack, 1993, p. 135.
18. Rang M: Children's Fractures, 2nd ed. Philadelphia, JB Lippincott, 1983.
19. Spiegel PG, Cooperman DR, Laros GS: Epiphyseal fractures of the distal ends of the tibia and fibula. J Bone Joint Surg 1978; 60A:1046.

41

Osteoid Osteoma

Richard M. Jay, D.P.M.

Osteoid osteoma is a well-recognized benign bone tumor in adolescents and young adults. It can be present in all the bones of the foot, the talus being the most common site.[1] The characteristic symptom is throbbing pain, which is more intense at night and may respond dramatically to aspirin. When the osteoid osteoma is in a juxta-articular location, the clinical picture is confounded by other joint symptoms such as stiffness, muscle atrophy, or loss of motion. The nidus is not always surrounded by sclerotic bone and is often not easy to identify in the complex radiologic anatomy of the joints. This atypical picture often leads to misdiagnosis and delayed definitive treatment.

Pain is the cardinal sign of osteoid osteoma, and it is transmitted by autonomic nerve fibers that accompany the blood vessels in the fibrous zone that surrounds the nidus of the lesion. Reports by Jaffe and Lichtenstein[2] suggest that lesions that appear in expansible bone may produce less pain, possibly owing to the fact that the cancellous bone matrix has the ability to yield under this vascular pressure.[3] This is also thought to be the reason for the referred pain associated with osteoid osteoma. Pain is not always localized at the exact site of the lesion, which makes localization of a suspected lesion difficult. Pain often develops when the child has been asleep for at least 1 to 2 hours. Aspirin can reduce the pain in about 25% of children.[4]

The atypical picture of osteoid osteoma often leads to misdiagnosis, including muscle fatigue, post-traumatic synovitis, rheumatoid arthritis, and even hysteria. In many cases patients undergo unnecessary treatment, such as immobilization with plaster casts, use of crutches for an extended period of time, joint injections, arthroscopy, and even psychoanalysis. Bone islands (enostosis), Brodie's abscess, and stress fractures should be considered in the differential diagnosis. Most researchers believe that this lesion is more common in males than females and the usual age at occurrence is 10 to 30 years old. Half of the lesions appear in the tibia or femur, further complicating early detection.[5]

It is important to note that often the nidus may not become apparent on imaging until almost 8 months after the first symptoms appear. When an osteoid osteoma is suspected in young patients with persistent undiagnosed joint pain, radiologic examination, bone scans, and computed tomography (CT) should be repeated 1 year after the onset of symptoms, since initially negative findings may become positive at a later date. Bone scintigraphy and computed tenography aid in the diagnosis. Scintigraphy identifies the affected joint, and CT assists in localizing the precise tumor site. This allows differentiation from osteochondritis, stress fracture, and Brodie's abscess.

RADIOGRAPHY

Radiologic studies have proved to be the most valuable diagnostic tool; however, in young children in whom the lesion is present in cancellous bone, the lesion is difficult to locate owing to the extensive hazy trabecular pattern of such bones. Additionally, there should be a dense sclerotic rim surrounding the lesion, and this, too, is not easily spotted in the very young child with an early developing lesion. The dense rim does not appear until late in the maturation of the lesion as it is vascularly compressed. If the lesion is in the spongy layer, it increases in size, causing referred pain, but does not consolidate a sclerotic rim about the central clear nidus[6] (Fig. 41–1).

It is recommended that young children presenting with this vague but classic type of pain should undergo further studies to identify a suspected lesion more clearly. Chil-

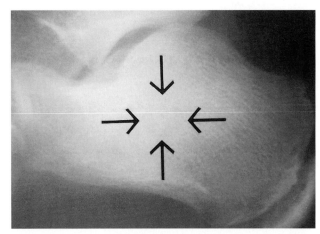

Figure 41–1. The lesion is difficult to locate in cancellous bone with its extensive hazy, trabecular pattern. A dense sclerotic rim surrounding the lesion is noted in this radiograph. This too is not easily spotted in the very young child with an early developing lesion. The dense rim does not appear until late in the maturation of the lesion as it is vascularly compressed. If the lesion is in the spongy layer, it increases in size and causes referred pain but does not consolidate a sclerotic rim about the central clear nidus.

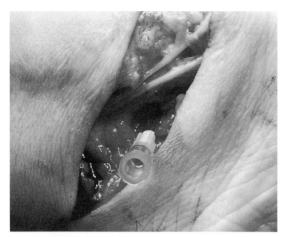

Figure 41–2. Visualization of the lesion can be aided by introducing a needle under fluoroscopic control.

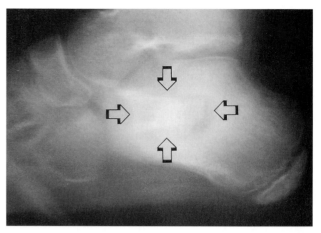

Figure 41–4. Radiograph of total en bloc resection with bone graft in place.

dren do not normally have pain. If pain is present, it must be seriously considered until a firm diagnosis is attained. The lesion can be located in cortical, cancellous, or subperiosteal bone. Cortical lesions usually appear as a radiolucent nidus with a sclerotic rim. Cancellous and subperiosteal bone lesions are more difficult to diagnose because the radiolucent nidus and sclerotic rim are less distinct and harder to see.

In the young child with osteoid osteoma the lesion is usually difficult to isolate during the surgical procedure.[7] Introduction of needles under fluoroscopy is recommended to better localize the lesion (Fig. 41–2). If the lesion is not fully resected, the remaining nidus will result in exacerbation of the original symptoms. Total excision of the lesion is the accepted procedure.[8] Since the depth and exact location may be difficult to determine, a wide and deep block excision should be performed (Figs. 41–3 and 41–4).

PROCEDURE

After the lesion has been located on radiographs and CT the exact measurements are taken to determine accu-

rately the area to be excised, on the bone in question. Four K-wires are used in each corner of a premeasured rectangle. The required depth is marked directly on the saw blade. Using a saw guide, the bone is cut to the required depth, and the four corners are connected. The wires are removed, and the cuts are continued to the corners, completing the rectangle. Using two thin osteotomes placed in the cuts opposite each another, the cortical shelf is gently teased from the underlying cancellous bone. Care is taken not to fracture this cortical covering. The deeper spongy bone is resected using a small curved osteotome until the desired depth is attained. If a good solid block is removed, a radiograph can be taken to ensure that the complete nidus has been removed. The surgeon should not be shocked if the block does not come out in one piece.

The cavity is then filled with cancellous bone chips, and the cortical shelf is replaced if it is not involved with the lesion. Depending on the bone site, use of a plate, wire, or cast may be needed (Figs. 41–5 to 41–8).

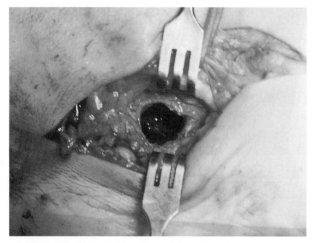

Figure 41–3. Resection of the spherical mass.

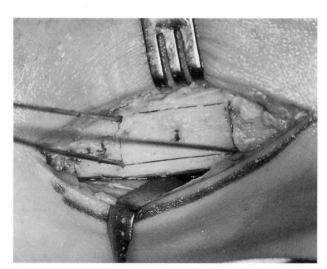

Figure 41–5. Osteoid osteoma of fibula. Four K-wires are placed in a rectangular fashion on the fibula. The wires are removed, and a sagittal saw is used to cut through the cortex to meet the four drill holes.

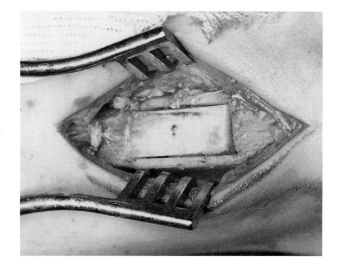

Figure 41–6. Once the rectangle is completed, the cortical shell is removed.

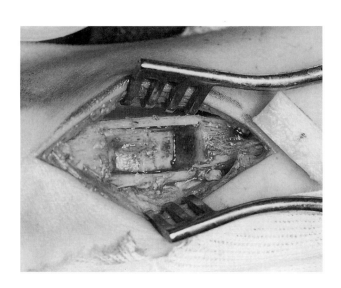

Figure 41–7. All of the deep cancellous bone is removed to the appropriate depth.

Figure 41–8. The nidus has been resected, and the area is packed with cancellous bone chips. If the nidus does not affect the cortical plate, this cortex is replaced. The graft is secured with wire or plate. The plate was involved in this child, and cortical allogenic bone was replaced over the chips and plated.

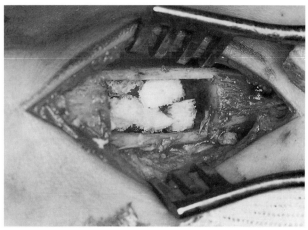

References

1. Capanna R, Van Horn JR, et al: Osteoid osteoma and osteoblastoma of the talus. Skeletal Radiol 1986; 15:360–364.
2. Jaffe HL, Lichtenstein L: Osteoid osteoma: Further experience with this benign tumor of bone. J Bone Joint Surg 1940; 22:645–682.
3. Lawrie TR, Aterman K, Patel FC, Sinclaire AM: Painless osteoid osteoma: A report of two cases. J Bone Joint Surg 1970; 52A:1357–1363.
4. Kenzora JE: Problems encountered in the diagnosis and treatment of osteoid osteoma of the talus. Foot Ankle 1981; 2:172–178.
5. Niwayama G, Resnick D: Diagnosis of Bone and Joint Disorders. Philadelphia, WB Saunders, 1981, p. 2656.
6. Havos AG: Bone Tumors: Diagnosis, Treatment, and Prognosis. Philadelphia, WB Saunders, 1979, p. 18.
7. Jay RM: Surgical treatment of osteoid osteoma in the adolescent. Foot Surg 1990; 29:495–498.
8. Shereff MJ, Cullivan WT: Osteoid osteoma of the foot. J Bone Joint Surg 1983; 65A:638–641.

42

Brodie's Abscess

Scott A. Alter, D.P.M.

Primary subacute pyogenic osteomyelitis, or Brodie's abscess, has received much attention since it was initially documented in the literature in 1832 by Sir Benjamin Brodie.[1] He described eight cases of osteomyelitis of the tibia in which the course of the infection was subacute or chronic rather than acute and the infection was arrested and well circumscribed. His recognition of "chronic abscess of the tibia" subsequently earned him a timeless recognition in the annals of medical literature.

Brodie's abscess has come to be known as one of the many clinical presentations of hematogenous osteomyelitis, an inflammation of bone caused by infectious bacteria that reach the bone through the patient's bloodstream. The most common offending organism is *Staphylococcus aureus* followed by *Streptococcus* sp.[2, 3] The organisms reach the bone from a site elsewhere in the body that may pose little or no threat of its own accord—for example, skin pustules, furuncles, impetigo, or infected blisters and burns.[4] It has even been suggested that the infection may be the outcome of as common an event as the "harmless" daily task of teeth brushing.[5] Narcotic addiction, hemodialysis, immunosuppressive therapy, sickle cell anemia, and leukocyte dysfunction have also been identified as predisposing factors for the development of hematogenous osteomyelitis.[6] Although hematogenous osteomyelitis is quite a different condition from the local osteomyelitis ("contiguous osteomyelitis") that develops around an infected focal lesion, the resultant pathology is very similar if the condition is misdiagnosed or untreated.

The sites most commonly affected by hematogenous osteomyelitis are the metaphyseal regions or growing ends of the long bones of the lower extremities such as the femur, tibia, and fibula as well as the humerus in the upper extremity.[1–5] Although relatively uncommon, the metatarsal bones of the foot have also been affected. A great deal of research has provided a multitude of theories that attempt to explain this generalization. Ultimately it is evident that this localization is dependent on the area's rather unique vascularization. Notably, other factors must be assumed to contribute to this tendency toward abscess formation. Fraser[7] suggested that the abundance of reticuloendothelial tissue present in the metaphyseal area of growing bone also contributes to the frequent localization of the infection to this area. He reasoned that since one of the most important functions of the reticuloendothelial system is that of defense against infection, the localization or fixation of infection in the metaphysis is the result of the defense activities of the

reticuloendothelial cells in this area in their efforts to correct a general infection.[7] This observation alone is not conclusive, but taken in conjunction with other researchers' contributions, it may be significant in understanding the localization of infection.

In 1921 Hobo proposed the theory that the vascular structures in the metaphysis make an abrupt loop as they approach the epiphyseal plate. He concluded that the diminished flow rate caused by this "loop" contributed to the metaphyseal localization.[8] Although this theory is frequently quoted as conclusive support for current theories, information obtained through electron microscopy has shown that these vessels are terminal.[9] There are fenestrations in these small distal arterioles that permit the egress of cells, including infectious bacteria. Because this vasculature closely approaches the epiphyseal area, which is devoid of phagocytic cells compared with the well-organized reticuloendothelial tissue in the metaphysis, localization at this point may occasionally involve the epiphysis.[10, 11]

PATHOGENESIS

Metaphyseal bone lacks the dense bone of the cortex in the diaphysis. The metaphysis is composed of a more densely organized area of trabecular bone, which during development contains the zones of growth and spongy bone.[12] The areas underlying the epiphyseal plate of a long bone are composed of calcified cartilage undergoing replacement by bone-forming osteoblasts.[5] Growth and remodeling occur to produce mature compact and spongy bone. Arterioles normally enter the calcified portion of the epiphyseal plate, form a loop, and then drain into the medullary cavity without establishing a capillary bed. This loop system slows the flow of blood in the area, allowing bacteria time to penetrate the walls of the microvasculature and establish an infective colony within the marrow. If the organisms are virulent and proliferate exponentially, they liberate exotoxins, which diffuse into the surrounding bone. The exotoxins then destroy and break down red cells, coagulate plasma, and cause the death of leukocytes.

Since this process occurs in tissue that is dense and hard it will increase the pressure on adjacent thin-walled vessels in its proximity because they lie in a closed space, the marrow cavity. As this situation progresses, defense cells have less opportunity to penetrate the inflammatory region to overcome the infection and assist the connective tissue cells in walling off the infection. Leukocytes appear in large numbers but are destroyed by the exotoxins, and a proteolytic ferment is liberated that autolyzes or destroys the dead bone. The subsequent increase in localized pressure further compromises additional vascular supply to the region as necrosis begins. The necrotic areas coalesce to form a larger avascular zone, allowing even further bacterial proliferation. At this point, the infection usually is contained through the modulation of marrow cells that become osteoblasts and osteoclasts and result in reactive new bone formation as well as bone resorption. This process is assisted through periosteal new bone formation, and the abscess configuration is completed.[5]

It should be noted that the formation of Brodie's abscess is merely one route that may be followed by this nidus of infection. Another possible course is the failure of endosteal bone to wall off this contamination. Obviously, this involves potentially serious complications with subsequent extension of the infection into the endosteal vascular channels that supply the cortex and spread throughout the Volkmann and haversian canals of the cortex.[5] Eventually, the infectious debris may follow the path of least resistance through the thin metaphyseal cortex, ultimately resulting in the characteristic changes of (1) necrosis of bone, (2) sequestration or throwing off of dead bone, and (3) new bone formation-involucrum.[13]

Gram-positive cocci are isolated in the vast majority of cases, although gram-negative organisms are isolated in up to 10% of cases. *Staphylococcus aureus* is by far the most frequently isolated gram-positive organism, occurring in at least 60% to 90% of cases, followed by streptococci, *S. epidermidis,* and *Hemophilus influenzae.*[14–16] Neonates are more likely to develop infection secondary to group B streptococci or gram-negative Enterobacteriaceae. Children between the neonatal period and age 3 often develop osteomyelitis secondary to *H. influenzae.* In children aged 3 or older with uncomplicated hematogenous osteomyelitis, the most common organism isolated is *S. aureus,* although streptococci are sometimes present. Patients with sickle cell anemia show a predisposition toward salmonellae, while *Pseudomonas aeruginosa* is isolated from skeletally mature intravenous drug abusers. Immunocompromised patients are susceptible to mycotic osteomyelitis, which may occur in the bones of the feet.[16]

Sex and Age Distribution

A discussion of the pathophysiology of this lesion would be incomplete without addressing its prevalence in terms of sex and age at presentation. Most studies suggest that the disease is classically described in children less than 5 years of age.[2, 10, 11, 14] Winters and Cohen reviewed 66 cases and ascertained that 23% of them were infants less than 1 year old.[3] Other research indicates that the majority of patients are in the 11- to 20-year age group with some degree of specificity. This same study, however, remains far from decisive about the most common age of onset because cases are reported in patients ranging from 1 year of age to more than 71 years of age. It may also be significant that there appears to be a higher incidence

of involvement of the vertebral bodies in adult patients for reasons yet to be elucidated.[2]

Sex distribution of the condition of osteomyelitis shows an approximate male-to-female ration of 2:1 regardless of the causative infectious agent.[14, 17] This ratio has been supported by several large studies and appears to be further skewed toward males when trauma to the area of affected bone preceded the infection.[14]

CLINICAL FEATURES

Minor local soft tissue swelling and erythema may or may not be evident on the initial patient examination. This is in contrast to the almost universal chief complaint of deep pain that has been present for weeks to months.[18] Most frequently, the pain presents in the lower extremity with no history of trauma to the affected area. The patient is typically afebrile at presentation, and the temperature is often normal for the duration of the illness except in patients with a fulminant actively spreading septicemia.[2] Obviously, the exact stage of the abscess formation or even its existence, for that matter, may elude the careless clinician.

LABORATORY AND RADIOGRAPHIC FINDINGS

In patients with subacute disease the total white blood cell count is usually normal, and the differential count is unremarkable. The erythrocyte sedimentation rate, though often normal, is more reliable than the white blood cell count. In some cases it has been reported to be over 50 mm in 1 hour in patients with staphylococcal infections.[18] It has not yet been explained why *Staphylococcus* produces an acute or fulminating illness in some patients and in others an illness that is mild or subacute. While many factors are assumed to play a role in this process, perhaps none is more individual than the patient's own immune status or the reduced virulence of the offending organism. The very nature of the abscess formation does not readily permit isolation of an organism via fine needle aspiration. For this reason, Lack and Towers proposed that staphylococcal antibody titers might be a better indicator of the diagnosis.[19] It should be noted, however, that a negative result does not exclude infection.

The most useful diagnostic tool to date remains the plain radiographic film. Radiographs taken during the first 1 to 2 weeks of infection may be completely unremarkable or may show only soft tissue manifestations of inflammation. Comparison views of the unaffected extremity may be helpful. Brodie's abscess typically presents as an area of central lucency surrounded by a sclerotic margin[20] (Fig. 42–1). Even more specific for abscess formation is the rather ill-defined and diffuse sclerotic margin that fades peripherally.[21] The period at which x-ray findings become positive varies with the age of the patient, the virulence and extent of the infection, and the density of the soft tissue overlying the bone. Additionally, owing to the subacute presentation of the disorder, x-ray diagno-

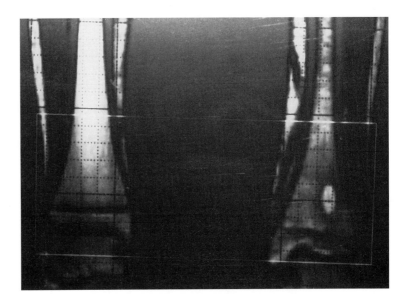

Figure 42–1. Magnetic resonance image of Brodie's abscess located in the distal and medial aspect of the tibia.

sis has become the rule rather than the exception. Harris and Kirkaldy-Willis noted that lesions may appear on radiographs without obvious abscess formation and may even resemble osteoid osteoma, Garré's sclerosing osteitis, or Ewing's sarcoma.[18] Technetium bone scans have demonstrated increased radioisotopic uptake in some cases of Brodie's abscess, but results are less dramatic than those seen in acute osteomyelitis.[11] Magnetic resonance imaging (MRI) and CT scans can further assist in the preoperative evaluation of the abscess. Differential diagnosis in a child who presents with acute or subacute bone pain and swelling should include trauma, fracture, acute rheumatic fever or arthritis, malignant bone tumor (e.g., Ewing's or osteogenic sarcoma), acute leukemia, and infantile cortical hyperostosis.

TREATMENT

The ultimate goals in the treatment of Brodie's abscess do not differ from those in the treatment of chronic osteomyelitis: to eradicate the infection by achieving a viable vascular environment, to stop tissue destruction, to prevent recurrence, and to achieve a normal functioning limb.[22] In children Brodie's abscess can usually be managed with specific intravenous antimicrobial therapy alone without surgical debridement. Surgical intervention is necessary for children who do not respond adequately within 48 hours to specific antimicrobial therapy or for those with evidence of joint sepsis or abscess. The specific treatment regimen employed is of course dictated by individual patient and lesion factors but should strictly adhere to the postulates of treatment for any infectious disease. The identification and sensitivity of the infectious organism are paramount in obtaining effective therapeutic result with the antibiotic selected. It is often not possible to identify the infectious organism or its antibiotic sensitivity prior to surgical intervention. Empiric antibiotic therapy is based initially on the patient's age group and the organism most likely to be isolated. In neonates the most common organism is group B *Streptococcus* or

gram-negative Enterobacter, and therefore these organisms require gram-negative coverage such as aminoglycosides or second- or third-generation cephalosporins. In neonates to 3-year-old toddlers the most common organism is *H. influenzae*. In children aged 3 and over the most common organism is *Staphylococcus aureus*. A beta-lactamase-resistant penicillin (nafcillin) or a first-generation cephalosporin provides adequate coverage. Definitive antibiotic therapy can proceed when the culture results are obtained through biopsy or blood cultures.

Treatment requires surgical drainage and curettage of the cyst contents and any necrotic tissue or bone. Surgical debridement is of vital importance to facilitate complete obliteration of the infection. The abscess must be incised and drained. This is accomplished by making a cortical window approximately 1 × 2 cm depending on the size of the abscess. The location of this window is determined through fluoroscopic guidance or marked preoperative radiographs. Abscesses are best treated by careful and thorough curettage, taking care to avoid periosteal stripping. All necrotic nonviable bone as well as any infectious granulation tissue must be removed to prevent reinfection. Cultures for aerobic and anaerobic organisms, acid-fast bacilli, and fungi should be obtained. It should be recalled that physical destruction of the tissue occurs as a sequelae of the host's inflammatory infiltration in response to invasion by the bacterial pathogen. This inflammatory response can be elicited by nonviable bacteria as well as by other microbial products released in their lysis. With this in mind, the degree of surgical debridement should err in favor of overzealous resection and lavage. Wounds are closed over a drain or packing (or both). Antibiotic therapy (parenteral or parenteral-oral) should be continued for at least 6 weeks after the incision and drainage. Subsequent bone grafting, if warranted, may occur when all signs of infection have subsided (Figs. 42–2 to 42–6).

DISCUSSION

The subacute presentation of a Brodie's abscess is masked by an absence of a definitive clinical syndrome.

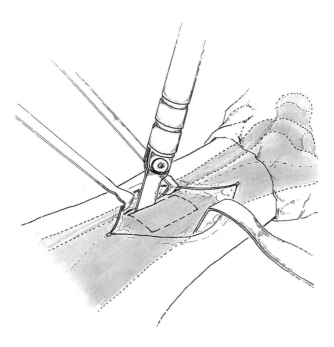

Figure 42–2. Sagittal saw (number 238) cuts into and through medial cortex of tibia. Safety drill holes are placed at each of the connecting right angles to protect against fracture.

Preoperative differential diagnosis includes unicameral bone cyst, osteoblastoma, fracture, osteosarcoma, aneurysmal bone cyst, Ewing's sarcoma, osteoid osteoma, reticulosarcoma, multiple myeloma, giant cell tumor, acute hematogenous osteomyelitis, and chronic osteomyelitis. A number of uncontrolled variables must be considered in the surgical or medical treatment of the disease. These include such factors as the age of the patient, the time of presentation, specific site of penetration, extent of bone involvement, presence of septicemia, the offending organism and its susceptibility to antibiotics, and the time and type of surgery. All of these are intricately involved in the patient's prognosis and the success of the treatment regimen.

SUMMARY

Regardless of the patient's age at presentation, the risk of pathologic fracture and subsequent acute osteomyelitis accompanies this disease. Aggressive surgical debridement and curettage and prolonged antibiotic use together

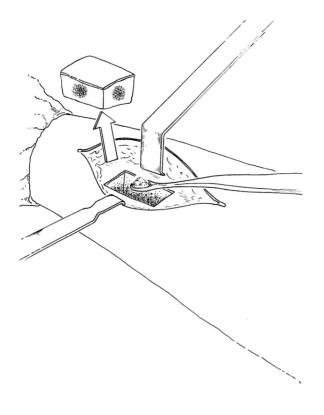

Figure 42–3. Block resection of cortex; cancellous bone including tumor is removed. Curettage of all surrounding cancellous bone is performed.

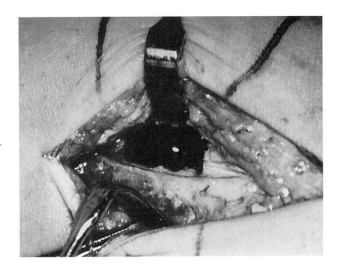

Figure 42–4. Excavated tibia, ready for implantation of graft.

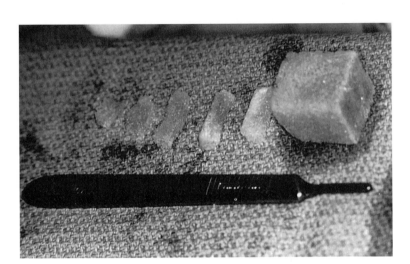

Figure 42–5. Graft measured and cut.

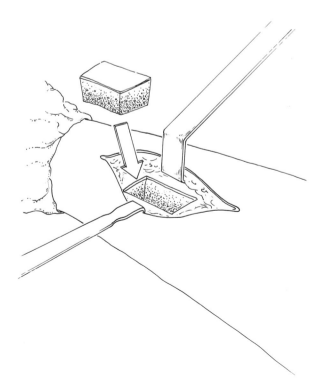

Figure 42–6. Insertion of graft.

have been highly successful in the treatment of Brodie's abscess. Variation in the size of the lesion obviously dictates the severity of the defect in bone subsequent to surgical intervention. If curettage results in a cavitation warranting bone grafting, the surgeon may opt for cancellous packing. Cancellous bone grafting is recommended as early as 5 to 10 days after the initial debridement when there is no evidence of infection or drainage and when healthy granulation has occurred. Usually the prognosis is favorable after reconstruction, and there are few complications. While recurrence following extensive surgical debridement is rare, cases have occurred, and these should be treated accordingly.

References

1. Brodie BC: An account of some cases of chronic abscess of the tibia. Trans Med Chir Soc 1832; 17:238–238.
2. Waldvogel FA: Osteomyelitis: A review of clinical features, therapeutic considerations and unusual aspects. N Engl J Med 1970; 282(4):198–206.
3. Winters JL, Cohen I: Acute hematogenous osteomyelitis: A review of 66 cases. J Bone Joint Surg 1960; 42A:691–704.
4. Dickson FD: Hematogenous osteomyelitis. Beaumont Foundation Lectures No. 23. Detroit, Wayne County Medical Society, 1944, p. 47.
5. Schiller AL: Bones and joints. *In* Rubin E, Farber JL (eds): Pathology. Philadelphia, JB Lippincott, 1988, pp. 1304–1393.
6. Velji AM, DeValentine SJ, Thornton CM: Infections of bones, joints, and soft tissues. *In* DeValentine SJ (ed): Foot and Ankle Disorders in Children. New York, Churchill Livingstone, 1992, pp. 601–608.
7. Fraser J: Acute osteomyelitis. Br Med J 1934; 2:539–541.
8. Hobo T: Zur Pathogenese de akuten haematogenen Osteomyelitis, mit berucksichtigung der vitalfarbungs Lehre. Translated by A. Seifen. Acta Scholar Med Kioto 1921; 4:1–29.
9. Schenk RK, Wiener J, Spiro D: Fine structural aspects of vascular invasion of the tibial epiphyseal plate of growing rats. Acta Anat 1968; 69:1–17.
10. Green NE, Beauchamp RD, Griffin PP: Primary subacute epiphyseal osteomyelitis. J Bone Joint Surg 1981; 63A:107–114.
11. Bogoch E, Thompson G, Salter RB: Foci of chronic circumscribed osteomyelitis (Brodie's abscess) that traverse the epiphyseal plate. J Pediatr Orthop 1984; 4:162–169.
12. Morrissy RT, Shore SL: Acute hematogenous osteomyelitis. *In* Gustilo RB, Gruninger RP, Tsukayama DT (eds): Orthopaedic Infection Diagnosis and Treatment. Philadelphia, WB Saunders, 1989, pp. 271–283.
13. Greenfield GB: The cardinal roentgen features. *In* Greenfield GB (ed): Radiology of Bone Diseases, 3rd ed. Philadelphia, JB Lippincott, 1975, pp. 369–514.
14. Dich VQ, Nelson JD, Haltalin KC: Osteomyelitis in infants and children. Am J Dis Child 1975; 129:1273–1278.
15. Jacobs JC: Acute osteomyelitis. NY State J Med 1978; 5:90.
16. Jackson MA, Nelson JD: Etiology and medical management of acute suppurative bone and joint infections in pediatric patients. J Pediatr Orthop 1982; 2:213.
17. Louw JH: Acute hematogenous osteomyelitis in childhood. Pediatr Dig 1967; 9:49–56.
18. Harris NH, Kirkaldy-Willis WH: Primary subacute pyogenic osteomyelitis. J Bone Joint Surg 1965; 47B:526–532.
19. Lack CH, Towers AG: Serological tests for staphylococcal infection. Br Med J 1962; 2:1227–1227.
20. Christman RA: The radiographic presentation of osteomyelitis in the foot. Clin Podiatr Med Surg 1990; 7(3):433–448.
21. Bonakdar-pour A, Gaines VD: The radiology of osteomyelitis. Orthop Clin North Am 1983; 14(1):21–48.
22. Gustilo RB: Management of chronic osteomyelitis. *In* Gustilo RB, Gruninger RP, Tsukayama DT (eds): Orthopedic Infection: Diagnosis and Treatment. Philadelphia, WB Saunders, 1989, pp. 155–165.

43

Iselin's Apophysitis

Richard M. Jay, D.P.M.

A traction apophysitis of the fifth metarsal base was first described by Iselin in 1912.[1] The disease occurs in active adolescents who place significant stress on the lateral aspect of the fifth metatarsal base where the peroneus brevis tendon inserts at a secondary ossification center. Repetitive microtrauma and overuse lead to osteochondrosis of the ossification center, where avascular necrosis may occur, leading to gradual resorption and recalcification.[2] Similar types of traction apophysitis occur in the lower extremity, including Osgood-Schlatter disease of the tibial tuberosity and Sever's disease of the posterior calcaneus.[3]

ETIOLOGY

A traction apophysitis is an aggravation of an ossification center at a place where a tendon inserts. The secondary ossification center of the fifth metatarsal base appears at approximately 12 years of age and reaches fusion at around 17 years of age. Iselin's apophysitis is most often seen in athletic teenagers or overweight children who

have adductovarus foot types that put excessive stress on the peroneus brevis tendon at its insertion. Overuse of the peroneus brevis tendon, the strongest pronator of the foot, can lead to irritation of the growth plate and osteochondrosis at the base or styloid process of the fifth metatarsal.[4]

In a typical scenario an athletic adolescent presents with continued pain along the lateral aspect of the foot after activity and experiences no relief from a change of shoe gear. On examination, there is tenderness on palpation at the lateral aspect of the base of the fifth metatarsal. The symptoms are aggravated by forced supination of the forefoot. Radiographs often reveal irregularities in density along the growth plate and enlargement of the fifth metatarsal base.[5]

DIFFERENTIAL DIAGNOSIS

The chief entity in the differential diagnosis is traumatic fracture from athletic activity. Although Iselin's disease can be aggravated by an inversion injury, an acute

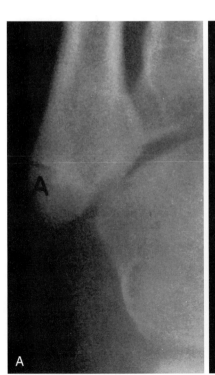
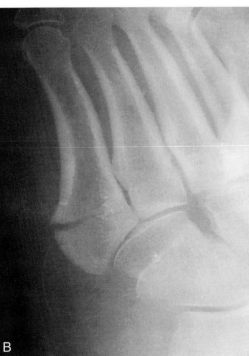

Figure 43–1. *A,* Perpendicularly placed fracture site (A). *B,* Transverse fracture of base of fifth metatarsal.

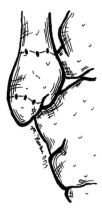

Figure 43–2. Fracture sites resting perpendicular to the shaft.

fracture of the fifth metatarsal tuberosity can be ruled out by careful radiographic evaluation. Avulsion fractures of the fifth metatarsal tuberosity tend to be oriented perpendicular to the long axis of the metatarsal and the pull of the peroneus brevis tendon (Figs. 43–1 and 43–2). The apophysis is oriented more parallel with the long axis of the metatarsal bone (Figs. 43–3 to 43–7). Furthermore, acute fractures are usually associated with edema, erythema, and ecchymosis. These signs are rarely present with a traction apophysitis.[6]

The other common consideration in the differential diagnosis is an accessory bone located just proximal to the fifth metatarsal base known as an os versalianum. This accessory ossicle is present in one of every thousand feet and is usually asymptomatic. Radiographic evaluation reveals that this bone is more spherical in shape and has smooth borders.

TREATMENT

Initial treatment begins with rest, ice, and elevation of the affected foot. Limitation of the aggravating activity is often adequate to calm the apophysitis. To limit the symptoms during the acute stage, a felt cutout is used just proximal to the base of the fifth metatarsal. This padding reduces only the direct pressure and is not intended for long-term therapy. The second step involves controlling the pronatory forces that lead to overuse of the peroneus brevis. Low Dye strapping and functional orthotics can limit the microtrauma caused by an overactive peroneus brevis tendon. A functional orthotic can limit the transverse and frontal plane motion associated with pronation. However, inversion of the rearfoot can create direct plantar pressure on the painful lateral metatarsal tuberosity. Therefore, a neutrally positioned, deep-seated orthotic is recommended to control excessive motion. An alternative method can be employed and has proved quite successful for acute and long-term treatment of the inflamed apophysis. A deep-seated orthotic similiar to the Dynamic Stabelizing Innersole System (DSIS; Langer Biomechanical Laboratories, Deer Park, NY) or Roberts plate is used, but instead of carrying the flange distally on the lateral side, it is cut short of the fifth metatarsal base (Fig. 43–8). A rearfoot varus post of 5 degrees is incorporated to control rearfoot motion and stability and to limit the pressure on the fifth metatarsal base caused by the buttressing effect of the flange.

In more severe cases, immobilization with a short leg cast helps to relieve tenderness and allows osseous growth to resume. Iselin's disease is a self-limiting process that ends when osseous growth finishes. The great majority of patients respond to conservative therapy. However, sev-

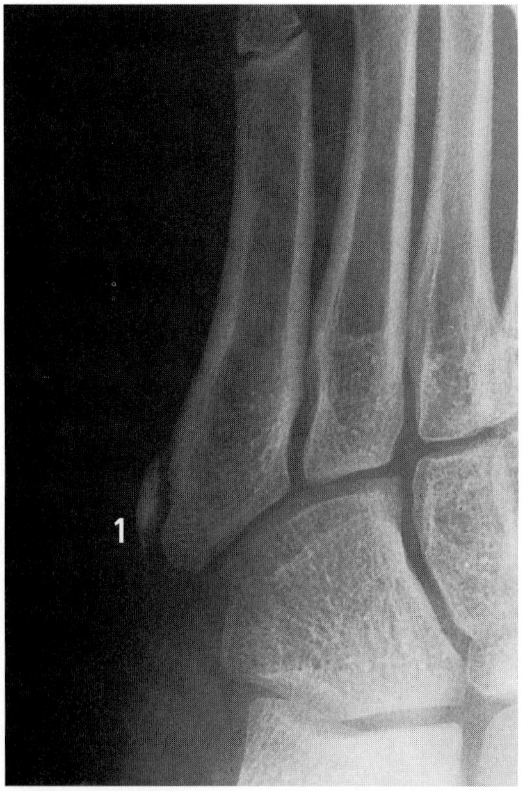

Figure 43–3. Apophysis at the base of the fifth metatarsal, anteroposterior view. The physis is parallel to the fifth metatarsal shaft as noted on the lateral, AP, and oblique views, as shown in Figs. 43–4 to 43–7.

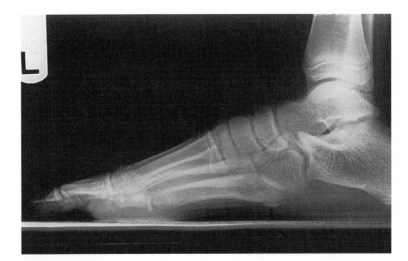

Figure 43–4. Apophysis at base of fifth metatarsal, lateral view.

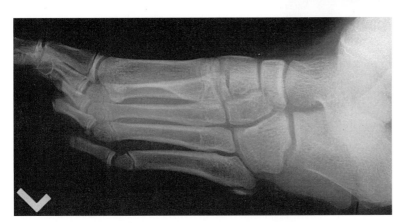

Figure 43–5. Apophysis at base of fifth metatarsal, oblique view.

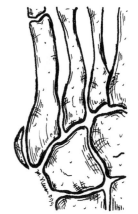

Figure 43–6. Drawing of apophysis at base of fifth metatarsal, AP view.

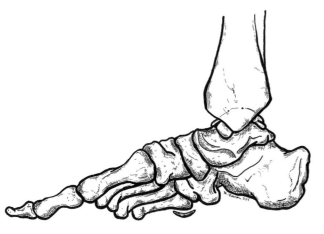

Figure 43–7. Drawing of apophysis at base of fifth metatarsal, lateral view.

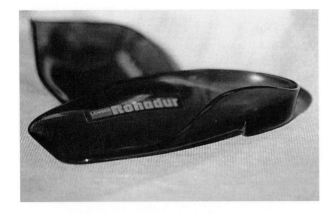

Figure 43–8. High-flanged orthotic cut at the base of the fifth metatarsal to act as a buttress protecting the inflamed fifth metatarsal base.

eral reports of nonunion persisting into early adulthood have been described; such cases require surgical intervention consisting of drilling to promote osseous fusion across the nonunion site.

References

1. Iselin H: Wachtumsbeschwerden zur Zeit dur Knochernen Entwicklung der Tuberositas metatarsi quint. Dtsch Zeit Chir 1912; 117:529–535.

2. Lehman RC, Gregg JR, Torg E: Iselin's disease. Am J Sports Med 1986; 14:494–496.
3. Micheli LJ: The traction apophysitis. Clin Sports Med 1987; 6:389.
4. Katz JF: Nonarticular osteochondroses. Clin Orthop 1981; 158:10.
5. Bunch WH: Decision analysis of treatment choices in the osteochondroses. Clin Orthop 1981; 158:91.
6. Schwartz B, Jay RM, Schoenhaus HD: Apophysitis of the fifth metatarsal base. J Am Podiatr Med Assoc 1991; 81:128–130.

44

Freiberg's Infraction

Richard M. Jay, D.P.M.

Freiberg's infraction can develop in the second, third, or fourth metatarsal bones. The condition can be traumatically induced or induced indirectly by a mechanical epiphyseal injury as occurs with chondral or osteochondral compression from the base of the proximal phalanx. The cause may be of single or multiple origin. Ischemia, trauma, and immaturity of the distal aspect of the metatarsal are the most common underlying causes. However, a resultant fracture of this distal epiphysis ties together the ischemia, trauma, and immaturity. A plausible theory for the failure of this articular epiphysis to heal is the result of constant compression. A delay in union results with poor endochondral ossification. The young immature epiphyses and the constant trauma change the mechanical efforts exerted on this joint. No longer does the joint rotate about the articular surface but rather experiences direct compression.[1, 2] The joint, if left unchecked, develops over the years into a rigid and painful osteoarthritic joint.

The metatarsal deformity can be treated according to a staging system. Smillie[3] described five stages of Freiberg's infraction. Stage 1 is a fissure type fracture that develops in the ischemic epiphyses. In stage 2 the articular surface is contoured and altered with a central portion of bone resorption. In stage 3 the central portion starts to sink further into the head as with resorption of the distal bone increases. The plantar aspect of the cartilage remains intact. Stage 4 develops with loose bodies that begin to separate, and finally in stage 5 there is a complete flattening of the distal head. Because of all these changes, it is obvious that no one procedure is indicated in the treatment of these varying stages. Treatment needs to be geared to the presenting radiographic and operative findings.

Several options are available for the treatment of Freiberg's infraction, and these should follow a certain order. The possible complications following the treatment can be worse than the deformity itself. A logical sequence of surgical procedures must be discussed with the parents.

RADIOGRAPHIC FINDINGS

The most obvious finding is a widening of the joint space. This occurs by the sixth week after symptoms begin. With progression of the condition, the density of the subchondral bone increases and the metatarsal head takes on the appearance of flattening. As the advanced stage develops in the older child, the ischemic epiphyseal bone and articular cartilage weaken and collapse. The collapsed bone creates fracturing within the joint, and loose bodies appear in the joint, resulting in pain. It is not unusual to see these fragments in the dorsal aspect of the joint space (Fig. 44–1).

TREATMENT

Loose Body Removal

It is not uncommon for pain to continue after all conservative approaches have been tried and exhausted. The least traumatic and certainly the most ambulatory type of surgery consists of removal of the fragment. Resecting the dorsal aspect of the metatarsal head allows an increase in the dorsal range of motion. This procedure is similar to that described for hallux limitus. One must

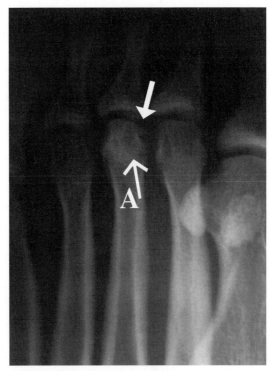

Figure 44–1. Radiograph of the third metatarsal head with stage 2 deformation. Central aspect (A) with bone resorption.

343

consider, however, that the mechanism of injury is still present—that is, constant compression with dorsiflexion of the proximal phalanx on the lesser metatarsal during propulsion.

Keller Type Procedure

Resection of the metatarsal to allow resection of the proximal phalanx base has been described and certainly decompresses the metatarsal head and usually decreases the symptoms. One must be aware that with this type of procedure, there is a risk of increased postoperative complications. With resection of the metatarsal head, the weight-bearing surface at propulsion will be shifted to the surrounding metatarsal head. In a young child this may not be of consequence because a large fat pad is present. In time, however, the child's weight increases, increasing the pressure on the surrounding metatarsal heads and creating a transfer lesion. With resection of the base of the proximal phalanx as well as the metatarsal head, the toe is obviously shortened, and this may have a psychological effect on the young child that neither the child nor the parent will accept.

Subchondral Drilling

Because there is a possibility of ischemia to the distal aspect of this fragile, rapidly growing epiphysis, one must realize that there is a different type of blood supply to the metatarsal in the adolescent and child than there is in the adult. A compromise in vasculature to the distal epiphysis may occur during the time the plate is open. Since this avascular area is being injured, it never has a chance to revascularize. The increase in constant trauma results in a form of aseptic necrosis at the end of the metatarsal. Perforating the subchondral surface by drilling is an option if it is considered early in the development of Freiberg's infraction. Penetration of the metatarsal head, epiphysis, and metatarsal shaft allows an increase in blood flow to the distal aspect. The result is a fibrocartilaginous surface that replaces the denuded aseptic surface. This may allow motion in the joint to take place without pain. However, if the defect is large or the compressive forces on the metatarsal head from the proximal phalanx are high, the symptoms will return.

Osteotomy

The metatarsal head in Freiberg's infraction can be staged in five categories according to Smillie.[3] In a patient with a plantar defect it may be advisable to consider an osteotomy to realign the metatarsal head. This would eliminate direct compression on the head from the plantar weight-bearing surface. In addition, rotating the head would decrease the retrograde force on the head from the phalanx.

The technique consists of joint debridement followed by intra-articular closed dorsal wedge osteotomy to bring the healthy plantar part of the metatarsal under direct vision to face the base of the proximal phalanx. The distal metatarsal is visualized by exposing the head on the medial and lateral sides. All loose bodies are removed, and the avascular portion of the head is debrided. A wedge is removed from the distal shaft and head, leaving the plantar cortical apex intact. The opened wedge is closed by dorsiflexing the capital fragment.[4] The method of fixation of the head to the shaft is the surgeon's preference. The use of Orthosorb (Johnson & Johnson Orthopaedics, Raynham, MA) pin fixation has reduced the operative time and obviated the need for pin placement through the digital epiphyses. In addition, it eliminates the need for pin removal. A slipper type cast is employed for 3 weeks, followed by a wedge shoe to offload the distal metatarsal osteotomy site. Certainly this is an appropriate procedure, but as with any shortening procedure, postoperative conservative control is mandatory to prevent the formation of transfer lesions and metatarsalgia (Fig. 44–2).

Resection

When the defect is too large or it is not logical or possible to rotate the head away from the joint to avoid a possible painful range of motion, it is acceptable to resect the metatarsal head in toto.[5] Resecting the head, with or without implant replacement, involves unpredictable long-term complications. The head must be resected

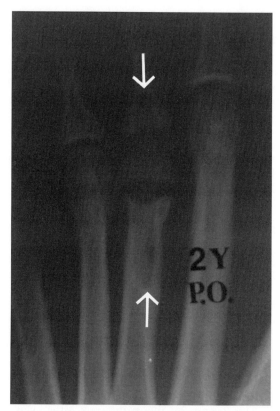

Figure 44–2. Intra-articular closed dorsal wedge osteotomy. The healthy plantar part of the metatarsal is plantarly dorsiflexed. A wedge is removed from the distal shaft and head leaving the plantar cortical apex intact. The opened wedge is closed by dorsiflexing the capital fragment.

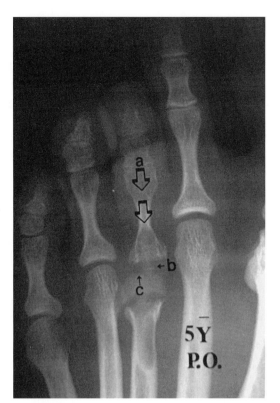

Figure 44–3. Increased compression (a) on the metatarsal implant dome (c) creates an increase in shear and the potential for stem fracturing (b).

completely, and unfortunately, this leads to a transfer of pressure to the adjacent metatarsal heads. Shortening and contracture are quite common with total head resections.

Implant

Joint destructive procedures in children should be avoided; however, if the pain is significant and damage to the articular portion is extensive, one may be led to resecting the metatarsal phalangeal joint completely or partially. To decrease the effects of a total resection, the alternative could be the use of implant arthroplasty. There are a number of implants that can be used in the metatarsal phalangeal joint.

The last option to be considered to maintain the alignment of the toe at the metatarsophalangeal joint in an extended position is the use of a double-stemmed implant. In using the implant the chances of shortening are also decreased as long as not too much of the metatarsal

head is removed. This does not mean that implants are not indicated; on the contrary, pain with this deformity in a child is exhausting to the child and to the parents, and if all else has failed, this radical approach is recommended. With late management of this deformity—that is, when the articular changes have produced a rigid and painful joint—the alternatives are few, and selection of a total joint replacement is recommended. Motion is restored with replacement of the joint; however, one must be aware that new problems will arise[2] (Fig. 44–3).

References

1. Douglas G, Rang M: The role of trauma in the pathogenesis of the osteochondroses. Clin Orthop 1981; 158:28–32.
2. Helal B, Gibb P: Freiberg's disease. Foot Ankle 1987; 8:94–102.
3. Smillie IS: Freiberg's infraction. J Bone Joint Surg 1957; 39B:580.
4. Kinnard P, Lirette R: Freiberg's infraction. Foot Ankle 1989; 9:226–231.
5. Hill J, Jimenez LA: Osteochondritis treated by joint replacement. J Am Podiatr Assoc 1979; 69:556–561.

45

Calcaneal Apophysitis

Richard M. Jay, D.P.M.

Calcaneal apophysitis or Sever's disease is an inflammation of the open apophysis of the calcaneus and is a self-limiting condition that is seen in active children. Boys are more commonly affected than girls. The age of onset ranges from 8 to 14 years. Calcaneal apophysitis is the most common cause of heel pain in children and is usually associated with muscle strain in the active or obese child.

Because the calcaneus is the first of the tarsal bones to ossify, it is the only tarsal bone that is continually under repetitive stress consisting of compression and tension. The calcaneus appears during the sixth fetal month, and the apophysis starts to ossify at 6 years of age in females and at 8 years in males. The apophysis does not finally fuse until the mid-teens. During this period of rapid growth and fusion of the bone the bone is under continual compression in the active child. To complicate matters, the tendo Achillis inserts in the posterior middle third of the calcaneus, surrounding this mobile fragment. Prior to fusion to the main body of the calcaneus, the apophysis is under continual traction from the tendo Achillis proximally and the plantar fascia distally[1–3] (Fig. 45–1).

Usually in active children there is an underlying cause of pronation secondary to an isolated tightness in the gastrocnemius or a combined equinus in the gastrocnemius-soleus. In either case, the calcaneus is under greatly increased tension. Add this to the factors operative in the active or obese child, and the result is heel pain to a varying degree. The amount of activity, equinus, and weight dictates the degree of deformity. The most common sports associated with this injury are soccer, track, and basketball.

Children complain of pain during and after activity. When the activity ceases, the pain usually subsides. The child perceives the pain in the entire heel and occasionally can pinpoint the discomfort to the exact location of the apophysis. When the heel is grasped by the examiner and medial and lateral compression is applied, the child feels pain throughout the heel. Pain may be present at the insertion of the tendo Achillis and may run proximally. By lightly pinching the distal Achilles tendon and advancing the fingers proximally, a mild tendinitis may also be demonstrated. It is not uncommon for such a child to walk in equinus to guard the tendon against increased motion during pronation.

In severe cases, hyperemia and edema are noticed around the heel. In this young age group hematogenous osteomyelitis, bone tumor, rheumatic fever, juvenile rheumatoid arthritis, calcaneal fracture, traumatic separation of the apophysis, and heel contusion must be ruled out.

The most commonly used diagnostic test is radiographic examination, and this should only be used to rule out bony disease. The apophysis may appear to be sclerotic, fragmented, and separated (Fig. 45–2), and this appearance does not confirm the presence or absence of apophysitis. Radiographs are not diagnostic of calcaneal apophysitis. Laboratory tests are used to rule out infectious processes and pain associated with diseases of rheumatologic origin (juvenile rheumatoid arthritis, Reiter's disease).[4]

TREATMENT

Treatment is directed toward the cause of the problem: overuse, pronation, equinus, or obesity. It is further determined by the degree of deformity: mild, moderate, or severe.

Mild Disease

The main thought to keep in mind when treating apophysitis is that it is usually self-limiting. With this basic premise in mind, treatment begins in the most conservative fashion. Simply raising the heel ½ to 1 inch decreases the proximal pull from the tight tendo Achillis

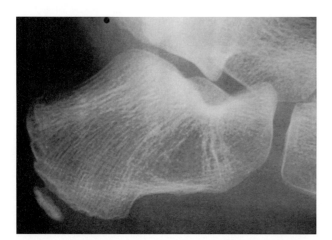

Figure 45–1. Early sign of the calcaneal apophysis. The tendo Achillis and plantar fascia pass through this body and are under direct assault from the longitudinal pull.

on the posterior calcaneus and also transfers weight to the forepart of the foot. The heel can be raised simply by fitting two pieces of ¼-inch felt in the heel seat of the shoe. A heel cup with felt incorporated onto the inferior surface also raises the heel nicely. The heel rise should be inserted into a heeled shoe or running shoe that already has a slight heel elevation. The child should now start stretching exercises. Although it is difficult to get children to institute a routine of exercises, they must perform these stretches and should be encouraged to do this before and after any sporting activity.

During treatment the child should be fitted for a cast for a neutral position orthosis[5] and should undergo a biomechanical examination. The orthotic device should maintain the heel in a neutral position, and if necessary a temporary heel raise may be incorporated. This must be removed after a few months to minimize the risk of inducing further equinus. A temporary prefabricated device can also be used to raise the heel.

Moderate to Severe Disease

The child who has an increased amount of pain that does not respond to the above treatment needs a more aggressive approach. The child must cease all activity for a minimum of 2 weeks and must be maintained in a Low Dye strapping. The strapping and heel raise must remove the pull from the tendo Achillis and the plantar fascia. If this cannot be fully accomplished with relief of pain, the child should be casted.

The cast is applied with the foot plantar-flexed at the ankle and midfoot. This removes all the tension on the heel. This, along with the non-weight-bearing status, usually causes the symptoms to resolve. The use of orthotics and physical therapy, including stretching of the tendo Achillis and plantar fascia, are very important post-treatment procedures.

Chronic Severe Apophysitis

On rare occasions the heel pain does not resolve even after all conservative approaches have been tried. Because

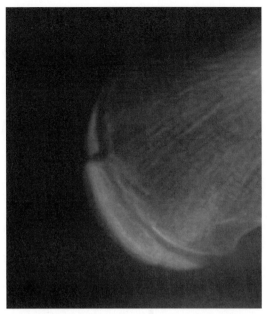

Figure 45–2. The apophysis can appear to be sclerotic, fragmented, and separated as noted in this 12-year-old child.

of the microtrauma to the rapidly closing growth site and the excessive pull on the heel, a tendo Achillis or gastrocnemius lengthening may be indicated. This procedure certainly reduces the deforming forces and should be considered if everything else has failed.

References

1. Andrish JT: Overuse syndrome of the lower extremity *In* Bouleau RA (ed): Youth Sports (Advances in Pediatric Sports). Champaign, IL, Human Kinetics Publishers, 1984, p. 189.
2. Brower AC: Osteochondroses. Orthop Clin North Am 1983; 14:99.
3. Katz JF: Nonarticular osteochondroses. Clin Orthop 1981; 158:70.
4. Micheli LJ, Sohn RS, Santopietro FJ: Athletic footwear modifications. *In* Nicholas JA (ed): Lower Extremity Injuries. St. Louis, Mosby, 1985, p. 584.
5. Micheli LJ: Prevention and management of calcaneal apophysitis in children. Pediatr Orthop 1987; 7:34–38.

46

Kohler's Disease

Richard M. Jay, D.P.M., and Michael Chung, D.P.M.

A disease process involving necrosis of the ossification center of the tarsal navicular bone was first described by Kohler in 1908.[1] Repetitive microtrauma and overuse lead to osteochondrosis of the ossification center, where avascular necrosis can occur with gradual bone resorption and recalcification. Radiographic characteristics include flattening, sclerosis, and fragmentation of the tarsal navicular bone (Figs. 46–1 and 46–2). Symptoms increase with activity and include tenderness, erythema, and edema of the medial midfoot. Kohler's disease is generally present in adolescent boys unilaterally and tends to resolve spontaneously over time. Like Freiberg's infarction of the second metatarsal head, this osteochondrosis is thought to result from compression.[2]

CLINICAL PRESENTATION

Kohler's disease generally presents as pain and swelling along the medial midfoot in an active teenage male. The patient may be limping and is unable to perform physical activity for any extended period of time because of the discomfort. Pain increases with weight bearing, and the child may supinate the foot to compensate for the pain on the medial side of the foot. Radiographic evaluation shows an irregularly ossifying navicular bone with sclerosis, flattening, and possible fragmentation of the ossification center. The bone shows increased density in patchy areas, or it may appear uniformly dense. Magnetic resonance imaging (MRI) reveals a homogeneous decrease in signal intensity on T1-weighted images.

ETIOLOGY

Unlike a traction apophysitis, Kohler's disease involves a necrosis of the ossification center secondary to the repetitive compressive forces imposed by weight-bearing

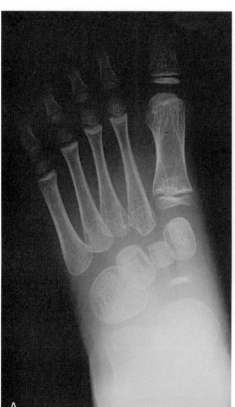

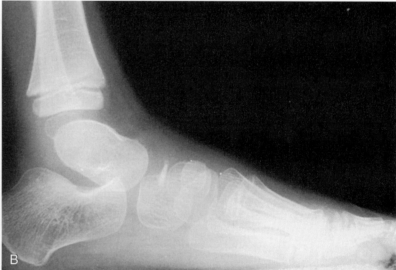

Figure 46–1. *A* and *B*, Osteochondrosis of the ossification center of the navicular. Avascular necrosis with gradual resorption and recalcification. Radiographic characteristics include flattening, sclerosis, and fragmentation of the tarsal navicular bone.

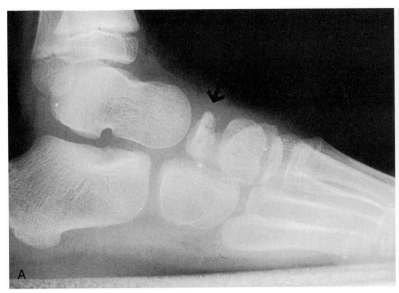

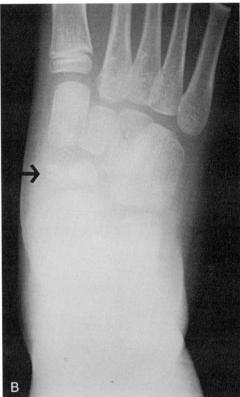

Figure 46–2. Kohler's disease. Lateral and anteroposterior views. Note the fragmentation and increase in sclerosis of the navicular.

activities. Therefore, young male athletes tend to be more commonly affected than females in a ratio of 6.5 to 1.[3]

The navicular bone generally begins to ossify between the ages of 18 and 36 months. Waugh found that the navicular ossifies later in boys than in girls.[4] Karp concluded that abnormalities of ossification occur more often in navicular bones that ossify later and therefore occur more often in boys.[3] Waugh also described the dense perichondral network of vessels on the nonarticular surfaces of the navicular with numerous arteries penetrating into the center in a radial manner. He believed that when the navicular ossifies later, after the child has grown larger, an increase in the stress of weight bearing causes an irregularity in the normal trabecular growth process. As a result, the navicular undergoes an ischemic episode secondary to disruption of the vascular network feeding the ossification center. However, the result is unlike avascular necrosis in the adult because the child's navicular consists mostly of cartilage, which prevents permanent damage.[4]

Scurran and colleagues[5] believe that Kohler's disease is actually a navicular compression fracture. They suggest that compression of the ossifying navicular causes a stress fracture, which becomes aggravated with further activity. It presents with the edema, erythema, and tenderness consistent with a stress fracture along with the radiographic signs of sclerosis, fragmentation, and possible flattening of the bony margins. These investigators believe that only a stress fracture would heal with limitation of activity and no permanent damage as is seen in avascular necrosis.

Microscopic examination of a bone biopsy has been reported to show scattered areas of necrosis, bone destruction, bone resorption, and areas of bone formation.[5]

TREATMENT

Initial treatment begins with rest, ice, and elevation of the affected foot. Limitation of the aggravating activity is often enough to calm the initial symptomatology. Several studies recommend short leg cast immobilization for approximately 2 months. The foot should be held in a plantar-flexed and inverted position.[6] Children placed in a cast for 2 months experience complete resolution of pain and return to normal activity within 2.5 months.[3] When the cast is removed, use of an accommodative device is recommended for approximately 2 more months. The medial side should be soft to limit pressure on the navicular. Permanent orthotics can be dispensed with when the child is asymptomatic. This is a self-limiting deformity and in most cases does not require any radical procedures. The great majority of patients with Kohler's disease experience no long-term sequelae. However, some patients do develop a distorted and sclerotic navicular leading to an arthritic talonavicular joint, which requires a midtarsal joint arthrodesis in adulthood.[7]

References

1. Kohler A: A frequent disease of individual bones in children, apparently previously unknown. Münch Med Wochenschr 1908;55:1923.
2. Williams GA, Cowell HR: Kohler's disease of the tarsal navicular. Clin Orthop 1981;158:53.

3. Karp MG: Kohler's disease of the tarsal scaphoid, an end result study. J Bone Joint Surg 1937;19:84.
4. Waugh W: The ossification and vascularization of the tarsal navicular and their relation to Kohler's disease. J Bone Joint Surg 1958;40B:765.
5. Scurran BL, Karlin JM, Stanton BK: Kohler's disease. J Am Pod Med Assoc 1992;82:625–629.
6. Ippolito E, Pollini PT, Falez F: Kohler's disease of the tarsal navicular: Long term follow-up of 12 cases. J Pediatr Orthop 1984;4:416–417.
7. Canale ST: Osteochondrosis or epiphysitis and other miscellaneous affections. *In* Crenshow AH (ed): Campbell's Operative Orthopaedics, 8th ed. St. Louis, CV Mosby, 1992, p. 1959.

47

Aneurysmal Bone Cyst

John H. Walter, Jr., D.P.M.

An aneurysmal bone cyst is neither a neoplasm nor a cyst. The current theory is that the lesion is an intraosseous arteriovenous malformation.[1] Since they were first described in 1942 by Jaffe and Lichtenstein,[2] aneurysmal bone cysts have been reported frequently in the literature. Aneurysmal bone cysts are benign blood-filled lesions with a cystlike wall composed predominantly of fibrous tissue and surrounded by a thin layer of periosteal new bone (Figs. 47–1 and 47–2).

INCIDENCE

Primary bone tumors in the lower extremity represent less than 1% of all tumors diagnosed in the United States each year, and it is estimated that only 1% to 2% of all these tumors occur in the foot and ankle area. Of these,

aneurysmal bone cysts represent only 6% to 8%.[3] Hence, the incidence in the foot and ankle bones is extremely low. The most frequent area in which aneurysmal bone cysts occur is the metaphyseal region of the long bones. Two other areas commonly involved are the pelvis and the spinal column. The majority of aneurysmal bone cysts occur in patients younger than 20 years of age. Most osseous tumors have a relatively equal sex distribution, but aneurysmal bone cysts have a slight predilection for the female sex.

PATHOGENESIS

The pathogenesis of aneurysmal bone cysts remains unclear, but there have been numerous postulations and

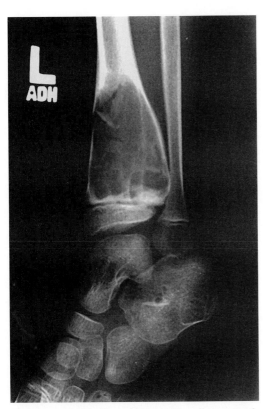

Figure 47–1. A massive fusiform dilation with well-circumscribed borders of the entire distal tibia. View shows cortical expansion and a thin lining. Multiple septal formations are noted with large lucent centers. The lesion shows the classic expansile lytic nature with numerous fine trabeculations coursing through the interior aspect of the lesion.

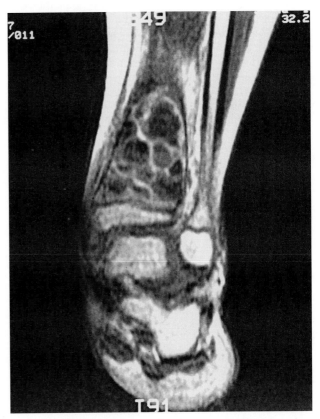

Figure 47–2. Magnetic resonance imaging scans clearly show a large multiloculated lesion with materials of high and low signal intensity occupying the distal tibia. The inferomedial aspect of the distal cortex also displays a pathologic fracture, which was not evident on the plain films.

theories over the years. Many investigators agree that aneurysmal bone cysts are the result of localized hemodynamic vascular changes, and this theory has been supported by angiographic findings. Even though the exact etiology remains speculative, most authors have concluded that two types of aneurysmal bone cyst must exist: (1) a primary type without a preexisting or coexisting lesion, and (2) a secondary form associated with some other lesion.[4]

DIFFERENTIAL DIAGNOSIS

1. Unicameral bone cyst
2. Giant cell tumor of bone
3. Chondroblastoma
4. Chondromyxoid fibroma
5. Fibrous dysplasia
6. Brown's tumor of hyperparathyroidism
7. Eosinophilic granuloma
8. Cavernous hemangioma
9. Nonossifying fibroma
10. Hydatid disease of bone

RADIOGRAPHIC FINDINGS

1. The neoplasm typically presents as an expansile lytic lesion with numerous fine trabeculation patterns producing the characteristic "soap-bubble" appearance.
2. The lesion extends beyond the normal confines of the bone and is outlined by a thin layer of subperiosteal new bone.
3. The lesion quickly enlarges to occupy the entire circumference of the affected bone.
4. The cyst is almost exclusively limited to the metaphysis in long bones.
5. The lesion displays an interior radiolucency.

Aneurysmal bone cysts have also been described as evolving through four radiologic stages: initial, active, stabilization, and healing.[5] In the initial phase the lesion is characterized by a well-defined area of osteolysis with a discrete elevation of the periosteum. This is followed by an active growth phase, in which the lesion grows rapidly, causing progressive destruction of bone and developing the characteristic "soap-bubble" appearance as a result of maturation of the bony shell. Finally, healing results in progressive calcification and ossification.[6]

SURGERY

The surgical plan should be total excision and curettage of the lesion with incorporation of an autogenous bone graft by a pediatric oncologist. The treatment of aneurysmal bone cyst is complicated by a high rate of recurrence after curettage alone and the possible risk of growth disturbance when the lesion is situated close to the physeal plate. Because of the expansile cystic nature of aneurysmal bone cysts, patients may sustain a pathologic fracture before presentation or during the immediate postoperative period. Reconstruction with polymethylmethacrylate can be considered for large metaphyseal lesions because it restores the strength of the bone and reduces the risk of fracture.

References

1. Mirra JM: Bone Tumors: Clinical, Radiologic and Pathologic Correlations. Philadelphia, Lea & Febiger, 1989, pp. 1233–1334.
2. Jaffe HL, Lichtenstein L: Solitary unicameral bone cyst, with emphasis on the roentgen picture, the pathologic appearance and the pathogenesis. Arch Surg 1942;44:1004.
3. Johnston MR: Epidemiology of soft tissue and bone tumors of the foot. Clin Podiatr Surg 1993;10:581.
4. Bonakdarpour A, Levy W, Aegerter E: Primary and secondary aneurysmal bone cyst: A radiological study of 75 cases. Radiology 1978;126:75.
5. Cory DA, Fritsch SA, Cohen MD: Aneurysmal bone cysts: Imaging findings and embolotherapy. Am J Roentgenol 1989;153:369–373.
6. Donaldson WF Jr: Aneurysmal bone cyst. J Bone Joint Surg 1962;441:25–40.

Six

Biomechanical Control

48

Orthotic Control

Richard M. Jay, D.P.M.

NORMAL FOOT FUNCTION

Static stance in the normal foot and leg is defined as follows: The distal third of the leg is vertical. The knee, ankle, and subtalar joints lie in the transverse plane, parallel to the supporting surface. The subtalar joint rests in its neutral position. The bisection of the posterior surface of the calcaneus is vertical. The midtarsal joint is locked in its maximally pronated position. The plantar forefoot plane parallels the plantar rearfoot plane, and both parallel the supporting surface. In this position, the sagittal bisection of the posterior surface of the calcaneus is perpendicular to the plantar plane of the foot. Metatarsals 2, 3, and 4 are in a totally dorsiflexed position, and the plantar surfaces of the metatarsal heads are in a common plane parallel to the supporting surface. Metatarsals 1 and 5 are maintained in such a position that the plantar surfaces of these heads lie in the same transverse plane as that of metatarsal heads 2, 3, and 4.

BIOMECHANICS OF THE SUBTALAR JOINT

The subtalar joint has been described as a triplane joint, incorporating motion in the sagittal, transverse, and frontal planes. The total range of subtalar motion in a normal foot is approximately 30 degrees. Twenty of the 30 degrees are supinatory, and 10 degrees occur in the direction of pronation. The normal subtalar neutral position is 0 degrees, or a bisection of the calcaneus relative to the lower third of the leg would show it to be parallel. In cases of hyperpronation, the calcaneus can be used as an indicator of how much motion is present. This is determined by measuring the deviation from the subtalar neutral position when the foot is in the resting calcaneal stance position. The resting calcaneal stance position represents the frontal plane position of the calcaneus after all compensation in the direction of pronation has taken place.

There are many causes of hyperpronation in the foot. Some are intrinsic to the foot, and some are extrinsic. Frontal, sagittal, and transverse plane motions of the subtalar joint can exert a negative influence on the frontal plane position of the calcaneus. The foot must attempt to compensate for deformity by pronating. The normal foot demonstrates approximately 4 to 6 degrees of subtalar motion in the direction of pronation during the walking cycle. By determining the subtalar joint neutral position and measuring the frontal plane position of the calcaneus when it is neutral, one can determine how much pronation has taken place. In this method of evaluation the uncompensated or neutral position calcaneus is composed with the compensated position of the calcaneus. One of two relationships can be observed. When the patient is in a weight-bearing position, the subtalar joint neutral position should be established. In this position, the posterior bisection of the calcaneus relative to the lower third of the leg can be measured. When the subtalar joint is relaxed and the foot is allowed to compensate for all inherent deformities, the frontal plane position of the calcaneus relative to the leg is again established.

In the other method of evaluation and use of appropriate reference points, the frontal plane position of the calcaneus relative to the ground is used. In this method the subtalar joint neutral position is compared to the frontal plane position of the calcaneus relative to the ground. This resting calcaneal stance position is the position of the calcaneus after all compensation has taken place.

It is well established that the subtalar joint has the ability to control the amount of motion that occurs at the midtarsal complex. Elfman explained the mechanism, describing the transverse tarsal joint as composed of the talonavicular and calcaneocuboid joints. When the hindfoot and midfoot are in supination, the axes of these joints are angled away from each other, and this part of the foot is "locked." After heel strike and eversion of the heel occur, this area "unlocks" to the limit of the range of the restricting ligaments.[1] Pronation in the range of 6 to 7 mm provides proper shock absorption for the stresses of standing, walking, jogging, and splinting. When pronation is restricted to less than 6 to 7 mm (as in the cavus foot), the forces of weight bearing, failing dissipation within the foot, are transmitted upward through the ankle joint, knee joint, hip joint, pelvis, and spine until they are dissipated.[1a] In closed kinetic chain pronation, the calcaneus everts and the talus adducts and plantar-flexes. The reactive force of gravity may then cause subluxation of the talonavicular or naviculocuneiform joint (or both), resulting in the midtarsal fault syndrome.[2] Parallelism of the longitudinal axis of the talonavicular and calcaneocuboid joints allows unlocking of the midtarsal joint with subsequent dorsiflexion of the forefoot on the rearfoot and hypermobility of the metatarsals during the propulsive phase of gait at a time when they should be stable.[3]

The end result of this chain of events is a painful pronated foot with multiple deformities and symptomatology of the forefoot. Disabling secondary deformities can result, the majority of which develop during childhood and are observable in adulthood. Hallux abducto valgus, plantar keratosis, metatarsalgia, hammer digit syndrome, neuromas, plantar fasciitis, heel spur syndrome, postural pains of the foot and leg, and arthrosis deformans of the midtarsal and subtalar joints may be directly related to the pronated foot.[4] The talonavicular joint is the first tarsal joint to be affected by arthritis. Hyperpronation inevitably develops, particularly in children who have static deformities in the legs, knees, or hips (e.g., internal tibial torsion, genu valgum). Tenosynovitis of the posterior tibial tendon frequently occurs and may ultimately result in partial or total rupture. The clinical pattern is predictable and consistent with either forefoot varus or subtalar valgus foot types. Compression forces retard longitudinal bone growth of the young bones according to the Heuter-Volkmann law.[5, 6] These compression forces are dorsal and lateral, and result in a decrease in longitudinal endochondral growth in these regions, with a relative increase in plantar and medial growth. If not treated, this imbalance leads to a structurally based and fixed pronated foot, probably a permanently pronated foot. As stated, the calcaneus everts, and the calcaneocuboid and talonavicular individual axes become parallel, maximizing motion at the midtarsal joint. Clinically, this is observed as a lowering of the longitudinal arch and a tendency for the calcaneus to evert from its neutral position. Often there is an abduction of the forefoot on the rearfoot as well. On occasion, the entire foot is observed in abduction relative to the motion and position of the talus. In closed kinetic chain pronation, the calcaneus everts while the talus plantar-flexes and abducts. The entire forefoot undergoes motion in the direction of dorsiflexion, eversion, and abduction.

ARCH INTEGRITY

Probably the greatest contributor to the integrity of the arch is the development of a satisfactory sustentaculum tali. Bony insufficiency results in instability of the subtalar joint. Harris and Beath[7] have shown that inadequate support of the head of the talus by the anterosuperior aspect of the calcaneus, including the sustentaculum tali, results in subtalar joint pronation. Often the talar neck is elongated, and the sustentaculum tali is a thin tongue-like structure that gives inadequate support. The end result is excessive subtalar joint pronation due to plantar flexion of the talus. The elongation of the talar neck and the absence of the anterior calcaneal facet is a common finding in patients with the flexible pes valgus

deformity. The second strongest factor in support of the arch is probably the integrity of the posterior tibial tendon. The deltoid ligament of the ankle, especially the deep portion, also helps to support the arch. A well-placed inferior calcaneonavicular ligament is supportive. The plantar aponeurosis, with its anchorage to the toes and the os calcis, creates a very strong fibrous windlass effect.[7]

Following a biomechanical examination and stance position measurements, the clinician can determine how much hyperpronation has occurred by observing the frontal plane position of the calcaneus. Controlling the frontal plane position of the calcaneus is essential to controlling midtarsal motion. In addition, we have observed that transverse plane control of the forefoot is essential, as is frontal plane control of the rearfoot.

THE BIOMECHANICAL ORTHOTIC DEVICE

Clinically, hyperpronation is identified by a forefoot and rearfoot that move in the transverse plane in the direction of abduction while the talus escapes from the talonavicular articulation and moves in the direction of adduction. Based on this basic concept, to control the rearfoot and the forefoot, a combination type of orthotic is necessary that controls not only frontal plane motion but also sagittal and transverse plane motion. Previous orthotic devices concentrated on frontal plane control in the hope that control of one plane of motion (i.e., the calcaneus) would control all three planes of subtalar motion. This idea was based on the concept that the subtalar axis deviates from all three planes, and therefore motion in one plane would allow motion in all three. If that premise were truly accurate, control of one plane of motion would also control the other two. Experience demonstrates, however, that control of the frontal plane of the calcaneus alone does not prevent lateral drift of the forefoot, as evidenced by talar escape medially and transverse plane deviation laterally.

In managing foot and ankle problems in children, the use of orthotics should:

1. Accommodate structural deformities intrinsic and extrinsic to the foot that may lead to untoward compensation in the musculoskeletal system and should also protect the foot during its growth period.[10]

2. Be rigid enough to provide control but must also be able to accommodate natural foot shape change during motion.

3. Create the proper postural alignment for the foot and lower extremity until the osseous, joint, and soft tissue structures have been established.

4. Create a proper patient-orthotic interface by optimizing orthotic materials and contour to prevent tissue breakdown in children.

Popular pediatric orthotics that have been almost satisfactory in regard to the aforementioned "ideal" characteristics include the Whitman-Roberts orthosis, the Schaffer plate, and the heel stabilizers.[11, 12] Each of these has significant drawbacks. The Whitman-Roberts orthosis, with its high medial and lateral flanges, was found to be useful only in children older than 9 years. The Schaffer plate orthosis has only a medial flange and thus does not control calcaneal eversion. Finally, although heel stabilizers have been claimed to control the foot better than the orthotics, just mentioned, they cannot be tolerated by children older than 8 to 10 years. None of these devices control transverse plane motion or allow for medial and lateral column function.[13, 14]

Dynamic Stabilizing Innersole System

The Dynamic Stabilizing Innersole System (DSIS; Langer Laboratories, Deer Park, NY) incorporates triplane control via mechanisms that actually allow for identification and control of motion in each plane. The offset position of the calcaneus maintains the subtalar joint in an inverted position, providing the necessary stabilization in the frontal plane. This stabilization is countered by medial and lateral flanges, which extend to the first and fifth metatarsal necks. These flanges prevent the lateral drift of the forefoot and rearfoot and talar escape medially at the talonavicular articulation. The transverse plane is a dominant plane that must be controlled, and this requires lateral stabilizing components.

Last, the sagittal plane is controlled by the calcaneal inclination angle, which is maintained by the elevated longitudinal arch. The relaxed calcaneal stance position should be compared with the controlled calcaneal stance position when the patient is wearing the DSIS. This is a simple means of determining the effectiveness of the DSIS. By controlling the frontal plane position of the calcaneus and the transverse position of the foot as well as offering sagittal plane control, the DSIS maintains the foot in a position close to neutral, which then allows normal rearfoot and forefoot motion. Maintaining the subtalar joint around its neutral position provides forefoot control and added stabilization.[8, 9]

The DSIS includes a deeply offset varus heel seat, which cups and maintains the calcaneus in 5 degrees of varus. It still allows normal pronation during the early stance phase of the gait cycle. This device also has high medial and lateral flanges that extend distally, just proximal to the first and fifth metatarsal heads. These flanges limit the transverse spread of the foot when weight is transferred from the rearfoot to the metatarsal heads. Also, the semi-rigid material of the DSIS is well tolerated by children. Too often, conventional orthotics have proved to be too hard and rigid to be tolerated by young patients with pronation[8] (Fig. 48–1). A modified version of the DSIS is available as a prefabricated product, the DFS (Langer Laboratories, Deer Park, NY). The design concept is the same; however, the material is more flexible, and the device can be used as a temporary insert (Figs. 48–2 and 48–3).

The cause of a flatfoot due to excessive subtalar joint pronation may be muscular, osseous, ligamentous, neurologic, or a combination of these.[4] Hyperpronation with arch flattening occurs in three planes (i.e., sagittal, frontal, and transverse). Frontal plane motion of the calcaneus is controlled by the deep offset heel seat of the DSIS that

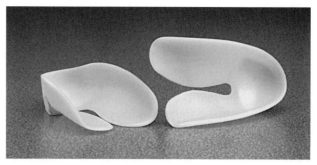

Figure 48–1. DSIS with medial and lateral flanges. The rearfoot has an offset 5-degree rearfoot varus post. The center of the orthosis is cut to limit transverse plane motion without creating pain on the medial flange. This is a prescription device made from a cast taken of the child's foot in the neutral position.

maintains the calcaneus in 5 degrees of varus. Sagittal plane talar drop is controlled by the raised flange on the medial side of the orthotic device. This flange limits talar plantar flexion and talar and navicular sag during hyperpronation. With frontal plane stability of the calcaneus controlled, the heel strikes the ground in a varus attitude, providing a stable lateral column. The midtarsal joint is locked, and the cuboid is stable. The peroneus longus tendon passing under the cuboid gains a mechanical advantage to plantar-flex the first ray. The normal ontogenous position of the first ray is a valgus, plantar-flexory direction. Due to the independent motion of the flanges in the DSIS, sagittal plane motion is allowed. The medial column of the DSIS works independently of the lateral column, allowing the first ray to gradually come down to the supporting surface. With rigid or fixed forefoot orthoses, the medial column is still in a varus attitude as the lateral column contacts the ground, thereby maintaining forefoot varus rather than letting the natural motion of the first ray occur with plantar flexion of the medial segment. Transverse plane flattening is very well controlled by the medial and lateral walled flanges. The high medial flange controls talar adduction, while the

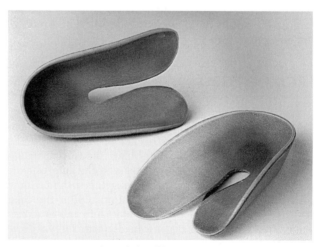

Figure 48–2. DFS with medial and lateral flanges. The rearfoot has an offset 5-degree rearfoot varus post. The center of the orthosis is cut to limit transverse plane motion without creating pain on the medial flange. This is a prefabricated product.

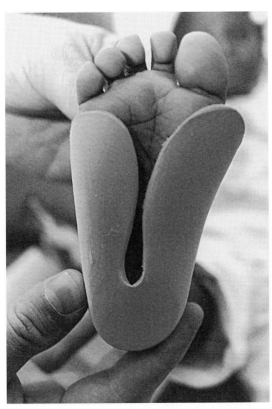

Figure 48–3. DFS maintains foot in neutral position. The device can extend far distally on the first and fifth metatarsal heads without exerting pressure due to the spring action of the flanges.

lateral flange limits abduction of the cuboid and fifth metatarsal. Standard functional orthoses do not achieve complete stabilization in this transverse plane without creating an increase in pressure on the talonavicular prominence or the fifth metatarsal base. The cutout section on the plantar aspect of the DSIS provides a spring action on the foot. The lateral and medial columns hold the foot securely in the shoe to limit abduction and adduction. As the pressure increases with further pronation, the spring action allows the orthosis to open gradually while still limiting excessive transverse motion.

The triplanar motion that occurs in hyperpronation is a unit motion in which each of the three motions works independently of each other. With limitation of motion in any one plane, however, a decrease in motion in the other two planes results. Considering the amount of control that each axis has on the other certainly explains how combined control in all planes can provide maximum support in a synergistic fashion.

Shoes and Flatfoot

Shoes may be detrimental to the development of a normal medial longitudinal arch. The critical age for the development of the longitudinal arch is before 6 years. Wearing shoes before the age of 6 predisposes the child to flatfoot, whereas if shoe-wearing is delayed until the child is older, the propensity for flatfoot is lower according to a study by Joseph,[19] in which 1846 subjects over the age of 16 years were evaluated. Assessment of the foot forms was based on the classification of static footprints obtained using the differential pressure footprint map of Harris and Beath (1947).[7] The height, weight, and duration of standing or walking each day were recorded. The body mass index was calculated, the presence of ligamentous laxity was noted, and the age at which shoes were first worn was recorded. The type of footwear used was also noted and the length of time the shoes were worn each day. Twenty-four footprints were analyzed on two separate occasions.

Of the 1846 subjects screened, 2.9% had flat feet, 10.5% had a high arch, and 88.6% had normal feet. The prevalence of flatfoot in those who started using footwear before the age of 5 years was 3.24%. It was 3.27% in those who began wearing shoes between the ages of 6 and 15 years and was 1.75% in those who first used shoes after the age of 16 years. Of the subjects who wore shoes before the age of 6 years, those who used them for longer then 8 hours each day in early childhood had a significantly higher prevalence of flatfoot than those who wore them for shorter periods. Subjects with ligamentous laxity and obese subjects had a significantly higher prevalence of flatfoot.

Age was not considered a variable in this study. Prolonged weight bearing was found to be unlikely to cause flatfoot; also, there was higher prevalence of flatfoot among adults who began using footwear in early childhood. The highest prevalence of flatfoot and the lowest prevalence of high-arched feet clearly occurred in early shoe-wearers. The author concluded that shoe-wearing has possible deleterious effects in children during development of the medial longitudinal arch, and the critical age for development of the arch is before 6 years. Joseph's study supports the fact that there is an association between shoe-wearing in early childhood and flatfoot, but prospective longitudinal studies are needed to confirm these impressions and to establish a causal relationship.

CLINICAL CONDITIONS ASSOCIATED WITH HYPERPRONATION

A flexible flatfoot deformity consists of a maximally pronated subtalar joint in closed kinetic chain. Abnormal pronation in the subtalar joint unlocks and destabilizes the midtarsal joint. In addition, the midtarsal joint and other distal joints become unstable and hypermobile. Hypermobility due to abnormal pronation can lead to symptomatology and frequently joint subluxation.[6] Joint subluxation in the child leads to permanent malpositioning, resulting in bunion formation, hallux limitus, hallux rigidus, and so on.[6] Intrinsic and extrinsic muscles (e.g., the tibialis posterior and peroneus longus) become inefficient and fatigued, resulting in a loss of stability. Muscles acting on the unstable forefoot may contribute to hammertoe deformities.

Transverse Axial Deformities

Transverse plane abnormalities in the axial segment (adduction or abduction) can cause compensatory flatfoot with hyperpronation. The various adduction deformities can cause an in-toeing gait.[7] To approximate a straight position, the child abducts the foot on the leg. This abduction is accomplished by pronating the subtalar and midtarsal joints. The abnormal correction leads to a pseudocorrection of the in-toeing gait and a secondary flatfoot. The talus is locked in the ankle mortise and follows the direction of the internally deviated tibia and fibula. The talus is maximally adducted; however, the calcaneus and the remainder of the foot abduct, thus increasing the subtalar and midtarsal joint pronation. Abduction deformities in the axial segment can result in a similar flatfoot. When the foot is excessively abducted from the line of progression, the child's body weight is medially displaced, aggravating the pronated position.

Primary gastrocnemius equinus produces a severe pronatory force on the foot because equinus prevents normal ankle dorsiflexion. As the talus assumes a more vertical and medial position, the calcaneus is forced to rotate posterolaterally from its position under the talus. The sustentaculum tali loses its supporting position beneath the neck of the talus as the calcaneus subluxates laterally. Because the hind part of the foot cannot be dorsiflexed, dorsiflexion occurs at the midfoot. A breech of the midpart of the foot or a rocker-bottom foot may result, with the hind foot in valgus angulation and the forefoot in abduction. Limitation of ankle joint dorsiflexion allows abnormal pronation at the subtalar and midtarsal joints.[15–17] Limited dorsiflexion of the ankle joint is translated into the subtalar and midtarsal joints.

Calcaneovalgus

Calcaneovalgus is a congenital deformity of osseous malpositon due to a deforming force in the direction of abduction and dorsiflexion. In the infant, application of a transverse abductory force at the level of the metatarsals causes all bones of the foot (except the talus) to move in the direction of abduction. The ankle joint is a strong mortise joint that primarily allows the talus to move in the sagittal plane (dorsiflexion and plantar flexion). Since the talus is locked into this ankle mortise, it cannot abduct. The navicular pivots on the head of the talus and comes to lie lateral to it. Other joints in the foot (i.e., the calcaneocuboid and metatarsocuboid joints) are strongly locked into their positions. Therefore, the calcaneus and the forefoot follow in the same direction. The net result is calcaneal abduction and pivoting under the talus, allowing the entire lateral column to abduct.

With the abductory drift of the calcaneus and the cuboid, the navicular abducts off the talar head. The spring ligament supports the head of the talus. When the navicular and calcaneus move laterally, they bring with them the spring ligament. Consequently, the talus plantarflexes since it is no longer supported. Now the entire foot is in an abducted position due to a transverse abductory force. Therefore, the transverse plane motion forces the entire lateral column to abduct, which in turn forces the calcaneus to abduct. Abduction of the calcaneus pulls on the spring ligament, which pulls the navicular laterally.

The talus further plantar-flexes because the spring ligament no longer supports it.

Control of Hyperpronation

Hyperpronation as a result of calcaneovalgus can be detected at childbirth. Casting and splints work well up to the age of ambulation. Torsional corrective casts and other torsional maintenance devices are used in children with transverse plane abnormalities. These rotational deformities can cause a secondary flatfoot deformity. Because hyperpronation in most children is undetected until the children are fully ambulatory and wearing shoes, the DSIS becomes an extremely important device in controlling hyperpronation and flatfoot in children. Children between the ages 2 and 16 years can benefit greatly from the DSIS because their bone and joint structures are still immature. The DSIS holds the foot in normal alignment and optimally changes the functionality of the soft tissues and osseous and joint structures over time. It is for this reason that I now use the DSIS frequently in the pediatric population.

Clinical signs of flatfoot include an excessively everted calcaneal stance (heel valgus), severe depression of the longitudinal arch, midtarsal subluxation, and medial talar head bulge. Hypermobility symptoms can include foot and heel pain, plantar fasciitis, excessive foot fatigue, and other similar complaints.[12] Evaluation of flatfoot deformity is accomplished by (1) evaluation of the position of the components of the foot, (2) evaluation of the motion of the components of the foot, and (3) roentgenographic studies of the foot in the standing weight-bearing position.

The flatfoot characteristic of the untreated calcaneovalgus foot is exacerbated by weight bearing. This is the point at which true deformity can occur. The increased pressure in the abnormal position of the foot will perpetuate the deformity as stated by Wolfe's law. Three structural deformities of the foot associated with the condition are: (1) abduction of the forefoot relative to the weight-bearing line, (2) supination of the forefoot, and (3) heel valgus. The flatfoot deformity may be caused by any one or a combination of these deformities. Generally, several are present, but at times only one component is seen. The talonavicular and the naviculocuneiform joints buckle, sag, or collapse during extreme pronation.[10]

Calcaneovalgus feet at birth that are not corrected, either with or without treatment, are subject to a resulting muscle imbalance at the ankle and continued weakness of the posterior tibial muscles; such feet may eventually result in hyperpronation and/or pes planus. If the condition is left untreated throughout life, a flexible flatfoot with severe long-term pronation about the subtalar joint and other joints can lead to a painful, joint-destructive, end-stage flatfoot syndrome along with associated forefoot, midfoot, rearfoot, and posterior leg symptoms.

The DSIS is a well-tolerated device that controls hyperpronation associated with primary and many secondarily induced flexible pes valgo planus deformities. This device, in studies by the author, has proved to be effective in children aged 2 and over to promote normal structural pedal alignment during growth.[8, 9] The DSIS has a rela-

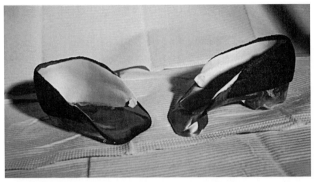

Figure 48–4. Roberts type orthosis with high medial and lateral flanges to control hyperpronation.

tively high patient and parent acceptance rate and offers a sound alternative to other conventional functional orthoses as well as popular pediatric orthoses.

Orthotics

A Roberts plate, calcaneal brace, rigid molded acrylic orthoses, or DSIS to stabilize the rearfoot is mandatory in the treatment of the child with flatfoot. The orthosis must extend far distally to secure the lateral column and at the same time stabilize the rearfoot in a slightly inverted 5-degree position. The lateral flange of the DSIS prevents the abductory transverse plane deformity that is seen in patients with flatfoot deformities. At the same time, the medial flange supports the medial column and prevents midtarsal and subtalar joint breakdown. The child should be fitted for the DSIS as early as possible. This orthosis can be placed directly into a running sneaker or shoe. Usually it will have to be replaced when the child's shoe size increases approximately two sizes. When the child becomes older and there is less fat around the heel and arch area, it may be necessary to reshape the deep-seated heel cup with the addition of a Plastizote or PPT flange to protect the font from irritation on the medial talar bulge (Figs. 48–4 to 48–9). When the child reaches approximately 7 or 8 years of age, he or she will not tolerate this very deep flanged orthosis and will need an orthosis that eliminates the far lateral flange and stops just short of the fifth metatarsal base. The younger child can tolerate the flange extending as far distally as the fifth metatarsal head because of the extra fat that is present. In the older child it is necessary to decrease the depth of the heel seat, but one should maintain an extra depth to

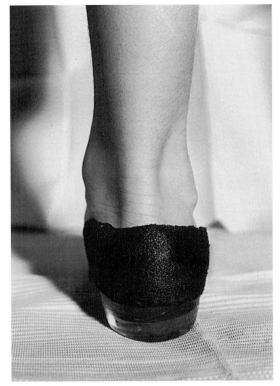

Figure 48–5. Calcaneal stance position maintained in high-flange Roberts type orthoses.

control the calcaneus in an inverted position. The DSIS device dynamically stabilizes both the rearfoot and the forefoot.[18]

Flatfoot Secondary to Tight Heel Cord

To control equinus flatfoot (tight heel cord) with an orthotic device, one must be cautious. Since the dorsiflexory component of gait is taken up at the midtarsal joint, the foot will pronate with great impact into the medial part of the orthosis, causing discomfort for the patient. If no dorsiflexion (upward foot motion on the leg) is available at midstance, the orthosis will probably fail, and the patient will most likely be a candidate for a leg-lengthening procedure. If, however, at least 5 degrees of dorsiflexion are available at the ankle joint, an orthosis can control this foot.

The orthosis may be casted with the patient's foot in a slightly pronated position. This eliminates the possibility

Figure 48–6. Rigid molded acrylic orthoses. *A*, Gait plate to encourage out toe. The lateral and distal aspects of the plantar surface of the orthotic extend distally to allow the first ray to increase its hypermobility and appearance of abduction. The rearfoot is stabilized with a rearfoot varus post of 5 degrees. *B*, Standard orthoses with rearfoot deep seat. *C*, A narrow-flanged Roberts plate. *D*, A deep-flanged Roberts plate with forefoot varus posting. *E*, A deep-flanged Roberts plate with forefoot varus posting.

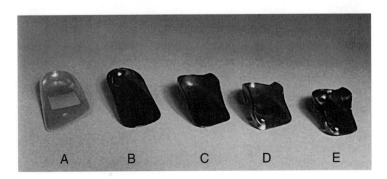

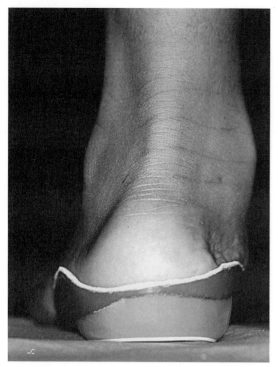

Figure 48–7. Rearfoot varus posts on flexible orthoses with deep-seated heel cup. Note the presence of forefoot abduction and minimal control of plantar flexion of talus. Calcaneus is mildly everted with an increase in Helbing's sign.

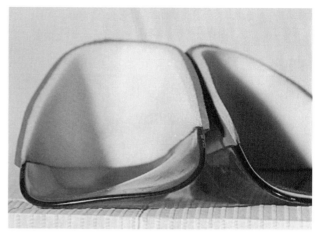

Figure 48–8. Deep-seated heel orthosis with medial and lateral flanges. Flanges are covered with PPT and Plastizote to increase height while minimizing irritation on the medial aspect of the foot.

of medial arch fatigue and allows the foot to pronate through gait but blocks the end range pronation. Dorsiflexion is allowed to occur at the midtarsal joint to a lesser degree. When a child is wearing a fully posted orthosis (with a rearfoot and forefoot post), stretching exercises should be encouraged. If length increases to the gastrocnemius-soleus complex, the pronatory effect that would otherwise be taken up by the subtalar and midtarsal joints will now take place as it should at the ankle joint. The subtalar and midtarsal joints remain in a neutral position,

and the cuboid remains stable and allows the peroneus longus tendon to plantar-flex the first ray. When this occurs, the forefoot post must be reduced gradually. It is easier to reduce extrinsic posts than to post the forefoot in varus intrinsically. Every month the forefoot post is ground down approximately 1 to 2 degrees. If this posting is not reduced, a first ray elevatus may develop. Some practitioners believe that it is necessary to completely recast the patient at 2-month intervals to capture the changing forefoot design. If cost is not a factor, this is the best approach; otherwise, gradual reduction of the extrinsic forefoot post is usually sufficient.

When there is concern that midtarsal joint breakdown might create pain from the orthosis medially, use of a more flexible sport orthotic device can be considered. The addition of compressible posts also creates some "give" in the orthotic in the direction of pronation. Remember, an orthotic device is not going to correct anything if the cause is not addressed. In this case, length

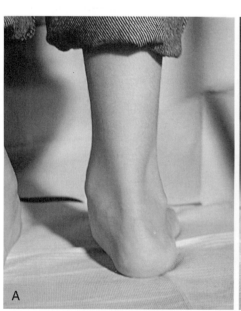
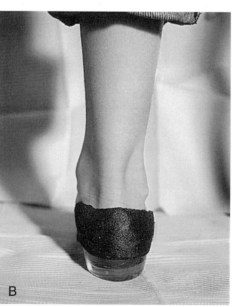

Figure 48–9. *A,* Transverse plane flatfoot with secondary equinus deformity. Note marked abduction of forefoot and plantar flexion of talus. *B,* Same child with flanged orthotic and rearfoot varus posting. A high crepe flange is used to maintain the transverse and sagittal plane.

must be obtained by either stretching exercises or a surgical lengthening procedure.

Flatfoot Secondary to In-Toe (Tibial Torsion)

In the child who is older than 6 years and still has an inward tibial torsion, the deformity probably will not decrease, and the sequelae of a flatfoot will increase. A flatfoot that is secondary to transverse plane abnormalities can become a fixed rigid flatfoot. A simple orthosis is recommended for these children. By maintaining the rearfoot in a subtalar neutral position, one can prevent the internal driving forces through the midtarsal joint and subtalar joint that create a flatfoot. It is often asked whether support of the subtalar and midtarsal joints in a supinated position will accentuate the toe-in. It will, but the support is needed to maintain a corrected position of the foot to avoid creating another problem as the child grows older—the flatfoot. This should be explained to the parent before treatment with an orthosis is begun. The orthosis still encourages removal of all the internal medial forces that are twisting the leg. When these forces are removed, the leg should go through its normal ontogenous process of external lateral growth.

Metatarsus Adductus with Flatfoot Compensation

In the ambulating child who presents with the complicated and compensated metatarsus adductus, an orthosis is needed for control. This orthotic device visually increases the apparent toe-in position; however, at the same time, it prevents the foot from pronating. Because the foot is maturing and the protective fat about the foot is decreasing, a device must be constructed that will control rearfoot pronation and also prevent the transverse drift of the forefoot that is commonly seen in the compensated metadductus deformity. If a concomitant internal axial deviation (internal tibial torsion, internal femoral position) occurs at the same time as the metadductus, the result is an internally positioned foot, which is controlled. It is imperative to explain the purpose of control by the orthosis as well as the visual effect of in-toe to the parent.

The child with a metatarsus adductus is prone to Iselin's apophysitis owing to the lateral prominence, which increases pressure and irritation. This pressure can be effectively decreased by the use of a rigid molded acrylic orthosis. This orthosis is a modified version of a Roberts plate, in which the flanges are kept low but the heel seat is deep. The lateral flange is cut proximally to the fifth metatarsal base. This orthotic device controls pronation and removes the direct pressure on the base. In patients with a healthy young fat pad this cut-out area is not necessary. The flange should be extended distally to just proximal to the fifth metatarsal head.

Flatfoot with Limb Length Discrepancy

A compensatory flatfoot develops in the child with an uneven limb length. The long limb pronates to shorten

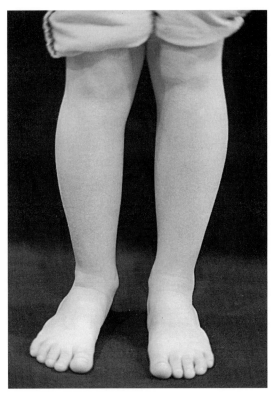

Figure 48–10. A 9-year-old child with a side limb length discrepancy. The right foot is abducting to accommodate the long side.

the affected side, and the foot abducts. The opposite short limb supinates to increase the height of that limb. A simple remedy is to increase the height of the shortened limb; however, care must be taken not to induce an equinus by elevating the heel height too much. I have found that a ½-inch heel rise along with a tapered ¼-inch forefoot 0-degree post does not affect the child adversely. If more elevation is needed, ¼-inch flat wedges can be placed in the running shoe. In patients with a great amount of shortening heel and sole wedges must be incorporated externally in the shoe. A molded orthosis with a 0-degree rearfoot post should be incorporated to prevent any unnecessary pronation (Fig. 48–10).

References

1. Elfman H: Torsion of lower extremity. Am J Physiol Anthropol 1945;3:255–265.
1a. Otman S: Energy cost of walking with flatfeet. Prosthet Orthot Int 1988;73:6.
2. Gamble FC, Yale I: Clinical Foot Roentgenology, 2nd ed. Huntington, NY, Robert Kreiger Publishing, 1975, pp. 209–212.
3. Steindler A: Kinesiology of the Human Body. Springfield, IL, Charles C Thomas, 1955, p. 413.
4. Root ML, Orien WP, Weed JH, et al: Biomechanical Examination of the Foot. Los Angeles, Clinical Biomechanical Corporation, 1971, p. 34.
5. Heuter C: Anatomische Studien an den extremita tengelenhen Neugeborener und erwach Sener. Virchow Arch 1862;25:572.
6. Volkmann R: Chirurgische Erfahrungan über Knochenverbiegurgen. Arch Pathol Anat 1862;24:512.
7. Harris RI, Beath T: Hypermobile flatfoot with short tendo Achillis. J Bone Joint Surg 1948;30A:116.

8. Jay RM, Schoenhaus HD: Hyperpronation control with a dynamic stabilizing innersole system. J Am Podiatr Med Assoc 1992;82:149–153.

9. Jay RM, Schoenhaus HD: The Dynamic Stabilizing Innersole System (DSIS): The management of hyperpronation in children. J Foot Ankle Surg 1995;34:124–131.

10. Tax HR: Orthotics and children. Podiatr Manage 1993;3:1251–1258.

11. Donatelli RA: Biomechanics of the Foot and Ankle. Philadelphia, F.A. Davis, 1990, pp. 201–208.

12. Root ML, Weed JH, Orien WP: Compensatory function of the foot. *In* Root ML, Weed JH, Orien WP (eds): Normal and Abnormal Function of the Foot, Vol. 2. Los Angeles, Clinical Biomechanics Corporation, 1977, pp. 115–122.

13. Doxey GE: Cinical use and fabrication of molded thermoplastic foot orthotic devices. Phys Ther 1985;65:1679–1682.

14. Smith LS: The effects of soft and semi-rigid orthoses upon rearfoot movement in running. J Am Podiatr Assoc 1986;227–233.

15. Schoenhaus HD, Jay RM: A modified gastrocnemius lengthening. J Am Podiatr Assoc 1978;68:31–37.

16. McGlamry ED, Banks AS, Downey MS: Pes planovalgus deformity. *In* Comprehensive Textbook of Foot and Ankle Surgery, Vol. 1, 2nd ed. St. Louis, C. V. Mosby, 1989, pp. 769–817.

17. Bowker P: Foot orthoses. *In* Biomechanical Basis of Orthotic Management. Oxford, Butterworth-Heinemann, 1993, pp. 88–89.

18. Jay RM: Pediatric orthoses. Biomechanics 1995;2:51–54.

19. Joseph B: The influence of footwear on the prevalence of flatfoot. J Bone Joint Surg 1994;77B:254–257.

49

Ankle-Foot Orthoses Following Surgery

Russell Volpe, D.P.M.

Ankle-foot orthoses (AFOs) are an important component in the management of foot and ankle problems in gait. They are used as either a follow-up treatment to a primary medical or surgical intervention or as an initial treatment of choice. The patient requiring foot and/or leg surgery often has a significant deformity that benefits from the level of maintenance of correction provided by ankle-foot orthoses. It is important to note that children requiring this combined therapeutic approach often have complex foot and ankle deformities. These may include congenital deformities, short or tight muscles, weakness, instability, or spasticity. Many of these children have neuromuscular deformities, and the special handling required in the use of postoperative orthoses in this population is considered later in this chapter.

Use of ankle-foot orthoses as an initial treatment of choice is indicated when more rigorous mechanical intervention is required clinically. These circumstances include functional muscular weakness or loss in the lower extremity of one or more muscle groups; upper or lower motor neuron disease or trauma with accompanying spasticity or loss of tone; or loss of sensory function in the lower extremity that would normally protect the leg from tissue breakdown. These clinical circumstances also often require surgical intervention either initially or after other primary treatments have proved to be no longer effective. The ankle-foot orthosis is an important adjunct to the postoperative management of many of these patients.

The design of the postoperative brace is very similar to the design of braces used for primary treatment. A major difference is the importance of padding or accommodation for incision sites, particularly if they lie over bony prominences.[1] It should be remembered that the role of any orthosis is to hold the foot in a position that can be passively attained during manual manipulation. As a general rule, if the foot and leg can be passively manipulated into the desired position, an adequate impression can be taken and a satisfactory device can be fabricated. It must be remembered that a brace or orthosis cannot by itself correct a deformity. These caveats are particularly noteworthy when discussing the use of bracing in the postoperative patient in whom the decision to operate may have been based in part on an inability to obtain a desired position with passive manipulation.

ANKLE-FOOT ORTHOSES—OVERVIEW

Ankle-foot orthoses are a group of devices designed to support, protect, or enhance the function of the foot and ankle during gait. Their role in providing these benefits is extremely valuable in the postoperative child. AFOs may be divided into two basic categories determined by their relationship to the shoe. An *extrinsic* AFO has an attachment to the outside of the shoe, whereas an *intrinsic* AFO is worn inside the shoe. These devices are further categorized by the function they perform—for example, ankle stabilization, foot-ankle immobilization, or dorsiflexion assistance.

The use of AFOs in the postoperative child may accomplish one of the following goals of orthotic function[2]:

1. Limit motion or weight bearing to reduce pain or load on a segment.
2. Immobilize and protect healing musculoskeletal segments.
3. Prevent recurrence of deformity.
4. Improve function.

The primary purpose of an orthosis applied in the immediate postoperative period is to maintain the desired corrected position during the healing process while allowing maximum functional ability during rehabilitation and return to normal activity. If the device is employed earlier in the postoperative period, it may be necessary to sacrifice some functional ability or mobility to ensure that the stable position is maintained during healing. Later in the therapeutic process, after healing has occurred, thus decreasing the need for stability of the surgical site, it may be feasible to design a device with greater mobility as a feature. This is an example of a serial approach to the use of AFOs in the postoperative patient.

The pediatric AFO may also be part of a serial therapeutic plan that incorporates different treatment options. The AFO may be used for a limited period with one objective, followed by another type of AFO to facilitate additional objectives made possible by the initial correction. A surgical procedure may be done as a component of this serial corrective approach, using the postoperative AFO to support, maintain, and encourage proper function. The rapid growth rate in children makes this serial approach to management ideal in this population. The timing of a second-stage AFO after a surgical correction may coincide with a recent growth spurt.

PREFABRICATED DEVICES

Practitioners may choose between prefabricated and custom-made ankle-foot orthoses. It has been stated that only 20% of the patient population can be successfully treated with prefabricated devices.[3] This statistic refers to the general population and does not take into account additional limitations on the use of prefabricated devices in the postoperative patient. These limitations include alterations in limb size due to fluctuating postoperative edema and the need to highly customize the design to meet specific needs dictated by the procedure performed and the desired postoperative role of the AFO. The efficacy of an AFO also depends in part on the quality of the fit to the patient's leg, and care should be taken to consider this before selecting a prefabricated device. Advantages of the use of prefabricated devices in the postoperative patient may include the relative ease of obtaining a device that may have only a temporary application for a defined time period and purpose. As in any clinical circumstance, the practitioner must weigh the advantages of expedience and cost in choosing a prefabricated device against the individualization and specificity of design in choosing a custom device.

EFFECTS OF ANKLE-FOOT ORTHOSES ON THE GAIT OF CHILDREN

A study of the effects of AFOs on the gait of children indicates that certain expectations should be considered before choosing an AFO for a child.[4] Normal children were studied wearing extrinsic and intrinsic or molded solid AFOs. In fast walking, speed and cadence were reduced when either type of AFO was worn. In fast walking, a significant decrease in speed was noted with the extrinsic type but not with the intrinsic type. Use of either brace reduced cadence in fast walking compared with no brace, but more so with the extrinsic type. Other findings included the consequences of the alteration of the ankle rocker caused by the fixed ankle position as described by Perry.[5] This fixed ankle position causes the tibia to be thrust forward as the foot comes flat to the floor, leading to increased demand and activity in the quadriceps muscles. Limitation of ankle dorsiflexion interferes with the normal advancement of the tibia over the planted foot, transmitting an external torque that tends to extend the knee during stance.

The weight of the braces also seemed to have an effect on gait. Greater muscular effort may be required to accomplish ground clearance in swing phase. This study found that hip flexion was increased when children wore braces compared with not wearing them.

The study concluded that extrinsic AFOs disrupt nor-mal walking in children more than intrinsic AFOs. This effect seemed to be due more to the additional weight in the extrinsic design than to any difference in restriction of ankle motion. Data on restriction of ankle motion were similar for both types of devices. The authors of the study recognized that the changes in walking resulting from wearing the braces may become less noticeable if the children wear the braces for a longer time. It should also be noted that this study was performed in normal children and not in children with pathologic conditions.

EXTRINSIC VERSUS INTRINSIC ANKLE-FOOT ORTHOSES

An intrinsic or molded AFO applied directly to the skin surface is closer to the center of force, which gives it a greater mechanical advantage, thereby making it more effective in altering function.[3] A further advantage of the intrinsic type is that it is considered more cosmetically acceptable. This type of device, also called an in-shoe device, can be largely hidden inside a shoe and under the pant leg. Intrinsic AFOs are considered less desirable when fluctuating or chronic edema is present. Chronic edema presents many challenges in casting and fitting the brace. Fluctuating edema, which may be present in a postoperative limb, may make sizing difficult and can create problems in maintaining proper fit of the device over time. Extrinsic devices, which are applied to the shoe, may be appropriate when these conditions limit the use of in-shoe AFOs. A Blucher-type shoe is usually chosen for extrinsic bracing because this type of shoe is designed for durability and support. In recent years, some practitioners have had success in using extrinsic AFOs with athletic footwear, but these shoes may not be able to withstand the high deforming forces put on them under these conditions. Two types of attachments are commonly used for extrinsic AFOs: stirrup and caliper. The most common is the double-upright stirrup.[3] Most extrinsic AFOs have an ankle-joint component to facilitate sagittal plane movement. This feature can be either spring-assisted to aid function or restrictive to block mo-tion that would reduce function.

Intrinsic AFOs are those molded to fit closely to the foot and leg and are worn inside the patient's shoe. They are generally made from thermoplastics that are pressed to positive models made from impressions or via com-puter-assisted design/computer-assisted manufacture (CAD-CAM) to produce specific shapes or design fea-tures. The most common design options include the static or rigid ankle device, often called a solid AFO; the semi-solid ankle form; the motion-assist form such as the poste-rior leaf spring (PLS) device; and the dynamic articulating or hinged form. Variations on these may include the supramalleolar orthosis, a type of solid ankle with a shorter leg segment, the floor reaction brace, and the patellar tendon bearing brace. It is essential to understand the basic design features and clinical indications for each of these braces before choosing them for use in the postoperative child. An understanding of how the devices work and the type of control, support, and assistance they provide enables the practitioner to prescribe them appropriately in highly individual postoperative circumstances.

TYPES OF ANKLE-FOOT ORTHOSES

Solid Ankle-Foot Orthoses

A solid AFO provides knee stability in the frontal and sagittal planes as well as stability at the ankle joint, its primary role. Significant numbers of patients who require assistance at the ankle benefit from this additional effect at the knee, particularly in postoperative circumstances when the relationship of synergistic muscle groups may have been altered by isolated procedures at a single joint level. If the ankle is placed in the proper position by the AFO, it will provide knee stability while minimizing knee flexion or extension moment at heel strike and early stance. A more plantarflexed ankle in the AFO will provide an extensor moment to the knee, whereas a more dorsiflexed ankle will provide a flexor moment to the knee (Fig. 49–1). Sankey and colleagues[6] described changes in the design of AFOs that included a more dorsiflexed position of the ankle joint when stretch on the Achilles tendon is desired in children with cerebral palsy. In a study of children with cerebral palsy with spastic equinus of the ankle, they found a marked decrease in the need for surgical lengthening of the heel cord in children who wore the AFO set in the dorsiflexed position. Of 10 children who went on to surgical lengthening, only one came from the group that wore the dorsiflexed AFO. This design feature, which may reduce the need for surgery in some children, may also be used after lengthening the tendo Achilles to encourage stretch on the tendon. This modification can be made by taking the impression cast in a more dorsiflexed ankle position or by altering the positive in the fabrication process. This modified solid device may be an alternative to a hinged AFO when

greater stability is desired. Shoes can be modified to adjust the angle made by the child's leg with the ground when the angle of the AFO has been altered.

Unless these increased knee moments or ankle effects are desired, the ankle should be placed in a neutral alignment to eliminate these effects. The need for controlled plantarflexion of the ankle can be provided by undercutting the heel or by using a solid ankle cushion heel (SACH) feature. Patients may change the shoe they wear with their AFO, recognizing that alterations in heel height will change the function of the orthosis. A negative heel environment mimics the effect of a plantarflexed ankle AFO by placing an extensor moment on the knee, whereas an elevated heel environment mimics the effect of a dorsiflexed ankle AFO by placing a flexor moment on the knee (Fig. 49–2). This fully supportive solid AFO is indicated in postoperative patients who require maximum support for the ankle-subtalar joint complex. If weakening of structures in this area has resulted from the surgery, this higher level of support is helpful in the immediate postoperative phase. Further, if pain with motion must be reduced, the high level of immobilization offered by this device is appropriate. In designing an AFO for the immediate postoperative period in a child the practitioner should consider that a solid AFO with anterior trim lines offering maximum control can be cut back and modified to reduce control as function improves over time.

Care should be taken to consider the role of the foot plate of any AFO. It is important to design the device to include a custom-contoured foot plate. This feature is most helpful when the distal joints are unstable and control or stability of these joints is desired. If the surgical procedure was performed for stabilization of the rearfoot or midfoot, as with a severe collapsing pes plano valgus, the ability to support and control motion in the foot is particularly important. In this case, the value of the carefully contoured foot plate, with intrinsic or extrinsic posting of the rearfoot and forefoot as needed, should be

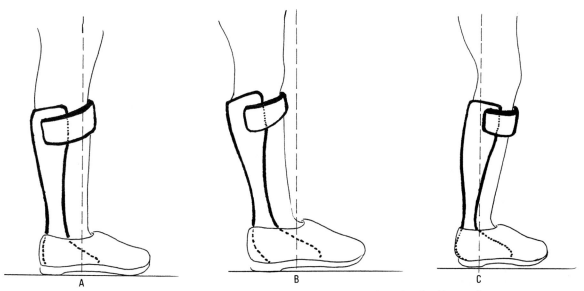

Figure 49–1. The effect of ankle position on the knee moment. *A,* Neutral ankle. *B,* plantarflexed ankle providing extensor moment to the knee. *C,* Dorsiflexed ankle providing flexor moment to the knee. (Modified from Drennan J: The Child's Foot and Ankle. New York, Raven Press, 1992.)

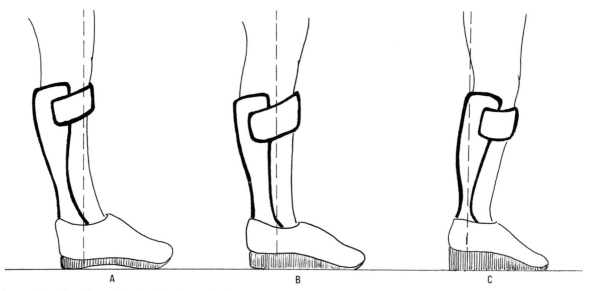

Figure 49–2. The effect of shoe heel height on the knee moment. *A,* Flat heel. *B,* Slight heel. *C,* High heel. (Modified from Drennan J: The Child's Foot and Ankle. New York, Raven Press, 1992.)

considered before a prefabricated device, which usually comes with a flat or minimally contoured foot plate, is chosen.

The ankle trimline of the AFO also affects the rigidity of the solid AFO (Fig. 49–3). Trimlines anterior to the malleoli increase the rigidity of the brace at the ankle, whereas trimlines cut posterior to the malleoli increase

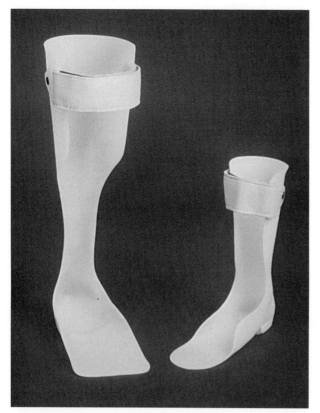

Figure 49–3. Solid ankle foot orthoses. Anterior trimline produces a more rigid solid AFO *(right).* Severe posterior trimline produces a posterior leaf spring (PLS) variation of a solid AFO *(left).*

the flexibility of the brace at the ankle. The location of the anterior trimline in a solid AFO should be determined by the need for mediolateral stability and the desired sagittal plane motion at heel strike. A trimline anterior to the malleoli, which is indicated for high mediolateral stability and restriction of sagittal plane ankle motion, is often needed to reduce pain or instability. In the immediate postoperative period in many patients who have undergone reconstructive foot and leg surgery, this level of control is necessary to provide support and allow healing while permitting minimum function. In a child who has undergone surgical lengthening for an equinus in the presence of high tone, hypotonic or weak medial and lateral ankle stabilizers may become evident after the surgery. Such a patient may need the additional support provided by a full-cut AFO to support the newly revealed weak supporting structures. Rehabilitative efforts directed at these structures may ensue over time. It should be remembered that a device designed with a more anterior trimline at the malleoli is more bulky and is cosmetically less appealing.

A solid AFO may also be employed as a night splint to maintain a plantigrade position obtained by surgical correction. Because this approach is most commonly used in the immediate postoperative period, it may be modified to include a more anterior trimline at the malleoli to provide increased support and additional padding for cushioning (Fig. 49–4).

Semi-Rigid Solid Ankle-Foot Orthoses

A solid AFO may be made more flexible at the ankle by cutting back the anterior trimline. When reduced mediolateral stability is required as postoperative stability improves, the trimline may be cut to bisect the malleoli. This design is most appropriate when minimal frontal plane ankle instability is present and sagittal plane knee motion during stance is under voluntary control.[7]

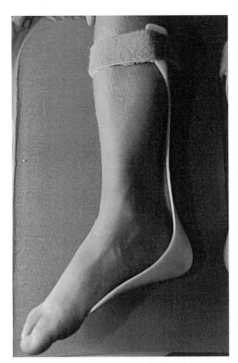

Figure 49–4. Solid ankle foot orthosis (MAFO) in plantarflexed position for use as a night splint to maintain correction.

When dorsiflexion assist at toe-off is needed, the trimline can be cut severely posterior to the malleoli. This is known as the posterior leaf spring (PLS) variation on the solid AFO (see Fig. 49–3). The severity of the trimline also determines whether the device can offer minimal plantarflexion and the degree of dorsiflexion assist provided in early swing. The more anterior the trimline, the greater the plantarflexion resistance provided. Such a

trimline also offers greater push-off assistance with dorsiflexion resistance. Progressive posterior trimming of the device was found to make the device less effective at push-off assistance but did provide adequate toe clearance in swing phase to aid with dropfoot.[8] The device can be modified to a slightly dorsiflexed position in patients with mild knee recurvatum to increase the flexor moment at the knee. It is important for the patient to have good quadriceps function in these cases in light of the reduced extensor moment in the AFO. This modification, however, may limit the effectiveness of the device in assisting with push-off.

Articulating or Hinged Ankle-Foot Orthoses

When maximum frontal plane stability is desired along with sagittal plane motion, the use of an articulating ankle-foot orthosis should be considered. The device incorporates features of the solid AFO in providing frontal plane stability and control of the rearfoot and forefoot while at the same time allowing maximum ankle motion in the sagittal plane (Fig. 49–5A). A plantarflexion stop may be incorporated in the device to limit genu recurvatum or to break up an extensor synergy pattern (Fig. 49–5B). The use of hinged AFOs are most appropriate in children with sufficient independent voluntary hip and knee movement. Voluntary knee extension with movement of the tibia during stance is a reliable indicator that the use of a hinged ankle device is appropriate. Care should be taken to monitor the balance of dorsiflexion and plantarflexion in the AFO. Limitation of dorsiflexion may decrease the effectiveness of push-off later in the stance phase. Excess plantarflexion may increase the demands of hip and knee flexion in swing phase.

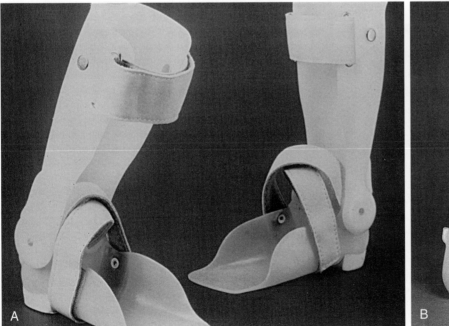
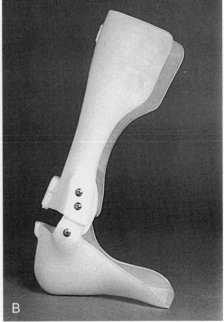

Figure 49–5. A, Articulating or hinged AFO with tibial and crossed-ankle straps. B, Articulating or hinged AFO with posterior stop to limit plantarflexion. (Courtesy of the Langer Biomechanics Group, Deer Park, NY.)

The indication for a hinged AFO is dorsiflexion of the ankle to 5 degrees with the subtalar joint in neutral. Fixed contractures of muscles that prevent dorsiflexion to this point are contraindications to the use of a hinged AFO. Hamstring or hip flexor tightness that contributes to crouch gait is also a contraindication to the use of hinged ankle-foot orthoses.

Clearly, the use of articulating AFOs in the postsurgical child is most appropriate when the tendo Achilles has been lengthened and the rehabilitative process includes gradually increasing use of the newly available ankle dorsiflexion. This device may follow the use of a solid AFO in the immediate postoperative period during the acute healing phase. The practitioner may want to consider the use of a prefabricated solid AFO in the immediate postoperative period while a custom-made hinged AFO is being fabricated. This is cost-effective because it enables the patient to make the transition from maximum support to maximum function quickly. The practitioner should avoid the excessive or prolonged use of solid AFOs in the child after tendo Achilles lengthening. Persistent blocking of ankle motion, while desirable in the immediate postoperative period, limits the long-term increase in range of motion at the ankle that was the indication for surgery in the first place. The use of a hinged device in rehabilitation encourages dynamic ankle dorsiflexion and is a valuable adjunct in the child needing supportive assistance in the postoperative period.

Supramalleolar Orthoses

Supramalleolar orthoses (SMOs), which have a trim-line above the malleoli, are an excellent option when control above the foot level is desired without the full height of an AFO (Fig. 49–6). They should be selected in children undergoing foot surgery in whom stability of

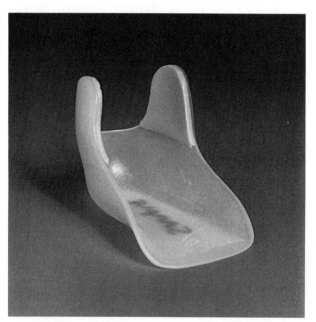

Figure 49–6. Low-cut supramalleolar orthosis (SMO) to provide control to the level of the malleoli.

the hindfoot and midfoot is needed in the frontal and transverse planes beyond that which can be expected from a submalleolar foot orthosis. In addition, while some control of sagittal plane ankle motion may be expected with an SMO, the design is such that sagittal plane motions needed for gait are allowed. The child undergoing a complex stabilization procedure for pes valgus, which exerts deforming forces on several body planes, may benefit from the use of an SMO postoperatively. While recognizing that the ultimate purpose of such stabilization procedures is to reduce or eliminate the need for such external stabilizing devices, it may be beneficial to prescribe these devices initially to reduce motion during healing while providing a minimum of external bulk and cosmetic baggage. SMOs can be easily cut down to submalleolar foot orthoses as the child's function and stability improve. The use of an SMO is a poor choice when sagittal plane control of the knee is needed owing to the short lever arm.

The SMO can also be fabricated with only a medial or lateral upright to provide extra support to only one side of the ankle joint (Fig. 49–7). This may be helpful in postoperative patients with residual weakness on the medial or lateral side after correction or during healing. It may also be an ideal option after talipes equinovarus or convex pes plano valgus surgery when medial or lateral instability or deformity may persist.

Patellar Tendon-Bearing Orthoses

The use of devices that have been designed to use the patellar tendon and tibial condyles to unweight below-knee amputees may be applied to other clinical circumstances in which this feature is desirable.[9] The patellar tendon-bearing orthosis (PTB) is ideal in cases in which reduced load on the distal leg and foot is required. These devices are designed so that the patellar tendon and the tibial condyles bear some of the load transmitted to the foot and leg in gait, thereby reducing distal load. The indication for these devices in the postoperative child is primarily the presence of complications such as persistent pain or delayed union or non-union of bone. They may also be useful for acquired loss of ankle function or sensation or avascular necrosis of the talar body. The PTB is more likely to be used in adults with chronic pain or dysfunction, and therefore, it has limited applications in pediatrics. Care should be taken in using this device in patients with fluctuating edema or in those with a history of intolerance to pressure distal to the knee.

Floor Reaction Ankle-Foot Orthoses

These devices are designed to stabilize the extremity without limiting knee motion. The device crosses in front of the proximal tibia/knee to deliver an extensor moment to the knee. It couples the plantarflexion floor reaction force to the anterior aspect of the proximal orthosis to assist in stabilizing the knee joint into full extension. It is indicated in children with cerebral palsy and dynamic knee flexion deformity due to overactive hamstring mus-

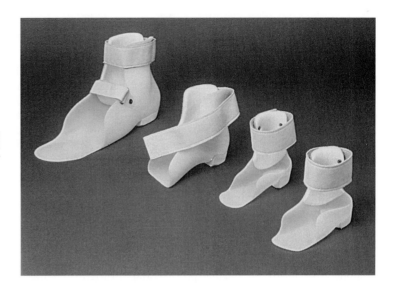

Figure 49–7. Supramalleolar orthoses (SMO) *(left to right)*: medial upright, lateral upright, double-upright metatarsal length, double-upright full length. (Courtesy of the Langer Biomechanics Group, Deer Park, NY.)

cles. Weak quadriceps muscles are also an indication for the use of this device. In the postoperative patient who has an overlengthened tendo Achilles, this device may be appropriate. The overlengthened heel cord may result in a crouch gait that requires the extensor moment effect of the floor reaction brace to stabilize the gait. An alternative to the floor reaction brace is a solid AFO with an anterior shell. This provides an extensor moment to the knee that stimulates the effect of a floor reaction brace. The floor reaction brace is contraindicated in patients with fixed flexion contractures of the hip or knee, poor hip extensor strength, or adductor spasticity.

LIFTS AND POSTS

Postoperative AFOs may benefit from the use of lifts and posts. These are materials applied to the external aspect of the plantar surface of the device to maintain a fixed angle of the foot or leg. In the child who has recently undergone a tendo Achilles lengthening, a heel lift might be placed under the AFO to maintain a plantar-flexed ankle position during the initial healing phase. Later, after initial healing has occurred, the lift could be reduced or removed to increase the function of the tendon in the newly corrected desired position. External lifts and wedges are excellent for this purpose because they are applied to the device with glue and are easily removed or modified. The use of angled posts should be considered when frontal plane deformity is present, particularly in the forefoot. Varus or valgus deformities of the forefoot may need post control to allow the AFO to be maximally effective. Extrinsic rearfoot posting on AFOs should be used primarily to stabilize the rear portion of the device in the shoe. These devices are already posted intrinsically in the rearfoot because the relationship between the rearfoot and the leg has been captured in the impression and is transmitted to the thermoplastic shell in the fabrication process.

USE OF ANKLE-FOOT ORTHOSES FOR SPECIFIC PEDIATRIC CONDITIONS

Equinus

Indications

Surgical correction of muscular or combined muscular-osseus equinus is indicated when conservative measures have failed. The purpose of the surgery is to provide relief of pain and a return to function.[10] In cases with an osseous block excision of the talotibial exostoses is necessary to achieve correction. The decision to operate on a patient with muscle shortening should be based on whether the shortening is dynamic or fixed (anatomic).[11] Dynamic shortening is reducible with loading of the segment returning the joint to neutral or beyond. A fixed or anatomic shortening cannot be brought to neutral even with load on the segment. Tendon lengthening is usually not appropriate to correct dynamic shortening because overlengthening is possible, leading to reciprocal deformities. An example of this is the crouch gait that may follow tendo Achilles lengthening when dynamic or fixed tightness in other muscles remains.

Mercer and Rang[11] recommend three level lengthenings in "spring-loaded" muscles. These usually include lengthening of the psoas, hamstrings, adductors, and heel cords. The procedure may include a lengthening or transfer of the rectus femoris to avoid a stiff-knee gait. Fixed muscle shortenings should be lengthened in a timely fashion to decrease the likelihood that compensatory changes will occur in the distal joints if the deformity persists. This is a significant possibility in the presence of joint laxity, and these patients are good candidates for preoperative and/or postoperative foot and ankle-foot orthoses to protect the distal structures. The patient with a fixed shortening that has been lengthened with no evidence of laxity is a candidate for postoperative bracing to facilitate rehabilitation and enhance function. Care should be taken to observe those children with dynamic deformities to monitor the progression to fixed deformities. Surgical release of a fixed muscle deformity will not necessarily allow a nonambulatory child with cerebral palsy to walk. Mercer and Rang[11] recommend placing the child in a kneeling position to see if he or she has the balance and ability to move. If he does, then lengthening of fixed contractures may aid in allowing a transition to a walker.

The postoperative period for a patient with a tendo Achilles lengthening usually begins with a cast for 4 to 6 weeks. The cast may be an above-knee cast first, which can be reduced to a below-knee cast after 3 to 4 weeks.[10] Rehabilitative exercises begin as early as several days postoperatively. Exercises can be facilitated by converting the cast to a bivalved cast that can be removed and reapplied. Bivalved casts can also serve as night splints in children to maintain correction. AFOs may be used as an alternative to bivalved casts as night splints or to facilitate rehabilitation during the healing process. Rapid progression to a postoperative AFO is facilitated by taking the impression for the AFO at the time of surgery.[1] The surgeon can place the limb in the desired position when the limb is anesthetized, and fabrication of the device can occur during the immediate postoperative casting period. Planning ahead in this manner aids greatly in moving patients into AFOs earlier in the rehabilitative process, enhancing their return to full function.

The use of a postoperative AFO after equinus surgery will depend on the particular clinical circumstances. In patients with nonneurologic equinus, a decision may be made to move from casting or cast alternatives such as walking braces directly to shoes. Therefore, an AFO may not be necessary. In these cases, a functional foot orthosis should be considered to prevent further destructive pedal changes that may have been initiated by the ankle equinus deformity.[10] If instability is present, or if related structures must be supported while active ankle dorsiflexion is encouraged, a hinged AFO may be an excellent option. In patients with spastic equinus of neurologic origin, postoperative management most often includes a brace such as an AFO. These children often have continued problems with balance, control, and function that persist even after surgical lengthening has increased available motion. The AFO in such a patient should encourage the use of the newly available motion while assisting the child to function to capacity.

Solid Versus Hinged Ankle-Foot Orthosis in Equinus Management

The child with equinus, who may present initially with toe-walking, is a candidate for bracing, serial casting, or surgery.[12] In managing these conditions in children with spastic equinus associated with cerebral palsy a solid AFO is often recommended. Alternatives such as a hinged AFO have traditionally been played down in some circles because of a concern that such devices do not provide enough control and that an ill-fitting hinged brace, because it allows more motion, will lead to irritation. Two studies have shown that hinged AFOs may give better mobility with adequate alignment than solid AFOs. Ricks and colleagues[13] found that hinged AFOs, solid AFOs,

and barefoot provided excellent alignment of the foot. Middleton and colleagues[14] found that hinged devices gave more desirable ankle joint motion and symmetry and limited excessive knee extension.

Carmick[12] cites a case of a toe-walking child with spastic equinus who, when placed in a solid AFO that blocked ankle plantarflexion, got up on his toes by swinging his arms forward and upward with a backward trunk movement to maintain balance.[12] The same child, after a physical therapy program in a hinged AFO increased ankle dorsiflexion to 5 degrees, was unable to get up on his toes using the same arm and trunk maneuver because the hinged device collapsed to plantigrade. Further, he demonstrated strong heel strike, reduced internal rotation, increased step length, and lower arm position. It was thought that the use of a hinged AFO in this case provided some stretch of the calf muscles during dorsiflexion and contraction during weight bearing, which may provide the stimulus necessary for growth.[15] In this case the hinged AFO after therapy increased the available ankle dorsiflexion and served as an alternative to surgical correction. The findings of improved posture, stability, and function with the hinged device can be extrapolated to suggest the value of this device after surgery in encouraging these same positive positions and functions.

Duchenne's Muscular Dystrophy

The benefit of bracing after surgery was demonstrated in a 1996 study by Vignos and associates,[16] who evaluated their program for the long-term treatment of Duchenne's muscular dystrophy at the University Hospital of Cleveland. Children with Duchenne's muscular dystrophy develop severe contractures of all weight-bearing joints. A typical problem caused by contractures of the ankle is difficulty in wearing normal shoes. This study found that a combined program of daily passive stretching exercises with prescribed time for standing, tenotomy of the Achilles tendon with posterior tibial tendon transfer, and application of knee-ankle-foot orthoses effectively controlled equinus contracture of the ankle.

A previous study reported on the effect of early surgery to extend the duration of the ability to walk without orthoses. Rideau and colleagues[17] reported that patients with Duchenne's muscular dystrophy who had early surgery walked *without orthoses* until they were a mean of 10.6 ± 1.69 years old. Vignos and associates[16] reported that patients who had orthoses or an operation and bracing walked *with braces* until they were a mean of 13.6 years old. This study documented that ambulation continued for a significantly longer period of time in children who wore orthoses as part of their comprehensive care.

Myelomeningocoele

A 1991 study on the effect of postoperative orthoses on patients with myelomeningocoele who had undergone transfer of the anterior tibial tendon to the calcaneus with Achilles tenodesis reported significant benefit from their use.[18] Molded polypropylene ankle-foot orthoses were prescribed primarily to protect the tendon transfer teno-desis, to improve rearfoot and midfoot support, and to protect the insensitive skin. Gait analysis, performed pre- and postoperatively with and without orthoses, revealed significant improvements in control, knee and ankle motion, single limb support, step length, and walking velocity with the orthosis. The authors concluded that continued orthotic support is beneficial both for protection and for improvement of long-term function.

THE ROLE OF POSTOPERATIVE ANKLE-FOOT ORTHOSES IN PREVENTING RECURRENCE

The surgeon operating on a child must be concerned with the possibility of recurrence of the deformity. An orthosis may be used to hold the previously hypertonic or contracted muscle in a neutral or corrected position. Persistent use of the brace will minimize the likelihood of recurrence and the need for further operations. Practitioners who do not use postoperative brace control have reported a higher recurrence rate of deformity.[19, 20] Although it is often desirable to discontinue the use of bracing over time in the postoperative patient, the possibility of recurrence may be reason enough to continue the use of bracing in some children. In the patient with cerebral palsy, the use of postoperative orthoses with intensive physical therapy is considered mandatory to maintain correction and facilitate optimum function.[21]

The nonambulatory patient with neuromuscular disease may be a candidate for surgical correction of fixed contractures of the ankle and foot to achieve a foot capable of wearing shoes that can rest plantigrade on the foot plate of the wheelchair and avoid excessive pressure areas on the foot. A study by Hsu and Jackson[22] reported in 1985 that the indications for surgical correction in these cases are (1) the presence of severe and unremitting pain, (2) skin breakdown and ulceration, and (3) an inability to fit and use shoewear. The authors concluded that these problems recurred if AFOs were not used after the surgical release. These nonambulatory children undergo surgical correction of fixed foot and ankle deformities primarily to reduce pain and skin breakdown or to enable them to wear shoes, and they benefit from the use of orthoses postoperatively to prevent recurrence. This highlights the importance of the use of AFOs in postoperative foot and ankle patients to prevent recurrence even if the patients are nonambulatory.

CASTING FOR ANKLE-FOOT ORTHOSES

Impression casting for an AFO in postoperative patients is similar to the process used when the AFO is the primary treatment modality. Depending on the purpose and position desired for the postoperative AFO, certain modifications in the casting or fabrication process can be made. The effect of a dorsiflexed or plantarflexed ankle on the knee moment has been discussed earlier and is an important consideration in determining the ankle position for casting.

Materials for casting include stockinette, one to two rolls of 4-inch elastic fast-setting plaster, one to two rolls of 4-inch fast-setting plaster, a ½-inch thick, 1-inch wide adhesive strip the length of the cast or lead strips to protect the leg. Other supplies needed include a utility knife or cast cutter for removal, a cast-marking pencil to note the bony prominences, bandage scissors, and warm water in a vessel. Drape sheets if the child is on the parent's lap for casting and for the floor are recommended.

The patient with nonneurologic disease is positioned with the hip and knee at or near 90 degrees of flexion to reduce resistance to neutral position casting. A patient with a neurologic component should be placed in a prone position to reduce extensor tone. The hip is extended, and the knee is flexed to 90 degrees during the cast application.

Next the malleoli, bony prominences, and the first and fifth metatarsal heads are marked with the pencil to assist in fabrication. The felt or lead strip is placed centrally on the tibia and dorsum of the foot. If a lead strip is used, tape can be used to fasten it to the leg. The foot and ankle are placed at 90 degrees or whatever position is desired for the foot-ankle relationship. Stockinette is applied to protect the skin from the plaster. The practitioner should practice placing the foot and ankle in the position desired for the cast at this point before the plaster is applied. Thought should be given to the purpose and design of the AFO, and efforts should be made to capture this desired position in the impression. Recommended positions include the subtalar neutral position with loading of the lateral column to resistance with sagittal plane pressure on the fourth and fifth metatarsal heads so as to lock the midtarsal joint. The forefoot hand should be used to set the ankle position at 90 degrees or at whatever angle is desired in the postoperative AFO.

The elastic plaster roll is applied first. The advantage of using elastic plaster first is that it provides improved contour of the foot and leg anatomy, which can improve the ultimate fit of the device. One roll of this plaster is usually sufficient, depending on the size of the limb. The plaster should be submerged for 20 to 30 seconds and wet thoroughly in warm water. Care should be taken not to wring out the roll too much because this will render the plaster too dry, making it difficult to unroll and laminate. The plaster is applied from the distal foot across the ankle and up the leg, stopping slightly above the level where the proximal trimline of the AFO will end. It is important to provide an impression that incorporates *at least* as much of the foot and leg as will be captured in the AFO. Lamination of the plaster as it is rolled on is important to ensure a smooth contour and fortify the cast with a minimum of plaster thickness. The second roll of nonelastic plaster is now applied in similar fashion and is laminated into the previous layer, taking care to smooth the contour of the arch, the tendo Achilles, and the malleolar region. The set position for the cast is now assumed to place the ankle and foot in the desired position.

The cast pencil should be used to draw horizontal lines

1 inch apart on the dorsum of the foot and leg to facilitate realignment during fabrication. The utility knife or cast cutter is carefully guided down the center of the cast over the felt pad or lead strip. The bandage scissor is used to cut any remaining plaster fibers and the stockinette. Once the plaster is fully set, the cast is opened in a clamshell fashion, sliding the cast backward on the leg, and removed.

In casting children efforts should be made to reduce the fear and anxiety associated with an unfamiliar experience. Preparing a sample or "dummy cast" for the child that will not be used can reduce this anxiety. A simplified, quick version of the real cast can be taken before the actual casts are taken, and this is then given to the child to hold. This maneuver may serve to reduce excessive tightness or motion induced by the child's fear of the unknown that may alter the quality of the impression. The child who is distracted by holding this sample cast will also be easier to cast because tone or tightness is often reduced when individuals are more relaxed. The child is offered the sample cast to take home as a souvenir of the experience. Pictures or drawings can be done at the end of a first or sample cast to calm or distract the agitated child, facilitating the application of the second or actual cast. This is also an option after the first leg has been casted in a child with bilateral deformity.

SUMMARY

The value and use of ankle-foot orthoses in the postoperative pediatric patient have been described. The opportunity to maximize the benefits of a surgical procedure through the use of orthoses may lead to an improved outcome. The tendency for certain conditions to recur after surgical corrections, particularly in the patient with neurologic disease, is another important indication for the use of these devices postoperatively. The procedure for casting for these devices and design features for the myriad variations on the ankle-foot orthosis have also been included. It should be remembered that a postoperative orthosis can only maintain the position attained by surgery. It cannot be expected to attain correction of the deformity by itself. As the practitioner gains more confidence and experience with the different types of orthoses, careful prescriptions can be written that build on the surgical correction and maximize the potential for the future.

ACKNOWLEDGEMENTS

My gratitude to Michael Smith, C.P.O., for his thoughts on this subject and for reviewing the manuscript. And thanks to Linda Grassia, of the Langer Biomechanics Group, for editorial support.

References

1. Smith M: Personal communication, 1997.
2. Redford J, et al (eds): Orthotics Etcetera. Baltimore, Williams & Wilkins, 1986, pp. 1–20.
3. Bumbo N: Ankle foot orthoses. *In* Valmassay R (ed): Clinical Biomechanics of the Lower Extremity. St. Louis, C.V. Mosby, 1996, pp. 391–403.
4. Brodke D, Skinner S, Lamoreux L, et al: Effects of ankle foot orthoses on the gait of children. J Pediatr Orthop 1989; 9:702.
5. Perry J: Gait analysis: Normal and pathological function. New York, McGraw-Hill, 1992.
6. Sankey RJ, Anderson DM, Young JA: Characteristics of ankle foot orthoses for management of the spastic lower limb. Dev Med Child Neurol 1989; 31:466.
7. Drennan J: The Child's Foot and Ankle. New York, Raven Press, 1992.
8. Lehmann JF, Esselman PC, Ko MJ, et al: Plastic ankle foot orthoses: Evaluation of function. Arch Phys Med Rehab 1983; 64:402.
9. McIllmurray WJ, Greenbaum WA: A below-knee weight-bearing brace. Orthot Prosthet 1974; 28:14.
10. Downey MS: Ankle equinus. *In* McGlamry ED, Banks AS, Downey MS (eds): Comprehensive Textbook of Foot Surgery, 2nd ed. Baltimore, Williams & Wilkins, 1992, pp. 687–729.
11. Wenger DR, Rang M: The Art and Practice of Children's Orthopedics. New York, Raven Press, 1993.
12. Carmick J: Managing equinus in a child with cerebral palsy: Merits of hinged ankle foot orthoses. Dev Med Child Neurol 1995; 37:1006.
13. Ricks NR, Eilert RE: Effects of inhibitory casts and orthoses on the bony alignment of the foot and ankle during weight-bearing in children with spasticity. Dev Med Child Neurol 1993; 35:11.
14. Middleton EA, Hurley GRB, McIllwain JS: The role of rigid and hinged polypropylene ankle foot orthoses in the management of cerebral palsy: A case study. Prosthet Orthot Int 1988; 12:129.
15. Rang M, Silver R, de la Garza J: Cerebral palsy. *In* Lovell WW, Winter RB (eds): Pediatric Orthopedics, Vol. 2, 5th ed. Philadelphia, J.B. Lippincott, 1986, pp. 345–390.
16. Vignos PJ, Wagner MB, Karlinchak B, Katirji B: Evaluation of a program for long-term treatment of Duchenne muscular dystrophy. Experience at the University Hospitals of Cleveland. J Bone Joint Surg 1996; 78A:1844.
17. Rideau Y, Glorion B, Duport G: Prolongation of ambulation in the muscular dystrophies. Acta Neurol 1983; 5:390.
18. Banta JV, Sutherland DH, Wyatt M: Anterior tibial transfer to the os calcis with Achilles tenodesis for calcaneal deformity in myelomeningocoele. J Pediatr Orthop 1981; 1:125.
19. Sharrad WJW: Paralytic deformity in the lower limb. J Bone Joint Surg 1967; 49B:731.
20. Truscelli D, Lespargot A, Tardieu G: Variation in the long-term results of elongation of the tendo Achilles in children with cerebral palsy. J Bone Joint Surg 1979; 61B:466.
21. Binder H, Eng G: Rehabilitation management of children with spastic cerebral palsy. Arch Phys Med Rehabil 1989; 70:482.
22. Hsu JD, Jackson R: Treatment of symptomatic foot and ankle deformities in the non-ambulatory neuromuscular patient. Foot Ankle 1985; 5:238.

50

Corrective Casting

Richard M. Jay, D.P.M.

When casting a child for metatarsus adductus, calcaneovalgus, talipes equinovarus, or torsional deformities, the degree of the deformity and the desired reduced position are determined prior to the actual application of the cast. There are three choices of casting materials: plaster of Paris, flexible fiberglass, and fiberglass. All these materials have advantages and disadvantages, and they should be used conservatively to correct these congenital deformities. Metatarsus adductus and talipes equinovarus require the use of plaster only. A highly moldable material such as plaster aids in obtaining a more controlled position of the foot. Reduction of the deformity by stabilizing the calcaneus is successfully accomplished by molding the plaster, and the entire foot can be maintained in a corrected position. Calcaneovalgus and torsion deformities may be casted in plaster or Scotchrap (3M Healthcare Products, St. Paul, MN). Reduction of calcaneovalgus is not as critical as it is in talipes equinovarus or metatarsus adductus. Fiberglass is a less desirable material because a noisy electric cast cutter must be used to remove the cast, thereby potentially traumatizing the child; it is the goal of the doctor to make the child's visit as relaxed and unstressful as possible.

Before any type of casting, the leg should be protected. Time is of the essence when casting because an infant will not tolerate a stationary position too long. An assistant should hold the foot in a neutral position while stockinette (Johnson and Johnson Orthopedics, Raynham, MA) and then Webril (Johnson and Johnson Orthopedics, Raynham, MA) padding are applied to the limb. Plaster application requires approximately 30 minutes for the material to set optimally; less time is needed with the flexible fiberglass.

Casting is generally recommended for the preambulatory child; otherwise, some minor adjustments must be made in the positioning of the ambulating child's foot. If an above-knee cast is applied and the child is expected to ambulate, the foot must be dorsiflexed and held in a neutral position when the knee is flexed. This enables the child to stand flat on the cast's plantar surface and walk properly. Plantarflexion of the cast is avoided in the ambulating child to prevent pressure sores (blisters) from developing on the dorsal surface of the toes.

CAST MATERIAL

Plaster of Paris

When applying plaster of Paris to children, a good foundation of stockinette and Webril is necessary. One-

or 2-inch stockinette pieces approximately 4 inches long are placed over the foot distally and the leg proximally. Webril is then placed over it firmly and not in excess. Small amounts of extra Webril must be placed over the bony prominences such as the malleoli and heels and also on the proximal segments of the leg. This firm foundation prevents the plaster from caving in and makes a stronger cast. If too much Webril is used, the plaster will have a soft foundation and motion will occur inside the cast, causing a loss of correction. Webril will compress over a period of a few days. If too much Webril is used on the foot and leg, the correction will be lost.

Next, the plaster is prepared. Water temperature should be maintained between 70° and 75°F. Since an exothermic reaction occurs with crystallization of the gypsum, a higher water temperature or a greater quantity of plaster will generate more heat. Water temperatures above 75°F will cause the plaster temperature to rise significantly. If one is applying a thick cast with warm water (above 75°F) on a young foot and leg, a thermal burn will result. Room temperature water must therefore be used, and it should be double-checked prior to cast application. The plaster roll is placed in the water for less than 30 seconds. Excess water is squeezed out at the ends. This allows the roll of plaster to take the shape of a cigar. A well-soaked roll allows the cast to be easily molded.

When applying the plaster, it is important to lay the layers smoothly on top of one another, overlapping by one half without wrinkling. The plaster should be rubbed to ensure that crystallization bonding takes place within the bandage itself. The stronger the bond, the better the lamination, and the less plaster is needed. Caution should be taken not to use excess plaster because this creates too much heat and too much weight for the child. When changing directions while the plaster is being rolled on, the plaster is tucked, folded, and rubbed in the desired direction. At one point, as the cast material is placed on the foot and leg, the stockinette should be rolled back on itself to pull back the Webril and create a cushion at the proximal tibia and the distal toes. This prevents the child from picking out the Webril and also provides a good barrier for protection and cushioning. The rolling of the cast material is then continued over the stockinette, completing the cast. When the last roll is applied a plaster tab is placed on the surface of the cast at the end of the roll. During the entire application of plaster, one's hands should be continually moving and rubbing the cast to minimize pressure indentations. Gentle and slow manipulation of the cast avoids leaving imprints of fingers in the plaster. The extremity is secured by holding the toes outside the cast and supporting the limb above the cast at the level of the thigh.

Fiberglass and Flexible Fiberglass

When applying fiberglass and flexible fiberglass Scotchrap on a child, the technique used is similar to that used with regular plaster of Paris application. However, the roll itself is more flexible, and it can be placed with less tension than with plaster. Each individual roll is opened separately and soaked in water between 70° and 75°F to begin the curing process. When removing the rolls from the water, too much water should not be squeezed out because this decreases the curing time and interferes with proper molding.

The fiberglass or Scotchrap is rolled in a continuous rolling motion against the leg, which has previously been covered with Webril and stockinette. The rolls extend from the toes to the proximal tibia. Rubbing and smoothing this material as one goes creates a better bond and a better laminated surface, which results in a stronger cast. Once curing begins and the Scotchrap becomes more rigid, the foot and leg are held in the desired position.

CAST REMOVAL

Removal of casts from children can be quite difficult. But with the newer flexible fiberglass materials, removal is as simple as unraveling stiff gauze. This flexible fiberglass does not need to be soaked or cut with a cast cutter. If, however, complete, rigid immobilization is needed, a rigid fiberglass or plaster cast is recommended. Removal of fiberglass warrants the use of a cast cutter. With at least the two layers of Webril and stockinette under the fiberglass, the risk of injury is markedly reduced. The cast cutter is stabilized on the cast to prevent jumping of the blade. Using an up-and-down, progressive motion of the blade, the cast is cut. This motion decreases the risk of the blade heating and possibly burning the child.

Plaster casts can be removed as described above with a cast cutter, or they can be soaked off. The physician instructs the parents how to soak and soften the cast. One ounce of vinegar is placed in warm water, and the child sits in a tub for 30 minutes. The parent then grasps the plaster tab and pulls, and the plaster roll unravels from the leg. The parents should be reminded to allow at least 1 hour for complete soaking and cast removal. No sharp instruments should be used to aid in removal. This procedure is used only on manipulative casts, not for casts used to maintain surgical procedures. Flexible fiberglass can be removed without water in the same fashion as the plaster cast.

Appendix

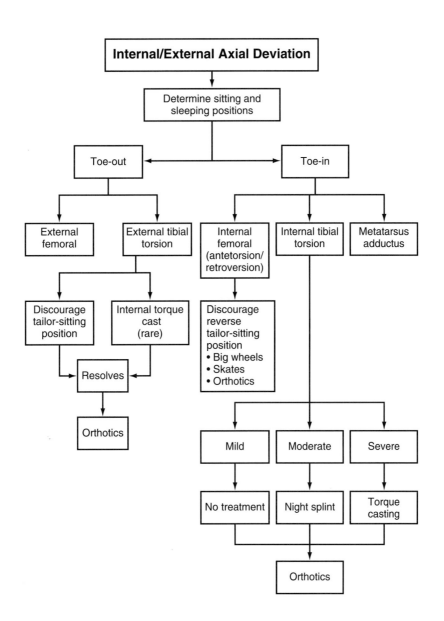

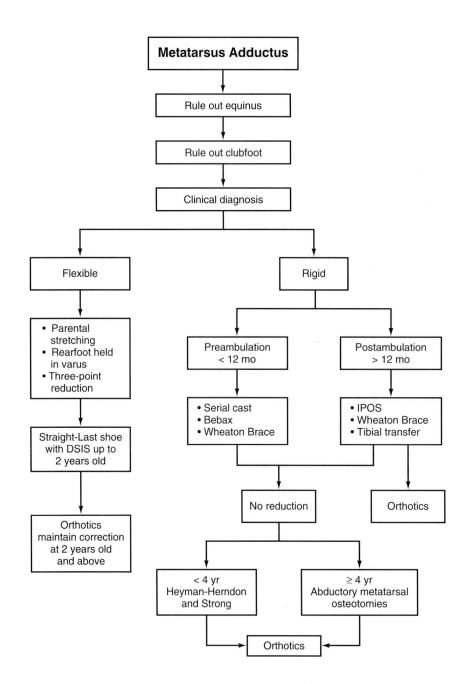

Metatarsus Adductus

Rule out equinus

Rule out clubfoot

Clinical diagnosis

Flexible

- Parental stretching
- Rearfoot held in varus
- Three-point reduction

Straight-Last shoe with DSIS up to 2 years old

Orthotics maintain correction at 2 years old and above

Rigid

Preambulation < 12 mo

Postambulation > 12 mo

- Serial cast
- Bebax
- Wheaton Brace

- IPOS
- Wheaton Brace
- Tibial transfer

No reduction

Orthotics

< 4 yr Heyman-Herndon and Strong

≥ 4 yr Abductory metatarsal osteotomies

Orthotics

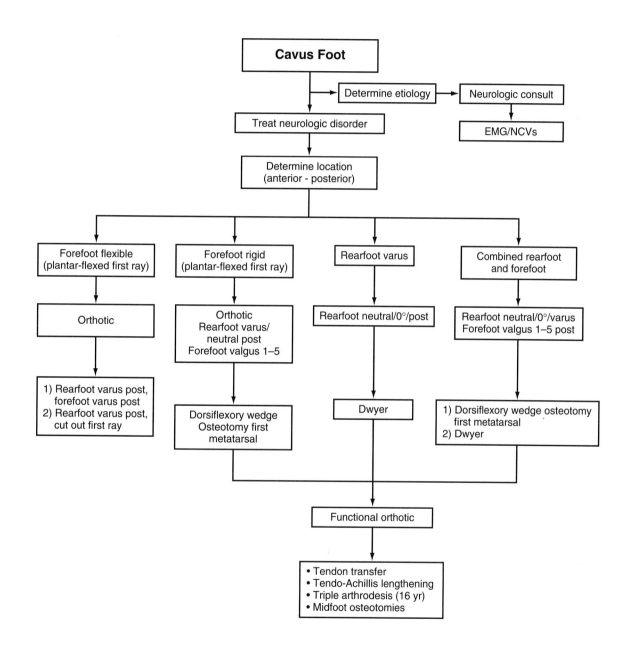

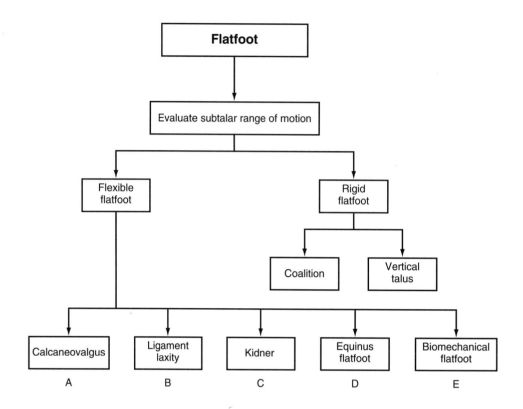

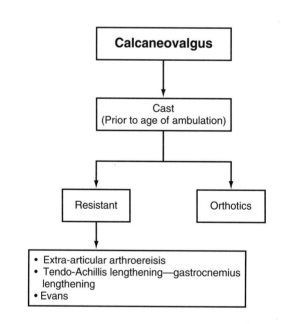

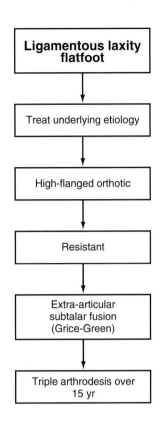

Ligamentous laxity flatfoot

↓

Treat underlying etiology

↓

High-flanged orthotic

↓

Resistant

↓

Extra-articular subtalar fusion (Grice-Green)

↓

Triple arthrodesis over 15 yr

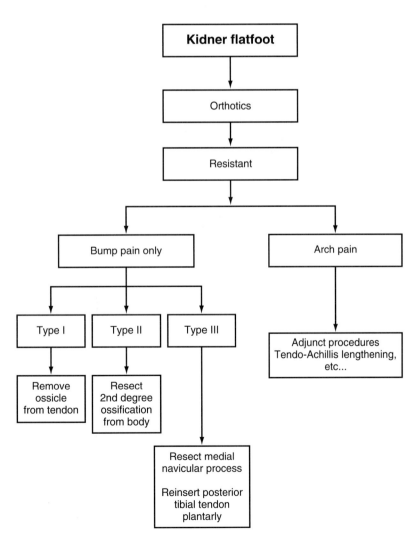

Kidner flatfoot

↓

Orthotics

↓

Resistant

Bump pain only | Arch pain

Bump pain only:
- Type I → Remove ossicle from tendon
- Type II → Resect 2nd degree ossification from body
- Type III → Resect medial navicular process / Reinsert posterior tibial tendon plantarly

Arch pain → Adjunct procedures Tendo-Achillis lengthening, etc...

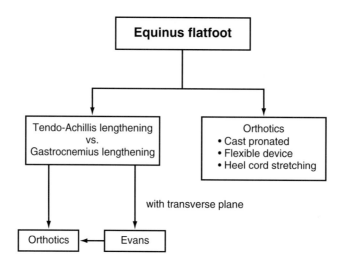

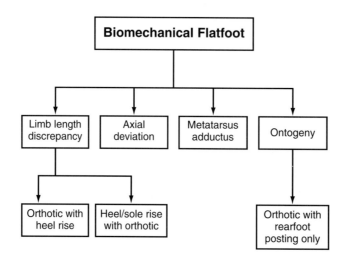

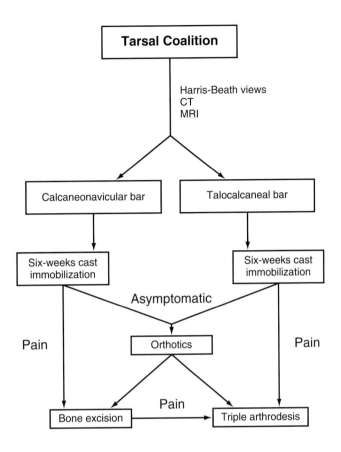

Tarsal Coalition

Harris-Beath views
CT
MRI

Calcaneonavicular bar

Talocalcaneal bar

Six-weeks cast immobilization

Six-weeks cast immobilization

Asymptomatic

Pain

Orthotics

Pain

Pain

Bone excision

Triple arthrodesis

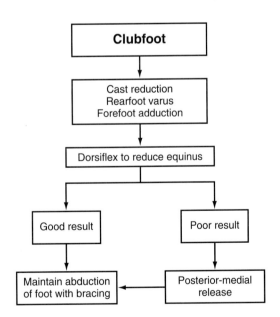

Clubfoot

Cast reduction
Rearfoot varus
Forefoot adduction

Dorsiflex to reduce equinus

Good result

Poor result

Maintain abduction of foot with bracing

Posterior-medial release

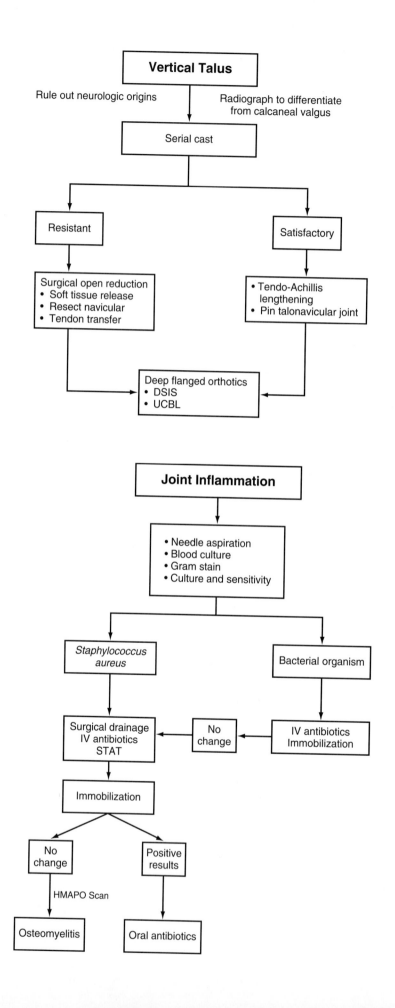

Vertical Talus

Rule out neurologic origins

Radiograph to differentiate from calcaneal valgus

Serial cast

Resistant

Satisfactory

Surgical open reduction
- Soft tissue release
- Resect navicular
- Tendon transfer

- Tendo-Achillis lengthening
- Pin talonavicular joint

Deep flanged orthotics
- DSIS
- UCBL

Joint Inflammation

- Needle aspiration
- Blood culture
- Gram stain
- Culture and sensitivity

Staphylococcus aureus

Bacterial organism

Surgical drainage IV antibiotics STAT

No change

IV antibiotics Immobilization

Immobilization

No change

Positive results

HMAPO Scan

Osteomyelitis

Oral antibiotics

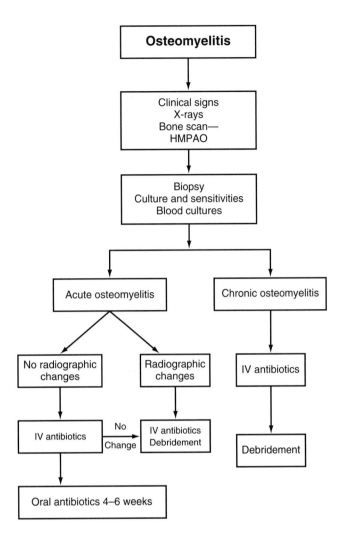

Index

Note: Page numbers in *italics* indicate illustrations; those followed by t indicate tables; those followed by b indicate boxed material.

ISBN 0-7216-7445-3

90038

9 780721 674452